Effective Care in Pregnancy and Childbirth

Effective Care in Pregnancy and Childbirth

Edited by Cora Bailey

hayle
medical

New York

Hayle Medical,
750 Third Avenue, 9th Floor,
New York, NY 10017, USA

Visit us on the World Wide Web at:
www.haylemedical.com

ISBN: 978-1-63241-618-6

Cataloging-in-Publication Data

Effective care in pregnancy and childbirth / edited by Cora Bailey.
   p. cm.
Includes bibliographical references and index.
ISBN 978-1-63241-618-6
1. Prenatal care. 2. Childbirth. 3. Pregnancy. 4. Maternal health services. I. Bailey, Cora.
RG940 .E34 2019
618.24--dc23

Contents

Chapter 25

Chapter 26

Preface

Pregnancy is the period in which an offspring develops within a woman's body. Childbirth occurs about 40 weeks from the last menstrual period. This period is typically divided into three trimesters. Prenatal care helps to improve pregnancy outcomes. It may include avoiding certain substances such as drugs, alcohol and nicotine, practicing healthy habits such as regular exercise and good nutrition, and opting for regular physical examinations, etc. Certain complications such as gestational diabetes, severe nausea and vomiting, and iron-deficiency anemia are fairly common in pregnancies. Nearly 10-15% of pregnancies end in miscarriages. This is because of obstructed labor, ectopic pregnancy, complications associated with ectopic pregnancy, bleeding, infections, etc. The newborn baby can also suffer from prematurity, birth trauma, infections and from a lack of oxygen at birth. Internal and external fetal monitoring can be done for the assessment of fetal well-being. This book is a valuable compilation of topics, ranging from the basic to the most complex principles and practices of care in pregnancy and childbirth. It presents the complex subject of pregnancy and childbirth in the most comprehensible language. The readers would gain knowledge that would broaden their perspective about these domains.

The information contained in this book is the result of intensive hard work done by researchers in this field. All due efforts have been made to make this book serve as a complete guiding source for students and researchers. The topics in this book have been comprehensively explained to help readers understand the growing trends in the field.

I would like to thank the entire group of writers who made sincere efforts in this book and my family who supported me in my efforts of working on this book. I take this opportunity to thank all those who have been a guiding force throughout my life.

Editor

Opium use during pregnancy and infant size at birth: a cohort study

Siavash Maghsoudlou[1,2]* ⓘ, Sven Cnattingius[1], Scott Montgomery[1,3,4], Mohsen Aarabi[5], Shahriar Semnani[6], Anna-Karin Wikström[1,7] and Shahram Bahmanyar[8]

Abstract

Background: The reported positive association between opiatic drug use during pregnancy and adverse pregnancy outcomes might be confounded by other factors related to high-risk behaviors, including the use of other harmful substances. In rural areas of Iran, opium use during pregnancy is relatively common among women who otherwise do not have a hazardous lifestyle, which reduces the risk of residual confounding and increasing the possibility to identify its effects. We aimed to examine the association of antenatal exposure to opium with risks of small for gestational age, short birth length, and small head circumference at birth.

Method: In this cohort study in the rural area of the Golestan province, Iran, we randomly selected 920 women who were exposed to opium during pregnancy and 920 unexposed women during 2008–2010. Log-binomial regression was used to estimate risk ratios (RR) and 95% confidence intervals (CI) for the associations between prenatal exposure to opium and risks of small for gestational age, short birth length, and small head circumference at birth.

Results: Compared with non-use of opium and tobacco during pregnancy, using opium only and dual use of opium and tobacco were associated with increased risks of small for gestational age at births (RR = 1.71; 95% CI 1.34–2.18 and RR = 1.62; 95% CI 1.13–2.30, respectively). Compared with non-use of opium and tobacco, exposure to only opium or dual use of opium and tobacco were also associated with more than doubled increased risks of short birth length, and small head circumference in term infants.

Conclusion: Maternal opium use during pregnancy is associated with increased risks of giving birth to a small for gestational age infant, as well as a term infant with short birth length or small head circumference.

Keywords: Birth size, Iran, Opium, Pregnancy, Small for gestational age

Background

There has been an epidemic of opioid abuse worldwide, including North America, UK, Australia, and Asian countries [1, 2]. Opium (Poppy tears, Lachryma Papaveris, Theriac) has traditionally been used in Middle-eastern and south Asian countries, such as Iran, Afghanistan, Pakistan, India, and China, even during pregnancy [3]. Opium obtained from the poppy plant, Papaver somniferous, contains morphine (10% of opium), Codeine (0.5%), Thebaine (0.2%), Papaverine (1%), and Noscapine (6%) [4].

Use of opioids during pregnancy, including heroin and methadone, has been associated with adverse pregnancy outcomes such as preterm delivery, low birth weight, SGA, and neonatal complications [5]. However, these studies were performed on drug addicts in high-income countries, and the reported effect of the opioid use on pregnancy outcomes might be confounded by social factors, lifestyle and other factors related to high-risk behaviors, including the use of other harmful substances [6]. Thus, differentiating the effects of opioid use from the effects of other risk factors has been difficult [7].

In Golestan province, northern Iran, some women use (mainly smoke) opium [8]. In this area, opium-using women are mostly homemakers, who otherwise do not have a hazardous lifestyle – such as homelessness and criminal behavior – which reduces the risk of residual

* Correspondence: siavashmaghsoudlou@hotmail.com;
shahram.bahmanyar@ki.se
[1]Clinical Epidemiology Unit, Department of Medicine, Karolinska Institute, Solna, Sweden
[2]Department of Obstetrics & Gynecology, McMaster University, 1280 Main Street West, room 3N52F, Hamilton, ON L8S 4K1, Canada
Full list of author information is available at the end of the article

confounding [9, 10]. In a cohort study from north-east Iran, we used prospectively collected information before and during pregnancy to examine the association of antenatal exposure to opium with anthropometric characteristics of the newborn infants, including weight, length, and head circumference at birth.

Methods

A detailed description of the study population and method appears elsewhere [11]. Briefly, we performed a cohort study in rural areas of Golestan province, in northeast Iran, between 2008 and 2010. The province has approximately 1, 700, 000 inhabitants. Around 50% are living in rural areas, where there are approximately 280, 000 women in reproductive age and 17, 000 births annually. Based on the national public health care system in Iran, each village has at least one rural health house, which is part of the primary health care organization and works under the authority of more specialized health care centers. The health houses are responsible for providing care and recording of health-related data, including medical information before and during pregnancy. Medical information including maternal drug use, cigarette smoking, alcohol use, and other high-risk behaviors are recorded both before and during pregnancy [9]. Opium is the most common drug in Golestan province and is usually smoked [12].

The exposed group included women with a self-reported history of using any of a variety of opiates during the index pregnancy. The unexposed group included women who did not use opium before or during pregnancy. We used the stratified random sampling method to select exposed and unexposed groups. Each of the 13 regions of the province was determined as a block, and the sample size of each block was estimated based on the population growth rate of the region. There were 30, 868 pregnancies during the study period. Exposed pregnancies were randomly selected, using computer-created random digits and the same number of women unexposed to opium during pregnancy were frequency-matched to the exposed women by the residential area (village). Information on pregnancies was abstracted from medical records and computerized. As a quality control, some 10% of the data was collected a second time. We recollected the data if there were more than 5% mismatches.

We selected a total of 920 opium users during pregnancy ("exposed" women) and 920 non-opium users ("unexposed" women). Thereafter, we excluded women with multiple births, miscarriages, and stillbirths, also women who gave up using opium in early pregnancy, used alcohol during pregnancy, and tobacco smokers among the unexposed group (15 unexposed and 33 exposed mothers). Finally, our study included 887 opium users (of whom 210 also smoked tobacco, and 677 only used opium) and 905 non-opium users with live singleton births.

Information on socioeconomic circumstances was based on the husband's profession (categorized as an unskilled manual worker, skilled manual worker, self-employed, farmer, other occupations, and unemployed). Agricultural production is the main economic sector in Golestan province. Gestational age was based on the time interval between the date of the first day of the last menstrual period and the date of delivery. Preterm delivery was defined as a delivery before 37 completed gestational weeks. Small for gestational age (SGA) was defined as a birth weight below the 10th percentile for gestational age, based on a sex-specific global reference for birth weight [13]. The 5th percentile of birth length (crown-heel length) and head (Occipito-Frontal) circumference among unexposed and term pregnancies were considered as cut-offs for short birth length (shorter than 47 cm) and small head circumference (smaller than 33 cm), respectively.

We used univariate and multivariate log-binomial regression models to estimate risk ratios (RRs) and 95% confidence intervals (CIs) for the associations between opium use during pregnancy and SGA, short birth length, and small head circumference. The models were adjusted for potential confounding factors, including the region of residence, maternal age, parity, height, body mass index, husband's occupation, and infant sex. Due to scarce data on preterm infants, we could not construct gestational-age specific curves for birth length and head circumference. We restricted the analyses of birth length and head circumference to term births (≥ 37 weeks), where we additionally also adjusted for gestational age (in weeks). Stratified analyses were performed to investigate the risks of SGA, short birth length, and small head circumference among opium-using mothers who smoked or did not smoke tobacco during pregnancy.

We used multiple imputation method with five imputations approach was used to provide data where there were missing values for maternal age (6 among mothers unexposed to opium and 5 among exposed mothers), infant sex (15 among mothers unexposed to opium and 10 among exposed mothers), husband's occupation (4 among unexposed and 9 among exposed), and mother's height (39 among unexposed and 17 among exposed). SAS software version 9.4 was used for all analyses.

Results

Table 1 shows maternal and births characteristics in unexposed, all exposed, exposed to opium only and exposed to both opium and tobacco. Among unexposed women, 28% were 30 years or older, and 59% were parous. For women exposed to opium corresponding figures were 44% and 78%, respectively. There were no differences between the cohorts regarding other maternal characteristics. Among infants prenatally unexposed and exposed to opium, 6.5% and 13.0% were shorter than 47 cm at birth, respectively,

Table 1 Characteristics of study subjects

	Unexposed [a]	Opium user		
		All	Opium user only	Tobacco and Opium user
	N (%)	N (%)	N (%)	N (%)
Maternal age (Years)				
≤ 19	134 (14.8)	49 (5.5)	40 (5.9)	9 (4.3)
20–24	250 (27.6)	161 (18.2)	133 (19.6)	28 (13.3)
25–29	260 (28.7)	278 (31.3)	210 (31.0)	68 (32.4)
30–34	187 (20.7)	251 (28.3)	181 (26.7)	70 (33.3)
≥ 35	68 (7.5)	143 (16.1)	108 (16.0)	35 (16.7)
Missing	6 (0.7)	5 (0.6)	5 (0.7)	0 (0)
Parity				
Nulliparous	372 (41.1)	199 (22.4)	155 (22.9)	44 (21.0)
Parous	533 (58.9)	688 (77.6)	522 (77.1)	169 (79.0)
Maternal height (cm)				
≤ 149	68 (7.5)	66 (7.4)	47 (6.9)	19 (9.0)
150–155	198 (21.9)	193 (21.8)	152 (22.5)	41 (19.5)
156–160	380 (42.0)	399 (45.0)	295 (43.6)	104 (49.5)
161–164	120 (13.3)	109 (12.3)	84 (12.4)	25 (11.9)
≥ 165	100 (11.0)	103 (11.6)	86 (12.7)	17 (8.1)
Missing	39 (4.3)	18 (2.0)	13 (1.9)	4 (1.9)
Maternal body mass index				
< 18.5	63 (7.0)	52 (5.9)	34 (5.0)	18 (8.6)
18.5 to < 25	439 (48.5)	474 (53.4)	356 (52.6)	118 (56.2)
25 to < 30	245 (27.1)	231 (26.0)	184 (27.2)	47 (22.4)
30 to < 35	91 (10.1)	91 (10.3)	72 (10.6)	19 (9.0)
≥ 35	28 (3.1)	21 (2.4)	18 (2.7)	3 (1.4)
Missing	39 (4.3)	17 (1.9)	13 (1.9)	5 (2.4)
Husband's occupation				
Unemployed	25 (2.8)	56 (6.3)	37 (5.5)	19 (9.0)
Non skill worker	400 (44.2)	419 (47.2)	312 (46.1)	107 (51.0)
Skill worker	91 (10.1)	70 (7.9)	58 (8.6)	12 (5.7)
Self-employed	111 (12.3)	101 (11.4)	89 (13.1)	12 (5.7)
Farmer	179 (19.8)	163 (18.4)	123 (18.2)	40 (19.0)
Other	95 (10.5)	69 (7.8)	52 (7.7)	17 (78.1)
Missing	4 (0.4)	9 (1.0)	6 (0.9)	3 (1.4)
Unemployed	25 (2.8)	56 (6.3)	37 (5.5)	19 (9.0)
Preterm delivery				
Term	850 (93.9)	798 (90.0)	616 (91.0)	182 (86.7)
Preterm	55 (6.1)	89 (10.0)	61 (9.0)	28 (13.3)
Infant sex				
Female	447 (49.4)	436 (49.2)	337 (49.8)	99 (47.1)
Male	443 (49.0)	441 (49.7)	331 (48.9)	110 (52.4)
Missing	15 (1.7)	10 (1.1)	9 (1.3)	1 (0.5)
Birth weight (gr)				
≤ 2500	43 (4.8)	99 (11.2)	75 (11.1)	24 (11.4)

Table 1 Characteristics of study subjects *(Continued)*

	Unexposed [a]	Opium user		
		All	Opium user only	Tobacco and Opium user
	N (%)	N (%)	N (%)	N (%)
2500–2999	139 (15.4)	179 (20.2)	134 (19.8)	45 (21.4)
3000–3299	205 (22.7)	203 (22.9)	143 (21.1)	60 (28.6)
3300–3599	269 (29.7)	193 (21.8)	154 (22.7)	39 (18.6)
≥ 3600	234 (25.9)	203 (22.9)	162 (23.9)	41 (19.5)
Missing	15 (1.7)	10 (1.1)	9 (1.3)	1 (0.5)
Birth length (cm)				
≤ 46	59 (6.5)	115 (13.0)	87 (12.9)	28 (13.3)
47–48	149 (16.5)	138 (15.6)	103 (15.2)	35 (16.7)
49–51	535 (59.1)	480 (54.1)	359 (53.0)	121 (57.6)
≥ 52	147 (16.2)	144 (16.2)	119 (17.6)	25 (11.9)
Missing	15 (1.7)	10 (1.1)	9 (1.3)	1 (0.5)
Head circumference (cm)				
≤ 32	56 (6.2)	119 (13.4)	88 (13.0)	31 (14.8)
33–34	242 (16.7)	337 (38.0)	252 (37.2)	85 (40..5)
35–36	476 (52.6)	362 (40.8)	281 (41.5)	81 (38.6)
≥ 37	116 (12.8)	59 (6.7)	47 (6.9)	12 (5.7)
Missing	15 (1.7)	10 (1.1)	9 (1.3)	1 (0.5)

[a]Unexposed includes mothers who are non-users of both opium and tobacco

while corresponding percentages for small head circumference (< 33 cm) were 6.2% and 13.4%, respectively (Table 1).

Compared with non-use of opium and tobacco, use of opium during pregnancy was associated with a 69% increased risk of birth of an SGA infant after adjusting for potential confounders. The risk of SGA was slightly higher in offspring of mothers who only used opium (RR = 1.71 and 95% CI; 1.34–2.18) than in offspring of mothers who both used opium and smoked tobacco during pregnancy (RR = 1.62 and 95% CI; 1.13–2.30). Meanwhile, when we restricted the analysis into the term pregnancies, the risk of SGA was almost identical in offspring of mothers who only used opium (RR = 1.58 and 95% CI; 1.22–2. 04), and offspring of dual user mothers (RR = 1.58 and 95% CI; 1.09–2.29) (Table 2).

Compared with prenatally unexposed term infants, term infants who were prenatally exposed to opium had a more than doubled risk of short birth length (< 47 cm). The risk of short birth length was essentially similar between those exposed to only opium (RR = 2.00 and 95% CI; 1.37–2.92) and those exposed to both opium and tobacco during pregnancy (OR = 2.40 and 95% CI; 1.20–3.48) (Table 3).

Compared with prenatally unexposed term infants, term infants who were prenatally exposed to opium had a 2.2-fold risk of the small head circumference at birth. The risk of a small head circumference was similar in infants

prenatally exposed to only opium and in infants exposed to both opium and tobacco (Table 4).

Discussion

This cohort study revealed an increased risk of SGA at birth among offspring of mothers who used opium during pregnancy. This study showed that prenatal opium exposure also increased the risks of a short birth length and a small head circumference in infants born at term.

Our findings are consistent and extend results of previous studies showing that infants of mothers using heroin, methadone, or other opiates during pregnancy intend to have a higher risk of low birth weight [14, 15]. Meta-analyses have shown that use of any kind of opiates during pregnancy is associated with a three-fold increased risk of perinatal mortality and a four-fold increased risk of low birth weight [16]. We found that infants prenatally exposed to opium were at increased risk of being born SGA, but the risk of SGA was similar among infants only prenatally exposed to opium and those exposed to both opium and tobacco. As maternal smoking is causally associated with fetal growth restriction, we expected a higher risk among infants exposed to both opium and tobacco [17]. We cannot explain the lack of additive effect of opium and tobacco on SGA. Residual confounding may be one possibility, but the lack of observed effect may also be due to chance [17].

Table 2 Risk ratios (RR) and 95% confidence intervals (CI) for the associations between opium and tobacco use during pregnancy and risk of small for gestational age at birth

	Pregnancies	Small for gestational age [a]	Crude	Adjusted [b]
	N	N (%)	RR (95% CI)	RR (95% CI)
Opium				
Unexposed	905	99 (10.9)	Reference	
Exposed	887	154 (17.4)	1.59 (1.26–1.99)	1.69 (1.34–2.13)
Tobacco and opium				
Unexposed	905	99 (10.9)	Reference	
Exposed to opium only	677	115 (17.0)	1.59 (1.22–2.06)	1.71 (1.34–2.18)
Exposed to tobacco and opium	210	39 (18.6)	1.58 (1.10–2.28)	1.62 (1.13–2.30)
Restricted to term pregnancies				
Opium				
Unexposed	850	93 (10.9)	Reference	
Exposed	798	132 (16.5)	1.46 (1.15–1.86)	1.58 (1.23–2.02)
Tobacco and opium				
Unexposed	850	93 (10.9)	Reference	
Exposed to opium only	616	97 (15.7)	1.43 (1.11–1.85)	1.58 (1.22–2.04)
Exposed to tobacco and opium	182	35 (19.2)	1.57 (1.10–2.24)	1.58 (1.09–2.29)

[a]Small for gestational age was defined as a birth weight below the 10th percentile for appropriate gestational age, based on a sex-specific global reference for birth weight [13]
[b]Adjusted for: maternal age, height, BMI, parity, husband's occupation, and residential place

Our study demonstrated that term infants who were exposed to opium had shorter birth length after adjusting for gestational age, sex and other potential confounders. An increased risk of a short birth length was also observed in studies investigating maternal heroin or methadone use during pregnancy [18]. Liu et al. reported that infants who

Table 3 Risk ratios (RR) and 95% confidence intervals (CI) for the associations between opium and tobacco use during pregnancy and risk of short birth length at term birth

	Pregnancies	Short birth length [a]	Crude	Adjusted [b]
	N	N (%)	RR (95% CI)	RR (95% CI)
Opium				
Unexposed	850	50 (5.9)	Reference	
Exposed	798	92 (11.5)	1.95 (1.38–2.75)	2.01 (1.40–2.89)
Tobacco and opium				
Unexposed	850	50 (5.9)	Reference	
Exposed to opium only	616	70 (11.4)	1.93 (1.36–2.73)	2.00 (1.37–2.92)
Exposed to tobacco and opium	182	22 (12.2)	2.03 (1.26–3.27)	2.04 (1.20–3.48)

[a]Birth length less than 47 cm (below the 5th percentile of birth length of unexposed and term live birth)
[b]Adjusted for: maternal age, height, BMI, parity, weeks gestational age, infant sex, husband's occupation, and residential place

were prenatally exposed to opium or methadone had shorter birth length compared with unexposed infants [15]. An ultrasonic investigation during pregnancy showed that fetuses exposed to opiates had shorter femur and humerus lengths compared with unexposed fetus [19].

In this study, we also found that opium exposure during pregnancy is associated with a reduced head circumference, which is consistent with results of previous studies on maternal heroin or methadone use during pregnancy [15]. Hunt et al. reported that neonates prenatally exposed to opiates on average had smaller head circumference at birth. However, the study included both term and preterm infants, and the exposed group were born at a lower gestational age than the unexposed group [20]. A Swiss study also documented a four-fold increased risk of the small head circumference at birth (smaller than the third percentile) among neonates of methadone-addicted mothers [21]. Previous studies reported children of mothers using opiate during pregnancy had higher risks of intentional disorders, impaired motors, and cognitive functions, at school ages which could be due to impaired neurodevelopment [20, 22]. The long-term effects of opium exposure in utero on psycho-behavioral dysfunctions in offspring have also been demonstrated in other studies [23].

Several explanations have been proposed for the associations of opiates exposures during pregnancy with risks of fetal brain development and growth restrictions. Using opiate during pregnancy is associated with risks of preeclampsia, premature labor, premature rupture of

Table 4 Risk ratios (RR) and 95% confidence intervals (CI) for the associations between opium and tobacco use during pregnancy and risk of small head circumference at term birth

	Pregnancies N	Small head circumference [a] N (%)	Crude RR (95% CI)	Adjusted [b] RR (95% CI)
Opium				
Unexposed	850	45 (5.3)	Reference	
Exposed	798	99 (12.4)	2.33 (1.64–3.32)	2.24 (1.55–3.24)
Tobacco and opium				
Unexposed	850	45 (5.3)	Reference	
Exposed to opium only	616	76 (12.3)	2.33 (1.61–3.36)	2.24 (1.53–3.29)
Exposed to tobacco and opium	182	23 (12.6)	2.36 (1.43–3.90)	2.23 (1.31–3.79)

[a]Small head circumference less than 33 cm (below the 5th percentile of head circumference of unexposed and term live birth)
[b]Adjusted for: maternal age, height, BMI, parity, husband's occupation, infant sex, weeks gestational age, and residential place

membranes, placental abruption, placental insufficiency and intrauterine death [24]. Maternal narcotic use induces hypoxia and asphyxia in the fetus, which is a consequence of fluctuating overdose-withdrawal cycles during pregnancy [25]. Moreover, animal studies showed a direct effect of opiates on the neural elements of the fetus [26]. It has also been suggested that factors such as parental psychopathology, maternal multiple drug abuse, poor prenatal care, dietary restriction, and disadvantaged socioeconomic circumstances could mediate associations between opiates exposures during pregnancy and risks of fetal brain development and growth restriction [27]. However, Pinto et al. reported that despite comprehensive antenatal care, drug-using women are at higher risk of giving birth to a low birth weight infant [5].

Opium has traditionally been used in southern Asia and middle-eastern countries such as Iran as a sedative and for pleasure. It has been shown that opium users have less psychiatric comorbidity, unemployment, homelessness, and criminal behavior compared with users of other narcotic drugs [10, 28]. In Iran, the socioeconomic profile of opium users was almost identical with the socioeconomic circumstance of the general population [8]. In rural areas of Golestan province, where most of them are housewives, their pregnancies are planned, and approximately 97% of all pregnant women have access to primary health service funded by the state [29].

Strengths of this study include the cohort design, using prospectively collected information from antenatal visits before and during pregnancy. The population was relatively homogeneous, and opium-exposed mothers had otherwise had a normal lifestyle and an acceptable level of care during pregnancy [10]. We excluded a small proportion of women who were exposed to alcohol and selected non-users of opium and tobacco as the reference group to increase internal validity. Potential limitations include a lack of detailed information on mothers' socioeconomic circumstances. However, we controlled for husband's occupation and

region of residence. Information on exposure to opium and smoking during pregnancy was based on self-reports during routine visits. There was no information on the frequency or dose of opium to estimate dose-response associations. If mothers did not report their drug use, this may have pushed our estimates toward the null. However, the reliability of self-reported opium use in rural Golestan has been reported as high [30]. Gestational age was estimated based on information on the first day of the last maternal menstrual period, which can be subject to error [31]. Finally, as the study was based on data on pregnancies in the rural area of Golestan province, there may be concern regarding the generalizability of the results.

Conclusions
Maternal opium use during pregnancy is associated with giving birth to small for gestational age infants, and with short birth length and small head circumference in term infants. It is unlikely that the observed associations are confounded by other factors related to high-risk behavior, such as the use of other harmful substances. Preventative intervention studies should be conducted in regions where opium use is common among young women.

Abbreviations
BMI: Body Mass Index; CIs: Confidence Intervals; cm: centimeter; RRs: Risk Ratios; SGA: Small for Gestational Age

Acknowledgments
We are indebted to the members of the primary health care system of Golestan University of medical sciences, particularly maternal health care units in the rural area of Golestan north of Iran. We value the administrative contribution of Dr. Mohammad Na'imi M.D., Mph, and Mr. Abbas Moghadami MSc, (both at Golestan University of medical sciences).

Funding
This work was entirely funded by internal funding of Karolinska Institute.

Authors' contributions

SC and SB planned and designed the study. SMaghsoudlou, SB, MA, and SS contributed in the data collection and provided access to the data. SMaghsoudlou, SC, and SB involved in the review of the raw data and directly involved in the analysis. SC, SB, SMontgomery, and AW supervised this process and provided analytical feedback based on aggregated results. SMaghsoudlou, SC, MA, SMontgomery, AW, and SB involved directly in interpreting the results, and substantively reviewed and commented on the multiple drafts. SMaghsoudlou drafted and wrote the manuscript. All authors read and approved the final manuscript.

Competing interests

All authors declare that they have no competing interests.

Author details

[1]Clinical Epidemiology Unit, Department of Medicine, Karolinska Institute, Solna, Sweden. [2]Department of Obstetrics & Gynecology, McMaster University, 1280 Main Street West, room 3N52F, Hamilton, ON L8S 4K1, Canada. [3]Clinical Epidemiology and Biostatistics, School of Medical Sciences, Örebro University, Örebro, Sweden. [4]Department of Epidemiology and Public Health, University College London, London, UK. [5]Faculty of Medicine, Mazandaran University of Medical Sciences, Sari, Iran. [6]Faculty of Medicine, Golestan University of Medical Sciences, Gorgan, Iran. [7]Department of Clinical Sciences, Karolinska Institute, Danderyd Hospital, Stockholm, Sweden. [8]Clinical Epidemiology Unit & Centre for Pharmacoepidemiology, Department of Medicine, Karolinska Institute, Solna, Sweden.

References

1. Fischer B, Jones W, Rehm J. Trends and changes in prescription opioid analgesic dispensing in Canada 2005–2012: An update with a focus on recent interventions. BMC Health Serv Res. 2014;14:90. Available from: https://www.ncbi.nlm.nih.gov/pmc/articles/PMC3941687/.

2. Knoppert D. The worldwide opioid epidemic: Implications for treatment and research in pregnancy and the newborn. Pediatr Drugs. 2011;13:277–9.

3. Macaleer B, Shannon J. Does HR planning improve business performance. Ind Manag. 2003;45(1):14.

4. Brunton LL, Knollmann BC, Hilal-Dandan R. Goodman & Gilman's the pharmacological basis of therapeutics [Internet]. Thirteenth. New York: McGraw Hill Medical; 2018. Available from: https://accessmedicine.mhmedical.com/book.aspx?bookid=2189.

5. Pinto SM, Dodd S, Walkinshaw SA, Siney C, Kakkar P, Mousa HA. Substance abuse during pregnancy: effect on pregnancy outcomes. Eur J Obstet Gynecol Reprod Biol. 2010;150:137–41. Available from: https://www.ejog.org/article/S0301-2115(10)00092-8/fulltext. Accessed 22 Aug 2017.

6. Bandstra ES, Morrow CE, Mansoor E, Accornero VH. Prenatal drug exposure: Infant and toddler outcomes. J Addict Dis. 2010;29:245–58. Available from: http://www.tandfonline.com/doi/abs/10.1080/10550881003684871.

7. Keegan J, Parva M, Finnegan M, Gerson A, Belden M. Addiction in pregnancy. J Addict Dis. 2010;29:175–91. Available from: http://www.tandfonline.com/doi/abs/10.1080/10550881003684723.

8. Khademi H, Malekzadeh R, Pourshams A, Jafari E, Salahi R, Semnani S, et al. Opium use and mortality in Golestan cohort study: prospective cohort study of 50,000 adults in Iran. BMJ. 2012;344:e2502. Available from: http://www.bmj.com/cgi/doi/10.1136/bmj.e2502.

9. Maghsoudlou S, Cnattingius S, Aarabi M, Montgomery SM, Semnani S, Stephansson O, et al. Consanguineous marriage, prepregnancy maternal characteristics and stillbirth risk: A population-based case-control study. Acta Obstet Gynecol Scand. 2015;94:1095-1101. Available from: https://doi.org/10.1111/aogs.12699. [Accessed 7 Feb 2017]

10. Rahimi-Movaghar A, Hefazi M, Davoli M, Amato L, Amin-Esmaeili M, Yousefi-Nooraie R. Pharmacological therapies for maintenance treatments of opium dependency. Cochrane Database Syst Rev. 2009; https://www.cochranelibrary.com/cdsr/doi/10.1002/14651858.CD007775.pub2/full.

11. Maghsoudlou S, Cnattingius S, Montgomery S, Aarabi M, Semnani S, Wikström AK, et al. Opium use during pregnancy and risk of preterm delivery: A population-based cohort study. PLoS One. 2017;12:1–11. Available from: https://journals.plos.org/plosone/article?id=10.1371/journal.pone.0176588. https://doi.org/10.1371/journal.pone.0176588.

12. Malekzadeh MM, Khademi H, Pourshams A, Etemadi A, Poustchi H, Bagheri M, et al. Opium Use and Risk of Mortality from Digestive Diseases: A Prospective Cohort Study. Am J Gastroenterol. 2013;108:1757–65. Available from: http://www.nature.com/doifinder/10.1038/ajg.2013.336.

13. Mikolajczyk RT, Zhang J, Betran AP, Souza JP, Mori R, Gülmezoglu AM, et al. A global reference for fetal-weight and birthweight percentiles. Lancet. 2011;377:1855–61.

14. Patel P, Abdel-Latif ME, Hazelton B, Wodak A, Chen J, Emsley F, et al. Perinatal outcomes of Australian buprenorphine-exposed mothers and their newborn infants. J Paediatr Child Health. 2013;49:746–53.

15. Liu AJW, Sithamparanathan S, Jones MP, Cook CM, Nanan R. Growth restriction in pregnancies of opioid-dependent mothers. Arch Dis Child Fetal Neonatal Ed. 2010;95:F258–62. Available from: http://fn.bmj.com/cgi/doi/10.1136/adc.2009.163105.

16. Hulse GK, Milne E, English DR, Holman CD. The relationship between maternal use of heroin and methadone and infant birth weight. Addiction. 1997;92:1571–9. Available from: http://www.ncbi.nlm.nih.gov/pubmed/9519499.

17. Cnattingius S. The epidemiology of smoking during pregnancy: Smoking prevalence, maternal characteristics, and pregnancy outcomes. Nicotine Tob. Res. 2004;6:125–40. Available from: https://doi.org/10.1080/14622200410001669187.

18. Minnes S, Lang A, Singer L. Prenatal tobacco, marijuana, stimulant, and opiate exposure: outcomes and practice implications. Addict Sci Clin Pract. 2011;6:57–70. Available from: https://www.ncbi.nlm.nih.gov/pubmed/22003423.

19. Visconti K, Hennessy K, Towers C, Hennessy M, Howard B. 128: opiate abuse/usage in pregnancy and newborn head circumference. Am J Obstet Gynecol. 2013;208:S67–8. Available from: https://www.ajog.org/article/S0002-9378(12)01376-2/fulltext.

20. Hunt RW, Tzioumi D, Collins E, Jeffrey HE. Adverse neurdevelomental outcome of infants exposed to opiate in-utero. Early Hum Dev. 2008;84:29–35.

21. Kashiwagi M, Arlettaz R, Lauper U, Zimmermann R, Hebisch G. Methadone maintenance program in a Swiss perinatal center: (I): management and outcome of 89 pregnancies. Acta Obstet Gynecol Scand. 2005;84:140–4.

22. Ranke MB, Krägeloh-Mann I, Vollmer B. Growth, head growth, and neurocognitive outcome in children born very preterm: methodological aspects and selected results. Dev Med Child Neurol. 2015;57:23–8.

23. Lester BM, Bagner DM, Liu J, LaGasse LL, Seifer R, Bauer CR, et al. Infant neurobehavioral dysregulation: behavior problems in children with prenatal substance exposure. Pediatrics. 2009;124:1355–62. Available from: http://pediatrics.aappublications.org/cgi/doi/10.1542/peds.2008-2898.

24. Kaltenbach K, Berghella V, Finnegan L. Opioid dependence during pregnancy: effects and management. Obstet Gynecol Clin North Am. 1998;25:139–51. Available from: http://www.sciencedirect.com/science/article/pii/S0889854505703624.

25. Kuczkowski KM. Anesthetic implications of drug abuse in pregnancy. J Clin Anesth. 2003;15:382–94.

26. Sakellaridis N, Mangoura D, Vernadakis A. Effects of opiates on the growth of neuron-enriched cultures from chick embryonic brain. Int J Dev Neurosci. 1986;4:293–302.

27. Cengiz H, Dağdeviren H, Karaahmet O, Kaya C, Yildiz S, Ekin M. Maternal and neonatal effects of substance abuse during pregnancy: a case report. Haseki

Tip Bul. 2013;51:76–8. Available from: http://www.hasekidergisi.com/archives/archive-detail/article-preview/maternal-and-neonatal-effects-of-substance-abuse-d/6200.

28. Ghaffari Nejad A, Ziaadini H, Banazadeh N. Comparative Evaluation of Psychiatric Disorders in Opium and Heroin Dependent Patients†This article has been published in the Journal of Rafsanjan University of Medical Sciences in Persian language. Addict Heal. 2009;1:20–3. Available from: https://www.ncbi.nlm.nih.gov/pmc/articles/PMC3905498/.

29. Rashidian A, Khosravi A, Khabiri R, Khodayari-Moez E, Elahi E, Arab M, et al. Islamic Republic of Iran's Multiple Indicator Demograpphic and Healh Survey (IrMIDHS) 2010. IrMIDHS. 2012;

30. Abnet CC, Saadatian-Elahi M, Pourshams A, Boffetta P, Feizzadeh A, Brennan P, et al. Reliability and validity of opiate use self-report in a population at high risk for esophageal cancer in Golestan, Iran. Cancer Epidemiol. Biomarkers Prev. AACR. 2004;13:1068–70.

31. Kramer MS, Platt RW, Yang H, Haglund B, Cnattingius S, Bergsjo P. Registration Artifacts in International Comparisons of Infant Mortality. Obstet Gynecol Surv. 2002;57:429–30. Available from: https://onlinelibrary.wiley.com/doi/abs/10.1046/j.1365-3016.2002.00390.x.

2

Antenatal influenza and pertussis vaccination in Western Australia: a cross-sectional survey of vaccine uptake and influencing factors

Donna B. Mak[1,2*], Annette K. Regan[1,3], Dieu T. Vo[1,4] and Paul V. Effler[1,5]

Abstract

Background: Influenza and pertussis vaccines have been recommended in Australia for women during each pregnancy since 2010 and 2015, respectively. Estimating vaccination coverage and identifying factors affecting uptake are important for improving antenatal immunisation services.

Methods: A random sample of 800 Western Australian women ≥18 years of age who gave birth between 4th April and 4th October 2015 were selected. Of the 454 (57%) who were contactable by telephone, 424 (93%) completed a survey. Data were weighted by maternal age and area of residence to ensure representativeness. The proportion immunised against influenza and pertussis was the main outcome measure; multivariate logistic regression was used to identify factors significantly associated with antenatal vaccination. Results from the 2015 study were compared to similar surveys conducted in 2012–2014.

Results: In 2015, 71% (95% CI 66–75) of women received pertussis-containing vaccine and 61% (95% CI 56–66) received influenza vaccine during pregnancy; antenatal influenza vaccine coverage was 18% higher than in 2014 (43%; 95% CI: 34–46). Pertussis and influenza vaccine were co-administered for 68% of the women who received both vaccines. The majority of influenza vaccinations in 2015 were administered during the third trimester of pregnancy, instead of the second trimester, as was observed in prior years. Women whose care provider recommended both antenatal vaccinations had significantly higher odds of being vaccinated against both influenza and pertussis (OR 33.3, 95% CI: 15.15–73.38). Of unvaccinated mothers, 53.6% (95% CI: 45.9–61.3) and 78.3% (95% CI: 70.4–85.3) reported that they would have been vaccinated against influenza and pertussis, respectively, if their antenatal care provider had recommended it.

Conclusions: Pertussis vaccination coverage was high in the first year of an antenatal immunisation program in Western Australia. Despite a substantial increase in influenza vaccination uptake between 2014 and 2015, coverage remained below that for pertussis. Our data suggest influenza and pertussis vaccination rates of 83% and 94%, respectively, are achievable if providers were to recommend them to all pregnant women.

Keywords: Maternal health, Vaccination, Influenza vaccine, Pertussis vaccine, Antenatal care

* Correspondence: donna.mak@health.wa.gov.au
[1]Communicable Disease Control Directorate, Department of Health, Shenton Park, Western Australia
[2]School of Medicine, University of Notre Dame, Fremantle, Western Australia
Full list of author information is available at the end of the article

Background

Antenatal influenza vaccination can protect pregnant women from serious complications of influenza and prevent severe, potentially fatal influenza and pertussis infections in young infants through maternal antibody transfer [1]. Vaccinating pregnant women for pertussis during the third trimester of pregnancy ensures maximum transfer of maternal antibodies from the vaccine to the child through the placental membrane, thereby protecting young infants from the life-threatening complications of pertussis [2, 3]. In Australia, antenatal influenza vaccination has been recommended to pregnant women at any trimester during their pregnancy during the flu season and funded through the national immunisation program since 2010 [4]. Acellular pertussis-diphtheria-tetanus vaccine has been recommended during the third trimester of every pregnancy since 2015 [5]. The Western Australian (WA) government has funded provision of antenatal pertussis vaccination since March 2015, following the death of a one-month old infant from pertussis [6, 7].

Despite the availability of free vaccine and the demonstrated effectiveness in pregnant mothers and infants under 6 months of age [8, 9], previous research has shown uptake of influenza vaccine during pregnancy to be sub-optimal [10]. A study in 2014 found that just 41% of pregnant women in WA received influenza vaccine during pregnancy [8] with lack of recommendation of the vaccine from health providers being a main barrier for uptake of the antenatal flu vaccine [10]. More than 40% of women were not recommended the vaccine during pregnancy. The majority of women reported that they would have been vaccinated if a healthcare professional had recommended the vaccine to them. The study also found that many women were vaccinated to protect their unborn child suggesting that promotional efforts should emphasize on the importance of the vaccine for the child [10]. A systematic review has also identified inadequate knowledge of influenza risk and concerns about the safety of the antenatal influenza as barriers to uptake [11].

As the introduction of the antenatal pertussis vaccination program is relatively recent compared to the antenatal influenza vaccination program, data on pertussis coverage in Western Australia is limited. However, factors influencing uptake of the antenatal pertussis vaccine in other Australian states have been documented. A 2016 survey of 136 Victorian pregnant women found recommendation of the pertussis vaccine by a health care provider and belief in protection for the unborn child against pertussis was a main determinant of vaccine uptake [12]. The importance of health care provider recommendation was also demonstrated in surveys of Aboriginal mothers in Western Australia [13] and women from culturally and linguistically diverse backgrounds in Melbourne [14].

The aim of this study was to: 1) measure influenza and pertussis vaccine coverage during pregnancy in the first year after introduction of an antenatal pertussis vaccination program; and 2) compare factors associated with the uptake of each vaccine.

Methods

Annual surveys of antenatal influenza vaccination uptake have been conducted by the WA Department of Health (WA DOH) since 2012 [10], and in 2015, this survey was expanded to include pertussis vaccination. A sample of women ≥18 years who had given birth to a live infant between 4th April and 4th October 2015 (i.e. the period when the 2015 seasonal influenza vaccine was readily available) were randomly selected from the state's perinatal birth dataset; the Midwives Notification System (MNS) is a mandatory data reporting program that captures > 99% of all births in the state [15]. Assuming at least 40% uptake of antenatal vaccines, a final sample of 450 respondents was required to estimate vaccine coverage with a precision +/− 4.5% at the standard 95% confidence interval. An initial sample size of 800 women was calculated after taking into consideration the proportion of women whom could be contacted by telephone in previous surveys of antenatal influenza vaccination uptake (~ 60%) and the participation rate among those contacted (> = 90%). Women selected at random from the MNS dataset were invited to participate via a letter sent from WA DOH and given the option to decline participation. The names and telephone number/s (as recorded in the MNS) of women who did not 'opt-out' were provided to WA DOH interviewers.

Participants were telephoned in December 2015 and asked to complete a 10-min telephone survey about whether they had been vaccinated against influenza and/or pertussis during their last pregnancy, and their reasons for being vaccinated/unvaccinated. Up to three telephone calls, at different times of day, were made to each woman; inability to make contact was recorded as 'no response'. At the beginning of the telephone call, verbal consent was obtained to proceed with the interview and women who declined were not asked any further questions. Consent or declination was documented. Women who agreed to be interviewed were informed that they could cease the interview at any time. Information obtained during the interview included the mother's age, education level, postcode of residence, the presence of chronic medical conditions, and the health care setting where the woman received the majority of her antenatal care. Because some women receive paper records of their vaccination, vaccinated women were asked for the date and batch number of the vaccine/s for verification purposes. Women who could not provide the batch number were asked for permission for WA DOH to retrieve details of the vaccination/s from their immunisation provider.

Data analysis

Statistical analyses were performed using SAS version 9.4. To ensure representativeness of survey results, analyses were weighted by maternal age group and area of residence. Vaccination uptake of influenza, pertussis and both vaccines, along with 95% confidence intervals (CIs), were calculated. Univariate analysis was used to identify factors associated with vaccination uptake and variables significant at $\alpha = 0.05$ were included in a hierarchical multivariate logistic regression model to control for potential confounding. Reasons for or against influenza or pertussis vaccination were compared using Pearson's chi square analysis. Data from the 2015 antenatal survey were compared to results of published studies conducted in a similar manner during 2012–2014 [10, 16, 17].

This study has received written approval from the WA DOH Human Research Ethics Committee (HREC# 2015/29).

Results

Twenty-three (2.9%) of the 800 randomly selected women declined to participate in the study after receiving a letter informing them of their eligibility to participate; of the 777 remaining, 323 (41.6%) could not be contacted via telephone after 3 attempts, 30 (3.9%) declined participation after being contacted by telephone, and 424 (54.6%) completed the telephone survey (Fig. 1). Three women (3.9%)

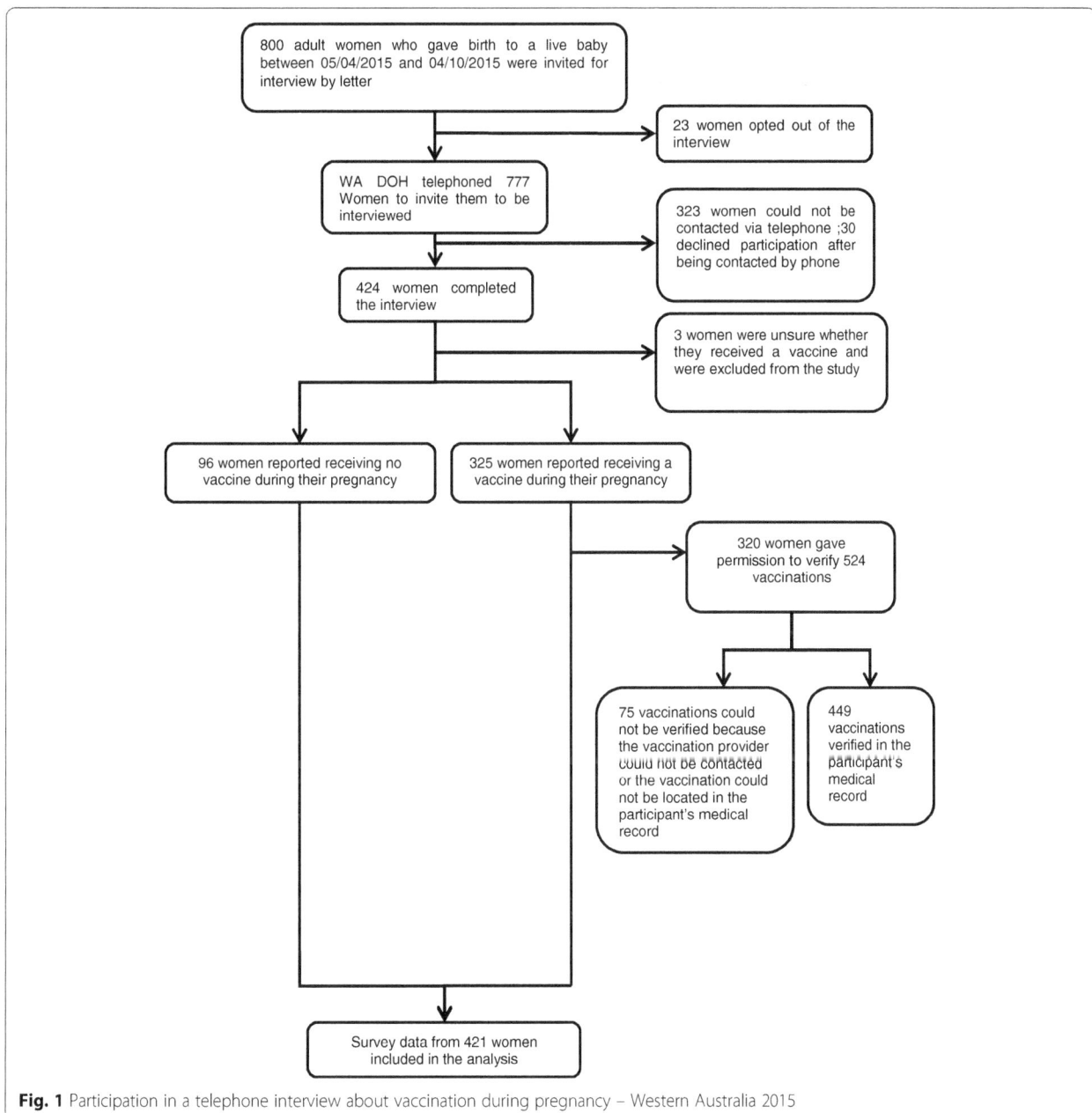

Fig. 1 Participation in a telephone interview about vaccination during pregnancy – Western Australia 2015

who were unsure whether they had received influenza or pertussis vaccine were excluded from the analysis.

The majority of survey participants (77.4%) lived in the Perth metropolitan area (Table 1); this is consistent with the proportion of births in the state in the Perth area (79.5%). However, slightly fewer participants were 18–24 years of age (10.9%) compared to all births during the study period (15.2%) and mothers 40 years and older were slightly over-represented (survey: 5.5%; state: 3.7%). Half of the women received most of their antenatal care at a public hospital antenatal clinic (49.6%), 30.4% from a private obstetrician, and 16.9% from a general practitioner. One in ten women (10.5%) had a chronic medical condition and about a third (31.3%) had a high school education or less.

The proportions of women who reported that their health care provider recommended that they receive the influenza, pertussis, or both vaccines, were 74.0% (95% CI: 69.7–78.3%), 72.4% (95% CI: 68.0–76.7%) and 63.2% (95% CI: 58.5–67.9%), respectively. There were no differences in the sociodemographic characteristics of women who were recommended and those who were not recommended influenza and/or pertussis vaccines ($p > .05$). The proportions of women who reported they had received influenza, pertussis and both influenza and pertussis vaccinations during their last pregnancy were 60.6% (95% CI: 56.0–65.6%), 71.0% (95% CI: 66.3–75.2%) and 54.5% (95% CI: 49.7–59.4%), respectively.

Influenza vaccine uptake increased significantly in 2015 with the annual antenatal vaccination survey from 2014 estimating coverage at 42.5% (95% CI: 38.8–46.3%). In addition, prior to 2015, the majority of women immunised against seasonal influenza received their vaccination in the second trimester (range: 54.3% [2013] to 58.9% [2012]); in 2015, this proportion declined to 28.1% while the proportion of immunised women who received their vaccination in the third trimester rose to 55.3% (Fig. 2). Most (90.1%) women immunised against pertussis received the vaccine in their third trimester and of the 211 women who received influenza and pertussis vaccine, 68.2% received both vaccines on the same day.

Of the 320 vaccinated women who gave permission for their immunisation record/s to be verified against medical records, 449 (85.7%) of the 524 reported vaccinations were confirmed (influenza: 79.6%, pertussis: 91.0%).

A total of 66.9% of women reported that they received their influenza vaccine at a general practice (GP), 17.9% at a public hospital antenatal clinic and 5.5% at their workplace; 68.6% of women reported receiving their pertussis vaccine at a GP, 20.9% at a public hospital antenatal clinic and 6.4% at a private hospital clinic.

Predictors of vaccination

On univariate analysis, a healthcare provider's recommendation ($p < .001$) was significantly associated with the uptake of either influenza or pertussis vaccine during pregnancy (Table 1). The impact of the healthcare provider's recommendation on vaccination appears to be vaccine specific, as women who were recommended pertussis vaccine (and not influenza vaccine) had a greater odds of pertussis (OR: 5.34, 95% CI: 1.23–13.00, $p = 0.005$) but not influenza, (OR: 1.56, 95% CI: 0.59–4.09, $p = 0.37$) vaccination. Similarly, women who were recommended influenza vaccine (and not pertussis vaccine) had greater odds of influenza (OR: 4.47, 95% CI: 1.89–10.59, $p < 0.001$) but not pertussis (OR: 0.94, 95% CI: 0.42–2.1, $p = .89$) vaccination compared to women not recommended to receive either vaccine. Women whose healthcare provider recommended both antenatal vaccinations had significantly higher odds of being vaccinated against both influenza and pertussis (OR 33.3, 95% CI: 15.15–73.38 $p < 0.001$). The existence of a chronic medical condition was negatively associated with pertussis vaccine uptake (OR 0.42, 95% CI: 0.22–0.80, $p < 0.05$) (Table 1). On multivariate analyses, a healthcare provider's recommendation was the only common independent predictor of the uptake of influenza, pertussis and both vaccines (Fig. 3).

Reasons for or against vaccination

Among vaccinated mothers, the most commonly reported reason they were immunised was to protect the baby (96.1% of mothers vaccinated against influenza and 98.6% of those vaccinated against pertussis). A significantly larger proportion of mothers vaccinated against pertussis vs influenza reported doing so because of influence of family, friends and media (73.7% vs 52.1%, $p < 0.001$) (Table 2).

Commonly reported reasons for not being vaccinated against pertussis included that vaccination had not been recommended by an antenatal care provider (43.9%) and concerns about vaccination harming the baby (23.0%). Common reasons women did not receive influenza vaccine included concerns about side-effects to the mother (37.1%), harming the baby (32.5%) and because the vaccine was not recommended by a health provider (33.6%) (Table 2). Concern about the side effects of the vaccine were more commonly reported for influenza vaccine than pertussis vaccine ($p = 0.04$).

Among unvaccinated women, 53.6% (95% CI: 45.9–61.3) and 78.3% (95% CI: 70.4–85.3) reported that they would have been vaccinated against influenza and pertussis, respectively, during their pregnancy if a health care provider had recommended it.

Discussion

This cross-sectional survey provides the first estimates of coverage and factors influencing uptake of both antenatal pertussis and influenza vaccines in Australia. A total of 72% of pregnant women received a pertussis

Table 1 Results of univariate logistic regression analysis estimating the odds of pertussis and/or influenza vaccines during pregnancy – Western Australia, 2015

	Adult women who gave birth to a live infant in WA, 05/04/2015–04/10/2015	Survey respondents	Percent vaccinated against influenza[a] (+/– pertussis vaccination)		Percent vaccinated against pertussis[c] (+/– influenza vaccination)		Percent vaccinated against pertussis and influenza[d]	
	n (unweighted %)	n (unweighted %)	n (weighted %)	OR (95% CI)[b]	n (weighted %)	OR (95% CI)[b]	n (weighted %)	OR (95% CI)[b]
Total	19,866	421 (100)	255 (60.6)	–	299 (71.0)	–	229 (54.4)	–
Age group								
18-24y	3010 (15.2)	46 (10.9)	32 (69.8)	Ref	33 (72.0)	Ref	28 (61.0)	Ref
25-29y	5713 (28.8)	109 (25.9)	61 (56.1)	0.55 (0.26–1.16)	71 (65.3)	0.73 (0.34–1.57)	55 (50.5)	0.55 (0.23–1.32)
30-34y	7049 (35.5)	164 (38.9)	98 (59.7)	0.64 (0.32–1.31)	124 (75.4)	1.20 (0.57–2.51)	89 (54.1)	0.90 (0.38–2.14)
35-39y	3368 (17.0)	79 (18.8)	54 (68.3)	0.94 (0.42–2.07)	57 (72.1)	1.01 (0.45–2.28)	48 (60.7)	0.95 (0.37–2.45)
≥40y	726 (3.7)	23 (5.5)	10 (43.5)	0.33 (0.12–0.95)	14 (60.9)	0.61 (0.21–1.75)	9 (39.1)	0.36 (0.10–1.21)
Residence								
Metropolitan	15,787 (79.5)	326 (77.4)	198 (60.9)	Ref	229 (70.2)	Ref	177 (54.4)	Ref
Non-metropolitan	4079 (20.5)	95 (22.6)	57 (60.6)	0.99 (0.61–1.60)	69 (72.9)	1.14 (0.67–1.64)	52 (55.00)	1.10 (0.60–2.00)
Educational attainment								
Primary/High School	–	132 (31.3)	79 (61.4)	Ref	92 (70.3)	Ref	72 (55.6)	Ref
TAFE[e]	–	98 (23.3)	59 (59.7)	0.93 (0.54–1.61)	66 (67.8)	0.89 (0.50–1.58)	52 (52.9)	0.89 (0.47–1.71)
University Undergraduate	–	102 (24.2)	63 (61.5)	1.00 (0.58–1.72)	77 (73.9)	1.20 (0.66–2.18)	56 (54.2)	1.24 (0.63–2.46)
University Postgraduate	–	89 (21.1)	54 (60.4)	0.96 (0.55–1.68)	64 (71.6)	1.07 (0.58–1.95)	49 (54.8)	1.04 (0.53–2.04)
Socioeconomic status[f]								
Quintile 1 and 2 (Lowest)	–	57 (13.5)	36 (63.0)	Ref	42 (72.7)	Ref	35 (61.0)	Ref
Quintile 3	–	117 (27.8)	66 (56.7)	0.77 (0.40–1.50)	72 (62.2)	0.59 (0.29–1.20)[h]	56 (48.6)	0.65 (0.30–1.41)
Quintile 4	–	89 (21.2)	52 (58.4)	0.83 (0.41–1.66)	66 (73.1)	0.97 (0.45–2.10)	48 (53.44)	0.97 (0.42–2.23)
Quintile 5 (Highest)	–	158 (37.5)	101 (64.5)	1.07 (0.56–2.03)	119 (75.0)	1.07 (0.53–2.17)	90 (57.2)	1.29 (0.60–2.77)
Chronic medical conditions[g]								
Yes	–	44 (10.5)	20 (48.9)	0.58 (0.30–1.10)	23 (52.8)	0.42 (0.22–0.80)[h]	15 (35.9)	0.40 (0.18–0.86)[h]
No	–	377 (89.5)	235 (62.3)	Ref	276 (73.0)	Ref	214 (56.8)	Ref
Antenatal care provider								
Private Obstetrician	–	128 (30.4)	86 (66.6)	1.57 (0.98–2.51)	104 (81.1)	2.42 (1.41–4.13)[h]	78 (60.3)	2.86 (1.51–5.42)[h]
General Practitioner	–	71 (16.9)	46 (65.5)	1.49 (0.84–2.65)	53 (75.3)	1.71 (0.92–3.18)	41 (59.1)	1.91 (0.93–3.92)
Private Practice Midwife	–	10 (2.4)	6 (67.7)	1.65 (0.44–6.14)	6 (67.7)	1.18 (0.32–4.39)	6 (67.7)	1.25 (0.33–4.70)
Public Hospital Antenatal Clinic	–	209 (49.6)	116 (56.0)	Ref	135 (64.1)	Ref	103 (49.3)	Ref
Other	–	3 (0.71)	1 (37.9)	0.48 (0.04–5.60)	1 (37.9)	0.34 (0.03–4.00)	1 (37.9)	0.362 (0.03–4.28)

Table 1 Results of univariate logistic regression analysis estimating the odds of pertussis and/or influenza vaccines during pregnancy – Western Australia, 2015 *(Continued)*

	Adult women who gave birth to a live infant in WA, 05/04/2015–04/10/2015	Survey respondents	Percent vaccinated against influenza[a] (+/– pertussis vaccination)		Percent vaccinated against pertussis[c] (+/– influenza vaccination)		Percent vaccinated against pertussis and influenza[d]	
	n (unweighted %)	n (unweighted %)	n (weighted %)	OR (95% CI)[b]	n (weighted %)	OR (95% CI)[b]	n (weighted %)	OR (95% CI)[b]
Recommendation by healthcare provider								
Recommended pertussis only	–	37 (8.8)	10 (25.4)	1.56 (0.59–4.09)	26 (73.8)	5.34 (2.19–13.00)[h]	10 (25.4)	3.73 (1.23–11.35)[h]
Recommended influenza only	–	44 (10.5)	21 (49.3)	4.47 (1.89–10.59)[i]	15 (33.3)	0.94 (0.42–2.11)	10 (22.3)	2.16 (0.78–6.03)
Recommended pertussis and influenza vaccines	–	268 (63.7)	211 (79.4)	17.66 (8.92–34.99)[i]	231 (86.4)	11.96 (6.53–21.91)[i]	197 (74.3)	33.34 (15.15–73.38)[i]
Not recommended either vaccine	–	72 (17.1)	13 (17.9)	Ref	26 (34.6)	Ref	12 (16.7)	Ref

[a] Woman received seasonal influenza vaccine during pregnancy +/– pertussis vaccination
[b] Odds of vaccination and corresponding 95% confidence intervals
[c] Woman received diphtheria-tetanus-acellular pertussis vaccine during pregnancy +/– influenza vaccination
[d] Woman received both influenza and pertussis vaccines during pregnancy
[e] TAFE, technical and further education qualification
[f] Socioeconomic level was determined based on postcode of residence and Socioeconomic Index for Areas (insert link to website)
[g] Chronic medical conditions included asthma, chronic heart disease, chronic lung conditions, and diabetes
[h] p < .05
[i] p < .001

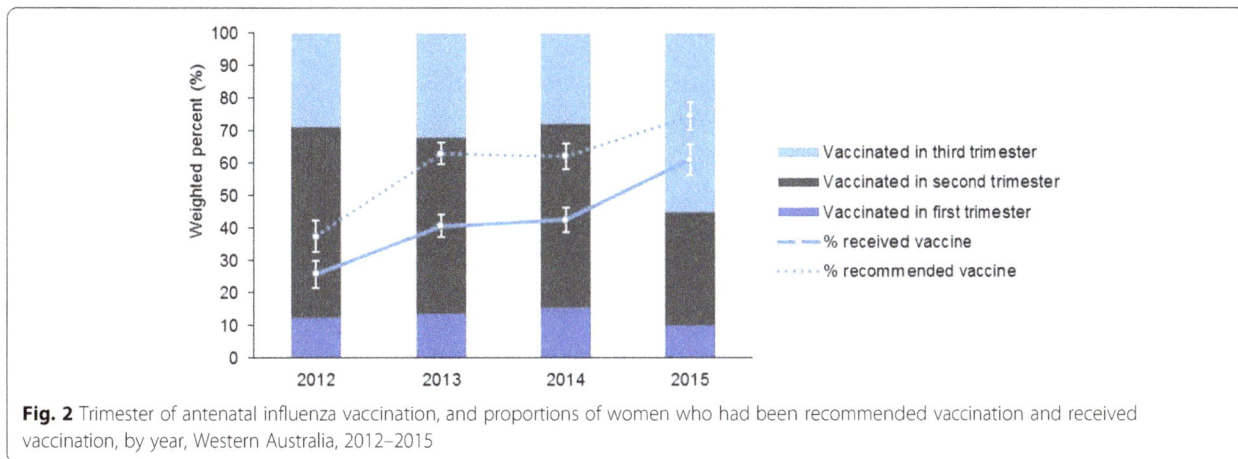

Fig. 2 Trimester of antenatal influenza vaccination, and proportions of women who had been recommended vaccination and received vaccination, by year, Western Australia, 2012–2015

vaccine; 61% received an influenza vaccine, an increase from 42% the previous year [16]. These results demonstrate that most women receive routinely recommended vaccines during pregnancy in Western Australia, but there is still room for improvement.

The introduction of the antenatal pertussis vaccination program in 2015 may have influenced seasonal influenza vaccination of pregnant women in terms of both uptake and trimester of vaccine administration. In contrast to previous years, 2015 was the first year that most women vaccinated against influenza received the vaccine in their third, rather than second trimester. As nearly 70% of women who vaccinated against both influenza and pertussis received them on the same day, it would seem that introduction of a recommendation for pertussis vaccination between weeks 28–32 of pregnancy may have had the effect of shifting the timing of the influenza vaccination to the third trimester as well as

increasing the coverage of antenatal influenza vaccination. While vaccinating for influenza during the third trimester of pregnancy is ideal for antibody transfer [1] to the unborn child, it leaves pregnant women potentially unprotected against influenza during their first two trimesters of pregnancy. This may have serious adverse consequences for women at high risk of developing complications of influenza.

WA's antenatal pertussis vaccination program was quite successful in its first year, given that in other settings less than 25% of women received a pertussis vaccine during pregnancy in the first year of their program [18, 19]. A recent study from the Northern Territory, Australia, found that 22.3% of women received a pertussis vaccination during pregnancy [18]. In the United Kingdom, the antenatal pertussis vaccination program was implemented for 4 years before a comparable coverage of antenatal pertussis vaccination was achieved (70%) [20]. Unpublished data from the

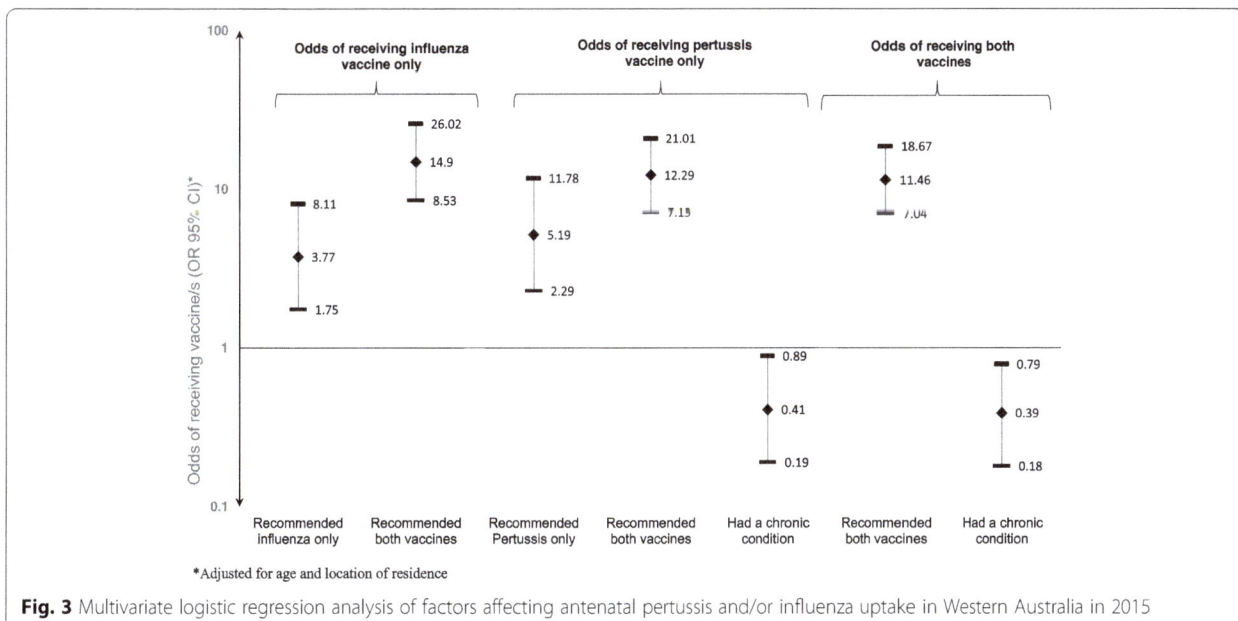

Fig. 3 Multivariate logistic regression analysis of factors affecting antenatal pertussis and/or influenza uptake in Western Australia in 2015

Table 2 Reasons why women received/did not receive an influenza or pertussis vaccination – Western Australia, 2015 (multiple responses allowed)

Reasons why vaccinated women received a vaccine during pregnancy	Influenza vaccine ($n = 256$)	Pertussis vaccine ($n = 299$)	p-value
	n (%)	n (%)	
Protect baby	247 (96.1)	296 (98.6)	.30
Influenced by family, friends and media	136 (52.1)	222 (73.7)	<.001
Antenatal care provider recommended it	229 (90.6)	265 (88.4)	.48
General practitioner recommended it	155 (61.3)	172 (57.9)	.83
Worried about pertussis/influenza	138 (53.7)	188 (63.2)	.03
Obstetrician recommended it	129 (49.1)	157 (52.4)	.25
Midwife recommended it	128 (49.6)	165 (55.9)	.02
To protect family	6 (2.2)	–	–
To protect herself	11 (4.2)	–	–
Normally get vaccine	115 (44.6)	–	–
Health care employee	8 (2.9)	–	–
Chronic medical condition	16 (6.4)	–	–
Reasons why unvaccinated women did not receive a vaccine during pregnancy	Influenza vaccine ($n = 165$)	Pertussis vaccine ($n = 122$)	p-value
	n (%)	n (%)	
No antenatal care provider recommendation	56 (33.6)	54 (43.9)	.64
Worried that it would harm the baby	54 (32.5)	28 (23.0)	.47
Worried about potential side effects	62 (37.1)	15 (11.9)	.04
Was advised against it	11 (6.9)	8 (7.8)	.92
Was too late in pregnancy	–	7 (5.9)	–
Vaccine not available	6 (3.7)	3 (2.5)	.58
Already received or planning to receive after pregnancy	7 (6.9)	11 (8.6)	.10
Not necessary	6 (3.4)	–	–
Don't normally get vaccine	56 (33.3)	–	–
First trimester of pregnancy	43 (25.8)	–	–

WA Department of Health indicates that antenatal pertussis coverage in WA has not only been sustained, but has continued to increase to almost 80% in 2016.

One factor which may have influenced this success in WA is the potential influence of the tragic death of a young infant in early March 2015. At that time the mother was pregnant, antenatal pertussis vaccination was not recommended in the Australian Immunisation Handbook and there was no government-funded pertussis vaccination program in WA in place [21]. The baby's death was well publicised and his family continue to promote the benefits of antenatal and childhood vaccination in Australia via mass- and social-media and parent and baby expos. The impact of their efforts is likely reflected in the high proportion of mothers who said they were vaccinated against pertussis because of the influence of family, friends and media (74%). This finding suggests that social-media and community-driven campaigns can be effective in promoting vaccinations among pregnant women.

Despite the success of WA's antenatal pertussis vaccination program and continued increases in antenatal influenza uptake, further improvement in uptake is achievable and should be pursued. Results from this survey and other studies have consistently identified the recommendation by a healthcare provider as the strongest predictor of antenatal vaccination [12–14, 16–18]. Although influenza and pertussis vaccination were standard antenatal care for women in our study, less than two-thirds were recommended both vaccines during their pregnancy. Data from unvaccinated women in this survey suggest that if 100% of women were recommended to be vaccinated in accordance with current standard-of-care obstetrical guidelines in Australia, coverage rates among pregnant women for influenza and pertussis vaccine could reach 82% and 94%, respectively.

Barriers to vaccination reported by the women in this survey reveal a need for additional education for pregnant mothers and their antenatal care providers. Over a third of women not vaccinated for influenza and 27% of women not vaccinated for pertussis cited concerns about side effects of the vaccination to themselves or harm to their babies as reasons for non-vaccination. Other reasons reported for not vaccinating include already being immunised for pertussis before pregnancy and/or plans to vaccinate post-partum. None of these reasons for not being vaccinated in pregnancy are evidence-based decisions [3, 8, 10, 22]. The results also suggest that further education would be beneficial for antenatal care providers given that 8% and 7% of women not vaccinated for pertussis and influenza respectively reported that a healthcare provider had advised them against vaccination.

A negative association between having a chronic medical condition and pertussis vaccination uptake even after controlling for healthcare provider's recommendation was unexpected. It is not clear why women with a chronic medical condition would be more likely than women without a chronic medical condition to refuse pertussis vaccination if it was offered.

There are several limitations to our study. First, assignment of vaccination status relied on self-report. Previous research has shown that vaccination coverage can be over-estimated based on self-report [23]. However, we were able to verify 86% of self-reported vaccinations directly with the immunisation provider, suggesting any bias introduced is likely to be small. Second, although women were selected at random to participate in the survey, there was some under-representation of mothers under the age of 25 years. To account for this under-representation, survey results were weighted by age and apart from this particular subset of women, age and geographic distribution of survey respondents was generally comparable with the population of women eligible for study selection. The response rate of 54.6% is considered satisfactory for a telephone survey [24]. Finally, this survey was conducted in WA and the views and opinions of mothers in this state may not represent those in other parts of Australia or other countries. Further assessments on the uptake of pertussis and influenza vaccines in other geographic settings are needed.

Conclusions

Almost three quarters of pregnant women were immunised in the first year of an antenatal pertussis vaccination program. Although increasing, antenatal influenza vaccine coverage remains lower than that for pertussis vaccine. A substantial proportion of unimmunised women indicated that they would have been vaccinated if it had been recommended to them by an antenatal care provider, suggesting that antenatal vaccination coverage approaching 90% could be achieved if providers universally recommended immunisation. Strategies for improving antenatal vaccination uptake should include education of pregnant women and their healthcare providers on the benefits and safety of influenza and pertussis vaccination during pregnancy.

Abbreviations
CI: Confidence interval; GP: General Practitioner; MNS: Midwives Notification System; WA DOH: Western Australian Department of Health; WA: Western Australia

Acknowledgements
The authors would like to acknowledge staff from the Department of Health Western Australia's Maternal and Child Health Unit and the Data Integrity Directorate for assisting in the selection of eligible participants and obtaining initial consent from participating women.

Funding
This study was funded by Communicable Disease Control Directorate, Department of Health Western Australia.

Data analysis
Statistical analyses were performed using SAS version 9.4. To ensure representativeness of survey results, analyses were weighted by maternal age group and area of residence. Vaccination uptake of influenza, pertussis and both vaccines, along with 95% confidence intervals (CIs), were calculated. Univariate analysis was used to identify factors associated with vaccination uptake and variables significant at $\alpha = 0.05$ were included in a hierarchical multivariate logistic regression model to control for potential confounding. Reasons for or against influenza or pertussis vaccination were compared using Pearson's chi square analysis. Data from the 2015 antenatal survey were compared to results of published studies conducted in a similar manner during 2012–2014 [10, 16, 17].
This study has received written approval from the WA DOH Human Research Ethics Committee (HREC# 2015/29).

Authors' contributions
DM wrote the study protocol and ethics application, undertook extensive revision of the first and subsequent drafts of this manuscript and contributed to data analysis. AR contributed to the study protocol and ethics application, led the data collection, and undertook the bulk of the data analysis presented in the manuscript. DV was involved in the data cleaning, contributed to data analysis and contributed to the initial drafting of the manuscript. PE oversaw the conception and implementation of this study and contributed to the study design and data analysis. All authors contributed to interpreting the study's findings, writing the manuscript and all approved the final manuscript.

Competing interests
The authors have no competing interests to declare.

Author details
[1]Communicable Disease Control Directorate, Department of Health, Shenton Park, Western Australia. [2]School of Medicine, University of Notre Dame, Fremantle, Western Australia. [3]School of Public Health, Curtin University,

Bentley, Western Australia. [4]School of Population Health, University of Western Australia, Crawley, Western Australia. [5]School of Pathology and Laboratory Medicine, University of Western Australia, Crawley, Western Australia.

References

1. Marshall H, McMillan M, Andrews R, Macartney K, Edwards K. Vaccines in pregnancy: the dual benefit for pregnant women and infants. Hum Vaccines Immunotherapeutics. 2016;12(4):848–56.
2. Abraham C, Pichichero M, Eisenberg J, Singh S. Third-trimester maternal vaccination against pertussis and pertussis antibody concentrations. Obstet Gynecol. 2018;131(2):364–9.
3. Munoz FM, Bond NH, Maccato M, Pinell P, Hammill HA, Swamy GK, et al. Safety and immunogenicity of tetanus diphtheria and acellular pertussis (Tdap) immunization during pregnancy in mothers and infants: a randomized clinical trial. JAMA. 2014;311(17):1760–9.
4. National Centre for Immunisation Research and Surveillance. History of influenza vaccination in Australia. National Centre for immunisation research and surveillance; 2016.
5. Australian Government Department of Health. The Australian Immunisation Handbook 10th Edition. In: Australian Government Department of Health, editor. Canberra 2015.
6. Cox N. WA health minister announces free whooping cough vaccines for expectant mums. WA today 2015.
7. Operational Directive: Influenza and pertussis vaccinations for pregnant women, F-AA-13121 (2015).
8. Benowitz I, Esposito DB, Gracey KD, Shapiro ED, Vázquez M. Influenza vaccine given to pregnant women reduces hospitalization due to influenza in their infants. Clin Infect Dis. 2010;51(12):1355–61.
9. Omer SB, Goodman D, Steinhoff MC, Rochat R, Klugman KP, Stoll BJ, et al. Maternal influenza immunization and reduced likelihood of prematurity and small for gestational age births: a retrospective cohort study. PLoS Med. 2011;8(5):e1000441.
10. Regan AK, Mak DB, Hauck YL, Gibbs R, Tracey L, Effler PV. Trends in seasonal influenza vaccine uptake during pregnancy in Western Australia: implications for midwives. Women Birth. 2016;29(5):423–9.
11. Yuen CYS, Tarrant M. Determinants of uptake of influenza vaccination among pregnant women – a systematic review. Vaccine. 2014;32(36):4602–13.
12. Naidu MA, Krishnaswamy S, Wallace EM, Giles ML. Pregnant women's attitudes toward antenatal pertussis vaccination. Aust N Z J Obstet Gynaecol. 2017;57(2):235.
13. Lotter K, Regan AK, Thomas T, Effler PV, Mak DB. Antenatal influenza and pertussis vaccine uptake among aboriginal mothers in Western Australia. Aust N Z J Obstet Gynaecol. 2017.
14. Krishnaswamy S, Cheng AC, Wallace EM, Buttery J, Giles ML. Understanding the barriers to uptake of antenatal vaccination by women from culturally and linguistically diverse backgrounds: a cross-sectional study. Hum Vaccines Immunotherapeutics. 2018;14:1591–598. https://doi.org/10.1080/21645515.2018.1445455.
15. Ballestas T. The 14th Report of the Perinatal and Infant Mortality Committee of Western Australia for deaths in the triennium 2008–2010. Perth: Western Australian Department of Health; 2014.
16. Mak DB, Regan AK, Joyce S, Gibbs R, Effler PV. Antenatal care provider's advice is the key determinant of influenza vaccination uptake in pregnant women. Aust N Z J Obstet Gynaecol. 2015;55(2):131–7.
17. Taksdal SE, Mak DB, Joyce S, Tomlin S, Carcione D, Armstrong PK, et al. Predictors of uptake of influenza vaccination: a survey of pregnant women in Western Australia. Aust Fam Physician. 2013;42(8):582.
18. Overton K, Webby R, Markey P, Krause V. Influenza and pertussis vaccination coverage in pregnant women in the Northern Territory in 2015—new recommendations to be assessed. NT Dis Control Bull. 2016;23:1–8.
19. Kharbanda EO, Vazquez-Benitez G, Lipkind H, Naleway AL, Klein NP, Cheetham TC, et al. Receipt of pertussis vaccine during pregnancy across 7 vaccine safety datalink sites. Prev Med. 2014;67:316–9.
20. Public Health England. Pertussis vaccination programme for pregnant women update: vaccine coverage in England, October to December 2016. Public Health England; 2017. Contract No.: 8.
21. Hughes C. Hughes C, editor. UNICEF: UNICEF. 2015. Available from: https://www.unicef.org.au/blog/stories/december-2015/light-for-riley.
22. Sukumaran L, McCarthy NL, Kharbanda EO, Weintraub E, Vazquez-Benitez G, McNeil MM, et al. Safety of tetanus, diphtheria, and acellular pertussis and influenza vaccinations in pregnancy. Obstet Gynecol. 2015;126(5):1069.
23. Jiménez-García R, Hernandez-Barrera V, Rodríguez-Rieiro C, Garrido PC, de Andres AL, Jimenez-Trujillo I, et al. Comparison of self-report influenza vaccination coverage with data from a population based computerized vaccination registry and factors associated with discordance. Vaccine. 2014; 32(35):4386–92.
24. Davern M, Call K, Ziegenfuss J, McAlpine D, Beebe T. Are low response rates hazardous to your health. American association of public opinion research. 2006.

3

Development of an integrated, district-wide approach to pre-pregnancy management for women with pre-existing diabetes in a multi-ethnic population

Maryam Sina, Freya MacMillan, Tinashe Dune, Navodya Balasuriya, Nouran Khouri, Ngan Nguyen, Vasyngpong Jongvisal, Xiang Hui Lay and David Simmons*

Abstract

Background: Poor diabetes management prior to conception, results in increased rates of fetal malformations and other adverse pregnancy outcomes. We describe the development of an integrated, pre-pregnancy management strategy to improve pregnancy outcomes among women of reproductive age with diabetes in a multi-ethnic district.

Methods: The strategy included (i) a narrative literature review of contraception and pre-pregnancy interventions for women with diabetes and development of a draft plan; (ii) a chart review of pregnancy outcomes (e.g. congenital malformations, neonatal hypoglycaemia and caesarean sections) among women with type 1 diabetes (T1D) ($n = 53$) and type 2 diabetes (T2D) ($n = 46$) between 2010 and 2015 (iii) interview surveys of women with T1D and T2D ($n = 15$), and local health care professionals ($n = 13$); (iv) two focus groups ($n = 4$) and one-to-one interviews with women with T1D and T2D from an Australian background ($n = 5$), women with T2D from cultural and linguistically diverse (CALD) ($n = 7$) and indigenous backgrounds ($n = 1$) and partners of CALD women ($n = 3$); and (v) two group meetings, one comprising predominantly primary care, and another comprising district-wide multidisciplinary inter-sectoral professionals, where components of the intervention strategy were finalised using a Delphi approach for development of the final plan.

Results: Our literature review showed that a range of interventions, particularly multifaceted educational programs for women and healthcare professionals, significantly increased contraception uptake, and reduced adverse outcomes of pregnancy (e.g. malformations and stillbirth). Our chart-review showed that local rates of adverse pregnancy outcomes were similarly poor among women with both T1D and T2D (e.g. major congenital malformations [9.1% vs 8.9%] and macrosomia [34.7% vs 24.4%]). Challenges included lack of knowledge among women and healthcare professionals relating to diabetes management and limited access to specialist pre-pregnancy care. Group meetings led to a consensus to develop a district-wide approach including healthcare professional and patient education and a structured approach to identification and optimisation of self-management, including contraception, in women of reproductive age with diabetes.

Conclusions: Sufficient evidence exists for consensus on a district-wide strategy to improve pre-pregnancy management among women with pre-existing diabetes.

Keywords: Pre-pregnancy care, Contraception, Type 1 diabetes, Type 2 diabetes, Intervention programs, Malformations

* Correspondence: Da.Simmons@westernsydney.edu.au
Western Sydney University, Sydney, NSW 2751, Australia

Background

Women with type 1 and type 2 diabetes have a high risk of adverse pregnancy outcomes, especially when conception is unplanned [1]. Uncontrolled hyperglycaemia before and during pregnancy leads to adverse maternal and foetal outcomes [2]. Pre-pregnancy care (PPC) includes services aimed at managing glycaemia, education on diabetes complications in pregnancy, screening and treatment of diabetic complications, management of medications, and the supplementation of higher-dose folic acid required by women of reproductive age to ensure higher chances of an uncomplicated pregnancy [3]. A meta-analysis in 2012 showed that across 12 studies, PPC was effective in reducing congenital malformation [Risk Ratio (RR) = 0.3 (95% CI 0.2, 0.4)] and perinatal mortality [RR = 0.3 (95% CI 0.2, 0.8)] [3]. PPC was associated with a lower HbA1c in the first trimester of pregnancy by an average of 1.9% (95% CI: – 2.1, – 1.8) or 20.8 mmol/mol (95% CI: – 23.0, – 19.7) [3].

However, these studies showing reduced malformations and perinatal mortality have come from clinics established for women who are planning pregnancy, and are willing and able to attend [4, 5]. Lack of information and practical constraints, such as commitment to work, are often major obstacles for those who do not attend pre-pregnancy clinics [6]. Furthermore, approximately 50% of pregnancies among women with pre-existing diabetes remain unplanned [7, 8], and many of these should therefore be seen as largely a failure of contraception rather than a failure of access to a pre-pregnancy clinic. However, a proportion of these 'unplanned' pregnancies occur among women who wish to maintain autonomy during the pregnancy process [9], and who would not attend a pre-pregnancy clinic. It is clear that a pregnancy in a woman with diabetes without PPC is often a failure of 'the system', although at times this may be due to the failure of clinicians to understand the perspective of women with diabetes. In fact, the term "PPC" could be misleading as it implies that women are planning pregnancy, when all that may be required is effective contraception or knowledge about the options and methods of their use. Therefore, we use the term 'pre-pregnancy management' (PPM), to emphasize the integrated approach required to improve contraception uptake and pregnancy outcomes in this population.

There have been a variety of interventions at a population level that could be used for PPM, including better contraception choices, in order to reach women who have not traditionally attended pre-pregnancy clinics [5, 10–13]. However, no population-based intervention program has been implemented in Australia. South West Sydney (SWS) is a home to women from culturally and linguistically diverse (CALD) backgrounds who may have different risks to women participating in previous population based approaches, requiring additional or different PPM [1, 14]. We now present the steps in the development of an intervention program for PPM, including enhanced contraception uptake, for the multiethnic district of SWS.

Methods

The development of the intervention involved: 1) a narrative literature review of PPC intervention programs used in women with type 1 diabetes (T1D) and type 2 diabetes (T2D); 2) chart review of women with T1D and T2D; 3) interview surveys with women with T1D and T2D and health care professionals (HCPs); 4) in-depth qualitative exploration of local pregnancies through focus groups one-to-one interviews with women with T1D and T2D and partners; 5) the preparation of a draft intervention plan with discussion at a local conference; and 6) a discussion of the intervention at two multidisciplinary meetings one, predominantly primary care (n = 15) and one predominantly secondary care (e.g. general practitioners, obstetricians, midwives, endocrinologists, diabetes educators, dietitians) (n = 17) to finalise the plan.

Narrative review

Google Scholar, PubMed and Medline databases were searched for randomised trials (including cluster and quasi-randomised trials), as well as cohort and case-control studies assessing the impact of PPC programs on women's knowledge of the components of PPC and the use of contraception and/or their pregnancy outcomes (Fig. 1). Studies investigating solely the effect of (a) pre-pregnancy clinics on pregnancy outcomes, as opposed to the effect of other interventions (e.g. leaflets, posters) were not included [3]. The search strategy included the following keywords: "pre-conception care" or "intervention programs" or "contraception" or "contraception uptake" or "pre-pregnancy care" AND "negative pregnancy outcomes" or "adverse pregnancy outcomes" or "pregnancy complications" AND "type 2 diabetes" or "type 1 diabetes" or "diabetes". Only full-text journal articles in English of studies that assessed the impact of PPC programs on women's knowledge and/or their pregnancy outcomes were included. Additional information was obtained from authors of publications where required.

Chart review

Hospital records (in electronic and paper formats) of pregnant women with pre-gestational T1D (n = 53) and T2D (n = 46) from Macarthur Diabetes in Pregnancy Clinic (MDPC), between 2010 and 2015, were reviewed. To minimise classification bias, medical records were re-reviewed. Data that were extracted from the charts included parity, age and body mass index (BMI), type of diabetes (type 1 vs. type 2 vs other), family history of diabetes, type of treatment (e.g. insulin, Metformin) at conception and during pregnancy, folate use, country of birth, third trimester HbA1c (%), mode of delivery (e.g. vaginal, caesarean section, vacuum and forceps), as well

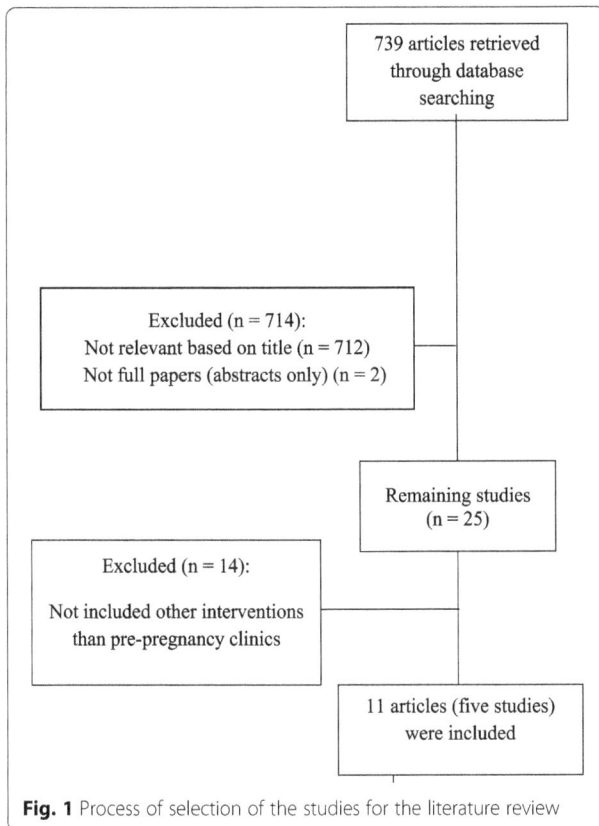

Fig. 1 Process of selection of the studies for the literature review

as pregnancy outcomes including neonatal hypoglycaemia, congenital malformations [15], macrosomia (birth-weight ≥ 4000 g or > 90% centile) [16], stillbirth, pre-eclampsia and hypertension (blood pressure ≥ 140/90 mmHg) [16].

Interview surveys

Fifteen women and 13 HCPs were asked about their current and previous experiences of pre-pregnancy diabetes care/management and for suggestions to improve care, using closed and open questions either face to face or over the telephone. HCPs included General Practitioners (GPs) ($n = 2$), endocrinologists ($n = 3$, private and 'public'), gynaecologists ($n = 3$), diabetes educators ($n = 2$), a dietitian ($n = 1$) and midwives ($n = 2$). Answers were summarised in relation to two identified over-arching key themes (contraception and PPM).

Focus groups and one to one interviews

Two separate focus groups were conducted involving two women with T1D, another including two women from CALD backgrounds (Muslim and Asian). Due to lack of flexibility in time for women and their partners to attend the focus-group sessions, 12 in-depth one-to-one interviews were also conducted using the same questions with women from an Australian background with T1D ($n = 2$) and T2D ($n = 1$), women with T2D of CALD background ($n = 5$) as well as partners of CALD women with T2D ($n = 3$), and an

Aboriginal woman with T2D ($n = 1$). Each focus group/interview was audio recorded and transcribed verbatim.

Development of a PPM plan

The development of a draft PPM intervention plan was based on the identified approaches from the narrative review, using the components of previous studies (e.g. East Anglia Study group for Improving Pregnancy Outcomes in women with Diabetes (EASIPOD) [5]) and was then amended addressing gaps identified from the results of the chart-review, interview surveys and focus groups/interviews (Table 3). The plan components were shared in a local conference comprising multi-disciplinary HCPs and researchers. The attendees voted for each component based on feasibility, practicality and sustainability. The draft proposal was then discussed in two face-to-face meetings using a Delphi approach [17, 18]. The first focussed on the perspective from primary care, including GPs ($n = 12$); a dietitian ($n = 1$) and endocrinologists ($n = 2$). Each proposed PPM/contraception component was evaluated using a pros and cons list.

The final meeting involved key stakeholders from across the district (each of the 5 hospital facilities and primary care) representing a range of views from endocrinologists ($n = 4$), a diabetes educator, midwives ($n = 5$), obstetricians/gynaecologists ($n = 2$), a GP, a dietician, a clinical manager and health economists ($n = 2$). The meeting was facilitated by an endocrinologist. Those present formed three groups: two hospital facility groups and 'the rest' to discuss possible components of the intervention that related to their facility/perspective (Fig. 2). Once all groups reached consensus for each component of the program, responses were debated across the meeting, creating an opportunity for open discussion and combining or modifying the group outcomes. The final plan arose from this meeting.

Analyses

In the chart review, demographic characteristics and pregnancy outcomes among women with T1D and T2D were compared using chi-squared (categorical data) and t-tests (numerical data). Multivariate analyses (logistic regression and linear regression) were performed to adjust for age to compare the differences in characteristics between women with T1D and T2D. All analyses were performed using Stata v14. All tests were 2-tailed and significance was taken as $P < 0.05$.

Qualitative data from the open-ended interview survey questions, focus groups and individual interviews were thematically analysed identifying topics and substantive categories within participants' accounts in relation to the study objectives. This helped to identify topical responses

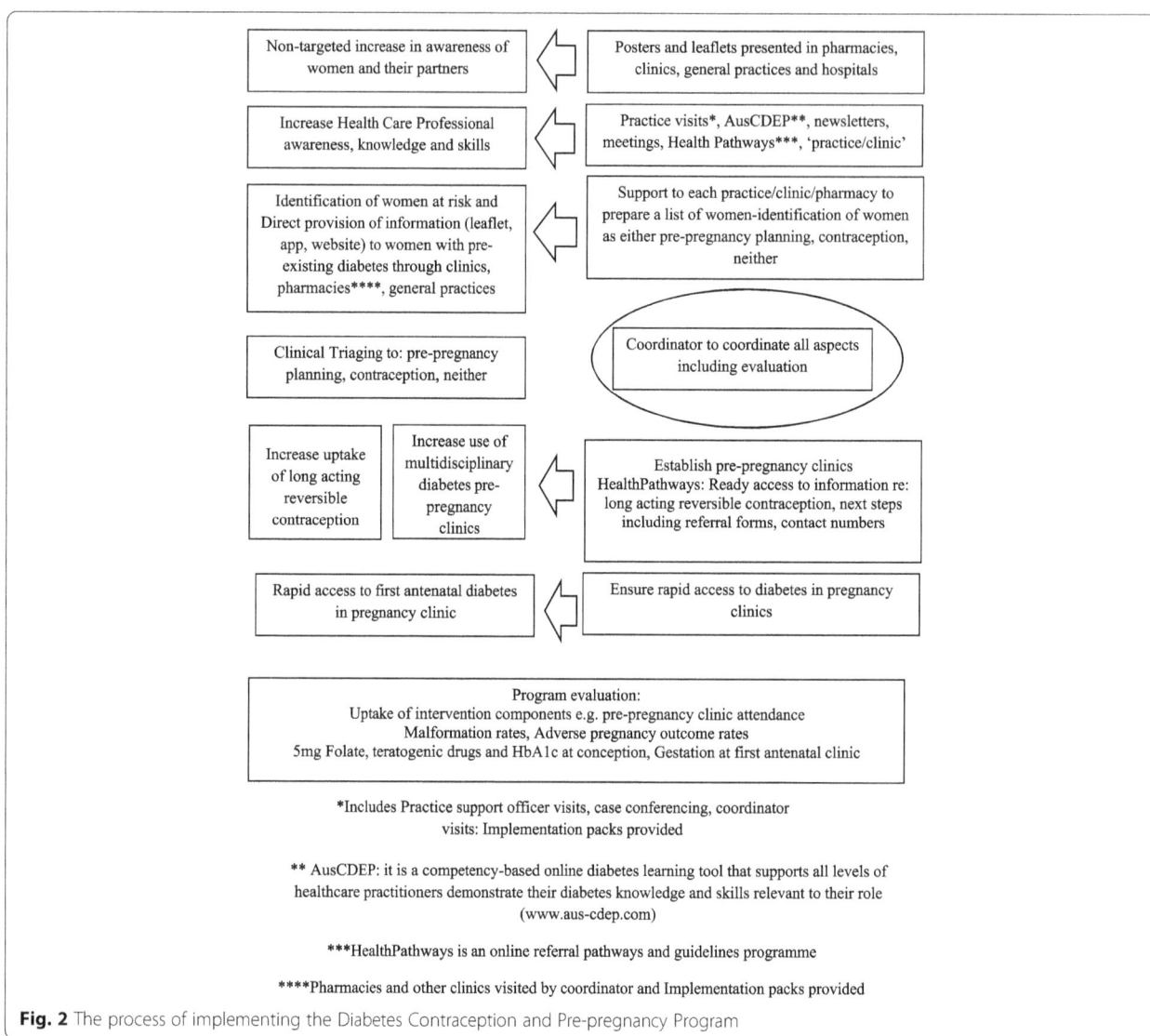

Fig. 2 The process of implementing the Diabetes Contraception and Pre-pregnancy Program

and emergent substantive categories, coding particularly for word repetition, direct and emotional statements and discourse markers including intensifiers, connectives and evaluative clauses. Responses and quotes from individuals participating in focus groups and interviews and responding to open ended questions from the interview surveys, are shown by alphanumeric coding, where women are labelled 'W' and men 'M' and the type of diabetes is indicated (e.g. W102- T1D = participant 102 who was a woman with type 1 diabetes).

Results

Narrative review

Figure 1 shows the number of studies identified and reasons for exclusion in the narrative review. As shown, from 739 studies, 714 studies were excluded in the first screening phase. One further publication emerged following the review [19]. As shown in

Table 1, five studies (published in 11 articles), which assessed different aspects of each type of intervention, were identified. Of the five studies, four used multi-faceted approaches (e.g. books, CD-ROM, posters, leaflets, HCP educational courses, counselling sessions, online learning materials for HCPs) [5, 9, 12, 19–22] and one used a mono-faceted approach (DVDs) [10, 13, 23, 24]. All approaches contained information on the importance of pregnancy planning, use of contraception, maternal and baby risk, and PPM components [10, 13, 19, 23, 24].

Table 1 summarises the impact of four approaches on adverse pregnancy outcomes and/or knowledge of PPM. DVDs, the READY-Girls and the EASIPOD interventions improved the knowledge of women in pregnancy planning and contraception use [21] [23], and in PPM [12, 13]. Multi-faceted interventions (i.e. EASIPOD and leaflets and posters in healthcare facilities) decreased the rate of

Table 1 Literature-review of pre-pregnancy programs

Studies and interventions	Region/Country	Program content	Specialist delivered the interventions	Centres	Results
DVD [10, 13, 23, 24]	Northern Island/UK	The importance of planning pregnancy and the role of contraception.	A diabetes specialist- nurse and -midwife, a dietitian, a GP, a clinical health Psychologist, an obstetrician, a nutritionist	**1** [10]: Two national health services **2** [13]:At their centre **3** [23]: Five diabetes care within the five health and social care trust and general practices; **4** [24]: At their centre	**1** [10]: The DVD significantly improved self-efficacy and reduced perceived barriers. Knowledge of pregnancy planning and pregnancy-related risks increased ($P < 0.001$). **2** [13]: The development process and outcome evaluation are an important point of reference for future educational programs **3** [23]: The viewed-DVD subgroup had lower first visit HbA1c ($P < 0.001$; increased planned pregnancy ($P < 0.001$); increased folic acid preconception ($P = 0.001$); and had improved HbA1c preconception ($P < 0.001$). **4** [24]: the development of an e-learning continuing professional development resource within the website.
EASIPOD a [5, 9, 19]: websites, workshops for HCP, Leaflets, structured audit with benchmarking, poster formal and informal patient education programs	East-Anglia/ UK	Planning a pregnancy and contact details for local PPC coordinator	Diabetes physician, specialist nurse, midwife or obstetrician	Primary-care teams in community settings, women with T1D: by specialist teams in hospital settings. Joint clinics.	**5** [5]: Women with PPC presented earlier ($P = 0.001$), were more likely to take 5 mg preconception folic acid ($P = 0.0001$) and had lower HbA1c ($P = 0.0001$). They had fewer adverse pregnancy outcomes $P = 0.009$). Lack of PPC was independently associated with adverse outcome (OR = 0.2; 95% CI 0.05–0.89). **6** [9]: Understanding PPC (90%); optimal glycaemic control (80%); risks of malformation (48%) and macrosomia (35%). 70% were not regularly using contraception (70%), stopped deliberately (45%), become less rigorous (28%) or experienced side effects (14%).
EASIPOD 2 a [19]: websites, workshops for HCP, Leaflets, structured audit with benchmarking, poster formal and informal patient education programs; GP software flags, online education program for HCPs	East-Anglia/UK	Planning a pregnancy and contact details for local PPC coordinator	Diabetes physician, specialist nurse, midwife or obstetrician	Primary-care teams in community settings, women with T1D: by specialist teams in hospital settings. Joint clinics.	**7** [19]: In those withT1D: improved gestational age at booking (7.6 vs 8.4 weeks), and in women with T2D: high rate of first HbA1c of < 6.5% < 48 mmol (58.5% vs 44.4%) and higher rate of preconception 5 mg folic acid (41.8% vs 23.5%).
READY-Girls [12, 20, 21]	Pittsburgh/ USA	Presents the effects of diabetes on reproductive health, puberty, sexuality, and pregnancy and the benefits of PPC and includes skill-building exercises for healthy decision making and communication with HCPs.	Specialised nurses and GPs	Major university-based diabetes clinics	**8** [20]: Improved knowledge about family planning and reproductive health issues. **9** [12]: Increased in knowledge after the first visit ($P < 0.001$) and being sustained for 9 months ($P < 0.05$). preconception counselling barriers decreased over time ($P < 0.001$), and intention and initiation of preconception counselling and reproductive health discussions increased ($P < 0.001$). **10** [21]: Stronger knowledge about PPC ($P = 0.003$) and seek PPC when planning a pregnancy ($P = 0.02$)
Leaflets and posters in out-patient waiting room [22]	Ireland	Patient education, a full medication review; assessment & treatment of diabetes-complications and thyroid status, commencement of folic acid 5 mg/d and focus on intensive glucose monitoring	Specialist and general practitioners	Antenatal care by Primary care clinicians, local endocrinologist, diabetes nurse specialist and dietitian	Attendees were more likely to take preconception folic acid ($P < 0.001$) and less likely to smoke ($P = .03$). Attendees had lower glycated haemoglobin levels ($P < .001$; third trimester HbA1c ($P = 0.001$), and their offspring had lower rates of serious adverse outcomes ($P = 0.007$)

a EASIPOD: East Anglia Study group for Improving Pregnancy Outcomes in women with Diabetes
Numbers in bold refer to different reports

smoking [21], reduced HbA1c [5, 9, 22]) and increased 5-mg folic-acid uptake [5, 9, 22] at conception. The rates of adverse pregnancy outcomes including congenital malformations (7.3% vs. 4.3%; $P =$ 0.04) [9]; (0.8% vs 5.2%; $P = 0.04$) [21] and perinatal mortality (1.8 vs. 3.7%, $P = 0.07$) [9] were also significantly reduced. A revised EASIPOD programme (EASIPOD 2), in which primary diabetes practitioners were far more engaged, in addition to secondary healthcare providers, showed an increased rate of pre-conception 5 mg folic-acid uptake (from 46 to 64%) in women with T1D as well as significant improvement of HbA1c at conception in women with T2D, with almost 60% of women reaching target (6.5% or ≤ 48 mmol/mol) [19].

Chart-review

Table 2 shows that overall, women with diabetes were often overweight/obese, parous with a strong family history of diabetes. Women with T1D were largely (78.3%) from Australia/ of European descent, with those with T2D from more varied backgrounds. High dose folic acid uptake was low, with no difference between women with Type 1 and Type 2 diabetes. Third trimester HbA1c was relatively high and several women (9.5%) with T2D were medicating with potentially fetotoxic diabetes medications. Recorded retinal screening during pregnancy was low particularly (but non-significantly) in women with T2D. Malformation rates were high with an overall rate of 12.4%. The overall rates of other pregnancy outcomes were also high including Caesarean section rates (57.5%), hypoglycaemia (24.5%), hypertension/preeclampsia (23.4%) and macrosomia (29.8%). While there were no stillbirths, women with T1D had a high miscarriage rate (8.0%).

Qualitative results (from interview surveys, focus groups and one to one interviews)

Patients

Early referral to the endocrinologist and clinic care (W102-T1D, W112-T2D), longer consultations and more frequent clinics (W105-T1D, W115-T1D), were highlighted as ways to improve the current service. Additional file 1 provides quotes reflecting each theme identified.Five women did not comment when asked how pre-pregnancy clinic care could be improved and a further three said no improvements were necessary.

Barriers to contraception and PPM included lack of awareness, limited motivation to change and/or a sense of information overload that reduced women's engagement with the education being provided to them. Most women took contraceptives until they were ready to become pregnant. However, they perceived the pre-pregnancy information they were provided was not pertinent until after they fell pregnant.

Women indicated that being aware of complications and having resources to assist them in leading a healthy life was important. Google was a common source of information that women felt was reliable (W109-T2D, W111-T2D, W103-T2D). However, those who solely relied on being educated by family and friends received incorrect information.

Partner support and investment were key to engagement with healthy lifestyle choices. Male partners were interested in enhancing their knowledge on pre-pregnancy diabetes management and contraception methods.

HCPs

HCPs utilised resources from a variety of sources to enhance their knowledge of PPM including specialists, self-education, information from professional organisations, meetings/seminars/conferences/ journal clubs, through personal experience and training courses. According to HCPs, the most common barriers to pre-pregnancy planning was lack of education/knowledge and unawareness of PPM in women.

Furthermore, HCPs suggested that advertisement and awareness of services (including mention of the power of word of mouth, use of TV screens in GP surgeries and leaflets distributed through pharmacies), incorporation of discussion about contraception and pregnancy planning with women with diabetes of child-bearing age, positive relationships with other HCPs, after-hours services, education of women from HCPs, support from the patient's partner, online services and more patient visits to GPs, could enhance PPM (Table 3). GPs highlighted the importance of referrals from primary to secondary care for PPM once women fall pregnant. GPs felt that the diabetes specialist services were best placed to provide the pre-pregnancy counselling.

Development of the plan

At the conference, HCPs agreed that all proposed components were practical and sustainable and should be included (Table 3). The subsequent HCP meetings led to reduced emphasis on any specially made media (e.g. DVD's) and GP checklist software (rather to include in existing software) due to their relatively high cost impact. Tables 4 and 5 show the items considered along with pros and cons of each component. The agreed core content for informational materials for both HCPs and women and their partners is shown in Table 6.

Figure 2 shows the final components for the district-wide "Diabetes Contraception and Pre-pregnancy Program" (DCAPP) including the required resources and activities to be undertaken for the different target groups (women of childbearing age with T1D or T2D, women's partners and HCPs). This included establishing pre-pregnancy clinics and referral pathways, disseminating educational materials relating to both planning pregnancy

Table 2 Characteristics and pregnancy outcomes of women with T1D and T2D from the chart review

Variables	T1D	T2D	P-value[*]	T1D Melbourne (n = 107) [29]	Background population in NSW[d] (2010) [28]
Age (years), mean (SD)	28.6 (5.6)	32.9 (5.2)	< 0.001	29.3 (5.3)	30.8
n = 99	n = 53	n = 46			
BMI[a] (Kg/m^2), mean (SD)[c]	25.8 (5.2)	35.4 (8.1)	< 0.001	27.3 (5.0) --	
n = 93	n = 48	n = 45			
Gravida, n (SD)[**]	2.6 (2.2)	3.1 (2.2)	0.17	–	
n = 98	n = 53	n = 45			
Parity, n (SD)[**]	1.0 (1.2)	1.5 (1.4)	0.09	–	
n = 98	n = 53	n = 45			
Country of birth, n (%)[**]			0.07[***]		
Australia	13 (35.1)	8 (19.1)		95 (89)	67.3%
European descent	16 (43.2)	12 (28.6)		–	–
India/Bangladesh	1 (2.7)	5 (11.9)		–	3.5%
Aboriginal	2 (5.4)	5 (11.9)		–	3.3%
Others	5 (13.5)	12 (28.6)		–	25.9%
n = 79	n = 37	n = 42			
Family history of diabetes, n (%)[**]	20 (66.7)	30 (83.3)	0.30	–	–
n = 66	n = 30	n = 36			
Third-trimester HbA1c[**]				–	–
%	7.0 (1.8)	6.5 (1.4)	0.4		
mmol/mol (SD)	53.0 (19.7)	47.5 (15.3)			
n = 76	n = 39	n = 37			
Folic acid, n (%)[**]			0.4[***]		
Nil	13 (36.1)	9 (30.0)			
< 5 mg	7 (19.4)	8 (26.7)			
5 mg	8 (22.2)	10 (33.3)			
Yes (dosage unknown)	8 (22.2)	3 (10.0)			
n = 66	n = 36	n = 30			
Treatment before pregnancy, n (%)[**]			< 0.001[***]		
Diet alone	0	4 (9.4)			
Tablets	0	11 (26.2)			
Metformin	0	8 (19.0)			
Gliclazide	0	3 (7.1)			
Janumet (Metformin + Sitagliptin)	0	1 (2.4)			
Insulin	51 (96.2)	16 (38.1)			
Insulin + Metformin	2 (3.8)	7 (16.7)			
Nil	0	4 (9.4)			
n = 95	n = 53	n = 42			
Treatment during pregnancy, n (%)[**]			0.003[***]		
Insulin	38 (92.7)	32 (78.1)			
Metformin	1 (2.4)	2 (4.9)			
Insulin & metformin	1 (2.4)	5 (12.2)			

Table 2 Characteristics and pregnancy outcomes of women with T1D and T2D from the chart review *(Continued)*

Variables	T1D	T2D	P-value[*]	T1D Melbourne (n = 107) [29]	Background population in NSW[d] (2010) [28]
CSII[b]	1 (2.4)	0			
Insulin only at labour	0	1 (2.4)			
Total	41 (100)	40 (97.6)			
n = 82	n = 41	n = 41			
Retinopathy screening, n (%)[**]			0.06[***]		
Yes	18 (64.3)	9 (39.1)			
No	10 (43.5)	14 (60.9)			
n = 55	n = 29	n = 26			
Thyroid disease, n (%)[**]			0.8[***]		
Yes	6 (12.0)	5 (11.9)			
No	42 (84)	36 (85.7)			
n = 89	n = 48	n = 41			
Delivery methods[b], n (%)[**]			0.005[***]		
Vaginal	12 (24.5)	18 (41.9)			
Elective CS[c]	17 (34.7)	13 (30.2)			
Emergency CS[c]	11 (22.5)	9 (20.9)			
Vacuum	3 (6.1)	4 (9.3)			
n = 87	n = 43	n = 44			
Pregnancy outcomes[φ], n (%)[**]					
Neonatal Hypoglycaemia	9 (36.0)	3 (12.5)	0.12	–	–
n = 49	n = 25	n = 24			
Any congenital malformations	4 (9.1)	7 (15.6)	0.25	4 (4)	775 (0.8)
Major	4 (9.1)	4 (8.9)	0.55	–	–
Minor	0	4 (8.9)	–	–	–
n = 89	n = 44	n = 45			
Hypertension	11 (24.4)	10 (22.2)	0.25	2 (2)	6357 (6.7)
n = 90	n = 45	n = 45			
Pre-eclampsia	6 (12.2)	4 (10.3)	0.84	5 (5)	–
n = 88	n = 49	n = 39			
Macrosomia (birthweight> 4000 g)	17 (34.7)	11 (24.4)	0.50[ϒ]	47 (44)	–
n = 94	n = 49	n = 45			
Stillbirth	0	0	–	7 (7)	555 (0.6)
n = 88	n = 48	n = 40	–		–
Miscarriage	4 (8.0)	0	–		
n = 94	n = 50	n = 44			

[a]*BMI* body mass index; [b]*CSII* continuous subcutaneous insulin infusion; [c]*CS* Caesarean section; [d]*NSW* New South Wales
[*]Age was included in all the statistical models;
[**]denominators vary due to missing values;
[***]Overall *P*-value
[φ] those with miscarriage were excluded from the analyses (n = 4);
[ϒ] adjusted for age, *BMI* and history of macrosomia

and avoiding unplanned pregnancies (contraception) for the woman, her partner and HCPs using a multitude of approaches including sending materials directly to the women, and establishing a programme to monitor uptake.

A key resource is the coordinator (may be more than one person), who will be appointed to oversee all aspects of the program including the educational program, data management and identifying/developing strategies to

Table 3 Current gaps in adherence to optimal care, possible interventions and actions required for developing the interventions in South Western Sydney based on HCPs[a] and women/partners inputs

Gaps (requirements)	Intervention programs used in the literature/ suggested by HCP's/women/partners	Actions required to implement the interventions
Lack of time for women/patients to attend diabetes clinic	Websites, leaflets, contact details of local HCPs[a] [5], social media	1) Providing after-hours clinics 2) Providing other educational resources (e.g. webpages, social media, and apps) 3) Reaching out to all patients and mailing them leaflets and information sheets on a regular basis
Lack of communication (miscommunication) between HCPs and patients	Workshops, newsletters, online learning resources,regular meetings and education programs [46]	1) Reminding HCPs about online resources and workshops 2) Adding techniques for communication to the existing learning materials
Lack of knowledge about PPM and contraception methods in women and their partners	Leaflets, posters, DVDs, PPM education programs and peer support	1) Developing a wide range of educational resources (e.g. posters, apps) 2) Increasing the accessibility of educational resources 3) Translating educational resources in most common languages
Disparities of preferences in receiving knowledge about PPM and contraception options	Use of a wide range of interventions (e.g. online resources, social media, leaflets and posters)	Raising awareness among patients and their partners about the ranges of interventions

[a]*HCPs*: Healthcare Professionals

address 'hard to reach' women. The coordinator will additionally visit hospital clinics, general practices, pharmacies and relevant clinics (e.g. fertility clinics), to deliver and discuss implementation packs tailored to each of the four settings. General practices will also be informed of the DCAPP through visits by the local Primary Health Network Practice Support Officers and local case-conferencing (where an endocrinologist visits practices to advise on the care of individual patients with diabetes). Pharmacies will also be visited by the DCAPP coordinator and medical students.

Implementation packs include asking HCPs at each venue to, display posters, have leaflets available, show DCAPP information on TV screens, if available, and undertake brief online training about pre-pregnancy planning (AusCDEP – a competency based online multiple choice based training tool). Practice and clinic staff will be given information on how to access Health-Pathways (the local online referral and clinical guideline portal) for diabetes contraception/pre-pregnancy information, patient/partner printable materials and referral advice. All staff will be asked to explain the DCAPP (briefly), offer a DCAPP leaflet to each woman of reproductive age with diabetes and ask the woman to enrol (by text, email, DCAPP website and Facebook or Instagram) to access further materials, for an annual DCAPP update and to receive any new information should it arise. How this occurs will vary by setting:

- Pharmacists will be asked to approach those picking up diabetes prescriptions.
- GP surgeries, private fertility and public diabetes clinics will be requested to make a list of the women

with T1D/T2D of reproductive age and provide the coordinator with this number. This may be facilitated by using practice software. The hospital clinics have been provided with BIOGRID database/ software [25] to facilitate this process. A clinic/ practice member will be identified as the contact person to provide/receive further information. General practice and diabetes clinic staff who see the women will be asked to record if a leaflet has been provided, and their assessment of whether the woman is

- planning to become pregnant (and therefore warrant pre-pregnancy management/referral to the pre-pregnancy clinics or private care)
- not planning to become pregnant and identify the form of contraception in place including abstinence or not required (e.g. hysterectomy, confirmed menopause)
- neither and listing reason including informed decision, religious reasons, not currently sexually active.

The contact person will be asked to maintain an internal register of leaflets provision, pre-pregnancy and contraception status and to provide a summary to the coordinator on a regular basis (quarterly). After the first round of approaches, the assessment would occur at each annual review (unless status changes beforehand).

All HCPs will also be invited to workshops/presentations run by their organisation/professional groups to allow further dissemination and discussion about the DCAPP (One of these has already occurred with 112 general practitioners attending).

Table 4 Evaluation of interventions proposed for enhancement of Pre-Pregnancy Management (PPM) based on weighing pros and cons items

Interventions	Content/ details	Places (to be implemented)	Pros	Cons	Included
Workshops for HCPs[a]	Interpersonal techniques for communicating with other HCPs and patients (including CALD[b] women), and PPM[c]	Primary and secondary care services	Motivational, Enhancing skills and knowledge	Lack of flexibility in time, expensive	Yes
DVD	'Risk of unplanned pregnancy, and effective contraception methods', 'local support team', 'blood glucose targets, hypos and ketoacidosis', 'diet, delivery' and 'post-birth'	Primary and secondary care services including pharmacies	Easily accessible and convenient	High cost, not sustainable (can be lost/or scratched)	No
Web-based education program	PPM information, links to pre-existing YouTube channels in multiple languages e.g. Arabic and Vietnamese	Websites and social media	Easily accessible and convenient, no limits in content	Passive	Yes
Courses for patients and their partners	The importance of PPM (e.g. glycaemic control, smoking cessation and physical activity) and use of effective contraception	Primary and secondary care services, women's health clinics	Motivational, they can ask questions	High cost, lack of flexibility in time	No
Posters presentation /T.V screen advertisement	The importance of PPM with information about available local services (contact details for local HCPs)	Waiting rooms of primary and secondary care services, pharmacies, women's health and fertility clinics	Easily visible, encourage an active response	Limited content	Yes
Peer support/web chat	Sharing experiences about diabetes in pregnancy and services they have used	DCAPP social media	Easily accessible and convenient	Possibility of inaccuracy (Vulnerable to (cognitive) biases)	Yes
Text message reminders	Links to the important websites, available resources (e.g. local pre-pregnancy clinics, social media)	Will be sent from the GP practices on regular bases (every six weeks)	Easily accessible and convenient	High cost	No
Leaflets	Links to useful websites, potential risks of unplanned pregnancy and risk factors for potential complications	Primary and secondary care services, mail, pharmacies and women's health clinics	Easy to access	High cost (if mailed), lack of interest (so common)	Yes
Apps	'Risk of unplanned pregnancy, and effective contraception methods', 'local support team', 'blood glucose targets, hypos and ketoacidosis', 'diet, delivery' and 'post-birth'	DCAPP website and social media, leaflets, and posters	Systematic approach, no cost to design (already existed)	Only available to smart-phone users	Yes
Social media	Useful websites (e.g. NDSS[d]), updates/posts on the importance of PPM and contraception, and YouTube channel	Online (i.e. Facebook and Instagram)	High chance of being visited regularly	Only available to DCAPP social media followers	Yes
Checklist software for general practitioners	Medication review, contraception advice, weight management strategies, importance of having optimal glycaemic control	GP surgeries	Systematic approach	High cost of design Needs to articulate with existing software	No

[a]*HCPs*: health care professionals
[b]*CALD*: culturally and linguistically diverse
[c]*PPM*: pre-pregnancy management
[d]*NDSS*: National Diabetes Service Scheme: An initiative of the Australian Government administered with the assistance of Diabetes Australia [47]

DCAPP Evaluation [26, 27]

Evaluation will include assessment of uptake of the various components, qualitative evaluation of the perspectives of women, their partners and HCPs, a health economic evaluation and a comparison of pregnancy preparation and outcome measures over the first 12–24 months with those from the prior 6 years.

Table 5 Interventions to increase contraception uptake- Pros and cons based on literature as well as conference and survey/focus group discussions

Interventions	Content/ details	Places (to be implemented)	Pros	Cons	Included
Workshops for HCPs[a] and pharmacies [48]	Available contraceptive methods for women with diabetes and insertion techniques for IUD[b]	Primary and secondary care services and pharmacies	Potentially motivates HCPs, updates their knowledge	Lack of flexibility in time, High cost	Yes
Courses for patients and their partners	The importance of planning for pregnancy and available contraception options for women with diabetes	Primary and secondary care services and pharmacies	Potentially motivates patients and their partners, they can ask questions	Lack of flexibility in time, High cost	No
Accessibility of contraception	Providing free condoms in health-care services (especially primary care centres)	Primary and secondary care services, dental clinics, women's health clinics, NDSS[c]	Easily visible, encourages people to use contraception	High cost	No
Leaflets women and their partners' awareness [49]	Importance of planning pregnancy and contraception uptake in women with diabetes	Primary and secondary care services, women's health clinics and NDSS[c]	Minimises potential conflicts which could exist within the couples	High cost if mailed	Yes
Mass-media, community and interpersonal channels [50]	Benefits of IUD, wide range of available contraception options, importance of optimised diabetes management prior to pregnancy	Primary and secondary care services, pharmacies and women's health clinics	Repetitions, accessible to the majority of population group	High cost, not usable/usable for CALD women	No
Web-based program including YouTube channel	The importance of planning for pregnancy and role of contraception, education of contraception options	The app will be addressed on leaflets, posters	Accessible anytime, pre-existed	Needs internet connection	Yes
Checklist software for HCPs	Contraception advice	The link will be available on leaflet and posters	Potentially motivates HCPs, updates their knowledge	High cost Needs to articulate with existing software	No

[a]*HCPs*: Health care professionals
[b]*IUD*: intrauterine device
[c]*NDSS*: National Diabetes Service Scheme [47]- An initiative of the Australian Government administered with the assistance of Diabetes Australia

Program uptake will be evaluated by detailed monitoring of HCP education (AusCDEP uptake, workshop attendance, case conferencing patients), number of HealthPathways visits/clicks, number of social media followers, leaflets sent, pharmacy registrations, practice/pharmacy/clinic participation, practice/clinic reports (leaflet distribution, assessment

Table 6 Agreed core content for informational materials for both HCPs and women and their partners

Why conception with poor glucose control and/or unsafe medications should be avoided

Contraception and family planning advice, with emphasis on the most effective contraception options (e.g. Long Acting Reversible Contraception and emergency contraception) to prevent unplanned pregnancies.

Emphasising the importance of glycaemic control using safe medications at least three months prior to conception

5 mg folic-acid uptake at least three months prior to pregnancy.

Avoidance/replacement of teratogenic drugs particularly for hypertension and dyslipidaemia

Importance of retinal, renal and vascular complication screening prior to conception

The risk of smoking during pregnancy

Online educational resources (e.g. National Diabetes Supply Scheme, Facebook and Instagram pages)

Contact details of local health services

status and long acting reversible contraception uptake reports), pre-pregnancy clinic attendance and gestation (weeks) at attendance of antenatal clinic once pregnant.

Measures of pregnancy preparation will be assessed from antenatal clinic records including: 5 mg folic acid uptake from at least 3-months preconception, whether this is a planned pregnancy or otherwise, use of potentially teratogenic medications at conception and gestational age at first visit. Other measures include first visit blood pressure, HbA1c, BMI and smoking status. Third trimester HbA1c will also be assessed.

Pregnancy outcomes will be collected from birth records including major and minor congenital malformations, stillbirths, neonatal trauma, emergency caesarean section, preeclampsia, prenatal mortality, miscarriage, preterm birth, small and large for gestational age, severe maternal hypoglycaemia, and gestational weight-gain [26, 27].

Process evaluation will include assessment of reach and the use of the DCAPP materials, through interviews in a purposeful sample of women of reproductive age with diabetes who have become pregnant (planned and unplanned) and received the materials, plus partners and HCPs. Interviews will include evaluation of the most effective mix of approaches (e.g. online and/or through pharmacies, hospital clinics and/or GP surgeries) for contacting and enrolling patients, identification of barriers and facilitators to implementation for each program component and aspects that both stimulate and obstruct use of DCAPP. Interviews will be repeated over time to facilitate continuous evaluation and quality management of the program.

Cost-effectiveness analysis will be conducted using the total intervention cost, summation of the different components, and benefits to New South Wales Health based on primary and secondary outcomes and their unit costs. An incremental analysis will be conducted for the women who had prior pregnancies. A full plan is currently under discussion.

Discussion

The rate of congenital malformations in this district (6.8–12.4%) [1] is higher than that of the background population (1.7%, from 2005 to 2010) [28], as well as the rates reported by two previous Australian studies conducted in Melbourne (4%) [29] and Adelaide (5%) [30] and several international studies from England, Wales, and Northern Ireland (4.6%) [31] and from north west England (9.4%) [32]. Similarly, the rate of preeclampsia is considerably higher in our study than that reported from Melbourne (12.2% vs. 5.0%). However, the rates of macrosomia (34.7%) and caesarean section (57.2%) are slightly lower in our study than those reported by the study done in Melbourne (44% and 62%, respectively) [28]. Our results showed few women (2.4%) with T1D were receiving continuous subcutaneous insulin infusions (CSII) in comparison with those in the United Kingdom (20%) [33, 34], which could be due to its out of pocket cost in Australia and HCP time requirements [35].A range of barriers have been identified, similar to those reported previously [36], that are likely to have contributed to limitations in clinical care and self-management. These in turn will have increased the likelihood of unplanned pregnancies and poor pregnancy outcomes (e.g. congenital malformations) [36, 37]. In view of the high rate of congenital malformations, and existing barriers to optimal care, the development and implementation of a district-wide contraception and pre-pregnancy program was considered to be an urgent initiative. The program does not address issues related to undiagnosed diabetes and its association with adverse pregnancy outcomes.

The DCAPP program is the first Australian diabetes pre-pregnancy intervention program based upon various research tools (comprehensive literature review, audits, interview surveys and in-depth focus-groups and interviews in addition to multidisciplinary meetings with HCPs). It has targeted women's partners who can potentially influence women's PPM and contraceptive uptake decision making [38]. Furthermore, the program is based upon principles of integrated care, with a primary-secondary care partnership, including aspects of clinical care within primary care, rather than simple specialist/hospital educational interventions. The program has been developed to allow both sustainability and scalability. In the few places where such a comprehensive program has been put into place, malformations in particular were (cardiac, spinal) has been estimated to have a lifelong cost of $1,000,000 [39].

As a program across a population of almost a million [40], over 450 general practices, 188 pharmacies and five hospitals with birthing facilities, DCAPP is faced with a range of challenges associated with large scale programs. As a result, the program will be implemented practice by practice, clinic by clinic and pharmacy by pharmacy with the support of other organisations including the Primary Health Network that supports all general practices across SWS. By including both general practices and pharmacies in the program, we expect to also reach those women with T1D/T2D who attend private providers (e.g. endocrinologists, educators) for their care. The degree of participation by those under the public and private sectors (and their pregnancy outcomes) will be included in the evaluation.

With such an extensive range of providers, the role of the coordinator, the DCAPP team and the within clinic/practice contacts will also be crucial in identifying those reached or otherwise by the roll out and in developing new strategies to reach women who are hard to reach. For example, women with T2D on diet management alone might not attend pharmacies and may need additional practice based strategies. Evaluation of the uptake of the clinic/practice contact and their reporting will be important to identify the need for any further support/incentives for this role.

SWS is characterised by its rich cultural diversity (represented by residents from East and South Asia, the Middle East and the Pacific Islands) [40]. Of particular interest, as the program is rolled out, will be the uptake of contraception among cultural groups who may have religious objections to pharmacological or barrier contraception methods. This is likely to require additional work (e.g. a targeted optimisation program, including avoidance of potentially teratogenic agents) among women with T2D not taking contraception.

Myths and misconceptions as well as lack of knowledge of emergency contraception, and their male partners' perspectives regarding contraception, are the most common barriers to utilising contraception for women (especially in those with lower levels of education) [41–44]. Previous studies [44, 45] have also highlighted the important role of social media and group-session workshops in raising and updating women's knowledge of contraception uptake. Methods to achieve this are included as part of the DCAPP.

Our chart reviews and interviews/focus groups were limited due to small sample size/number of participants, leading to wide limits for the pregnancy outcomes and possible under-reporting the participants' comments and suggestions. Nevertheless, our results have shown the severity of poor pregnancy outcomes in women living in SWS, emphasising the need for an intervention program in this district.

Conclusions

With the high rates of congenital malformations and high ethnic diversity in this district of Sydney, it is hoped that this program will sustainably reduce adverse pregnancy outcomes in women with pre-existing T1D/T2D. DCAPP is based upon formative research, current best practice, a partnership across primary and secondary care, with new facets including social media and information for partners that have not been included in previous PPM programs. The role of implementation, outcome and cost-effectiveness monitoring will be crucial to assess whether the program should be continued and extended to other areas.

Abbreviations

BMI: Body mass index; DCAPP: Diabetes Contraception and Pre-pregnancy Program; EASIPOD: East Anglia Study group for Improving Pregnancy Outcomes in women with Diabetes; GP: General practitioner; HCP: Health care professional; PPC: pre-Pregnancy Care; PPM: Pre-Pregnancy Management; SWS: South Western Sydney; T1D: Type 1 diabetes; T2D: Type 2 diabetes

Acknowledgements

We thank patients and their partners, health care professionals and other health staff for their input. We thank Professor Helen Murphy and Deborah Hughes for the documentation from EASIPOD and EASIPOD2.

Funding

This project has been funded by South Western Sydney Local Health District with support from South Western Sydney Primary Health Network and the Sydney Partnership for Health Education Research and Enterprise.

Authors' contributions

MS drafted the manuscript and conducted the literature-review, contributed to the quantitative data collection, data management and data analysis, performed focus-groups, some of the one-to-one interviews and contributed to the qualitative analysis. FM supervised interviews and performed focus-groups and part of the qualitative analysis. TD conducted the qualitative analysis for the focus-groups and interviews. NB, NN, NK, VJ and XHL carried out data-collection. DS conceived the overall program, chaired group meetings, supervised the work of MS, NB, NK, NN, VJ and XHL, designed Fig. 2 and revised the manuscript. All authors read and approved the final manuscript.

Competing interests

The authors declare that they have no competing interests.

References

1. Wong VW, Suwandarathne H, Russell H. Women with pre-existing diabetes under the care of diabetes specialist prior to pregnancy: are their outcomes better? Aust N Z J Obstet Gynaecol. 2013;53(2):207–10.
2. Simmons D. Epidemiology of diabetes in pregnancy. London: Blackwell publishing; 2010.
3. Wahabi HA, Alzeidan RA, Esmaeil SA. Pre-pregnancy care for women with pre-gestational diabetes mellitus: a systematic review and meta-analysis. BMC Public Health. 2012;12:792.
4. Kikuchi K, Okawa S, Zamawe COF, Shibanuma A, Nanishi K, Iwamoto A, Saw YM, Jimba M. Effectiveness of continuum of care—linking pre-pregnancy care and pregnancy care to improve neonatal and perinatal mortality: a systematic review and meta-analysis. PLoS One. 2016;11(10):e0164965.
5. Murphy HR, Roland JM, Skinner TC, Simmons D, Gurnell E, Morrish NJ, Soo SC, Kelly S, Lim B, Randall J, et al. Effectiveness of a regional prepregnancy care program in women with type 1 and type 2 diabetes: benefits beyond glycemic control. Diabetes Care. 2010;33(12):2514–20.
6. O'Higgins S, McGuire BE, Mustafa E, Dunne F. Barriers and facilitators to attending pre-pregnancy care services: the ATLANTIC-DIP experience. Diabet Med. 2014;31(3):366–74.
7. Henshaw SK. Unintended pregnancy in the United States. Fam Plan Perspect. 1998;30(1):24–46.
8. Janz NK, Herman WH, Becker MP, Charron-Prochownik D, Shayna VL, Lesnick TG, Jacober SJ, Fachnie JD, Kruger DF, Sanfield JA, et al. Diabetes and pregnancy. Factors associated with seeking pre-conception care. Diabetes Care. 1995;18(2):157–65.
9. Murphy HR, Temple RC, Ball VE, Roland JM, Steel S, Zill EHR, Simmons D, Royce LR, Skinner TC. Personal experiences of women with diabetes who do not attend pre-pregnancy care. Diabet Med. 2010;27(1):92–100.
10. Holmes VA, Spence M, McCance DR, Patterson CC, Harper R, Alderdice FA. Evaluation of a DVD for women with diabetes: impact on knowledge and attitudes to preconception care. Diabet Med. 2012;29(7):950–6.
11. Charron-Prochownik D, Ferons-Hannan M, Sereika S, Becker D. Randomized efficacy trial of early preconception counseling for diabetic teens (READY-girls). Diabetes Care. 2008;31(7):1327.
12. Fischl AFR, Herman WH, Sereika SM, Hannan M, Becker D, Mansfield MJ, Freytag LL, Milaszewski K, Botscheller AN, Charron-Prochownik D. Impact of a preconception counseling program for teens with type 1 diabetes (READY girls) on patient-provider interaction, resource utilization, and cost. Diabetes Care. 2010;33(4):701.
13. Spence M, Harper R, McCance D, Alderdice F, McKinley M, Hughes C, Holmes V. The systematic development of an innovative DVD to raise awareness of preconception care. Eur Diabetes Nurs. 2013;10(1):7–12b.
14. Malin M, Gissler M. Maternal care and birth outcomes among ethnic minority women in Finland. BMC Public Health. 2009;9(1):84.
15. Landon MB, Spong CY, Thom E, Carpenter MW, Ramin SM, Casey B, Wapner RJ, Varner MW, Rouse DJ, Thorp JM Jr, et al. A multicenter, randomized trial of treatment for mild gestational diabetes. N Engl J Med. 2009;361(14):1339–48.
16. Feig DS, Corcoy R, Jensen DM, Kautzky-Willer A, Nolan CJ, Oats JJ, Sacks DA, Caimari F, McIntyre HD. Diabetes in pregnancy outcomes: a systematic review and proposed codification of definitions. Diabetes Metab Res Rev. 2015;31(7):680–90.
17. Gazing into the oracle. The Delphi method and its application to social policy and public health. London: Jessica Kingsley Publishers; 1996.
18. Sinha IP, Smyth RL, Williamson PR. Using the Delphi technique to determine which outcomes to measure in clinical trials: recommendations for the future based on a systematic review of existing studies. PLoS Med. 2011;8(1):e1000393.

19. Yamamoto JM, Hughes DJF, Evans ML, Karunakaran V, Clark JDA, Morrish NJ, Rayman GA, Winocour PH, Hambling C, Harries AW, et al. Community-based pre-pregnancy care programme improves pregnancy preparation in women with pregestational diabetes. Diabetologia. 2018;61(7):1528–37.

20. Charron-Prochownik D, Ferons-Hannan M, Sereika S, Becker D. Randomized efficacy trial of early preconception counseling for diabetic teens (READY-girls). Diabetes Care. 2008;31:1327–30.

21. Charron-Prochownik D, Sereika SM, Becker D, White NH, Schmitt P, Powell AB 3rd, Diaz AM, Jones J, Herman WH, Fischl AF, et al. Long-term effects of the booster-enhanced READY-girls preconception counseling program on intentions and behaviors for family planning in teens with diabetes. Diabetes Care. 2013;36(12):3870–4.

22. Egan AM, Danyliv A, Carmody L, Kirwan B, Dunne FP. A Prepregnancy care program for women with diabetes: effective and cost saving. J Clin Endocrinol Metab. 2016;101(4):1807–15.

23. Holmes VA, Hamill LL, Alderdice FA, Spence M, Harper R, Patterson CC, Loughridge S, McKenna S, Gough A, McCance DR. Effect of implementation of a preconception counselling resource for women with diabetes: a population based study. Prim Care Diabetes. 2017;11(1):37–45.

24. Gough A, McCance D, Alderdice F, Harper R, Holmes V. Preconception counselling resource for women with diabetes. BMJ Qual Improv Rep. 2015; 4(1):u209621–w3984.

25. BioGrid Australia-health through information. In. BioGrid Australia.

26. Egan AM, Galjaard S, Maresh MJA, Loeken MR, Napoli A, Anastasiou E, Noctor E, de Valk HW, van Poppel M, Todd M, et al. A core outcome set for studies evaluating the effectiveness of prepregnancy care for women with pregestational diabetes. Diabetologia. 2017;60(7):1190–6.

27. Kekalainen P, Juuti M, Walle T, Laatikainen T. Pregnancy planning in type 1 diabetic women improves glycemic control and pregnancy outcomes. J Matern Fetal Neonatal Med. 2016;29(14):2252–8.

28. Centre for Epidemiology and Evidence. New South Wales Mothers and Babies 2010. Sydney: NSW Ministry of Health; 2012.

29. Abell SK, Boyle JA, de Courten B, Knight M, Ranasinha S, Regan J, Soldatos G, Wallace EM, Zoungas S, Teede HJ. Contemporary type 1 diabetes pregnancy outcomes: impact of obesity and glycaemic control. Med J Aust. 2016;205(4):162–7.

30. Sharpe PB, Chan A, Haan EA, Hiller JE. Maternal diabetes and congenital anomalies in South Australia 1986–2000: a population-based cohort study. Birth Defects Res Part A: Clin Mol Teratol. 2005;73(9):605–11.

31. Macintosh MCM, Fleming KM, Bailey JA, Doyle P, Modder J, Acolet D, Golightly S, Miller A. Perinatal mortality and congenital anomalies in babies of women with type 1 or type 2 diabetes in England, Wales, and Northern Ireland: population based study. BMJ. 2006;333(7560):177.

32. Casson IF, Clarke CA, Howard CV, McKendrick O, Pennycook S, Pharoah POD, Platt MJ, Stanisstreet M, van Velszen D, Walkinshaw S. Outcomes of pregnancy in insulin dependent diabetic women: results of a five year population cohort study. BMJ. 1997;315(7103):275–8.

33. Egan AM, Murphy HR, Dunne FP. The management of type 1 and type 2 diabetes in pregnancy. QJM. 2015;108(12):923–7.

34. Pickup JC. Insulin-pump therapy for type 1 diabetes mellitus. N Engl J Med. 2012;366(17):1616–24.

35. Xu S, Alexander K, Bryant W, Cohen N, Craig ME, Forbes M, Fulcher G, Greenaway T, Harrison N, Holmes-Walker DJ, et al. Healthcare professional requirements for the care of adult diabetes patients managed with insulin pumps in Australia. Intern Med J. 2014;45(1):86–93.

36. Simmons D, Weblemoe T, Voyle J, Prichard A, Leakehe L, Gatland B. Personal barriers to diabetes care: lessons from a multi-ethnic community in New Zealand. Diabet Med. 1998;15(11):958–64.

37. Nam S, Chesla C, Stotts NA, Kroon L, Janson SL. Barriers to diabetes management: patient and provider factors. Diabetes Res Clin Pract. 2011;93(1):1–9.

38. Forde R, Patelarou EE, Forbes A. The experiences of prepregnancy care for women with type 2 diabetes mellitus: a meta-synthesis. Int J Women's Health. 2016;8:691–703.

39. Kruse M, Michelsen SI, Flachs EM, Bronnum-Hansen H, Madsen M, Uldall P. Lifetime costs of cerebral palsy. Dev Med Child Neurol. 2009;51(8):622–8.

40. Draft South West District Plan. In: Our vision –south West District 2036. Edited by Turnbull HL; 2016.

41. Salisbury P, Hall L, Kulkus S, Paw MK, Tun NW, Min AM, Chotivanich K, Srikanok S, Ontuwong P, Sirinonthachai S, et al. Family planning knowledge, attitudes and practices in refugee and migrant pregnant and post-partum women on the Thailand-Myanmar border – a mixed methods study. Reprod Health. 2016;13(1):94.

42. Richmond DM, Sabatini MM, Krueger H, Rudy SJ. Contraception: myths, facts, and methods. Dermatol Nurs. 2001;46(2):19–26.

43. Ezeanolue EE, Iwelunmor J, Asaolu I, Obiefune MC, Ezeanolue CO, Osuji A, Ogidi AG, Hunt AT, Patel D, Yang W, et al. Impact of male partner's awareness and support for contraceptives on female intent to use contraceptives in Southeast Nigeria. BMC Public Health. 2015;15:879.

44. Ochako R, Mbondo M, Aloo S, Kaimenyi S, Thompson R, Temmerman M, Kays M. Barriers to modern contraceptive methods uptake among young women in Kenya: a qualitative study. BMC Public Health. 2015;15:118.

45. Cupples JB, Zukoski AP, Dierwechter T. Reaching young men: lessons learned in the recruitment, training, and utilization of male peer sexual health educators. Health Promot Pract. 2010;11(3):19S–25S.

46. Rajashree KC. Training programs in communication skills for health care professionals and volunteers. Indian J Palliat Care. 2011;17(Suppl):S12–3.

47. National Institute for clinical Excellence (NICE) (Great Britain). Diabetes in pregnancy. In: Management of diabets and its complications from preconception to the postnatal period. London: PROG Press; 2015.

48. Simmons KB, Rodriguez MI. Reducing unintended pregnancy through provider training. Lancet. 2015;386(9993):514–6.

49. Phiri M, King R, Newell JN. Behaviour change techniques and contraceptive use in low and middle income countries: a review. Reprod Health. 2015;12:100.

50. Rattan J, Noznesky E, Curry DW, Galavotti C, Hwang S, Rodriguez M. Rapid contraceptive uptake and changing method mix with high use of long-acting reversible contraceptives in crisis-affected populations in Chad and the Democratic Republic of the Congo. Global health, science and practice. 2016;4(2):S5–s20.

4

Postpartum quality of life in Indian women after vaginal birth and cesarean section: a pilot study using the EQ-5D-5L descriptive system

Stefan Kohler[1,2]* , Kristi Sidney Annerstedt[2], Vishal Diwan[2,3,4], Lars Lindholm[5], Bharat Randive[3,5], Kranti Vora[6] and Ayesha De Costa[2]

Abstract

Background: There has been little evaluation of the postpartum quality of life (QOL) of women in India and its association with the mode of birth. This study piloted the use of the generic EQ-5D-5L questionnaire to assess postpartum QOL experienced by rural Indian women.

Methods: A convenience sample of rural women who gave birth in a health facility in Gujarat or Madhya Pradesh was recruited into this pilot study. QOL was measured during three interviews within 30 days of birth using the EQ-5D-5L questionnaire. Patient-level quality-adjusted life days (QALDs) were estimated. Multivariate regression was used to adjust for selected baseline characteristics.

Results: Forty-six women with cesarean section and 178 with vaginal birth from 17 public and private health facilities were studied. Postpartum QOL in both groups improved between interviews 1 and 3. Comparing between vaginal and cesarean births indicated that the vaginal birth group had a higher QOL (0–3 days postpartum: 0.28 vs. 0.57, 3–7 days postpartum: 0.59 vs. 0.81; $P < 0.001$) and was more likely to report no or slight problems in 4 of 5 health dimensions (mobility, self-care, usual activities, pain or discomfort; $P \leq 0.04$) during interviews 1 and 2. Postpartum QOL converged, but still differed between groups by the time of interview 3 (21–30 days postpartum: 0.85 vs. 0.93; $P < 0.001$). While most women reported no problems by the end of the first postpartum month, the difference in the ability to perform usual activities persisted ($P = 0.001$). In result, fewer QALDs were attained by women in the cesarean section group between day 1 and day 21 postpartum (13.1 vs. 16.6 QALDs; $P < 0.001$). Subgroup analysis showed that having had an episiotomy during vaginal birth was also associated with reduced QOL postpartum, but to a lesser extent than cesarean section. Similar results were obtained when adjusting for socioeconomic, pregnancy and birth characteristics, but postpartum QOL already ceased to be statistically different between groups before interview 3.

Conclusions: Vaginal births, even with episiotomy, were associated with a higher postpartum QOL than cesarean births among the Indian women in our pilot study. Finding these expected results suggests that the EQ-5D-5L questionnaire is a suitable instrument to assess postpartum QOL in Indian women.

Keywords: India, Quality of life, Postpartum period, Vaginal delivery, Episiotomy, Caesarean section, Pilot study

* Correspondence: stefan.kohler@uni-heidelberg.de
[1]Heidelberg Institute of Global Health, Heidelberg University, Heidelberg, Germany
[2]Division of Global Health, Department of Public Health Sciences, Karolinska Institutet, Stockholm, Sweden
Full list of author information is available at the end of the article

Background

The postpartum period is sometimes referred to as the fourth stage of labor. It begins after having given birth and may extend up to six months after giving birth [1]. Returning to the prepregnant state, women who gave birth experience physiological and psychological changes and continue to have increased health risks, particularly during the first weeks of the postpartum period. Postpartum health risks include physical health risks, like anemia, infections or wound healing complications, as well as mental health risks, like anxiety, depression, fatigue or stress [1, 2], which can bring about various degrees of morbidity in the postpartum period.

The number of women experiencing pregnancy related morbidity in the postpartum period is estimated to be magnitudes greater than the number who die [3]. Yet, there is little reliable information on the prevalence of maternal morbidity and postpartum quality of life (QOL), specially from low income settings [4–6].

In India, despite the implementation of large programs focused on intrapartum care, an emphasis on the provision of postpartum care and its evaluation is lacking. The latter has partly been due the absence of appropriate measuring instruments until quite recently, when the Mother Generated Index (MGI) and the Maternal Postpartum Quality of Life (MAPP-QOL) questionnaires have become available [7, 8]. However, the MGI is qualitative in nature and requires an educated trained health worker to administer the questionnaire. The MAPP-QOL, in turn, is a self-administered, paper and pencil questionnaire that requires women to be able to read and write. These characteristics limit the usability of the existing, specific postpartum QOL questionnaires in large-scale studies and among women with low levels of literacy.

In the absence of validated simple-to-implement instruments for measuring the QOL of pregnant or postpartum women, multiple studies have assessed the QOL of pregnant and postpartum women using generic instruments. Most of these studies were conducted in high income countries [4].

We used the generic EQ-5D questionnaire with five levels (EQ-5D-5L) for assessing the postpartum QOL experienced by rural Indian women in a pilot study. Our aims were to determine the feasibility of applying the EQ-5D-5L questionnaire to postpartum women in rural India and to explore whether the instrument can detect differences in postpartum QOL among rural Indian women who delivered vaginally or by caesarean section. Specific objectives were, first, to measure the QOL of Indian women in the first month postpartum; second, to examine which dimensions of QOL have been affected and, third, to assess postpartum health based on quality-adjusted life days (QALDs).

Methods

Study design and setting

This was a prospective pilot study of the QOL of postpartum women living in rural areas of the Indian states of Gujarat and Madhya Pradesh. Postpartum women were recruited in the two purposively selected districts of Ujjain in Madhya Pradesh and Surendranagar in Gujarat. Only women who lived within these district were included into the study to facilitate follow-ups in their community after discharge from hospital.

Women from Ujjain district in Madhya Pradesh who gave birth in April 2016 were recruited either in the government district hospital or the non-governmental teaching medical hospital of the district. In Gujarat, women who gave birth between July and November 2014 were recruited in a community health center and 14 private hospitals of Surendranagar district. Women were purposively selected to include vaginal births and cesarean sections in the sample. Vaginal births included vaginal births with episiotomies, but no forceps or vacuum assisted births. Cesarean sections included both emergency and elective procedures.

Women were approached three times after giving birth. Visits for an interview occurred 0–3 days, 3–7 days, and 21–30 days postpartum. The first administration of the EQ-5D-5L questionnaire was in the health facility. During the first interview socioeconomic, pregnancy and birth characteristics of the women were elicited. Follow-ups were conducted in women's homes for discharged women, or in the health facilities for a minority of women who were still in the health facility at the scheduled follow-up times. At all visits, women were interviewed by the same research assistant.

The study was part of the MATIND research projected, which evaluated two large scale demand side financing programs for maternal health in India – the Chiranjeevi Yojana (CY) scheme and the Janani Suraksha Yojana (JSY) scheme [9]. Early stage MATIND research demonstrated that many women accessing the CY and JSY schemes lack formal education and are part of traditional Indian societies [10, 11], in which women often have low levels of autonomy and freedom of expression.

Quality of life measurement

Health-related QOL was assessed based on women's responses to the EQ-5D-5L questionnaire. The EQ-5D is a two-part instrument. Part one, the so-called descriptive system, is a self-assessment of today's health along 5 pre-specified dimensions: mobility, self-care, usual activity, pain or discomfort, and anxiety or depression. For each dimension, the respondent selects one of 5 levels of incapacitation in the 5L version: no, slight, moderate, severe, or extreme problems. The combination of answers can result in $5^5 = 3125$ possible health states. Part two of the EQ-5D consists of a visual analogue scale (VAS) which can be used to obtain a visually guided self-rating of today's health on a scale from 0 (worst) to 100 (best). Both parts of the EQ-5D instrument should be used together [12], but women in the pilot study women had difficulties to assess their health using a VAS. Thus, use of the EQ VAS was ceased within the pilot study.

Data collection and analysis

We used the Hindi version of EQ-5D-5L health questionnaire with permission from the EuroQoL Group [13, 14]. The questionnaire was intended to be administered to each recruited woman by a trained research assistant at three points in time: 1, 7 and 21 days after birth or as close as possible to these dates. In practice, the first interview occurred between 0 and 3 days postpartum, the second interview between 3 and 7 days postpartum, and the final interview between 21 and 30 after women gave birth. Women's characteristics were obtained at baseline from hospital records and staff as well as by interviewing women. Interviews took place in a language understood by both the woman and the research assistant. No sample size calculation was made for this pilot study.

Problem levels, reported by the postpartum women through answering the descriptive system of the EQ-5D-5L at three different points in time, were mapped to QOL weights based on a value set obtained from the general population in the United Kingdom by time trade-off valuation techniques. We used the United Kingdom value set due to the lack of an EQ-5D population norm for India [15]. Furthermore, we used a crosswalk value set that allows to link responses to the EQ-5D-5L with the existing value sets for the EQ-5D-3L [16], as only value sets for the 3-level version of the EQ-5D were available at the time of analysis.

Quality-adjusted life time was calculated based on days (QALDs) rather than years (QALYs) due to the brief postpartum period studied. QALDs were estimated on the individual-level by applying the area-under-the-curve method [17, 18]. The area-under-the-curve method was implemented summing up, by birth mode and episiotomy status, the areas of under the curves obtained from linearly connecting each woman's QOL values from day 1 to day 21 postpartum.

To obtain comparable QALDs, despite some variation in the postpartum days when QOL data was collected, we standardized the reference period for which QALDs are reported to days 1 to 21 postpartum. For women surveyed in Gujarat, we used recorded interview dates to impute QOL weights for days 1 and 21 postpartum based on linear interpolation. In one instance, interpolation led to a QOL weight greater than one and was set to one, the weight for the best health status. For women surveyed Madhya Pradesh, we assumed that all interviews took place exactly 1, 7 and 21 days after birth.

In the descriptive analysis, differences in continuous variables were assessed using Wilcoxon rank-sum and two-sample t-tests. Differences in proportions were compared using Pearson's chi-squared tests. Hypotheses about regression coefficients were assessed based Wald tests. Generalized estimating equation was used to estimate the adjusted association between time and QOL, assuming a Gaussian distribution of QOL, an identity link function and unstructured correlation between the data obtained over three interview visits. Linear regression was used to examine the association between birth mode and QALDs, controlling for characteristics that may affect postpartum QOL.

Results

Participant characteristics

In total, 231 women were recruited into the pilot study: 60 in Ujjain district of Madhya Pradesh and 171 in Surendranagar district of Gujarat. Seven women were excluded from the analysis: one woman who gave birth on the way to a hospital, two women who experienced a still birth or neonatal death, and four women who could not be contacted for follow-up interviews.

The final sample included 224 women, of which 178 (79%) gave vaginal birth and 46 (21%) gave birth by cesarean section. Socioeconomic, pregnancy and birth characteristics of these women are shown in Table 1. Women were aged 18 to 36 years. Those who had a vaginal birth were more likely to belong to a socially and educationally disadvantaged group and a poorer household. The state specific Indian poverty line considers several other factors than income, and similar portions of women in both birth groups were below poverty line.

The number of previous pregnancies ranged from 0 to 7 in both birth groups with the same median of one previous pregnancy. An episiotomy was reported by 67% of the women who gave vaginal birth and by one woman with a cesarean section. In the vaginal birth group, 10% of women experienced one or more of the following complications during their birth or pregnancy: premature rupture of membranes, preeclampsia signs, obstructed labor, malpresentation, oligohydramnios, previous cesarean section. By contrast, 87% of the women with a cesarean section had at least one of these complications that increase the likelihood of cesarean section. No women in the sample was diagnosed with eclampsia or had convulsions. Similar portions of 87% and 91% of the newborns were healthy in both groups 2–3 days postpartum. Cesarean sections were more likely to

Table 1 Socioeconomic, pregnancy and birth characteristics of women in the pilot study by birth mode

	Vaginal birth	Cesarean section	P
Socioeconomic characteristics			
Mother's age			0.49
18–20	39 (21.9%)	6 (13.0%)	
21–24	84 (47.2%)	23 (50.0%)	
25–29	46 (25.8%)	13 (28.3%)	
30–36	9 (5.1%)	4 (8.7%)	
Years of schooling			0.007
None	53 (29.8%)	8 (17.4%)	
Primary (1–5)	35 (19.7%)	4 (8.7%)	
Secondary (6–12)	87 (48.9%)	30 (65.2%)	
Higher (> 12)	3 (1.7%)	4 (8.7%)	
Caste of woman			< 0.01
Scheduled Caste/Tribe	45 (25.3%)	7 (15.2%)	
Other Backward Caste	125 (70.2%)	31 (67.4%)	
General Caste	8 (4.5%)	8 (17.4%)	
Household income			0.01
0–2499 INR	16 (9.0%)	1 (2.2%)	
2500–4999 INR	49 (27.5%)	5 (10.9%)	
5000–9999 INR	68 (38.2%)	20 (43.5%)	
10,000–60,000 INR	45 (25.3%)	20 (43.5%)	
Below poverty line			0.84
No	40 (22.5%)	11 (23.9%)	
Yes	138 (77.5%)	35 (76.1%)	
Pregnancy and birth characteristics			
Previous pregnancies			0.42
None	23 (12.9%)	10 (21.7%)	
1–2	125 (70.2%)	31 (67.4%)	
3–4	24 (13.5%)	4 (8.7%)	
5–7	6 (3.4%)	1 (2.2%)	
Woman reported episiotomy			< 0.001
No	58 (32.6%)	45 (97.8%)	
Yes	120 (67.4%)	1 (2.2%)	
Risk factors for cesarean section[1]			< 0.001
No	160 (89.9%)	6 (13.0%)	
Yes	18 (10.1%)	40 (87.0%)	
Ante- or postpartum hemorrhage			0.40
No	169 (94.9%)	45 (97.8%)	
Yes	9 (5.1%)	1 (2.2%)	
Prolonged labor, anemia or fever			0.72
No	151 (84.8%)	40 (87.0%)	
Yes	27 (15.2%)	6 (13.0%)	
Baby's health (2–3 days postpartum)			0.43
Healthy	155 (87.1%)	42 (91.3%)	
Sick	23 (12.9%)	4 (8.7%)	

Table 1 Socioeconomic, pregnancy and birth characteristics of women in the pilot study by birth mode *(Continued)*

	Vaginal birth	Cesarean section	P
Length of hospital stay after birth, median (IQR)	2.0 (1.0, 2.0)	3.0 (3.0, 5.0)	< 0.001
Length of hospital stay			< 0.001
Below median duration for birth mode	81 (45.5%)	7 (15.2%)	
Of median duration for birth mode	81 (45.5%)	23 (50.0%)	
Above median duration for birth mode	16 (9.0%)	16 (34.8%)	
Birth place			0.02
Community health center	55 (30.9%)	6 (13.0%)	
District hospital	39 (21.9%)	8 (17.4%)	
Private hospital	84 (47.2%)	32 (69.6%)	
N	178	46	

[1]Risk factors for cesarean section include premature rupture of membranes, preeclampsia signs, obstructed labor, malpresentation, oligohydramnios, and previous cesarean section
INR Indian Rupee, *IQR* interquartile range
P-values of Wilcoxon rank-sum test or Pearson's chi-squared test

happen in a private hospital, associated with longer hospital stays, and all performed by a medical doctor.

Feasibility of using the EQ-5D

The pilot study started administering both parts of the EQ-5D-5L questionnaire. We observed early in the study that participating women had difficulties with the VAS component of the EQ-5D questionnaire. Given the standard instructions, several respondents were uncertain of where to place a mark on the VAS. Therefore, a decision was made to pursue the pilot study further using only the descriptive system of the EQ-5D-5L questionnaire through which we obtained the results presented below.

Postpartum quality of life
Descriptive analysis

Postpartum women rated each of five health dimensions (mobility, self-care, usual activities, pain or discomfort, and anxiety or depression) in the EQ-5D-5L questionnaire as associated with no problems = 1, slight problems = 2, moderate problems = 3, severe problems = 4, unable to/extreme problems = 5. Assuming the numbers assigned to these problem levels are such that numerically equal differences in ratings represent equal differences in the levels of problems, Fig. 1 shows the mean levels of incapacitation for each dimension, by birth mode and the time passed since giving birth. On average, women with cesarean section perceived stronger problems than women with vaginal birth in 4 out of 5 health dimensions assessed by the EQ-5D. The level of reported problems with anxiety or depression was low across birth modes. Receiving an episiotomy during vaginal birth reduced postpartum QOL in the same health dimensions as having a cesarean section, but, overall, to

a lesser extent. For all birth modes, reported problems decreased in the observed postpartum period.

The percentages of women reporting problem levels 1 to 5 for each of the five dimensions of the EQ-5D-5L are shown in Table 2. Within the first three days of birth, the portions of women reporting no problems were substantially higher, in both birth groups, for anxiety or depression ($\geq$74%) than for the other four dimensions (self-care, mobility, usual activities, and pain or discomfort; <47%, P < 0.001) The respective severity of problems varied significantly with the birth mode in all of the latter four dimensions up to 3–7 days after birth ($P \leq 0.04$). By the time of the last interview 21–30 days postpartum, $\geq$ 89% of women, regardless of the mode of their recent birth, reported no problems with mobility, self-care, pain or discomfort, and anxiety or depression, regardless of the mode of their recent birth. No women indicated extreme problems during the last interview, $\leq$0.6% severe problems, $\leq$2.2% moderate problems, and <20% slight problems in any of the EQ-5D health dimensions.

Only the ability to perform usual activities continued to be significantly different between women with vaginal and cesarean births towards the end of the first postpartum month (96 vs. 80% without problems; P = 0.001). Anxiety or depression was the only dimension for which the data did not indicate a difference by birth mode throughout the whole first month postpartum ($P \geq 0.51$). The highest shares of extreme problems for the dimensions of mobility, self-care, usual activities, and pain or discomfort as well as most severe problems occurred in the cesarean section group shortly after birth.

For an overall assessment of the health problems reported in the five dimensions assessed by the EQ-5D, the reported problem levels were mapped into to QOL weights. Table 3 compares the unadjusted QOL weights

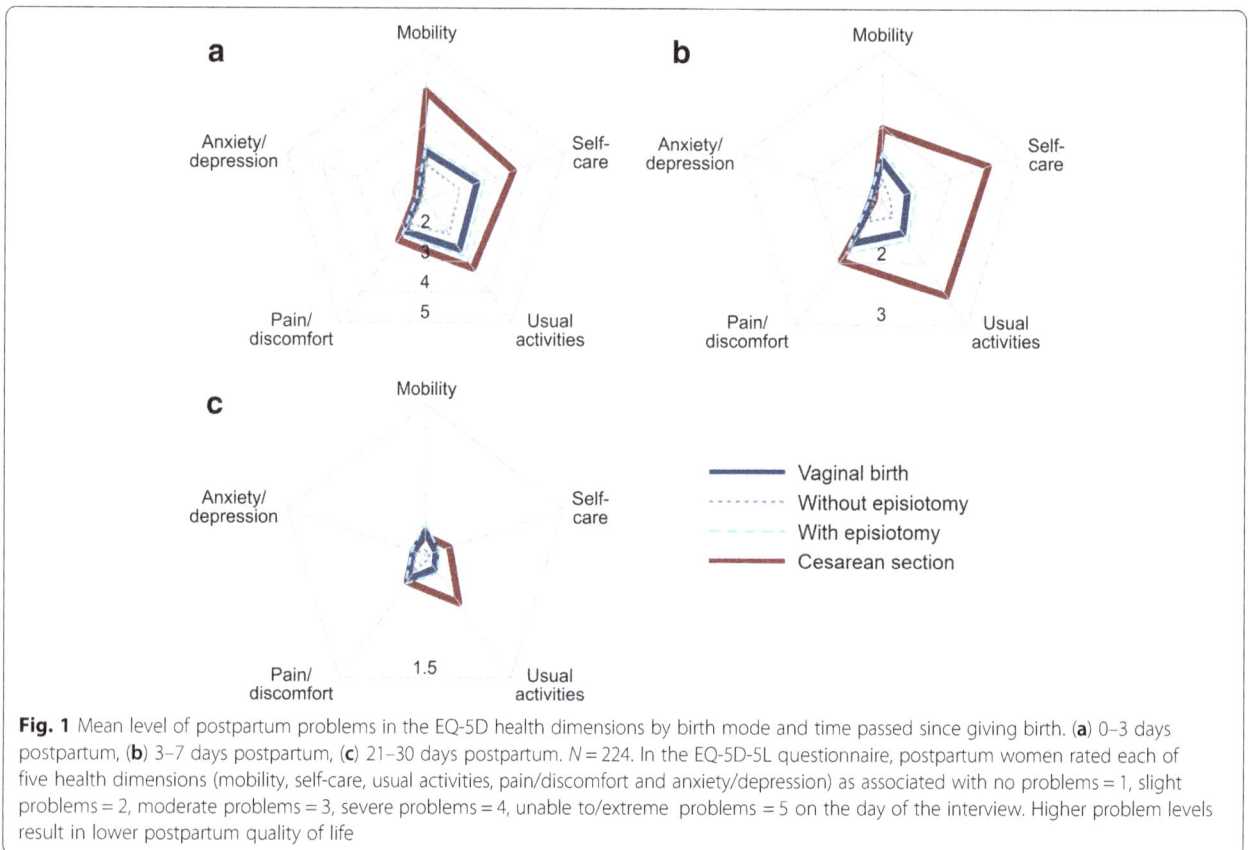

Fig. 1 Mean level of postpartum problems in the EQ-5D health dimensions by birth mode and time passed since giving birth. (**a**) 0–3 days postpartum, (**b**) 3–7 days postpartum, (**c**) 21–30 days postpartum. $N = 224$. In the EQ-5D-5L questionnaire, postpartum women rated each of five health dimensions (mobility, self-care, usual activities, pain/discomfort and anxiety/depression) as associated with no problems = 1, slight problems = 2, moderate problems = 3, severe problems = 4, unable to/extreme problems = 5 on the day of the interview. Higher problem levels result in lower postpartum quality of life

between vaginal and cesarean births. The QOL weights quantify how postpartum QOL improved between interviews 1 and 3 in both groups, and they indicate that the vaginal birth group had a higher QOL throughout in comparison to women after cesarean section. In result, fewer QALDs were attained by women in the cesarean section group between day 1 and day 21 postpartum (13.1 vs. 16.6 QALDs, $P < 0.001$; see Fig. 2a). Subgroup analysis showed that having had an episiotomy during vaginal birth was also associated with reduced postpartum QOL in comparison to a vaginal birth without episiotomy (16.0 vs. 18.0 QALDs; $P < 0.001$), but to a lesser extent than giving birth by cesarean section (13.1 vs. 18.0 QALDs, $P < 0.001$; see Fig. 2b).

Multivariate analysis

Results similar to those of the descriptive analysis were obtained when adjusting for selected baseline characteristics. Table 4 presents generalized estimating equation models 2 of the QOL weight at the postpartum interview times and linear regression models 2 of the QALDs in the first 21 postpartum days. Models (a) compare women who gave vaginal birth and women who gave birth by cesarean section. Models (b) further distinguish whether an episiotomy was performed during vaginal

birth. All regression models adjusted for the socioeconomic, pregnancy and birth characteristics reported in Table 1.

In models 1, the lowest QOL weights were estimated immediately after birth, irrespective of the birth mode and whether an episiotomy was performed or not. On average, QOL improved for all women between interviews 1 and 3 as indicated by significantly increasing QOL coefficients from 0–3 days to 21–30 days postpartum for both birth modes. Women with a vaginal birth, for instance, had an average QOL weight of 0.40 at the time of interview 1, which significantly increased to 0.64 at the time of interview 2 and to 0.76 at the time of interview 3 ($P < 0.001$). An episiotomy significantly lowered the estimated QOL weights after vaginal birth in comparison to a vaginal birth with no episiotomy until the time of interview 2 (3–7 days postpartum; $P \leq 0.008$) but not afterwards.

How the estimated differences in women's postpartum QOL weights accumulate over time is captured by the QALDs outcome in models 2. On average, women had more QALD during the first 21 postpartum days after vaginal birth than after cesarean section (14.6 vs. 11.3 QALDs; $P < 0.001$). A vaginal birth with an episiotomy was associated with significantly fewer QALDs in the first 21 postpartum days than a vaginal birth without episiotomy (15.3 vs. 17.1 QALDs; $P < 0.001$), but with

Table 2 Comparison of problems by EQ-5D health dimension in women with vaginal birth and cesarean section within the first month postpartum

Health dimension	Problem level	0–3 days postpartum			3–7 days postpartum			21–30 days postpartum		
		VB (%)	CS (%)	P	VB (%)	CS (%)	P	VB (%)	CS (%)	P
Mobility	No problems	24.7	4.3	< 0.001	53.4	39.1	0.004	93.3	93.5	0.75
	Slight problems	48.3	17.4		39.3	39.1		5.6	6.5	
	Moderate problems	11.2	4.3		6.2	13.0		1.1		
	Severe problems	5.1	34.8		1.1	2.2				
	Unable to	10.7	39.1		0.0	6.5				
Self-care	No problems	23.0	2.2	< 0.001	69.7	23.9	< 0.001	96.1	91.3	0.18
	Slight problems	52.2	32.6		27.0	50.0		3.9	8.7	
	Moderate problems	1.7	17.4		1.7	0.0				
	Severe problems	0.6	6.5		0.0	0.0				
	Unable to	22.5	41.3		1.7	26.1				
Usual activities	No problems	20.8	19.6	0.01	60.1	28.3	< 0.001	95.5	80.4	0.001
	Slight problems	46.6	23.9		35.4	39.1		3.9	19.6	
	Moderate problems	8.4	10.9		1.1	8.7				
	Severe problems	1.1	6.5		1.1			0.6		
	Unable to	23.0	39.1		2.2	23.9				
Pain or discomfort	No	27.0	28.3	0.008	47.8	28.3	0.04	92.1	89.1	0.28
	Slight	48.9	30.4		39.3	47.8		5.6	10.9	
	Moderate	21.3	26.1		11.8	23.9		2.2		
	Severe	2.2	13.0		1.1					
	Extreme	0.6	2.2							
Anxiety or depression	No	82.6	73.9	0.51	88.2	91.3	0.83	96.6	97.8	0.51
	Slight	15.2	23.9		9.0	6.5		2.2		
	Moderate	0.6			1.7	2.2		1.1	2.2	
	Severe	1.7	2.2		1.1					
	Extreme									
N		178	46		178	46		178	46	

VB vaginal birth, *CS* cesarean section

Table 3 Comparison of quality of life weights and quality-adjusted life days in women with vaginal birth and cesarean section within the first month postpartum

	Vaginal birth			Cesarean section
	All	No episiotomy	Episiotomy	
	Mean (95% CI)	Mean (95% CI)	Mean (95% CI)	Mean (95% CI)
QOL weight				
0–3 days postpartum	0.57 (0.52, 0.61)	0.68 (0.6, 0.75)	0.51 (0.46, 0.56)	0.28 (0.18, 0.38)
3–7 days postpartum	0.81 (0.78, 0.84)	0.9 (0.87, 0.93)[a]	0.76 (0.73, 0.8)	0.59 (0.51, 0.67)
21–30 days postpartum	0.93 (0.92, 0.94)	0.96 (0.95, 0.98)[a]	0.92 (0.9, 0.93)	0.85 (0.82, 0.89)
QALDs (1–21 days postpartum)	16.6 (16.2, 17.0)	18.0 (17.5, 18.5)	16.0 (15.5, 16.4)	13.1 (12.0, 14.2)
N	178	58	120	46

QALDs quality-adjusted life days, *QOL* quality of life
Two-sample *t*-tests and Wilcoxon rank-sum tests indicate significant differences in the means and distributions of the QOL weights and QALDs in the following comparisons: all vaginal births vs. cesarean section, no episiotomy vs. episiotomy, no episiotomy vs. cesarean section, and episiotomy vs cesarean section; $P < 0.001$. QOLs weights increased significantly with the time passed since birth in each of the four birth groups distinguished; $P < 0.001$ for all comparisons between visits, except for the following comparison: [a] $P = 0.04$

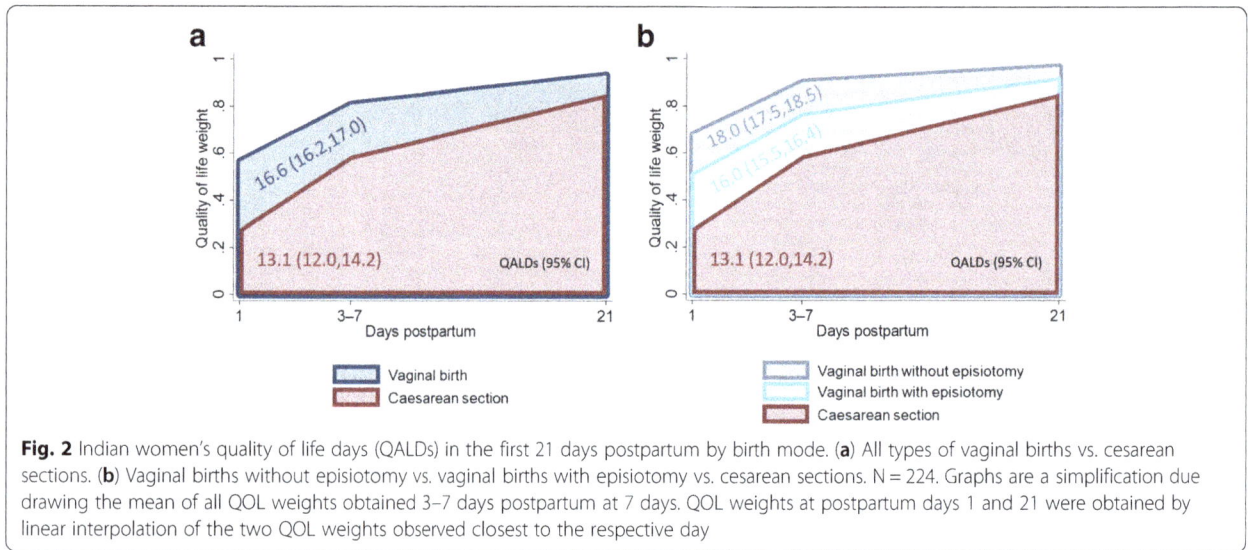

Fig. 2 Indian women's quality of life days (QALDs) in the first 21 days postpartum by birth mode. (**a**) All types of vaginal births vs. cesarean sections. (**b**) Vaginal births without episiotomy vs. vaginal births with episiotomy vs. cesarean sections. N = 224. Graphs are a simplification due drawing the mean of all QOL weights obtained 3–7 days postpartum at 7 days. QOL weights at postpartum days 1 and 21 were obtained by linear interpolation of the two QOL weights observed closest to the respective day

significantly more QALDs in the first 21 postpartum days than a cesarean section (15.3 vs. 12.5 QALDs; $P < 0.001$).

Discussion

Motivation for piloting the EQ-5D questionnaire with rural Indian postpartum women

As health care becomes more patient-centered, patient-reported outcomes such as QOL are becoming increasingly important [19, 20]. The few studies that assessed postpartum QOL in India prior to our study have used the MGI questionnaire [21, 22]. Related to a lack of research on postpartum QOL in Indian women [23], there is limited knowledge and experience on choice of a suitable questionnaire for the study postpartum QOL in India.

We tested using the generic EQ-5D questionnaire for postpartum QOL assessment in India by interviewing a convenience sample of rural women three times with the EQ-5D-5L descriptive system in their first month postpartum. The rationale behind testing the EQ-5D questionnaire for postpartum QOL assessment in rural Indian women was that existing specific instruments for postpartum QOL, like the MGI or MAPP-QOL questionnaire, can be impractical for large-scale use in low-literacy populations and in settings in which women have low levels of autonomy and freedom of expression.

The MGI measures subjective QOL and, unlike the EQ-5D, does not consist of a predefined checklist of problems. Specifically, the MGI consist of three steps during which a woman generates her own QOL index. Step 1 requires a woman to identify up to eight most important areas of her life that have been affected by having a baby, and to indicate if she thinks these areas are positive, negative, both or neither of these. Step 2 asks a woman to

score, on a visual analogue scale from 0 to 10, how she has been affected in each identified area over the past month. Step 3 requires a woman to allocate 20 points across the identified areas, according to how important an area is to her QOL. Thus, applying the MGI requires settings in which women are able, have time and are given time to think about and articulate such issues. In studies including larger numbers of women with low levels of education and/or from conservative rural settings, applying the MGI could become difficult. Use of the MGI may, for instance, require significant time and prompting from skilled counsellors to support women in expressing their postpartum experience [24]. At the same time, counsellors need to avoid influencing the women's choices and expression.

An exploratory study that evaluated the use of the MGI in urban India found that all interviewed women identified only 2 to 5 areas of their life that had been affected by their pregnancy, after much suggestion and stimulation by the counsellors. The women in the study were perceived to have conceptual difficulty in identifying any areas or aspects of life which were positively affected by the birth [22]. The MAPP-QOL questionnaire, in turn, another specific instrument for postpartum QOL assessment, is self-administered and requires women to be able to read and write, but in our pilot study 45% of women had no or at most five years of schooling.

As we deemed the use of the MGI and MAPP-QOL instruments unfeasible for data collection on postpartum QOL within the MATIND project, we tested the use of the EQ-5D-5L questionnaire with rural Indian postpartum women in the states of Gujarat und Madhya Pradesh. Choosing the EQ-5D tool for postpartum QOL measurement was a pragmatic choice: Firstly, the EQ-5D

Table 4 Adjusted comparison of quality of life weights and quality-adjusted life days in women with vaginal birth and cesarean section within the first month postpartum

	QOL weight		QALDs (1–21 days postpartum)	
	Model 1a	Model 1b	Model 2a	Model 2b
	Coef. (95% CI)	Coef. (95% CI)	Coef. (95% CI)	Coef. (95% CI)
Vaginal birth (all)				
0–3 days postpartum	0.39 (0.27, 0.52)[a]		14.6 (12.3, 16.9)[m]	
3–7 days postpartum	0.64 (0.52, 0.76)[b]			
21–30 days postpartum	0.76 (0.65, 0.88)[c]			17.1 (14.6, 19.6)[n,o]
Vaginal birth (no episiotomy)				
0–3 days postpartum		0.52 (0.35, 0.7)[d,e]		
3–7 days postpartum		0.75 (0.61, 0.89)[f,g]		
21–30 days postpartum		0.81 (0.67, 0.95)[h,i]		15.3 (131, 17.6)[n,p]
Vaginal birth (episiotomy)				
0–3 days postpartum		0.41 (0.27, 0.54)[d,j]		
3–7 days postpartum		0.66 (0.53, 0.79)[f,k]		
21–30 days postpartum		0.81 (0.69, 0.94)[h,l]		
Cesarean section				
0–3 days postpartum	0.15 (0.01, 0.29)[a]	0.2 (0.05, 0.35)[e,j]	11.3 (8.94, 13.7)[m]	12.5 (10.1, 14.8)[o,p]
3–7 days postpartum	0.46 (0.33, 0.59)[b]	0.51 (0.37, 0.65)[g,k]		
21–30 days postpartum	0.73 (0.62, 0.83)[c]	0.77 (0.65, 0.89)[i,l]		
Mother's age (ref. = 21–24)				
18–20	0.03 (−0.02, 0.08)	0.03 (−0.02, 0.08)	0.49 (−0.49, 1.48)	0.36 (−0.61, 1.33)
25–30	−0.01 (−0.07, 0.04)	−0.02 (−0.07, 0.03)	−0.52 (−1.6, 0.56)	−0.6 (−1.64, 0.45)
30–36	0.04 (−0.03, 0.11)	0.03 (−0.04, 0.11)	0.89 (−0.68, 2.45)	0.64 (−0.96, 2.24)
Years of schooling (ref. = secondary: 6–12)				
None	0.06 (0.01, 0.11)	0.06 (0.01, 0.1)	0.33 (−0.66, 1.32)	0.3 (−0.65, 1.25)
Primary (1–5)	0.06 (0.01, 0.12)	0.06 (0.01, 0.11)	0.756 (−0.332, 1.83)	0.69 (−0.36, 1.75)
Higher (> 12)	−0.13 (−0.23, −0.02)	−0.13 (−0.23, −0.02)	−2.22 (−4.44, −0.002)	−2.18 (−4.53, 0.17)
Caste of woman (ref. = Other Backward Caste)				
Scheduled Caste/Tribe	0.02 (−0.02, 0.06)	0.02 (−0.02, 0.06)	−0.17 (−1.06, 0.72)	−0.14 (−0.99, 0.71)
General Caste	0.14 (0.04, 0.23)	0.13 (0.04, 0.22)	1.75 (−0.23, 3.74)	1.64 (−0.27, 3.54)
Household income (ref. = 2500–4999 INR)				
0–2499 INR	0.1 (0.03, 0.18)	0.09 (0.02, 0.17)	1.13 (−0.19, 2.44)	0.85 (−0.37, 2.08)
5000–9999 INR	0.06 (0.01, 0.12)	0.05 (0.001, 0.11)	0.66 (−0.35, 1.68)	0.48 (−0.52, 1.47)
10,000–60,000 INR	0.03 (−0.01, 0.08)	0.03 (−0.01, 0.08)	0.08 (−0.92, 1.07)	0.09 (−0.88, 1.07)

Table 4 Adjusted comparison of quality of life weights and quality-adjusted life days in women with vaginal birth and cesarean section within the first month postpartum (Continued)

	QOL weight		QALDs (1–21 days postpartum)	
	Model 1a	Model 1b	Model 2a	Model 2b
	Coef. (95% CI)	Coef. (95% CI)	Coef. (95% CI)	Coef. (95% CI)
Above poverty line	0.04 (−0.01, 0.09)	0.03 (−0.02, 0.08)	0.8 (−0.24, 1.85)	0.6 (−0.42, 1.61)
Previous pregnancies (ref. = 1–2)				
None	0.08 (−0.01, 0.16)	0.04 (−0.05, 0.13)	1.11 (−0.39, 2.61)	0.25 (−1.22, 1.73)
3–4	0.14 (0.04, 0.25)	0.08 (−0.03, 0.2)	2.05 (0.15, 3.96)	0.49 (−1.51, 2.49)
5–7	0.05 (−0.08, 0.17)	−0.02 (−0.16, 0.12)	1.27 (−1.31, 3.85)	−0.42 (−3.06, 2.22)
Risk factors for cesarean section[1]	−0.003 (−0.06, 0.06)	−0.00108 (−0.06, 0.06)	0.36 (−0.85, 1.56)	0.4 (−0.76, 1.56)
Ante- or postpartum hemorrhage	−0.03 (−0.12, 0.07)	−0.02 (−0.11, 0.07)	−0.69 (−2.39, 1.02)	−0.52 (−2.07, 1.02)
Prolonged labor, anemia or fever	0.03 (−0.02, 0.08)	0.03 (−0.02, 0.08)	0.33 (−0.56, 1.22)	0.35 (−0.53,1.23)
Baby is sick (2–3 days postpartum)	−0.01 (−0.04, 0.01)	−0.02 (−0.05, 0.01)	−0.27 (−0.89, 0.34)	−0.39 (−1.01, 0.23)
Length of hospital stay (ref. = median duration for birth mode)				
< Median duration for birth mode	−0.03 (−0.09, 0.02)	−0.03 (−0.08, 0.03)	0.33 (−1.02, 1.69)	0.45 (−0.87, 1.77)
> Median duration for birth mode	−0.04 (−0.11, 0.04)	−0.04 (−0.11, 0.03)	0.04 (−1.45, 1.54)	−0.06 (−1.47, 1.35)
Health facility (ref. = private hospital)				
Community health center	0.05 (−0.02, 0.11)	0.05 (−0.02, 0.11)	0.29 (−1.24, 1.82)	0.37 (−1.12, 1.87)
District hospital	0.12 (0.04, 0.21)	0.09 (0.003, 0.18)	1.09 (−0.41, 2.59)	0.24 (−1.33, 1.82)
R^2			0.97	0.97
N	224 × 3	224 × 3	224	224

[1]Risk factors for cesarean section include premature rupture of membranes, preeclampsia signs, obstructed labor, malpresentation, oligohydramnios, and previous cesarean section

[a] $P < 0.001$, [b] $P = < 0.001$, [c] $P = 0.30$, [d] $P = 0.01$, [e] $P < 0.001$, [f] $P = 0.008$, [g] $P < 0.001$, [h] $P = 0.91$, [i] $P = 0.28$, [j] $P < 0.001$, [k] $P = 0.002$, [l] $P = 0.20$, [m] $P < 0.001$, [n] $P < 0.001$, [o] $P < 0.001$, [p] $P < 0.001$. QOL weights increased significantly with the time passed since birth in each of the four birth groups distinguished; $P < 0.001$ for all comparisons between interview visits

QALDs quality-adjusted life days, QOL quality of life. Models 1 generalized estimating equation of QOL weights, models 2 linear regression of QALDs. Sampling weights were used to resemble a population with an equal number of normal vaginal deliveries and cesarean sections. R^2 from linear regression models without intercept

instrument is available in many languages. Secondly, it can be administered in a number of modes, including face-to-face and telephone interviews. Thirdly, the EQ-5D questionnaire is relatively easy and quick to apply in comparison to the MGI or MAPP-QOL instruments. In addition, there had been some experience with using the EQ-5D questionnaire to evaluate postpartum QOL, yet mostly from high income countries [25–28].

Appropriateness of using the EQ-5D an the Indian setting

The findings of the pilot study at hand indicate that the descriptive system of the EQ-5D-5L was able to depict and differentiate early postpartum QOL in Indian women by birth mode and over time. On average, at least 75% of the women in our study reported slight to extreme problems in four of the five health dimensions assessed by the EQ-5D-5L. The median woman who gave vaginal birth reported slight problems with mobility, self-care, usual activities, and pain or discomfort in the first interview 0–3 days after birth. At a similar postpartum time, the median woman who gave birth by cesarean section reported slight problems only with pain or discomfort and extreme problems with mobility, self-care and usual activities. No problems with anxiety or depression were reported by the median women in both birth groups, and less than 3% of the women interviewed ever reported more than slight problems with anxiety or depression. Among the women who gave vaginal births, the EQ-5D based QOL measure was lower for women who reported to have had an episiotomy during birth in comparison to those women who did not have this oftentimes discomforting procedure. Differences in the level of problems, and consequently QOL weights, between women with vaginal births and women with cesarean sections were highest at the time of the first interview which took place within the first three days postpartum. As time progressed, differences in QOL between women with vaginal and cesarean births narrowed and ceased to be statistically discernible at the time of the last follow-up interview when adjusting for socioeconomic, pregnancy and birth characteristics. Estimating the overall QOL in the first 21 days postpartum, vaginal births were associated with significantly more QALDs than cesarean sections.

The differences and trends in the postpartum QOL of Indian women, which were measured using the EQ-5D-5L in this pilot study, reflect plausible outcomes that are consistent with the findings of prior studies of postpartum QOL, conducted in other settings and/or using other QOL instruments [4–6]. Anxiety or depression was the EQ-5D dimension that was least affected by problems in our study. A recent systematic review and meta-analysis of postpartum depression in India, which included mostly studies that have used depression

specific instruments, suggests a prevalence of postpartum depression of 22% (95% CI: 19%, 25%) overall and of 17% (95% CI: 14%, 21%) in rural areas [29]. In our study of the first postpartum month, 17% of women after vaginal birth and 26% after cesarean section reported slight to severe problems with anxiety or depression at the time of the first interview. By the end of our one-month pilot study, 97% of all women interviewed reported no problems with anxiety or depression. A decrease in the prevalence of possible depression within the first weeks postpartum is also suggested by the most comparable study, in terms of state and timing, of postpartum depression in the systematic review and meta-analysis. Using the Edinburgh Postnatal Depression Scale (EPDS), a prevalence of depression of 11%, 7% and 3% was found on postpartum days 1 and 6 and postpartum week 6, respectively, among randomly selected postpartum women in the Government Medical College in Gujarat [30], the state in which we recruited 74% of the women in our pilot study.

The fact that mostly slight if any problems with anxiety or depression were reported in our pilot study raises the question if the EQ-5D descriptive system is sensitive enough to detect changes in postpartum problems with anxiety or depression relevant to the QOL of Indian women. A systematic review of the EQ-5D responsiveness classified the overall responsiveness of the instrument to anxiety and depression disorders as small to large [31]. Future research might therefore need to study the existence and relevance of a possible lack of sensitivity in the anxiety or depression dimension when using the EQ-5D for postpartum QOL assessment in rural Indian women. Stigma expressing postpartum anxiety or stress, particularly when interviewed at home rather than in a hospital environment, could be a possible limitation to assessing problems with anxiety or depression in India [29]. Besides, difficulties to differentiate between postpartum blues and postpartum depression in the early postpartum period [29] might confound early postpartum period responses to questions about anxiety or depression. On the other hand, some researchers argue that postpartum stress in India can be low due strong extended family support during seminal moments in life like childbirth [32].

Strengths and limitations

To our knowledge, this study was the first to assess postpartum QOL using the EQ-5D in a low resource setting. As a pilot study, this study has several limitations. Only part the EQ-5D questionnaire (the descriptive system) was assessed, and no validation whether the EQ-5D descriptive system measured postpartum QOL in Indian women accurately and consistently was performed. We can therefore not exclude that the descriptive system of the generic EQ-5D instrument failed to measure or inadequately measured health-related problems of Indian women in the postpartum period (see [33]). Further, due to the unavailability of an EQ-5D population norm, which would reflect the preferences over health states of the general public for India, a United Kingdom value set was used as an approximation to obtain QOL weights from the gathered problem levels. Finally, the pilot study's sample, sample size and time horizon were pragmatic choices. Districts, health facilities and women were selected such that they could be reached well by research assistants. Applying a convenient sampling procedure resulted in a sample in which, for instance, the majority of women gave birth in a private health facility and all women with a cesarean section were primipara. While we adjusted for selected baseline differences in a multivariate analysis, there may be other confounders and lack of variation or statistical power in the data that influenced the results. The study was restricted to 4 weeks for logistical reasons even though the immediate postpartum period is commonly defined as up to 6 weeks after birth. However, 87% of all women in the study reported no problems in all five EQ-5D domains during the last interview. Therefore, impairments to QOL in the immediate postpartum period that can be measured with the EQ-5D-5L descriptive system appear to have been measured to a large extent in this pilot study. Changes in later postpartum QOL, beyond the immediate postpartum period, have not been studied.

Conclusions

Postpartum QOL data from India is scarce, partly because of difficulties with implementing existing, specific postpartum QOL instruments in common Indian settings. We explored the feasibility of applying the generic EQ-5D-5L health questionnaire to postpartum women in India, of whom many had little or no formal education. We found that only the use of the descriptive part of the EQ-5D, which asks about the level of problems experienced in five generic areas of health, was feasible and acceptable to the rural women participating in our pilot study.

Subgroup analyses of problem levels, reported by women who gave birth in different ways, showed significant differences between the QOL of women who had a vaginal birth without episiotomy, those who had a vaginal birth with episiotomy and those who gave birth by cesarean section. As time progressed, postpartum QOL converged and ceased to be differed between groups by or before the end of the first postpartum month. Summing up the estimated QOL over the first 21 postpartum days, most QALDs were attained by women who gave vaginal birth without having an episiotomy. Significantly fewer QALDs were estimated for women who had

an episiotomy during their vaginal birth, and again fewer for women who gave birth by cesarean section.

Differences and changes in the five health dimensions assessed by the EQ-5D-5L, as well as the estimated postpartum QOL and OALDs, reflect plausible health effects and recovery paths from vaginal and cesarean births. Finding results that are consistent with our expectations and many other studies of postpartum QOL suggests that measuring health-related QOL in the immediate postpartum period with the descriptive part of the generic EQ-5D-5L instrument can support assessments of maternal QOL in the postpartum period in India.

Abbreviations

CS: cesarean section; CY: Chiranjeevi Yojana; EPDS: Using the Edinburgh Postnatal Depression Scale; EQ-5D-5L: EuroQoL-5 dimensions-5 levels; INR: Indian Rupee; IQR: interquartile range; JSY: Janani Suraksha Yojana; MAPP-QOL: Maternal Postpartum Quality of Life; MGI: Mother Generated Index; QALDs: quality-adjusted life days; QALYs: quality-adjusted life years; QOL: quality of life; VAS: visual analogue scale; VB: vaginal birth

Acknowledgements

The authors thank the women who took part in this pilot study. We are further grateful to the MATIND research and field staff at R.D. Gardi Medical College and the Indian Institute of Public Health in Gandhinagar for their tireless efforts during data collection and entry. Finally, we would like to acknowledge the National Rural Health Mission of the Government of Madhya Pradesh in Bhopal, the Department of Health and Family Welfare of the Government of Gujarat, and financial support by Deutsche Forschungsgemeinschaft and Ruprecht-Karls-Universität Heidelberg within the funding programme Open Access Publishing.

Funding

The study was conducted as a part of the MATIND project which is financially supported by the European Community's Seventh Framework Program under grant agreement no. 261304.

Authors' contributions

KSA, BR, LL and ADC conceptualized the study and designed the data collection tools. VD and KV facilitated the data collection. KSA and BR performed the first analysis of the data. SK performed the presented, new and extended analysis of the data. SK and ADC drafted the manuscript together. ADC and KSA helped with data interpretation and the manuscript revision. All authors read and approved the final manuscript.

Competing interests

The authors declare that they have no competing interests.

Author details

[1]Heidelberg Institute of Global Health, Heidelberg University, Heidelberg, Germany. [2]Division of Global Health, Department of Public Health Sciences, Karolinska Institutet, Stockholm, Sweden. [3]Department of Public Health and Environment, R. D. Gardi Medical College, Ujjain, India. [4]International Centre for Health Research, Ujjain Charitable Trust Hospital and Research Centre, Ujjain, India. [5]Epidemiology and Global Health, Department of Public Health and Clinical Medicine, Umeå University, Umeå, Sweden. [6]Indian Institute of Public Health, Ahmedabad, India.

References

1. Romano M, Cacciatore A, Giordano R, La Rosa B. Postpartum period: three distinct but continuous phases. J Prenat Med. 2010;4:22–5.
2. Brockington I. Postpartum psychiatric disorders. Lancet. 2004;363:303–10.
3. Firoz T, Chou D, von Dadelszen P, Agrawal P, Vanderkruik R, Tunçalp O, et al. Measuring maternal health: focus on maternal morbidity. Bull World Health Organ. 2013;91:794–6.
4. Mogos MF, August EM, Salinas-Miranda AA, Sultan DH, Salihu HM. A systematic review of quality of life measures in pregnant and postpartum mothers. Appl Res Qual Life. 2013;8:219–50.
5. Rezaei N, Tavalaee Z, Sayehmiri K, Sharifi N, Daliri S. The relationship between quality of life and methods of delivery: a systematic review and meta-analysis. Electron Physician. 2018;10:6596–607.
6. Rezaei S, Salimi Y, Zahirian Moghadam T, Mirzarahimi T, Mehrtak M, Zandian H. Quality of life after vaginal and cesarean deliveries: a systematic review and meta-analysis. Int J Hum Rights Healthc. 2018;11:165–75.
7. Symon A. The mother-generated index: a new approach to assessing maternal quality of life. In: Martin C, editor. Perinatal mental health: a clinical guide. Keswick: M&K Update Ltd.; 2012. p. 325–34.
8. Hill PD, Aldag JC, Hekel B, Riner G, Bloomfield P. Maternal postpartum quality of life questionnaire. J Nurs Meas. 2006;14:205–20.
9. Sidney K, de Costa A, Diwan V, Mavalankar DV, Smith H. An evaluation of two large scale demand side financing programs for maternal health in India: the MATIND study protocol. BMC Public Health. 2012;12:699.
10. Sidney K, Iyer V, Vora K, Mavalankar D, De Costa A. Statewide program to promote institutional delivery in Gujarat, India: who participates and the degree of financial subsidy provided by the Chiranjeevi Yojana program. J Health Popul Nutr. 2016;35:2.
11. Sidney K, Diwan V, El-Khatib Z, de Costa A. India's JSY cash transfer program for maternal health: who participates and who doesn't - a report from Ujjain district. Reprod Health 2012;9:2.
12. van Reenen M, Oppe M. EQ-5D-5L user guide: basic information on how to use the EQ-5D-5L instrument. Rotterdam: EuroQol Research Foundation; 2015.
13. Herdman M, Gudex C, Lloyd a, Janssen M, Kind P, Parkin D, et al. Development and preliminary testing of the new five-level version of EQ-5D (EQ-5D-5L). Qual Life Res. 2011;20:1727–36.
14. Janssen MF, Pickard a S, Golicki D, Gudex C, Niewada M, Scalone L, et al. Measurement properties of the EQ-5D-5L compared to the EQ-5D-3L across eight patient groups: a multi-country study. Qual Life Res. 2013;22:1717–27.
15. Szende A, Williams A. Measuring Self-Reported Population Health. An international perspective based on EQ-5D. Rotterdam: EuroQol Group; 2004.
16. van Hout B, Janssen MF, Feng Y-S, Kohlmann T, Busschbach J, Golicki D, et al. Interim scoring for the EQ-5D-5L: mapping the EQ-5D-5L to EQ-5D-3L value sets. Value Heal. 2012;15:708–15.
17. Matthews JN, Altman DG, Campbell MJ, Royston P. Analysis of serial measurements in medical research. BMJ. 1990;300:230–5.
18. Manca A, Hawkins N, Sculpher MJ. Estimating mean QALYs in trial-based cost-effectiveness analysis: the importance of controlling for baseline utility. Health Econ. 2005;14:487–96.
19. Gregory KD, Korst LM, Saeb S, Fridman M. The role of patient-reported outcomes in women's health. OBG Manag. 2018;30:18–48.
20. Laine C, Davidoff F. Patient-centered medicine. A professional evolution. JAMA. 1996;275:152–6.
21. Bodhare TN, Sethi P, Bele SD, Gayatri D, Vivekanand A. Postnatal quality of life, depressive symptoms, and social support among women in southern India. Women Health. 2015;55:353–65.
22. Nagpal J, Dhar R, Sinha S, Bhargava V, Sachdeva A, Bhartia A. An exploratory study to evaluate the utility of an adapted mother generated index (MGI) in assessment of postpartum quality of life in India. Health Qual Life Outcomes. 2008;6:107.
23. Bele S. Postnatal quality of life: a neglected research area in India. Perspect Med Res. 2014;2:1–2.
24. Vissandjée B, Abdool SN, Dupéré S. Focus groups in rural Gujarat, India: a modified approach. Qual Health Res. 2002;12:826–43.
25. Ride J, Lorgelly P, Tran T, Wynter K, Rowe H, Fisher J. Preventing postnatal maternal mental health problems using a psychoeducational intervention: the cost-effectiveness of what were we thinking. BMJ Open. 2016;6:e012086.
26. Petrou S, Kim SW, McParland P, Boyle EM. Mode of delivery and long-term health-related quality-of-life outcomes: a prospective population-based study. Birth. 2017;44:110–9.
27. Gerard Jansen AJ, Duvekot JJ, Hop WCJJ, Essink-Bot M-L, Beckers EAMM, Karsdorp VHMM, et al. New insights into fatigue and health-related quality of life after delivery. Acta Obstet Gynecol Scand. 2007;86:579–84.
28. Shorten A, Shorten B. The importance of mode of birth after previous cesarean: success, satisfaction, and postnatal health. J Midwifery Womens Health. 2012;57:126–32.
29. Upadhyay RP, Chowdhury R, Salehi A, Sarkar K, Singh SK, Sinha B, et al. Postpartum depression in India: a systematic review and meta-analysis. Bull World Health Organ. 2017;95:706–717C.
30. Gokhale AV, Vaja A. Screening for postpartum depression. Gujarat Med J. 2013;68:46–51.
31. Payakachat N, Ali MM, Tilford JM. Can the EQ-5D detect meaningful change? A systematic review. PharmacoEconomics. 2015;33:1137–54.
32. Wasan AD, Neufeld K, Jayaram G. Practice patterns and treatment choices among psychiatrists in New Delhi, India. Soc Psychiatry Psychiatr Epidemiol. 2009;44:109–19.
33. Chen T-H, Li L, Kochen MM. A systematic review: how to choose appropriate health-related quality of life (HRQOL) measures in routine general practice? J Zhejiang Univ Sci B. 2005;6:936–40.

5

Is the socioeconomic status of immigrant mothers in Brussels relevant to predict their risk of adverse pregnancy outcomes?

Mouctar Sow[1,2]* (iD), Judith Racape[3], Claudia Schoenborn[1] and Myriam De Spiegelaere[1]

Abstract

Background: Understanding and tackling perinatal health inequities in industrialized countries requires analysing the socioeconomic determinants of adverse pregnancy outcomes among immigrant populations. Studies show that among certain migrant groups, education is not associated with adverse pregnancy outcomes. We aim to extend this analysis to further dimensions of socioeconomic status (SES) and to other settings. The objective of this study is to identify sociodemographic characteristics associated with adverse pregnancy outcomes, according to the origin of mothers residing in Brussels.

Methods: We analysed all singleton live births in Brussels between 2005 and 2010 ($n = 97,844$). The data arise from the linkage between three administrative databases. Four groups of women were included according to their place of birth: Belgium, EU, North Africa, and Sub-Saharan Africa. For each group, logistic regression was carried out to estimate the odds ratios of low birthweight (LBW) and small for gestational age (SGA) according to SES indicators (household income, maternal employment status, maternal education) and single parenthood.

Results: Three key findings emerge from this study: 1) 25% of children were born into a household under the poverty threshold. This proportion was much higher for mothers born outside of the EU. 2) For North African immigrants, SES indicators didn't influence the pregnancy outcomes, whereas their risk of LBW increased with single parenthood. 3) For Sub-Saharan Africans the risk of LBW increased with low household income.

Conclusion: In a region where immigrant mothers are at high poverty risk, we observe a classic social gradient in perinatal outcomes only for mothers born in Belgium or the EU. In the other groups, SES influences perinatal outcomes less systematically. To develop interventions to reduce inequities from birth, it's important to identify the determinants of perinatal health among immigrants and to understand the underlying mechanisms in different contexts.

Keywords: Health inequalities, Perinatal health, Immigrants, Adverse birth outcomes, Poverty, Socioeconomic status

Background

The reduction of health inequities at birth is a major challenge for public health and society. Giving a better start in life to new-borns belonging to vulnerable communities helps break the vicious cycle of poverty and reduce social inequities in health [1–3]. In industrialized

* Correspondence: mamasow@ulb.ac.be;
mamadoumouctar.sow@umontreal.ca
[1]Research centre in Health Policies and Health Systems, Ecole de Santé Publique, Université Libre de Bruxelles (ULB), Route de Lennik 808, 1070 Bruxelles, Belgium
[2]Department of social and preventive medicine , Ecole de Santé Publique, Université de Montréal, Montréal, Québec H3N 1X9, Canada
Full list of author information is available at the end of the article

countries, the analysis of determinants influencing adverse pregnancy outcomes should not only consider the socioeconomic dimension, but also the parents' migration patterns. Indeed, several studies show that the parents' socioeconomic level and their migration patterns constitute two interrelated dimensions which may influence perinatal health differently depending on the contexts [4, 5]. Some authors argue for a framework of social inequities in health that takes into account the relation between socioeconomic determinants and migration [6–8]. Furthermore, in several western countries, immigrants constitute an important part of the population [9].

The relation between the socioeconomic status (SES), migration and perinatal health varies depending on health issue, socioeconomic indicator, migrant and comparative groups, and adjustment variables considered [4, 5, 10, 11]. Studies carried out on the subject can be divided into two types, mainly: a) those which focus on the influence of ethnic or geographical origin (place of birth) on perinatal health, by adjusting for socioeconomic factors [5, 10, 12–15] and b) those which identify socioeconomic factors that influence perinatal health specifically among migrants [4, 16–19]. There are many studies using the first approach, showing different results, sometimes contradictory ones. Although certain groups of migrants or ethnic groups have a higher risk of suffering adverse pregnancy outcomes, other groups show more favourable perinatal health indicators even if they are socioeconomically vulnerable. The example of mothers of Mexican origin living in the United States, also known as the Mexican paradox, is the most cited [12]. In Belgium, mothers from Maghreb are in a similar situation. They show lower rates of low birth weight and preterm births despite a low SES [13, 20, 21]. In a previous study, we analysed in detail the risk of adverse pregnancy outcomes according to the place of birth of mothers residing in Brussels [21].

Studies focusing on the influence of SES on adverse pregnancy outcomes among immigrant populations are lower in numbers. Conducted mainly in North America, they show that the relation between socioeconomic factors and perinatal health varies according to maternal origin. If SES helps predict the risk of adverse pregnancy outcomes in the overall population and among native mothers, it does not influence pregnancy outcomes among certain groups of migrants, i.e. for Latino-Americans living in the United States, particularly those of Mexican origin. In this group the risk of adverse pregnancy outcomes does not differ according to education [16–18, 22, 23]. As the authors point out, education is often the only socioeconomic indicator examined. It would be appropriate to consider other indicators. Indeed, education is not always a good proxy for the material living conditions. For recent immigrants, for example, income and employment status might be more relevant [22, 24–26]. In other words, irrespective of their educational level, immigrants are at greater risk of being unemployed and living in a low-income household. This can lead to stressful situations that can have a negative impact on the progress of the pregnancy, and on the health of mother and new-born. It would also be appropriate to extend the analysis to other contexts, with other characteristics (migration policies, social protection systems and healthcare programs).

Brussels is a very diverse city from a sociocultural standpoint. Three quarters of births occur in families with an immigrant background [27]. As far as we know,

no study specifically analyses the socioeconomic factors associated with perinatal health among migrants in Brussels. The objective of this study is to identify socioeconomic factors associated with the risk of adverse birth outcomes, according to the origin of mothers residing in Brussels. It is in continuity with previous studies in perinatal health in Belgium [13, 20, 21, 27]. Three indicators of SES (income, employment status, education) and single parenthood are considered.

Methods
Study population and data
Three administrative databases have been linked: the birth and death statistical reports for Brussels residents, the national registry and the "Banque carrefour de la sécurité sociale" (BCSS, Crossroads Bank for Social Security). In Belgium, all births and neonatal deaths must be recorded from 22 weeks of gestation as well as all live births weighing more than 500 g. The quality of the birth and death statistical reports is ensured by two perinatal epidemiology centres, in collaboration with maternity wards and civil registration services [28]. The BCSS electronically gathers the socioeconomic data originating from social security organizations in Belgium. Each organization is in charge of recording and updating their own information. The BCSS shares data on various socioeconomic aspects (income, unemployment, welfare, etc.), which can then be communicated to administrative services or researchers based on very strict authorizations [29]. The national registry is a centralized file that contains the identification data of the Belgian citizens residing in Belgium or abroad and of any other individual who legally resides in Belgium, as well as some information on the people who have requested a refugee status. Each individual is identified with a unique number [30]. This number has allowed linking the three databases. This linkage was done by the Directorate General Statistics and Economic Information and by the BCSS, after obtaining the approval of the Privacy Protection Commission. This is the first data-linking of its kind in Brussels. The analyses focused on the births to mothers residing in Brussels between 2005 and 2010.

Definitions of the exposures and outcomes
Outcomes
The analysis presented covers two pregnancy outcomes: low birth weight (LBW), and small for gestational age (SGA). A low birth weight means a weight less than 2500 g. SGA means a birth weight below the 10th percentile for gestational age. Without a reference curve based on the births in Belgium, the revised curve by Fenton et al. has been used as a reference. This curve has the advantage of being developed from a meta-analysis including studies carried out in six developed countries [31]. Preterm births

(before 37 weeks of gestation) were also analysed. LBW, preterm birth, and SGA can have a negative impact on the child's development, and on their health in childhood and adulthood [2, 32, 33]. They may be caused by different types of determinants (medical, social, etc.) [34, 35] whose influence varies according to the outcome, hence the importance of studying each of these outcomes. The results of the analyses concerning preterm births are broadly similar to those of LBW. To lighten the text, they were not presented and discussed (See additional file 1). Previous studies on perinatal health in Brussels also show similar results between these two indicators [13, 20].

Explanatory variables

Maternal place of birth: Based on maternal native country (as recommended [36]), immigrant mothers were distinguished from those of Belgian origin. This variable was grouped into 5 categories according to maternal region of birth: Belgium, European Union outside of Belgium (EU), Maghreb, Sub-Saharan Africa, and other countries. The proposed categorisation takes into account the mapping of the various parts of the world, the distribution of births in Brussels and the results of previous studies on perinatal health in Brussels [20, 21]. Maghreb is the North African region excluding Egypt. In Belgium, North African immigration comes mainly from the Maghreb. So, the interpretation of the results will refer to North Africa. The 'other countries' category is very heterogeneous, so it is not reported in the results.

Household income covers earned income and replacement incomes collected yearly. Real estate and movable incomes are not considered. It is the annual taxable gross income (after deduction of social security contributions). To be able to compare households, the household income is established by factoring in the size of the household (household equivalent income) according to the OECD-modified scale [37]. In the database, we have the equivalent income for households, by deciles. These deciles are based on the distribution of income for all the Belgian households. They have been categorized by quintile. We can therefore know in which quintile (or decile) a household living in brussels is, compared to all the Belgian households, but not the exact amount of the income. To identify the households with an equivalent income below the risk-of-poverty threshold, we have compared the equivalent risk-of-poverty threshold (60% of the median income) to the threshold of the income quintiles. The threshold of the poorest quintile (Q5) is close to the risk-of-poverty threshold. This is why we approximate that households with incomes in the lowest quintile are "at risk of poverty". Based on income quintiles, three categories of

households were identified: households at risk of poverty (Q5), median income households (Q4 and Q3), and high-income households (Q1 and Q2).

The mother's employment status is based on the nomenclature of the socioeconomic position of the DWH (Datawarehouse) [38]. It relates to the situation during the last trimester before birth. This situation broadly represents the mothers' activity during pregnancy [27]. The variable distinguishes: a) mothers who had a job during this trimester, b) those who received social assistance of last resort (any financial aid from a public social welfare centre), c) other situations of off-duty status (unemployment, transition after studies, career interruption, work incapacity...); (d) an 'other' category, which includes people who do not contribute to a social security scheme in Belgium (e.g. officials and international diplomats, housewives). This category is rather large in Brussels. The last two categories are very heterogeneous. The comparison and interpretation of the results will mainly focus on the first two categories: mothers who have held a job versus those who benefited from social welfare. Social welfare recipients are a particularly vulnerable group who experiences increased poverty and an important risk of social precariousness. The negative impact of these conditions on health can be important [39, 40].

Maternal education was categorised into four groups, as in previous studies [21]: superior (university or higher education), upper secondary (completed secondary school), lower secondary or less (up to the third completed year of secondary), completed primary or less, and other. This last category mainly concerns mothers for whom educational level is unknown.

Household situation is based on the LIPRO (Lifestyles Projections) position [41, 42]. The new-born's LIPRO position makes it possible to distinguish children whose parents live in a couple (married or not) to those born in a single-parent household.

Statistical analysis

Logistic regression was used to estimate odds ratios (ORs) of the association between the perinatal indicators (LBW and SGA) and the mother's demographic characteristics (household income, education, employment status, household situation). Initially, unadjusted models have been developed to estimate the crude association between adverse pregnancy outcomes and each of the mother's characteristics. These analyses were first performed for all births, then for each group, depending on maternal origin. Later, adjusted multivariate models have been developed. For LBW, we considered parity, maternal age, infant sex and birth cohort (year of birth) as adjustment variables. For SGA, the same variables were considered, with the exception of infant sex, since the reference curve to estimate

SGA factors it in. Crude and adjusted ORs derived from the logistic regression and the *p*-value of the Wald test (with a significance level set at 5%) are presented (Tables 2 & 3). The Hosmer et Lemeshow test was used to check the suitability of the models. Analyses were processed through Stata, version13.

Results
Maternal characteristics
Table 1 shows the distribution of maternal sociodemographic characteristics according to their place of birth. The analysis looked at 97844 Brussels single live births over the period of 2005–2010. 40% of the mothers were born in Belgium, 14% in another country of the European Union, 19% in North Africa and 7% in sub-Saharan Africa. The LBW and SGA rates vary according to maternal origin. Mothers from the European Union and North Africa have the lowest prevalence while those from sub-Saharan Africa show a higher prevalence of LBW and SGA. A large proportion of the births occurs in precarious households. This situation is even more pronounced for new-borns whose mothers are of non-European origin (North Africa and sub-Saharan Africa). These are significantly more disadvantaged. Proportionally, more of them live in a household at risk of poverty, their mothers do not work and have a low level of education. Approximately six out of ten births occur in a household living under the risk of poverty threshold, which means more than two times more than for the mothers born in Belgium. Conversely, very few mothers from North Africa or sub-Saharan Africa (respectively 4 and 8%) live in a high-income household, compared to 39% of the Belgian natives. The situation of non-European immigrants in the job market is also rather striking. While 60% of mothers born in Belgium are employed only 17 and 23% of those from North Africa or sub-Saharan Africa, respectively, have a job. Among mothers from sub-Saharan Africa, three in ten received social welfare assistance during pregnancy, this proportion largely exceeds that observed for the other three groups.

Regarding educational level, the proportion of less educated women is almost twice as high among non-European immigrants (about 40%) compared to the mothers born in Belgium. There is a significant proportion of lone-parenthood among the mothers from sub-Saharan Africa (36%). This proportion does not exceed 15% for the other groups.

Relation between the mothers' characteristics and the adverse pregnancy outcomes
The analysis of the risk factors associated with adverse pregnancy outcomes shows differences according to the mother's region of birth (Tables 2 & 3). Three different profiles stand out: Belgium or another EU country, Maghreb and Sub-Saharan Africa.

Belgium or another European Union country
These two groups have similar profiles. Several factors influence the risk of LBW and SGA. Among women born in Belgium, being a recipient of social assistance, being less educated, or a single parent are risk factors of LBW, in the fully adjusted model. Income, education, and lone-parenthood are significantly associated with SGA (Table 3). Among women from EU, a low level of education and single-parenthood are risk factors for LBW, after adjustment for all variables. The same factors and being recipient of social assistance have an effect on the risk of SGA (Table 3).

North Africa
None of the socioeconomic indicators (income, education, employment status) are associated with LBW or SGA, before and after adjustment for all variables (Tables 2 & 3). The prevalence of LBW according to household income shows a reverse gradient. In fact, the rate of LBW increases as the household income level increases. However, these differences are not significant (Table 2). Among mothers from North Africa, lone-parenthood is a risk factor for LBW (Tables 2 & 3).

Sub-Saharan Africa
Household income influences the risk of LBW for this group. This risk decreases considerably among the richest households (Tables 2 & 3). The other SES indicators and single-parenthood are not associated with LBW. The prevalence of LBW increases as education level increases. However, these differences are not significant. After adjustment for all variables, maternal educational level is the only factor associated with SGA (Table 3).

Discussion
Findings
Three key findings emerge from this study: 1) 25% of children were born into a household under the poverty threshold. This proportion was much higher among immigrants from non-European countries. 2) For North African immigrants, SES (education, occupation, and income) didn't influence the pregnancy outcomes, whereas their risk of LBW increased with single parenthood. 3) For Sub-Saharan Africans, the risk of LBW increased with low household income.

One of the substantial contributions of this article relates to the fact that household income and maternal employment status help assess new-born's precariousness and analyse its links with pregnancy outcomes. This is seldom possible because comprehensive data on household income are often difficult to obtain [25, 43].

Table 1 Characteristics of mothers and new-borns according to maternal birth place

N	All births	Belgium	EU27	North Africa	SS Africa
	97,844*	39,591	14,195	18,797	6812
% of births	100	40.5	14.5	19.2	7.0
Household income (n)	88,655	38,638	11,132	18,286	5756
high (%)	24.85	38.75	31.77	4.06	8.01
median (%)	33.75	34.88	31.69	36.05	29.90
low (at risk of poverty) (%)	41.40	26.36	36.53	59.89	62.09
Employed (n)	97,844	39,591	14,195	18,797	6812
Yes (%)	40.91	60.49	42.86	17.75	22.97
No - social recipient (%)	6.98	3.24	3.13	6.33	30.49
No - other (%)	19.60	29.18	7.93	17.10	11.44
Other (%)	32.51	7.09	46.08	58.82	35.10
Maternal education (n)	97,142	39,369	14,109	18,582	6749
Superior (%)	29.29	38.28	41.89	10.09	17.44
secondary superior (%)	32.53	33.10	30.41	32.77	33.47
< = secondary inferior (%)	30.69	22.81	22.55	45.90	40.41
Other	7.49	5.80	5.16	11.24	8.68
Living alone (n)	92,975	38,909	13,417	18,414	6154
No - married (%)	61.45	52.53	65.92	84.46	41.45
No - not married (%)	17.16	26.56	20.50	1.94	12.58
Yes (%)	15.78	15.70	10.66	9.70	37.16
Unknown	5.61	5.21	2.92	3.90	8.81
Parity (n)	97,234	39,381	14,144	18,645	6771
0 (%)	47.70	52.09	53.74	36.66	44.75
1–2 (%)	43.70	41.73	42.32	47.19	44.22
3 (%)	8.60	6.18	3.94	16.14	11.03
Maternal age (n)	97,844	39,591	14,195	18,797	6812
< 20 (%)	2.39	2.39	1.74	2.01	3.27
20–40 (%)	93.29	94.68	92.74	91.24	93.09
> = 40 (%)	4.31	2.92	5.52	6.75	3.64
Infant sex (n)	97,844	39,591	14,195	18,797	6812
Female	48.73	48.89	48.85	48.18	48.61
LBW (n)	96,813	39,155	14,060	18,616	6742
(%)	4.64	5.08	3.98	3.29	5.75
Preterm (n)	95,490	38,670	13,830	18,428	6657
(%)	5.22	5.48	4.95	4.09	5.65
SGA (n)	94,650	38,306	13,725	18,280	6601
%	10.56	11.40	9.97	8.62	12.33

*: "other birth country" ($n = 15,529$) and missing ($n = 2920$) included

Interpretations

A concentration of risk factors among mothers of Belgian origin

The influence of SES on pregnancy outcomes is clearly stronger among mothers born in Belgium. This result is consistent with previous studies which show that among new-borns in disadvantaged groups, those whose mothers are of Belgian origin are the most vulnerable. They present a greater risk of LBW than children of immigrant mothers of comparable SES [21, 27]. The specific profile of Belgian disadvantaged mothers may help explain these results. An important part of them live in a situation of intense poverty and may have been in this situation for a long time, through the intergenerational transmission of

Table 2 Unadjusted ORs (95% CI) of the association between maternal characteristics and pregnancy outcomes

	All Births		Belgium		EU27		North Africa		Sub-Saharan Africa	
	%	OR (95% CI)	%	OR (95% CI)	%	OR (95% CI)	%	OR (95% CI)	%	OR (95% CI)
					LBW					
Household income										
high	4.13	1	4.31	1	3.71	1	3.67	1	2.84	1
median	4.64	1,12 (1,03-1,23)[b]	5.06	1,18 (1,05-1,32)[b]	3.80	1,02 (0,80-1,31)	3.38	0,91 (0,61-1,38)	5.91	2,15 (1,19-3,86)[a]
low (at risk of poverty)	4.66	1,13 (1,04-1,23)[b]	5,59	1,31 (1,17-1,47)[c]	4.51	1,22 (0,97-1,54)	3.02	0,81 (0,54-1,21)	5.99	2,18 (1,23-3,84)[b]
Employed										
Yes	4.61	1	4.73	1	3.88	1	3.79	1	5.66	1
No - social recipient	6.65	1,47 (1,32-1,63)[c]	9.54	2,12 (1,74-2,58)[c]	7.82	2,09 (1,44-3,05)[c]	3.91	1,03 (0,73-1,45)	6.05	1,07 (0,81-1,42)
No - other	5.16	1,12 (1,03-1,21)[b]	5.41	1,04 (1,04-1,27)[b]	5.31	1,38 (1,03-1,85)[a]	3.29	0,86 (0,66-1,45)	7.13	1,28 (0,90-1,81)
Other	3.92	0,84 (0,78-0,90)[c]	4.73	0,99 (0,82-1,20)	3.58	0,91 (0,76-1,10)	3.07	0,80 (0,65-0,99)	5.11	0,89 (0,67-1,18)
Maternal education										
Superior	4.08	1	4.10	1	3.35	1	3.38	1	6.01	1
secondary superior	4.81	1,19 (1,09-1,29)[c]	5.23	1,28 (1,15-1,44)[c]	4.21	1,26 (1,03-1,55)[a]	3.53	1,04 (0,78-1,39)	5.66	0,93 (0,69-1,26)
< = secondary inferior	4.80	1,18 (1,09-1,28)[c]	6.27	1,56 (1,39-1,75)[c]	4.49	1,34 (1,08-1,68)[b]	2.99	0,88 (0,66-1,16)	5.39	0,88 (0,66-1,19)
other	5.34	1,32 (1,17-1,49)[c]	5.76	1,42 (1,17-1,73)[c]	5.03	1,52 (1,06-2,19)[a]	3.89	1,16 (0,82-1,62)	6.91	1,15 (0,77-1,73)
Living alone (n)										
No - married	3.75	1	3.97	1	3.30	1	3.02	1	4.85	1
No - not married	5.33	1,44 (1,32-1,56)[c]	5.70	1,46 (1,31-1,63)[c]	4.45	1,36 (1,10-1,69)[b]	2.55	0,84 (0,43-1,63)	4.82	0,99 (0,68-1,44)
Yes	6.19	1,69 (1,56-1,83)[c]	6.43	1,66 (1,46-1,88)[c]	6.26	1,95 (1,53-2,50)[c]	4.81	1,62 (1,28-2,05)[c]	6.68	1,40 (1,09-1,74)[b]
Unknown	5.50	1,49 (1,31-1,69)[c]	5.96	1,53 (1,25-1,87)[c]	5.44	1,68 (1,07-2,65)[a]	3.23	0,85 (0,53–135)	6.00	1,25 (0,83-1,87)
					SGA					
Household income (n)										
high (%)	9.88	1	10.24	1	9.60	1	8.39	1	9.21	1
median (%)	10.68	1,09 (1,03-1,15)[b]	11.76	1,16 (1,08-1,26)[c]	10.06	1,05 (0,89-1,23)	8.73	1,04 (0,79-1,37)	11.92	1,33 (0,93-1,89)
low (at risk of poverty) (%)	10.71	1,09 (1,03-1,15)[b]	12.46	1,24 (1,15-1,35)[c]	10.69	1,12 (0,96-1,31)	8.38	0,99 (0,76-1,30)	12.65	1,42 (1,01-1,99)[a]
Employed (n)										
Yes (%)	10.27	1	10.89	1	9.83	1	8.15	1	9.64	1
No - social recipient (%)	12.48	1,24 (1,14-1,34)[c]	16.28	1,59 (1,36-1,86)[c]	16.90	1,86 (1,42-2,43)[c]	8.53	1,05 (0,82-1,33)	12.82	1,37 (1,11-1,70)[b]
No other (%)	11.21	1,10 (1,04-1,16)[c]	12.15	1,13 (1,05-1,21)[c]	12.67	1,33 (1,09-1,62)[b]	7.97	0,97 (0,81-1,16)	13.01	1,40 (1,06-1,84)
Other (%)	10.13	0,98 (0,93-1,03)	10.50	0,96 (0,84-1093)	9.16	0,92 (0,82-1,04)	8.95	1,10 (0,96-1,28)	13.45	1,45 (1,18-1,79)
Maternal education (n)										
Superior (%)	9.99	1	10.45	1	9,41	1	9.35	1	10.90	1
secondary superior (%)	10.77	1,08 (1,03-1,14)[b]	11.73	1,13 (1,05-1,22)[c]	10.02	1,07 (0,93-1,22)	8.82	0,93 (0,78-1,12)	11.22	1,02 (0,81-1,28)
< = secondary inferior (%)	10.84	1,09 (1,03-1,15)[c]	12.51	1,22 (1,12-1,33)[c]	10.70	1,15 (0,99-1,33)	8.22	0,86 (0,72-1,03)	13.41	1,25 (1,01-1,55)[a]
other	10.84	1,09 (1,01-1,19)[a]	11.18	1,08 (0,93-1,24)	11.27	1,22 (0,95-1,57)	9.21	0,98 (0,79-1,22)	14.29	1,35 (1,01-1,82)[a]
Living alone (n)										
No - married (%)	9.43	1	9.80	1	8.85	1	8.35	1	12.10	1
No - not married (%)	11.66	1,26 (1,19-1,34)[c]	12.16	1,27 (1,18-1,37)[c]	11.70	1,36 (1,18-1,57)[c]	8.31	0,99 (0,67-1,46)	9.38	0,75 (0,57-0,98)
Yes (%)	12.54	1,37 (1,29-1,45)[c]	14.19	1,52 (1,39-1,66)[c]	13.20	1,56 (1,31-1,86)[c]	9.56	1,15 (0,97-1,37)	13.12	1,09 (0,92-1,30)
Unknown	12.70	1,39 (1,28-1,52)[c]	14.46	1,55 (1,36-1,78)[c]	11.67	1,36 (0,98-1,88)	8.54	1,25 (0,97-1,60)	11.63	0,95 (0,71-1,28)

[a] ≤ 0.05
[b] ≤ 0.01
[c] ≤ 0.001

poverty [2, 44]. This situation experienced in the very long run, and in the context of social exclusion (school failure, family breakdown, etc.), can have a stronger impact on the health of mothers and new-borns. Moreover, for mothers born in Belgium, having only a primary or lower secondary diploma can be indicative of significant psycho-social vulnerability, involving a particularly difficult or complex schooling experience in the context of compulsory education up to 18 years. This is not the case for immigrant mothers, who come from countries where the enrolment rate remains low for women.

Breakdown of the link between SES and pregnancy outcomes among immigrant mothers, particularly those from North Africa

For North African mothers, SES does not influence LBW and SGA. We also observe that LBW rates increase as household income increases. However, the difference is not significant. This finding is similar to that of mothers from Mexican origin living in the United States. Less educated women show comparable prevalence of LBW, sometimes lower, than those more educated [18, 22]. Various assumptions can explain the lack of association and the absence (or weakness) of a social gradient in the link between SES and perinatal health among migrants.

More favourable pregnancy outcomes among low SES immigrants Mothers with a low SES who are from Mexican origin show better or similar indicators of perinatal health than white American natives with the same level of education. A similar situation is observed for immigrants in other countries [19, 21]. In Brussels, low SES immigrant mothers have a significantly lower risk of LBW compared to low SES mothers of Belgian origin [21]. Among Mexican women, one of the assumptions made to explain this fact is the selection effect [22, 45]. Regarding mothers born in North Africa, protective factors around pregnancy might be more present among disadvantaged mothers which would explain the lack of association between SES and adverse pregnancy outcomes. For example, cultural factors such as significant family and community support surrounding the pregnancy, as well a less risky lifestyle (lower smoking and alcoholism rates) can play a role [46, 47]. Furthermore, nearly 60% of mothers from North Africa do not contribute to the Belgian social security system ('other' category of the employment status), which is largely constituted by housewives. This category presents a lower risk of adverse pregnancy outcomes. The fact of not being confronted with difficult working conditions (which is often the case of low-skilled groups) could explain these results.

SES indicators do not reflect immigrants' living conditions? The breakdown of the link between SES and pregnancy outcomes among migrants could be explained by the breakdown of the link between SES and living conditions (quality of housing, working conditions, etc.). Indeed, the influence of the socioeconomic position on health is partly explained by its impact on the quality of life (physical and psychological). As socioeconomic position increases, quality of life increases, accompanied by a decline of risk factors of disease and an increase of protective factors. Among migrants, one may wonder if the indicators typically used to define SES are good proxies of their living conditions. Indeed, educational level may badly reflect unemployment situations or working conditions. Also working status and income level are not always a good proxy of working conditions. Migrants are much more likely to be unemployed, to hold (and accumulate) precarious jobs, regardless of their educational level. In Belgium, non-European workers are concentrated in the lower segments of the labour market, with a risk of higher unemployment, poorer working conditions and a greater job instability [48, 49].

Discrimination: A major determinant of health inequities More recently, some authors emphasize discrimination as a major factor explaining health inequities linked to migration. Discrimination and its consequences (stigma, unemployment, lack of access to employment and to services, impact on living conditions, etc.) experienced over the long-term by migrants, regardless of their socioeconomic level could erode the mechanisms that link socioeconomic status and health [50–53].

"Imported" social gradient in health The social gradient in health in the migrants' country of origin may be different, and sometimes even reverse. The explanatory mechanism might be a reverse gradient for health-related lifestyle factors. For example, the most disadvantaged show a lower prevalence of smoking than those with high SES [18, 23, 54]. The mechanisms underlying this observation might continue to be active in the host country.

Outcome specific process

The relation between SES indicators and perinatal health varies according to the health issue. The pregnancy outcomes appear to be "sensitive" in a different way to the determinants studied. For example, among mothers from sub-Saharan Africa, education is not associated to LBW, whereas it is a predictor of SGA. While the differential influence of SES indicators according to pregnancy outcome is well documented [4, 55–59], the explanatory mechanisms are unclear. A possible explanation concerns the combination of two factors [55]. On one hand, a SES indicator may better reflect a particular intermediate factor

Table 3 Adjusted ORs (95% CI) of the association between maternal characteristics and pregnancy outcomes

	All births OR (95% CI)	Belgium OR (95% CI)	EU27 OR (95% CI)	North Africa OR (95% CI)	SS Africa OR (95% CI)
			LBW		
Household income					
high	1	1	1	1	1
median	1,15 (1,05-1,27)[b]	1,10 (0,97-1,25)	0,97 (0,74-1,27)	1,00 (0,65-1,53)	2,28 (1,25-4,17)[b]
low (at risk of poverty)	1,11 (0,99-1,24)	1,07 (0,91-1,26)	1,05 (0,79-1,39)	0,90 (0,58–140)	2,28 (1,22-4,22)[b]
Employed					
Yes	1	1	1	1	1
No - social recipient	1,17 (1,02-1,34)[a]	1,49 (1,17-1,91)[c]	1,37 (0,87-2,16)	0,91 (0,62-1,35)	1,03 (0,72-1,49)
No - other	1,02 (0,93-1,12)	1,03 (0,90-1,16)	1,09 (0,78-1,51)	0,91 (0,68-1,21)	1,17 (0,80-1,72)
Other	0,85 (0,72-0,93)	1,02 (0,82-1,25)	0,94 (0,74-1,19)	0,92 (0,721,17)	0,82 (0,58-1,15)
Maternal education					
Superior	1	1	1	1	1
secondary superior	1,17 (1,07-1,28)[c]	1,27 (1,12-1,44)[c]	1,20 (0,93-1,55)	1,09 (0,80-1,48)	0,77 (0,55-1,08)
< = secondary inferior	1,27 (1,15-1,40)[c]	1,61 (1,39-1,86)[c]	1,35(1,01-1,79)[a]	0,99 (0,73-1,34)	0,86 (0,61-1,20)
other	1,28 (1,12-1,47)[c]	1,34 (1,08-1,65)[b]	1,32 (0,86-2,04)	1,21 (0,84-1,74)	1,03 (0,66-1,62)
Living alone (n)					
No - married	1	1	1	1	1
No - not married	1,36 (1,24-1,48)[c]	1,37 (1,19-1,58)[c]	1,25 (0,98-1,59)[c]	0,69 (0,35-1,37)	1,00 (0,68-1,47)
Yes	1,44 (1,31-1,58)[c]	1,43 (1,27-1,60)[a]	1,91(1,42-2,57)	1,43 (1,08-1,90)[a]	1,19 (0,89-1,60)
Unknown	1,29 (1,12-1,49)[c]	1,21 (0,98-1,49)	1,03 (0,59-1,82)	0,85 (0,53–135)	1,40 (0,84-2,32)
			SGA		
Household income					
high	1	1	1	1	1
median	1,13 (1,06-1,20)[c]	1,18 (1,08-1,28)[c]	1,03 (0,87-1,23)	1,09 (0,82-1,47)	1,22 (0,84-1,76)
low (at risk of poverty)	1,13 (1,05-1,22)[c]	1,16 (1,03-1,29)[b]	1,05 (0,87-1,27)	1,10 (0,81-1,48)	1,20 (0,82-1,75)
Employed					
Yes	1	1	1	1	1
No - social recipient	1,03 (0,93-1,14)	1,18 (0,98-1,42)	1,56 (1,14-2,13)[b]	0,96 (0,73-1,25)	1,22 (0,92-1,61)
No - other	1,06 (0,99-1,13)	1,04 (0,95-1,13)	1,19 (0,96-1,48)	1,06 (0,87-1,29)	1,41 (1,05-1,88)[a]
Other	0,99 (0,92-1,05)	1,01 (0,86-1,16)	0,87 (0,74-1,02)	1,23 (1,05-1,46)[a]	1,35 (1,06-1,72)[a]
Maternal education					
Superior	1	1	1	1	1
secondary superior	1,07 (1,01-1,14)[a]	1,10 (1,01-1,20)[a]	1,14 (0,96-1,35)	0,90 (0,75-1,10)	0,92 (0,71 1,10)
< secondary inferior	1,23 (1,15-1,32)[c]	1,32(1,19-1,45)[c]	1,36 (1,13-1,64)[c]	0,94 (0,78-1,13)	1,31 (1,02-1,67)[a]
other	1,05 (0,95-1,16)	0,99 (0,85-1,15)	1,23 (0,92-1,64)	0,96 (0,76-1,22)	1,12 (0,78-1,59)
Living alone (n)					
No - married	1	1	1	1	1
No - not married	1,23 (1,16-1,32)[c]	1,30 (1,18-1,44)[c]	1,30 (1,04-1,61)[a]	1,12 (0,92-1,37)	1,00 (0,81-1,23)
Yes	1,18 (1,11-1,26)[c]	1,19 (1,10-1,29)[c]	1,23 (1,05-1,43)[b]	0,93 (0,62-1,37)	0,74 (0,57-0,97)
Unknown	1,17 (1,06-1,29)[c]	1,24 (1,07-1,43)[c]	0,99 (0,69-1,43)	0,96 (0,74-1,27)	0,83 (0,55-1,26)

LBW: OR's adjusted for parity, mother age, infant sex and birth cohort
SGA: OR's adjusted for parity, mother age, and birth cohort
[a] ≤ 0.05
[b] ≤ 0.01
[c] ≤ 0.001

influencing the occurrence of adverse pregnancy outcomes. For example, maternal education can better represent her lifestyle habits during pregnancy (such as smoking) than household income does. Maternal occupation would be a better proxy for stressful situations linked to precarious working conditions during pregnancy. This relationship between an SES indicator and an intermediate factor may vary across population groups (depending on race, ethnicity or origin). On the other hand, a given factor may have a greater impact on a particular pregnancy outcome. For example, stress during pregnancy would have a greater influence on LBW and preterm birth than on intrauterine growth restriction [60, 61]. The same reasoning can be applied to other determinants of adverse pregnancy outcomes [62, 63]. In addition, the causes of the same pregnancy outcome may differ according to the population group [64].

It should be noted that in our study population, there is an important link between preterm birth and LBW. Nearly 60% of LBW infants are also preterm. By comparison, only 5% SGA infants are preterm. This could explain some differences between LBW and SGA. Future studies should help to better understand the mechanisms underlying the observed differences.

Non-European immigrant women: Similarities, but also differences

Although North African and sub-Saharan African mothers present similar SES profiles, there are significant differences in the impact of SES on pregnancy outcomes between these 2 groups: for sub-Saharan Africans, household income influences LBW and education is associated with SGA. This is consistent with studies that show that the excess of worse perinatal health risk found for this group in Brussels is explained mainly by its socio-economic disadvantage [21, 27]. Among women of North African origin, lone-parenthood is the only risk factor found. It is associated with LBW. Lone-parenthood is also associated with adverse pregnancy outcomes for Belgians and European women. Living alone may be associated with life situations (e.g. living with relatively lower income than a couple, isolation) and with an increased risk of stress, which can have a negative impact on the course of pregnancy and on the new-born's health. In the communities of Northern Africa, this situation may be exacerbated by the influence of cultural factors. Maternity out of wedlock can be a source of stigma within the community [65].

Limits

One of the limitations of the study relates to the available data which does not allow further exploration of certain assumptions. For instance, we had no data on the mother's health behaviours during pregnancy (smoking, alcohol) or on maternal obesity. Also, regarding immigrant populations,

length of residence has not been considered. Another limitation concerns the indicators used. Indeed, if administrative data show certain benefits compared to survey data, they also have some limitations. They are collected for other purposes, which implies some constraints. For example, the definition of household (used for LIPRO position) is based on the residence. The persons registered at the same address are considered to belong to the same household. This can lead to reporting biases concerning single parenthood situations. In fact, two parents could live as a couple while being registered under different addresses. Furthermore, the level of certain social benefits is linked to the lone-parenthood status. This could lead to an overstatement of single-parenthood. Also, some people remain unknown to social security institutions, the estimated number of these people in Brussels is high. This group is diverse and covers different realities depending on maternal origin. For mothers born in Belgium and the EU, it covers mainly European officials, whereas for the mothers from the Maghreb or sub-Saharan Africa, it covers mainly housewives or persons awaiting a residence permit. These groups could not be analysed separately. Another limitation concerns the classification of maternal region of birth. The proposed groups can hide some disparities. For example, sub-Saharan Africa includes countries with very disparate realities and covers various migratory patterns (migration to study, refugees, economic migration, etc.). Along the same line, regarding pregnancy outcomes, the curve used to describe SGA does not consider maternal origin. This could cause a classification bias of SGA in immigrant populations [66]. Moreover, we cannot exclude that the measure of gestational age contains more errors in the immigrant populations because of the risk of late initiation of prenatal care [67].

Conclusion

The association between socioeconomic factors and adverse pregnancy outcomes varies according to maternal origin. In a region where immigrants are at high poverty risk, we observe a classic social gradient in perinatal outcomes only for mothers born in Belgium or in another EU country. Among non-European immigrants, SES influences perinatal outcomes less systematically. The relationship between socioeconomic indicators, migration and pregnancy outcomes is complex. It is important to consider the specificity of different groups of migrants in order to better analyse the determinants of inequities in perinatal health. Quantitative and qualitative studies would be useful to better identify the risk factors for adverse pregnancy outcomes among migrants and help understand the mechanisms leading to the observed results. Such studies would help implementing interventions that address the causes of the causes of perinatal health inequities.

Abbreviations

BCSS: Banque carrefour de la Sécurité sociale ("Crossroads Bank for Social Security"); LBW: Low Birth Weight; SES: Socioeconomic status; SGA: Small for gestational age

Acknowledgements

We would like to thank Statistics Belgium (DGSIE) for providing the data.
Thanks to Dr. Tanis Fenton for providing the calculator for SGA.
This article is published with the support of the "Fondation Universitaire de Belgique".

Funding

This study is funded by the National Fund for Scientific Research (Fonds National de la Recherche Scientifique - FNRS).

Authors' contributions

MS performed the design of the study, the statistical analysis and wrote the draft of the manuscript. JR, CS and MDS have been involved in revising the manuscript and have made substantial contributions to the interpretation of data. All authors read and approved the final version of the article.

Competing interests

The authors declare that they have no competing interests.

Author details

[1]Research centre in Health Policies and Health Systems, Ecole de Santé Publique, Université Libre de Bruxelles (ULB), Route de Lennik 808, 1070 Bruxelles, Belgium. [2]Department of social and preventive medicine , Ecole de Santé Publique, Université de Montréal, Montréal, Québec H3N 1X9, Canada. [3]Research centre in Epidemiology, Biostatistics and Clinical research, Ecole de Santé Publique, Université Libre de Bruxelles(ULB), CP598. Route de Lennik 808, 1070 Bruxelles, Belgium.

References

1. Saunders M, Barr B, McHale P, Hamelmann C. Key policies for addressing the social determinants of health and health inequities. Copenhagen: WHO Regional Office for Europe (WHO Health Evidence Network Synthesis Reports); 2017. http://www.ncbi.nlm.nih.gov/books/NBK453566/. Accessed 12 Nov 2017.
2. Aizer A, Currie J. The intergenerational transmission of inequality: maternal disadvantage and health at birth. Science. 2014;344(6186):856–61.
3. Marmot M, Bell R, Donkin A (2013). Tackling structural and social issues to reduce inequities in children's outcomes in low and middle countries, Innocenti discussion papers. https://www.unicef-irc.org/publications/708. Accessed 10 Oct 2017.
4. Blumenshine P, Egerter S, Barclay CJ, Cubbin C, Braveman PA. Socioeconomic disparities in adverse birth outcomes. Am J Prev Med. 2010;39(3):263–72.
5. Urquia ML, Glazier RH, Blondel B, Zeitlin J, Gissler M, Macfarlane A, et al. International migration and adverse birth outcomes: role of ethnicity, region of origin and destination. J Epidemiol Community Health. 2009;64(3):243–51.
6. Acevedo-Garcia D, Sanchez-Vaznaugh EV, Viruell-Fuentes EA, Almeida J. Integrating social epidemiology into immigrant health research: a cross-national framework. Soc Sci Med. 2012;75(12):2060–8.
7. Acevedo-Garcia D, Almeida J. Special issue introduction: place, migration and health. Part Spec Issue Place Migr Health. 2012;75(12):2055–9.
8. Bauer GR. Incorporating intersectionality theory into population health research methodology: challenges and the potential to advance health equity. Soc Sci Med. 2014;110:10–7.
9. OECD. Foreign-born population. 2014. http://www.oecd-ilibrary.org/social-issues-migration-health/foreign-born-population/indicator/english_5a368e1b-en. Accessed 02 Oct 2017.
10. Gagnon AJ, Zimbeck M, Zeitlin J. Migration to western industrialised countries and perinatal health: a systematic review. Part Spec Issue Women Mothers HIV Care Resour Poor Settings. 2009;69(6):934–46.
11. Kim D, Saada A. The social determinants of infant mortality and birth outcomes in Western developed nations: a cross-country systematic review. Int J Environ Res Public Health. 2013;10(6):2296–335.
12. Page RL. Positive pregnancy outcomes in Mexican immigrants: what can we learn? J Obstet Gynecol Neonatal Nurs. 2004;33(6):783–90.
13. Racape J, De Spiegelaere M, Alexander S, Dramaix M, Buekens P, Haelterman E. High perinatal mortality rate among immigrants in Brussels. Eur J Pub Health. 2010;20(5):536–42.
14. Moore S, Daniel M, Auger N. Socioeconomic disparities in low birth weight outcomes according to maternal birthplace in Québec. Canada Ethn Health. 2009;14(1):61–74.
15. Acevedo-Garcia D, Soobader M-J, Berkman LF. The differential effect of foreign-born status on low birth weight by race/ethnicity and education. Pediatrics. 2005;115(1):e20–30.
16. Gould JB, Madan A, Qin C, Chavez G. Perinatal outcomes in two dissimilar immigrant populations in the United States: a dual epidemiologic paradox. Pediatrics. 2003;111(6 Pt 1):e676–82.
17. Madan A, Palaniappan L, Urizar G, Wang Y, Fortmann SP, Gould JB. Sociocultural factors that affect pregnancy outcomes in two dissimilar immigrant groups in the United States. J Pediatr. 2006;148(3):341–6.
18. Kimbro RT, Bzostek S, Goldman N, Rodriguez G. Race, ethnicity, nd the education gradient in health. Health Aff. 2008;27(2):361–72.
19. Auger N, Luo Z-C, Platt RW, Daniel M. Do mother's education and foreign-born status interact to influence birth outcomes? Clarifying the epidemiological paradox and the healthy migrant effect. J Epidemiol Community Health. 2008;62(5):402–9.
20. Racape J, De Spiegelaere M, Dramaix M, Haelterman E, Alexander S. Effect of adopting host-country nationality on perinatal mortality rates and causes among immigrants in Brussels. Eur J Obstet Gynecol Reprod Biol. 2013; 168(2):145–50.
21. Racape J, Schoenborn C, Sow M, Alexander S, De Spiegelaere M. Are all immigrant mothers really at risk of low birth weight and perinatal mortality? The crucial role of socio-economic status. BMC Pregnancy Childbirth. 2016;16:75.
22. Goldman N, Kimbro RT, Turra CM, Pebley AR. Socioeconomic gradients in health for white and Mexican-origin populations. Am J Public Health. 2006; 96(12):2186–93.
23. Acevedo-Garcia D, Soobader M-J, Berkman LF. Low birthweight among US Hispanic/Latino subgroups: the effect of maternal foreign-born status and education. Soc Sci Med. 2007;65(12):2503–16.
24. Galobardes B. Indicators of socioeconomic position (part 1). J Epidemiol Community Health. 2006;60(1):7–12.
25. Krieger N, Williams DR, Moss NE. Measuring social class in US public health research: concepts, methodologies, and guidelines. Annu Rev Public Health. 1997;18:341–78.
26. Ribet C, Melchior M, Lang T, Zins M, Goldberg M, Leclerc A. Characterisation and measurement of social position in epidemiologic studies. Rev Dépidémiologie Santé Publique. 2007;55(4):285–95.
27. Sow M, Feyaerts G, De Spiegelaere M. Profil des nouveau-nés bruxellois et impact sur la santé périnatale. In: Lahaye W, Pannecoucke I, Vranken J, Van Rossem R, editors. Pauvreté en Belgique: Annuaire 2017. Bruxelles; 2017. p. 147–67.

28. Minsart A-F, Buekens P, De Spiegelaere M, Van de Putte S, Van Leeuw V, Englert Y. Missing information in birth certificates in Brussels after reinforcement of data collection, and variation according to immigration status. A population-based study. Arch Public Health. 2012;70(1):25.

29. BCSS. https://www.ksz-bcss.fgov.be/fr. Accessed 12 Nov 2017.

30. Description du fichier du Registre national des personnes physiques. http://www.ibz.rrn.fgov.be/fileadmin/user_upload/fr/rn/fichier-rn/fichier-RN.pdf. Accessed 10 Oct 2017.

31. Fenton TR, Kim JH. A systematic review and meta-analysis to revise the Fenton growth chart for preterm infants. BMC Pediatr. 2013;13(1):59.

32. Nam H-K, Lee K-H. Small for gestational age and obesity: epidemiology and general risks. Ann Pediatr Endocrinol Metab. 2018;23(1):9–13.

33. Datar A, Jacknowitz A. Birth weight effects on Children's mental, motor, and physical development: evidence from twins data. Matern Child Health J. 2009;13(6):780–94.

34. Kramer MS. The epidemiology of adverse pregnancy outcomes: an overview. J Nutr. 2003;133(5 Suppl 2):1592S–6S.

35. Misra DP, Guyer B, Allston A. Integrated perinatal health framework. A multiple determinants model with a life span approach. Am J Prev Med. 2003;25(1):65–75.

36. Urquia ML, Gagnon AJ. Glossary: migration and health. J Epidemiol Community Health. 2011;65(5):467–72.

37. OECD. What are equivalence scales? http://www.oecd.org/eco/growth/OECD-Note-EquivalenceScales.pdf. Accessed 12 Oct 2017.

38. Variable: Nomenclature de la position socio-économique. https://www.bcss.fgov.be/fr/dwh/dwh_page/content/websites/datawarehouse/about/structure/nomenclaturede-la-position-socio-economique.html. Accessed 12 Nov 2017.

39. Naper SO. All-cause and cause-specific mortality of social assistance recipients in Norway: a register-based follow-up study. Scand J Public Health. 2009;37(8):820–5.

40. Løyland B, Miaskowski C, Paul SM, Dahl E, Rustøen T. The relationship between chronic pain and health-related quality of life in long-term social assistance recipients in Norway. Qual Life Res Int J Qual Life Asp Treat Care Rehabil. 2010;19(10):1457–65.

41. Variable: position LIPRO. https://www.bcss.fgov.be/fr/dwh/variabledetail/registre-national-et-registre-bcss/Variables/position-lipro.html. Accessed 12 Nov 2017.

42. Van Imhoff E. LIPRO: a multistate household projection model. In: van Imhoff E, Kuijsten A, Hooimeijer P, van Wissen L, editors. Household demography and household modeling the plenum series on demographic methods and population analysis. Boston: Springer; 1995. p. 273–91.

43. Turrell G. Income non-reporting: implications for health inequalities research. J Epidemiol Community Health. 2000;54(3):207–14.

44. Cheng TL, Johnson SB, Goodman E. Breaking the intergenerational cycle of disadvantage: the three generation approach. Pediatrics. 2016;137(6):e20152467.

45. Bostean G. Does selective migration explain the Hispanic paradox? A comparative analysis of Mexicans in the U.S. and Mexico. J Immigr Minor Health. 2013;15(3):624–35.

46. Saurel-Cubizolles M-J, Saucedo M, Drewniak N, Blondel B, Bouvier-Colle M-H. Santé périnatale des femmes étrangères en France. Bulletin Epidémiologique Hebdomadaire. 2012:30–4.

47. Reiss K, Breckenkamp J, Borde T, Brenne S, David M, Razum O. Smoking during pregnancy among Turkish immigrants in Germany-are there associations with acculturation? Nicotine Tob Res Off J Soc Res Nicotine Tob. 2015;17(6):643–52.

48. Corluy V, Marx I, Verbist G. Employment chances and changes of immigrants in Belgium: the impact of citizenship. Int J Comp Sociol. 2011;52(4):350–68.

49. OECD. International Migration Outlook 2013. OECD Publishing; 2013. http://www.oecd-ilibrary.org/social-issues-migration-health/international-migration-outlook-2013_migr_outlook-2013-en. Accessed 09 Oct 2017.

50. Dominguez TP. Race, Racism, and Racial Disparities in Adverse Birth Outcomes. Clin Obstet Gynecol. 2008;51(2):360–70.

51. Viruell-Fuentes EA, Miranda PY, Abdulrahim S. More than culture: structural racism, intersectionality theory, and immigrant health. Part Spec Issue Place Migr Health. 2012;75(12):2099–106.

52. Alhusen JL, Bower KM, Epstein E, Sharps P. Racial discrimination and adverse birth outcomes: an integrative review. J Midwifery Womens Health. 2016;61(6):707–20.

53. Phelan JC, Link BG. Is racism a fundamental cause of inequalities in health? Annu Rev Sociol. 2015;41(1):311–30.

54. Buttenheim A, Goldman N, Pebley AR, Wong R, Chung C. Do Mexican immigrants "import" social gradients in health to the US? Soc Sci Med. 2010;71(7):1268–76.

55. Parker JD, Schoendorf KC, Kiely JL. Associations between measures of socioeconomic status and low birth weight, small for gestational age, and premature delivery in the United States. Ann Epidemiol. 1994;4(4):271–8.

56. Rodrigues T, Barros H. Comparison of risk factors for small-for-gestational-age and preterm in a Portuguese cohort of newborns. Matern Child Health J. 2007;11(5):417–24.

57. Abrams B, Newman V. Small-for-gestational-age birth: maternal predictors and comparison with risk factors of spontaneous preterm delivery in the same cohort. Am J Obstet Gynecol. 1991;164(3):785–90.

58. Daoud N, O'Campo P, Minh A, Urquia ML, Dzakpasu S, Heaman M, et al. Patterns of social inequalities across pregnancy and birth outcomes: a comparison of individual and neighborhood socioeconomic measures. BMC Pregnancy Childbirth. 2014;(1):14, 393.

59. Sadovsky ADI, Matijasevich A, Santos IS, Barros FC, Miranda AE, Silveira MF. LBW and IUGR temporal trend in 4 population-based birth cohorts: the role of economic inequality. BMC Pediatr. 2016;16(1):115.

60. Torche F. The effect of maternal stress on birth outcomes: exploiting a natural experiment. Demography. 2011;48(4):1473–91.

61. Dunkel Schetter C, Tanner L. Anxiety, depression and stress in pregnancy: implications for mothers, children, research, and practice. Curr Opin Psychiatry. 2012;25(2):141–8.

62. Pfinder M, Kunst AE, Feldmann R, van Eijsden M, Vrijkotte TGM. Preterm birth and small for gestational age in relation to alcohol consumption during pregnancy: stronger associations among vulnerable women? results from two large Western-European studies. BMC Pregnancy Childbirth. 2013;13(1):49.

63. Horta BL, Victora CG, Menezes AM, Halpern R, Barros FC. Low birthweight, preterm births and intrauterine growth retardation in relation to maternal smoking. Paediatr Perinat Epidemiol. 1997;11(2):140–51.

64. Kempe A, Wise PH, Barkan SE, Sappenfield WM, Sachs B, Gortmaker SL, et al. Clinical determinants of the racial disparity in very low birth weight. N Engl J Med. 1992;327(14):969–73.

65. Cadart M-L. La vulnérabilité des mères seules en situation de migration. Dialogue. 2004;163(1):60–71.

66. Urquia ML, Berger H, Ray JG. For the Canadian curves consortium. Risk of adverse outcomes among infants of immigrant women according to birth-weight curves tailored to maternal world region of origin. Can Med Assoc J. 2015;187(1):E32–40.

67. Beeckman K, Louckx F, Putman K. Predisposing, enabling and pregnancy-related determinants of late initiation of prenatal care. Matern Child Health J. 2011;15(7):1067–75.

6

Neonatal near miss determinants at a maternity hospital for high-risk pregnancy in Northeastern Brazil: a prospective study

Telmo Henrique Barbosa de Lima[1,2,5*], Leila Katz[3], Samir Buainain Kassar[1] and Melania Maria Amorim[3,4]

Abstract

Background: To investigate the associations of maternal variables – sociodemographic, obstetrical and maternal near miss (MNM) variables – with neonatal near miss (NNM) using the new concept of NNM formulated by the Centro Latino-Americano de Perinatologia (CLAP) and the corresponding health indicators for NNM.

Methods: An analytical prospective cohort study was performed at maternity hospital for high-risk pregnancy in Northeastern Brazil. Puerperal women whose newborn infants met the selection criteria were subjected to interviews involving pretested questionnaires.
Statistical analysis was performed with the Epi Info 3.5.1 program using the Chi square test and Fisher's exact test when appropriate, with a level of significance of 5%. A bivariate analysis was performed to evaluate differences between the groups. All the variables evaluated in the bivariate analysis were subsequently included in the multivariate analysis. For stepwise logistic regression analysis, a hierarchical model was plotted to assess variable responses and adverse outcomes associated with MNM and NNM variables.

Results: There were 1002 live births (LB) from June 2015 through May 2016, corresponding to 723 newborn infants (72.2%) without any neonatal adverse outcomes, 221 (22%) NNM cases, 44 (4.4%) early neonatal deaths and 14 (1.4%) late neonatal deaths. The incidence of NNM was 220/1000 LB. Following multivariate analysis, the factors that remained significantly associated with increased risk of NNM were fewer than 6 prenatal care visits (odds ratio (OR): 3.57; 95% confidence interval (CI): 2.57–4.94) and fetal malformations (OR: 8.78; 95% CI: 3.69–20.90). Maternal age older than 35 years (OR: 0.43; 95% CI: 0.23–0.83) and previous cesarean section (OR: 0.45; 95% CI: 0.29 0.68) protected against NNM.

Conclusion: Based on the large differences between the NNM and neonatal mortality rates found in the present study and the fact that NNM seems to be a preventable precursor of neonatal death, we suggest that all cases of NNM should be audited. Inadequate prenatal care and fetal malformations increased the risk of NNM, while older maternal age and a history of a previous cesarean section were protective factors.

Keywords: Neonatal near miss, Neonatal mortality, Fetal death, Maternal near miss

* Correspondence: thbl@uol.com.br
[1]Health Sciences University of Alagoas (UNCISAL), Maceió, Brazil
[2]Health Sciences, Federal University of São Paulo (UNIFESP), São Paulo, Brazil
Full list of author information is available at the end of the article

Background

One of the United Nations (UN) Millennium Development Goals (MDGs) was to reduce the child mortality rate by two-thirds. Brazil met this goal before 2015, with a more considerable reduction in postneonatal mortality and a slower reduction in early neonatal mortality; early neonatal mortality is currently the main component of child mortality [1].

As part of the UN Agenda for Sustainable Development, the goal for the period from 2016 to 2030 is to end preventable deaths of newborns and children under 5 years of age. For this purpose, all the countries that signed the UN document committed to reducing neonatal mortality to at least 12 per 1000 live births (LB) [2].

To assess and improve the quality of the care delivered to this population, reliable assessment instruments are necessary. Child mortality rate has long been used as a classic indicator of social development, economics and healthcare quality [3]. However, for each child who dies, many others survive serious complications; as in the case of maternal health, application of the near miss concept to the neonatal setting might be useful to detect risk factors for death, investigate the quality of care delivered to this population, strengthen the healthcare system and reduce the child mortality rate [4].

However, until recently, there has not been a standardized definition or any international criteria for detecting neonatal near miss (NNM) that would allow performing comparisons within the same institution over time or between different institutions in various regions or countries. In response to this scenario, in 2015, the Latin American Centre of Perinatology (Centro Latino-Americano de Perinatologia - CLAP) led discussions and proposals aiming at establishing a standardized definition of NNM [5] based on the results of previous studies on the subject [4–6]. The CLAP suggests defining NNM as any newborn infant who exhibited pragmatic and/or management criteria and survived the first 27 days of life.

Two studies have described the impact of maternal near miss (MNM) on fetal and neonatal mortality and associated factors and concluded that fetal and neonatal death rates are high among MNM patients [7, 8]. It would seem logical for MNM to be strongly associated with NNM because their determinants – socioeconomic variables, demographic variables, reproductive history, health conditions during pregnancy, prenatal care and labor care – might be associated. However, we were not able to identify any study that investigated the association between these two conditions.

Therefore, the aim of the present study was to investigate the associations of maternal variables – sociodemographic, obstetrical and MNM variables – with NNM using the new concept of NNM formulated by the CLAP and to evaluate the corresponding health indicators for NNM.

Methods

The present prospective, analytical cohort study was conducted at Santa Monica Maternity School Hospital (Maternidade Escola Santa Mônica - MESM), which is located in Maceió, the capital of the state of Alagoas, in northeastern Brazil. MESM had the lowest Human Development Index (HDI) of 0.631 in the country in 2016. MESM is a public maternity hospital for women with high-risk pregnancies. It is the main obstetrical and neonatal referral center for highly complex cases in Alagoas, and approximately 50% of women with high-risk pregnancies in the state receive care at MESM.

Data collection was performed from June 2015 through May 2016 by the principal investigator and research assistants who were students of an undergraduate medical course and had received specific training for the study. The study was approved by the Human Research Ethics Committee of Universidade Estadual de Ciências da Saúde de Alagoas (UNCISAL) (CAAE no. 37977014.0.0000.5011). All the included women or their legally responsible parties were approached on the day after delivery by the researcher or one of the assistants and invited to participate in the study. They were included only after voluntarily agreeing to participate and signing an informed consent form.

The outcome variable was NNM, and the exposure variables were age, race, marital status, education level, origin, family income, prenatal care, number of prenatal visits, prenatal care performed at the hospital, household visits, current pregnancy, previous cesarean section, referral for childbirth, previous pregnancies, maternal admission to an intensive care unit (ICU), fetal presentation, smoking history, fetal malformations, comorbidities and MNM.

NNM was defined as a neonate who had suffered a life-threatening condition but survived the first 27 days of life [5]. Two sets of criteria that are recommended by the CLAP were used to identify newborn infants at a high risk of death at birth: pragmatic criteria (gestational age at birth less than 33 weeks; birth weight < 1750 g; and 5-min Apgar score < 7) and management criteria (parenteral antibiotics for up to 7 days before 28 days of age; use of a continuous positive airway pressure (CPAP) device; any intubation lasting for up to 7 days before 28 days of age; phototherapy within the first 24 h of life; cardiopulmonary resuscitation; use of vasoactive drugs, anticonvulsants, surfactant, or blood-derived products or use of steroids to treat refractory hypoglycemia; and any surgical procedure) [5].

Some indicators of perinatal care quality were calculated [5]: early neonatal mortality rate (ENMR), neonatal mortality rate (NMR), neonatal near miss rate (NNMR), early severe neonatal outcome rate (ESNOR), severe neonatal outcome rate (SNOR), and lethality ratio.

MNM was defined as a woman who survived a severe, life-threatening complication during pregnancy, childbirth or within 42 days of termination of pregnancy and met any of the clinical, laboratory or management criteria formulated by the World Health Organization (WHO) [9].

Puerperal women whose newborn infants met the selection criteria were subjected to interviews involving pretested questionnaires; other relevant information was obtained from medical records. The data for the newborn infants were collected during the immediate postpartum period and from their medical records. A second interview (by phone call or a home visit) was performed 42 days after childbirth to assess maternal and neonatal outcomes.

Data were collected on printed forms that were stored in the hospital until the final maternal and neonatal outcomes were assessed. Data were then entered into a database created specifically for this purpose in the statistical program Epi Info 3.5.1 (Atlanta, GA), in which the statistical analysis was performed. The data were entered twice and compared, and inconsistencies were corrected. In the bivariate analysis, NNM was the outcome variable, and the aforementioned exposure variables were dichotomized as yes/no variables. The risk ratio (RR) was estimated as a measure of risk, with the corresponding 95% confidence interval (95% CI). The Chi square test or Fisher's exact test was used as necessary.

All the variables considered for the bivariate analysis were included in a multiple logistic regression analysis to identify the variables that were most strongly associated with NNM, and the adjusted risk was calculated. A hierarchical model was plotted for multiple regression analysis; the variables were included in blocks according to risk categories, and biological and socioeconomic variables including race/skin color (nonwhite), educational level (less than 8 years of schooling), origin (inner state), income (less than the minimum wage), age (younger than 20 years old), age (older than 35 years old) and marital status (without a partner) were the most distal factors. In the intermediate level, variables corresponding to prenatal and labor care were included: no prenatal care, fewer than 6 prenatal care visits, prenatal care not performed at the hospital where the study was conducted, no referral to a maternity hospital for childbirth, previous cesarean section, nulliparity, noncephalic presentation, maternal admission to an ICU and smoking history. Variables that were considered to be closest to the outcome of NNM were included in the proximal level: comorbidities, MNM (clinical, laboratory and management criteria) and fetal malformations.

Stepwise logistic regression was performed; at the end of each block, the variables associated with the outcome at a 20% significance level were selected, followed by those that remained associated with the outcome at a 5% significance level. A final regression analysis was then performed to determine the adjusted risk for NNM for each of the variables that were significantly associated with the outcome at a 5% significance level. Odds ratios (ORs) and corresponding 95% CIs were calculated for these variables.

Results

From June 2015 to May 2016, 1149 women were admitted to the maternity ward. Thirty-four had miscarriages, and 21 delivered stillborn infants. The initial interview was performed with 1094 women on the first postpartum day, and when they were invited, all of them consented to participate. After initial inclusion, during the follow-up period, 44 newborns (4.4%) were early neonatal deaths, and 14 (1.4%) were late neonatal deaths. Of the 1002 LB that could be analyzed, 58 newborns were lost to follow-up; thus, 723 babies that did not exhibit any neonatal adverse outcomes (72.2%) and 221 (22%) NNM cases were included (Fig. 1).

Indicators of perinatal care quality were calculated for the aforementioned period, resulting in 220 NNM cases/1000 LB, a SNOR of 278/1000 LB and an NMR of 57/1000 LB (Table 1).

A total of 131 newborn infants met the pragmatic criteria for NNM, corresponding to an incidence of 131/1000 LB. Among the pragmatic criteria, gestational age younger than 33 weeks (47.5%) was the most commonly identified criterion, with an incidence of 105/1000 LB.

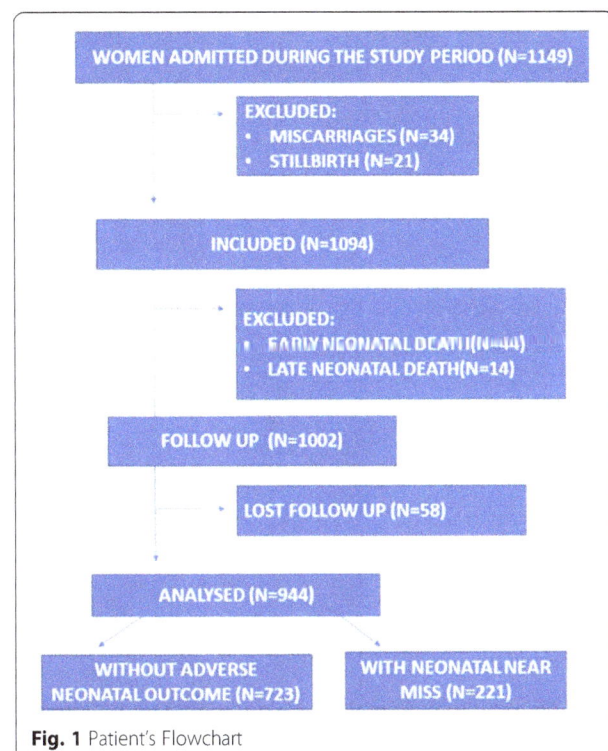

Fig. 1 Patient's Flowchart

Table 1 Indicators of perinatal outcomes

Indicators	No.	Rate
Number of live births	1002	
Early neonatal deaths	44	
Late neonatal deaths	14	
Newborn infants with neonatal near miss	221	
Neonatal near miss rate		220/1000 LB
Early severe neonatal outcome rate		264/1000 LB
Severe neonatal outcome rate		278/1000 LB
Early neonatal mortality rate		44/1000 LB
Neonatal mortality rate (early + late)		57/1000 LB
Lethality ratio	3.8	

All 221 newborn infants met the management criteria, corresponding to an incidence of 220/1000 LB; the use of a nasal CPAP device was the most commonly identified criterion (62.9%), with an incidence of 139/1000 LB (Table 2). Ninety newborn infants presented only the management criteria, while the remaining infants had both pragmatic and management criteria.

In the hierarchical bivariate analysis, the sociodemographic, obstetrical and MNM variables that exhibited statistically significant associations with NNM were age younger than 20 years (RR = 1.58; 95% CI = 1.25–1.99), age older than 35 years (RR = 0.37; 95% CI = 0.21–0.64), fewer than 6 prenatal care visits (RR = 2.63; 95% CI = 2.08–3.33), no referral for childbirth (RR = 1.49; 95% CI = 1.15–1.94), history of a previous cesarean section

Table 2 Criteria for neonatal near miss

Criteria	No.	%	Incidence of neonatal near miss/1000 LB
Pragmatic criteria	131	59.3	131.2
Gestational age < 33 weeks	105	47.5	105.2
Weight (< 1750 g)	99	44.8	99.1
5-min Apgar score (< 7)	15	6.8	15.0
Management criteria	221	100.0	220.0
Nasal continuous positive airway pressure	139	62.9	139.2
Surfactant	100	45.2	100.2
Intubation	84	38.0	84.1
Parenteral antibiotics	67	30.3	67.1
Blood-derived products	41	18.6	41.0
Phototherapy during the first 24 h	22	10.0	22.0
Vasoactive drugs	11	5.0	11.0
Surgical procedures	11	4.9	11.0
Anticonvulsants	7	3.2	7.0
Cardiopulmonary resuscitation	05	2.3	5.1
Steroids for hypoglycemia	01	0.5	1.0

(RR = 0.52; 95% CI = 0.37–0.73), nulliparity (RR = 1.31; 95% CI = 1.04–1.65), noncephalic presentation (RR = 1.78; 95% CI = 1.30–2.44), maternal admission to an ICU (RR = 1.64; 95% CI = 1.17–2.28), fetal malformations (RR = 3.07; 95% CI = 2.32–4.08), MNM (RR = 1.94; 95% CI = 1.31–2.89), clinical criteria for MNM (RR = 1.99; 95% CI = 1.32–2.98) and management criteria for MNM (RR = 1.86; 95% CI = 1.12–3.1) (Table 3).

All the variables assessed in the bivariate analysis were included in a multivariate analysis involving a logistic regression model with hierarchical levels. The factors that remained significantly associated with a higher risk of NNM were fewer than 6 prenatal care visits (OR = 3.57; 95% CI = 2.57–4.94) and the presence of fetal malformations (OR = 8.78; 95% CI = 3.69–20.90), while maternal age older 35 years (OR = 0.43; 95% CI = 0.23–0.83) and history of a previous cesarean section (OR = 0.45; 95% CI = 0.29–0.68) were protective against NNM (Table 4).

Discussion

In this study, the incidence of NNM was 220/1000 LB. Following multivariate analysis, the factors that remained significantly associated with a higher risk of NNM were fewer than six prenatal care visits and the presence of fetal malformations, while maternal age older than 35 years and previous cesarean section were protective factors against NNM.

We conducted an active search of the PubMed, Biblioteca Regional de Medicina (BIREME) and Scopus databases. This study is the first to analyze the association between MNM and the severe neonatal condition NNM with prospectively collected data and the use of the 2015 CLAP criteria [5] to define NNM in an attempt to standardize the definition of NNM and to facilitate comparisons of NNM rates between different regions and countries.

In our study, NNM accounted for 79.2% of the adverse perinatal outcomes; this NNM rate was 3.8 times higher than the NMR. In other studies, the NNM rate varied from 2.6- to 8-fold higher than the NMR, even when the same criteria and markers were used [4, 6, 10, 11].

The high NNM rate (220/1000 LB) and NMR (57/1000 LB) found in the present study differ from those in other reports (21.4–72.5/1000 LB and 6.3–11.1/1000 LB, respectively) [4, 6, 10, 11]. These differences might be attributable to the fact that the present study considered the associations of pragmatic (59.3%) and management (40.7%) criteria. Several studies have shown that the combination of these criteria exhibits better performance than either set of criteria used alone, with sensitivities and specificities of almost 93% [5, 12]; the use of this combination of criteria allowed us to assess a larger number of surviving newborn infants. Another reason that might explain the high NNM rate and NMR found in the present study is that other authors employed

Table 3 Associations of sociodemographic and obstetrical variables and maternal near miss with neonatal near miss

	Neonatal near miss		RR (95% CI)	P
	Yes, n (%)	No, n (%)		
Distal factors				
Race/skin color (nonwhite)	170(76.9)	583(80.6)	0.84 (0.64–1.10)	0.22
Education level (< 8 years)	121(54.8)	385(53.3)	1.04 (0.83–1.32)	0.69
Origin (inner state)	116(52.5)	359(49.7)	1.09 (0.86–1.37)	0.46
Income (< minimum wage)	185(83.7)	571(79.0)	1.27 (0.92–1.75)	0.12
Age (< 20 years old)	86(38.9)	185(25.6)	1.58 (1.25–1.99)	0.0001
Age (> 35 years old)	12(5.4)	114(15.8)	0.37 (0.21–0.64)	0.00007
Marital status (without a partner)	54(24.4)	141(19.5)	1.24 (0.95–1.61)	0.11
Intermediate factors				
No prenatal care	6(2.7)	11(1.5)	1.52 (0.79–2.92)	0.18*
< 6 prenatal care visits	133(60.2)	211(29.2)	2.63 (2.08–3.33)	< 0.0000001
Prenatal care at service	179(81.0)	544(75.2)	1.30 (0.96–1.75)	0.07
No household visits	219(99.1)	698(96.5)	3.22 (0.84–12.29)	0.04
No referral for childbirth	160(72.4)	441(61.0)	1.49 (1.15–1.94)	0.002
Current pregnancy (cesarean section)	165(74.7)	548(75.8)	0.95 (0.73–1.24)	0.73
Previous cesarean section	35(15.8)	214(29.6)	0.52 (0.37–0.73)	0.00004
Nulliparity	112(50.7)	302(41.8)	1.31 (1.04–1.65)	0.01
Noncephalic presentation	28(12.7)	43(6.0)	1.78 (1.30–2.44)	0.0009
Admission to an intensive care unit	25(11.3)	43(5.9)	1.64 (1.17–2.28)	0.006
Smoker	9(4.2)	20(2.7)	1.33 (076–2.33)	0.32
Proximal factors				
Fetal malformation	19(8.6)	9(1.2)	3.07 (2.32–4.08)	< 0.0000001
Comorbidities	78(35.3)	306(42.3)	0.79 (0.62–1.01)	0.06
Maternal near miss	15(6.7)	19(2.6)	1.94 (1.31–2.89)	0.003
Maternal near miss clinical criteria	14(6.3)	17(2.3)	1.99 (1.32–2.98)	0.003
Maternal near miss laboratory criteria	05(2.2)	9(1.2)	1.53 (0.75–3.13)	0.42*
Maternal near miss management criteria	09(4.0)	12(1.7)	1.86 (1.12–3.1)	0.07*

*Analysis performed with Fisher's exact test

Table 4 Multivariate analysis of neonatal near miss determinants

	OR	95% CI	P
Distal factors			
Age (> 35 years old)	0.43	0.23–0.83	0.0118
Intermediate factors			
Previous cesarean section (yes)	0.45	0.29–0.68	0.0002
< 6 prenatal care visits	3.57	2.57–4.94	0.0000
Proximal factors			
Fetal malformation (yes)	8.78	3.69–20.90	0.0000

population databases [4, 6, 10, 11], while the present study used only data from a maternity hospital that is a referral center for women with high-risk pregnancies; this sample selection was a source of bias that resulted in high frequencies of adverse outcomes. In addition, the observation period in our study was 28 days, while in other studies, it varied from 3 to 28 days after birth [4, 6, 10, 11] thus limiting the assessment of the quality of late neonatal care and neonatal mortality. By selecting a prospective design in which neonatal complications were monitored on a daily basis, we possibly avoided the losses that might occur in studies involving retrospective databases. Finally, the high NNM rate and NMR found might be related to the socioeconomic status of the state of Alagoas, which has the lowest HDI in Brazil.

Currently, comparison of the NNM rates of different hospitals is difficult due to the lack of a universally accepted definition of NNM, as there is for MNM [9]. In response to this scenario, in 2015, the CLAP guided a series of discussions and proposals to develop a consensus definition of NNM based on pragmatic and management criteria [5].

The management criteria for NNM cannot be used to compare the quality of healthcare between different hospitals because the NNM rate might be influenced by the technological complexity of the services provided [12], unless a general complexity index is developed and included in the statistical analysis [11]. Thus, the best option to detect NNM cases in hospitals with more substantial resources, such as ICUs and neonatal ICUs, as in the maternity hospital where the present study was conducted, is to combine the pragmatic and management criteria [5, 12].

As NNM is known to be a useful assessment of the quality of obstetrical and neonatal care [4–6, 10, 11], we sought to investigate whether maternal variables (sociodemographic, obstetrical and MNM variables) were related to NNM.

Multivariate analysis provided two results that diverged from those of other reports in the literature in terms of age extremes. First, age younger 20 years did not exhibit an association with NNM, although adolescent pregnancy is usually associated with poorer maternal and perinatal outcomes including prematurity, low birth weight and occurrence of 5-min Apgar scores of less than 7, than pregnancy in adult women [3, 13–15]. Other mechanisms that are not biological might mediate the relationships between adolescence and adverse obstetric/perinatal outcomes, which previous studies failed to detect.

Age older than 35 years exhibited a statistically significant association with NNM in the multivariate analysis, demonstrating evidence of a protective effect. This finding is in clear contrast with those of previous reports on age extremes and perinatal outcomes [3, 15]. The data on the risk associated with pregnancy at an age older than 35 years are conflicting due to the presence of other variables, such as parity and pre-existing diseases, which impair assessment of the risk associated with maternal age alone [16]. However, in the present study, we ruled out confounding variables; thus, the results might be explained by the fact that currently, most pregnancies among women older than 35 years are planned, and prenatal and required care are prioritized, leading to consequent improvement in perinatal outcomes. Alternatively, when caring for older pregnant women with or without associated diseases, healthcare providers might be more alert and intervene earlier in these women than in younger pregnant women, thus preventing adverse outcomes. Therefore, the results described here might pave the way for new studies.

Prenatal care is important. In theory, more prenatal visits might mean higher odds of receiving care, especially in the case of high-risk pregnancy, which is associated with poor maternal and perinatal outcomes. In Brazil, the prenatal care coverage and number of visits have increased over the past 15 years [17]. However, studies conducted in the country have still revealed flaws in prenatal care, such as difficult access to care, late onset of care, an inadequate number of visits and incomplete performance of procedures, all of which impact perinatal outcomes [18–20]. Such outcomes are below the country's potential and reflect unfavorable living and healthcare conditions, in addition to historical regional and socioeconomic inequalities [3].

Our findings confirm the deleterious effects of inadequate prenatal care. Attending fewer than 6 prenatal care visits was statistically significantly associated with NNM, increasing the risk of NNM by 4-fold. The nationwide hospital-based survey Birth in Brazil, which was conducted in 2014, analyzed neonatal mortality profiles and found high NNM rates among mothers who received inadequate prenatal care [3]. The underlying causes of most neonatal deaths are maternal obstetrical problems that were not resolved prenatally [21]. Therefore, the prenatal care coverage needs to be broadened, and the quality of the care delivered improved, especially for women with high-risk pregnancies.

Women with a history of a previous cesarean section are more often subjected to a second cesarean section because many obstetricians still base their decision-making on a principle that was formulated in 1916, according to which "once a C-section, always a C-section," and fear rupture of uterine scars [22]. However, there is no scientific evidence supporting this alleged risk, as uterine scar rupture occurs in approximately 1% of patients [23]. In our study, 94.3% of women with a history of a previous cesarean section were again subjected to cesarean section. In the multivariate analysis, this variable was protective against NNM. The presence of a previous uterine scar might have led to the decision to perform a cesarean section early in the course of labor, and some of the newborn infants might have benefited from the fact that 33.9% of the mothers had high-risk pregnancies that required urgent resolution. Adverse events derived from the lack of rigorous monitoring during labor, which is essential in women with a history of a previous cesarean section, might have been avoided; thus, cesarean section was a protective factor because maternal complications that contribute to the occurrence of adverse perinatal outcomes were prevented.

In one study published in 2017, the survival of newborn infants born to mothers without severe complications was better than that of infants born to mothers with eclampsia, intrapartum hemorrhage or other complications requiring ICU admission [15]. In the multivariate analysis performed in the present study, maternal ICU admission did not remain associated with NNM. Perhaps this marker of maternal severity is not always a marker of neonatal severity and vice versa. For instance, conditions such as puerperal sepsis or hemorrhage do not affect the newborn infant, even though the mother needs to be admitted to an ICU; in the case of spontaneous premature labor, the infant might be an NNM case, although the mother is not an MNM case.

Newborn infants with congenital malformations exhibited a 9-fold increased risk of NNM; this result remained unchanged after controlling for confounding variables. This finding was expected because fetal malformations increase neonatal morbidity and mortality. The literature shows that despite high-quality interventions, in most of these infants, neonatal death due to several fetal malformations cannot be avoided [12]. This variable has been rarely investigated in previous studies [5, 12] and seems to be a relevant marker for characterizing NNM cases; thus, it should be employed in future studies as a defining criterion for NNM.

Studies on MNM are abundant in the literature [24, 25], especially after 2009, following a publication on the definition of and criteria for MNM formulated by the WHO [9]. However, we were not able to locate any study reporting an association between MNM and NNM.

Two studies investigated the relationship between MNM and adverse perinatal outcomes (fetal and neonatal deaths) [7, 8]. In the first study performed in 2013, the authors found high frequencies of fetal and neonatal deaths among MNM cases, and the main factors associated with outcomes were severe pre-eclampsia, placental abruption, prematurity and endometritis; there was also an association between laboratory criteria and adverse outcomes [7]. These results were corroborated by a second study that was performed in 2017 [8].

It would seem logical for NNM to be strongly associated with MNM because the determinants (socioeconomic variables, demographic variables, reproductive history, health status during pregnancy, prenatal care and labor care) might also be associated. However, the multivariate analysis did not reveal an association between MNM variables and NNM outcomes. A possible explanation is that many of the conditions that lead to the classification of a woman as an MNM case are so severe that they lead to early resolution of pregnancy thus sparing the fetus from complications. Alternatively, many of the conditions for which a woman is classified as an MNM case, such as puerperal hemorrhage and sepsis, occur after birth, again sparing the fetus from complications.

Among the strengths of the present study are its prospective cohort design and the fact that a multiple regression model that accounted for the mutual interrelationships of variables was used; thus, potential confounding variables were controlled. In addition, this is one of the first studies to employ the CLAP criteria to define NNM and to investigate the impact of maternal factors on NNM and the association between MNM and NNM, both of which have rarely been analyzed in the literature.

Some limitations of the present study are derived from the fact that NNM was assessed at a hospital for women with high-risk pregnancies; thus, the study sample is not representative of the population of pregnant women in Alagoas. In addition, the data corresponding to socioeconomic variables and access to healthcare were collected in interviews conducted with the participants and might be subject to recall bias.

Conclusion

Based on the large differences between the NNM rate and NMR found in the present study and the fact that NNM seems to be a preventable precursor of neonatal death, we suggest that all cases of NNM should be audited. Inadequate prenatal care and fetal malformations increased the risk of NNM, while older maternal age and a history of previous cesarean section were protective factors.

Abbreviations

CLAP: Latin American Centre of Perinatology (Centro Latino-Americano de Perinatologia); ENMR: Early neonatal mortality rate; ESNOR: Early severe neonatal outcome rate; HDI: Human Development Index; ICU: Intensive care unit; LB: Live births; MDGs: Millennium Development Goals; MESM: Santa Monica Maternity School Hospital (Maternidade Escola Santa Mônica); MNM: Maternal near miss; NMR: Neonatal mortality rate; NNM: Neonatal near miss; NNMR: Neonatal near miss rate; OR: Odds ratio; RR: Risk ratio; SNOR: Severe neonatal outcome rate; SUS: Unified Heath System (Sistema Único de Saúde); UN: United Nations; UNCISAL: State University of Health Sciences of Alagoas (Universidade Estadual de Ciências da Saúde de Alagoas); WHO: World Health Organization

Acknowledgments

To all the women who agreed to participate in the study with their newborn infants, for believing in the potential of research to transform everyday clinical practice, our most sincere thanks.
Study conducted at Maternidade Escola Santa Mônica, Avenida Comendador Leão, SN, Poço, Maceió/AL, Brazil.

Funding

The present study did not have any specific funding.

Authors' contributions

THBL and SBK designed the initial project, which was revised by LK and MMA. THBL was responsible for the data collection. SBK, THBL and LK performed the statistical analysis. THBL wrote the manuscript draft, which was revised by LK, SBK and MMA. All authors read and approved the final version of the manuscript.

Competing interests

The authors declare that they have no competing interests.

Author details

[1]Health Sciences University of Alagoas (UNCISAL), Maceió, Brazil. [2]Health Sciences, Federal University of São Paulo (UNIFESP), São Paulo, Brazil. [3]Postgraduate Program, Fernando Figueira Institute of Integral Medicine (IMIP), Obstetric Intensive Care Unit, IMIP, Recife, Brazil. [4]Federal University of Campina Grande (UFCG), Campina Grande, Brazil. [5]Maternidade Santa Mônica, Maceió, Brazil.

References

1. Brasil, Ministério da Saúde. Reduzindo a mortalidade perinatal [Reducing perinatal mortality]; 2016. [cited 2016 Dec 17]. Available from: http://brasil.evipnet.org/wp-content/uploads/2016/07/Mortalidade_perinatal_WEB_jul.pdf
2. WHO - World Health Organization. Maternal mortality. Fact sheet no.348; 2015. [cited 2015 Dec 17] Available from: http://www.who.int/mediacentre/factsheets/fs348/en/.
3. Lansky S, Friche AADL, Silva AAMD, Campos D, Bittencourt SDDA, Carvalho ML, et al. Pesquisa nascer no Brasil: perfil da mortalidade neonatal e avaliação da assistência à gestante e ao recém-nascido [Birth in Brazil survey: neonatal mortality, pregnancy and childbirth quality of care]. Cad Saude Publica. 2014;30(suppl 1):S192–207.
4. Pileggi C, Souza JP, Cecatti JG, Faúndes A. Neonatal near miss approach in the 2005 WHO global survey Brazil. J Pediatr. 2010;86(1):21–6.
5. Santos JP, Cecatti JG, Serruya SJ, Almeida PV, Duran P, Mucio B, et al. Neonatal near miss: the need for a standard definition and appropriate criteria and the rationale for a prospective surveillance system. Clinics. 2015;70(12):820–6.
6. Pileggi-Castro C, Camelo JS, Perdoná GC, Mussi-Pinhata MM, Cecatti JG, Mori R, et al. Development of criteria for identifying neonatal near-miss cases: analysis of two WHO multicountry cross-sectional studies. BJOG. 2014;121(Suppl 1):110–8.
7. Oliveira LC, Costa AAR. Óbitos fetais e neonatais entre casos de near miss materno [fetal and neonatal deaths among cases of maternal near miss]. Rev Assoc Med Bras. 2013;59(5):487–94.
8. Nardello DM, Guimarães AMDAN, Barreto IDC, Gurgel RQ, Ribeiro ERO, Gois CFL. Fetal and neonatal deaths of children of patients classified as near miss. Rev Bras Enferm. 2017;70(1):98–105.
9. Say L, Souza JP, Pattinson RC. Maternal near miss – towards a standard tool for monitoring quality of maternal health care. Best Pract Res Clin Obstet Gynaecol. 2009;23(3):287–96.
10. Avenant T. Neonatal near miss: a measure of the quality of obstetric care. Best Pract Res Clin Obstet Gynaecol. 2009;23(3):369–74.
11. Silva AAMD, Leite ÁJM, Lamy ZC, Moreira MEL, Gurgel RQ, Cunha AJLA, et al. Morbidade neonatal near miss na pesquisa nascer no Brasil [neonatal near miss in the birth in Brazil survey]. Cad Saude Publica. 2014;30(suppl 1):S182–91.
12. Santos JP, Pileggi-Castro C, Camelo JS, Silva AA, Duran P, Serruya SJ, et al. Neonatal near miss: a systematic review. BMC Pregnancy Childbirth. 2015;15(1):320.
13. Morcillo AM, Carniel EDF, Zanolli MDL, Moreno LZ, Antonio MÂRGM. Caracterização das mães, partos e recém-nascidos em Campinas, São Paulo, 2001 e 2005 [Characterization of mothers, mode of deliveries and newborns in Campinas, São Paulo, 2001 and 2005]. Rev Paul Pediatr. 2010;28(3):269–75.
14. Partridge S, Balayla J, Holcroft C, Abenhaim H. Inadequate prenatal care utilization and risks of infant mortality and poor birth outcome: a retrospective analysis of 28,729,765 U.S. deliveries over 8 years. Am J Perinatol. 2012;29(10):787–94.
15. Anggondowati T, El-Mohandes AAE, Qomariyah SN, Kiely M, Ryon JJ, Gipson RF, et al. Maternal characteristics and obstetrical complications impact neonatal outcomes in Indonesia: a prospective study. BMC Pregnancy Childbirth. 2017;17(1):100.
16. Takagi MM, Jorge SRPF, Rodrigues LDP, Yamano LM, Piato S, Aoki T. Perinatal results in pregnant women with more than 35 years. Arq Med Hosp Fac Cienc Med Santa Casa São Paulo. 2010;55(3):108–14.
17. Viellas EF, Domingues RMSM, Dias MAB, Gama SGND, Filha MMT, Costa JVD, et al. Assistência pré-natal no Brasil [Prenatal care in Brazil]. Cad Saude Publica. 2014;30(suppl 1):S85–100.
18. Saavedra JS, Cesar JA. Uso de diferentes critérios para avaliação da inadequação do pré-natal: um estudo de base populacional no extremo Sul do Brasil [Use of different criteria to assess inadequate prenatal care: a population-based study in Southern Brazil]. Cad Saude Publica. 2015;31(5):1003–14.
19. Domingues RMSM, Hartz ZMDA, Dias MAB, Leal MDC. Avaliação da adequação da assistência pré-natal na rede sus do município do Rio de Janeiro, Brasil [Adequacy of prenatal care in the national health system in the city of Rio de Janeiro, Brazil]. Cad Saude Publica. 2012;28(3):425–37.
20. Nunes JT, Gomes KRO, Rodrigues MTP, Mascarenhas MDM. Qualidade da assistência pré-natal no Brasil: revisão de artigos publicados de 2005 a 2015 [Quality of prenatal care in Brazil: review of published papers from 2005 to 2015]. Cad Saude Colet. 2016;24(2):252–61.
21. Pedrosa LDCO, Sarinho SW, Ordonha MR. Análise da qualidade da informação sobre causa básica de óbitos neonatais registrados no sistema de informações sobre mortalidade: um estudo para Maceió, Alagoas, Brasil, 2001–2002 [Quality of information analysis on basic causes of neonatal deaths recorded in the mortality information system: a study in Maceióa, Alagoas State Brazil, 2001–2002]. Cad Saude Publica. 2007;23(10):2385–95.
22. Ugwumadu A. Does the maxim "once a caesarean, always a caesarean" still hold true? PLoS Med. 2005;2(9):e305.
23. Nair M, Soffer K, Noor N, Knight M, Griffiths M. Selected maternal morbidities in women with a prior caesarean delivery planning vaginal birth or elective repeat caesarean section: a retrospective cohort analysis using data from the UK obstetric surveillance system. BMJ Open. 2015;5(6):e007434.
24. Domingues RMSM, Dias MAB, Schilithz AOC, Leal MDC. Factors associated with maternal near miss in childbirth and the postpartum period: findings from the birth in Brazil national survey, 2011–2012. Reprod Health. 2016;13(S3):115.
25. Tunçalp Ö, Hindin MJ, Souza JP, Chou D, Say L. The prevalence of maternal near miss: a systematic review. BJOG. 2012;119(6):653–61.

7

Lithuania's experience in reducing caesarean sections among nulliparas

Justina Kacerauskiene[1]*[iD], Meile Minkauskiene[1], Tahir Mahmood[2], Egle Bartuseviciene[1], Dalia R. Railaite[1], Arnoldas Bartusevicius[1], Mindaugas Kliucinskas[1], Ruta J. Nadisauskiene[1], Kastytis Smigelskas[1], Kornelija Maciuliene[3], Grazina Drasutiene[4] and Diana Ramasauskaite[4]

Abstract

Background: To evaluate the role of the TGCS to reduce the caesarean section (CS) rate among nulliparas (Robson groups 1 and 2) and to find out which group of women have reduced the CS rate by using this tool.

Methods: The Robson classification was introduced in Lithuanian hospitals prospectively classifying all the deliveries in 2012. The CS rate overall and in each Robson group was calculated and the results were discussed. The analysis was repeated in 2014 and the data from the selected hospitals were compared using MS EXCEL and SPSS 23.0.

Results: Nulliparas accounted for 43% (3746/8718) and 44.6% (3585/8046) of all the deliveries in 2012 and 2014 years, respectively. The CS rate among nulliparas decreased from 23.9% (866/3626) in 2012 to 19.0% (665/3502) in 2014 ($p < 0.001$).The greatest decrease in absolute contribution to the overall CS rate was recorded in groups 1 ($p = 0.005$) and 2B ($p < 0.001$). Perinatal mortality was 3.5 in 2012 and 3.1 in 2014 per 1000 deliveries ($p = 0.764$).

Conclusion: The TGCS can work as an audit intervention that could help to reduce the CS rate without a negative impact on perinatal mortality.

Keywords: Caesarean section, Rate, Robson classification, Intervention, Nulliparas

Background

The caesarean section (CS) rate had been increasing for several decades worldwide [1]. In Lithuania it has increased from 9.49% in 1995 to 24.71% in 2010 [2]. Similar rates were reported in Canada (27%), the USA (33%), Brazil (50%) or Australia (31%) [1]. On the other hand, northern European countries, such as Finland (16%) or Norway (17%), are known for lower rates [1]. Caesarean section not only increases societal economic burden but also has huge impact on the future fertility potential of the woman. This has led to debate among obstetricians and gynaecologists, health care policy makers and service users to define strategies in order to reduce the rate of primary CSs. As a consequence, various strategies have been recommended to improve the antenatal and intrapartum care of women, to increase normal vaginal delivery rates, thus reducing the incidence of primary CS rates [3–7]. Most of these strategies are either quality improvement tools or audit and feedback processes [3]. One such approach, proposed by the World Health Organization [8], is to use the Robson classification (also known as the 10-group classification system (TGCS)) as an audit tool [9]. It helps to identify the groups of women who are responsible for the increasing CS rate the most (Table 1), so that corrective solutions could be put in place to reduce the CS rates.

It is well-known that nulliparous women are a special group in labour as they represent almost a half of all the deliveries. They have a greater risk of adverse outcomes during their delivery compared with multiparas [10]. On the other hand, the mode of delivery is of great importance, because it would influence on planning for a subsequent pregnancy and mode of delivery. It has been reported that women whose deliveries end by an operation have a risk of at least 50–60% of delivering by CS in a subsequent delivery [11]. Nulliparous women make up the first, the second and the sixth and might be a part of the eight, the ninth and the tenth

* Correspondence: jusbra@hotmail.com
[1]Lithuanian University of Health Sciences, Eiveniu str. 2, 50167 Kaunas, Lithuania
Full list of author information is available at the end of the article

Table 1 The 10-group classification system

No.	Group
Group 1	Nulliparous, single cephalic, 37 weeks, in spontaneous labour
Group 2A	Nulliparous, single cephalic, 37 weeks, induced labour
Group 2B	Nulliparous, single cephalic, 37 weeks, CS before labour
Group 3	Multiparous (excluding prev. CS), single cephalic, 37 weeks, in spontaneous labour
Group 4A	Multiparous (excluding prev. CS), single cephalic, 37 weeks, induced labour
Group 4B	Multiparous (excluding prev. CS), single cephalic, 37 weeks, CS before a labour
Group 5A	Previous CS, single cephalic, 37 weeks, induced labour
Group 5B	Previous CS, single cephalic, 37 weeks, CS before labour
Group 5C	Previous CS, single cephalic, 37 weeks, in spontaneous labour
Group 6	All nulliparous breeches
Group 7	All multiparous breeches (including prev. CS)
Group 8	All multiple pregnancies (including prev. CS)
Group 9	All abnormal lies (including prev. CS)
Group 10	All single cephalic, ≤ 36 weeks (including prev. CS)

groups according to the TGCS. But only groups 1 and 2 are not influenced by the number of foetuses, their presentation or gestation favourable to the caesarean section. Therefore, these important groups of patients should be studied carefully as regards conduct of labour and the interventions they had during labour.

The aim of this study was to evaluate the role of the implementation of the TGCS as a national audit intervention to reduce the CS rate among nulliparous women, with a singleton pregnancy, cephalic presentation at term pregnancy either in spontaneous or induced labour or had a planned elective CS (Robson groups 1 and 2). Our objective was to find out which group of women has reduced the CS rate by using the TGCS, which might be beneficial for other countries looking where to start from.

Methods

This paper presents results of one part of a multifaceted intervention that was performed in 2012–2016 in Lithuania. This intervention consisted of three parts:

- the implementation of the Robson classification nationally (2012–2014),
- a national educational course (2015) and
- an audit performed in some randomly selected hospitals (2016).

The Robson classification has been used for this two phase study (Table 1).

Before the national interventional study, the Lithuanian obstetricians and gynaecologists were made aware of the usefulness of the Robson classification as a quality improvement tool. However it had not been formally endorsed nationally and was not used in everyday practice. In 2011, the Lithuanian Society of Obstetricians and Gynaecologists (LSOG) organised a special meeting to which obstetricians and gynaecologists and the authorities of all Lithuanian hospitals were invited. The Caesarean Section Working Group of the LSOG revisited the principles of the TGCS and encouraged the participants of the meeting to classify the deliveries routinely. All the participants were invited to join the study and to send relevant data to the study coordinators.

The study spanned over two periods. During the first period (from January 1 to December 31 of 2012), in the vast majority of Lithuanian hospitals all the deliveries were classified by their clinicians and summary data were sent to the study investigators. Continuous assistance was provided by study investigators where difficulties in classifying a woman arose. In 2013 all the data from the hospitals were analysed and a conference was organised specifically for this project. The attendees of the conference included administrators of the participating hospitals, members of the LSOG, the Lithuanian Health Ministry and the members of the Lithuanian Parliament. During the conference, the overall CS rates and the CS rates in different groups according to the TGCS were assessed and compared between different hospitals [12]. This has led to a conclusion that the CS rate overall and in different groups of women is higher than recommended [11] and can be lowered. No specific recommendations or interventions were proposed and no special groups of women were singled out. Another purpose of the conference was to send a message to all hospitals that the CS rates were important at national level and they would be analysed in the future.

During the second period (from January 1 to December 31 of 2014), the classification of deliveries according to the Robson classification was recorded and the data were sent to the study investigators.

At the time of the study, there were 33 hospitals providing obstetrical care in Lithuania. The inclusion criteria for hospitals were: that there should be at least 300 deliveries per year before national intervention was conducted and no other programs dedicated to reduce the CS rate had to be performed during the intervention. On the whole, 26 hospitals admitted these inclusion criteria.

The maternity hospitals within Lithuania are currently categorized as follows:

Level IIA hospitals, which provide health care services to women with low-risk pregnancies and deliveries. In 2012, there were 25 level IIA hospitals with 9554 deliveries. The inclusion criteria were met by 18 of them;

Level IIB hospitals, which provide health care services to women with low- and high- (not requiring tertiary-level care, for example, a preterm delivery after 34 gestational weeks) risk pregnancies and deliveries. At the beginning of the study, there were 6 level IIB hospitals with 11,966 deliveries;

Level III hospitals, which provide health care services to women with pregnancies and deliveries of all risk levels. In 2012, there were 2 level III hospitals with 7157 deliveries in Lithuania.

The necessary number of hospitals for inclusion in the study was calculated according to the number of deliveries in them. It had to be sufficient to represent the national data overall and in each stratum (level IIA, level IIB and level III hospitals). Therefore, three level IIA hospitals (with 1635 deliveries in total in 2012 and 1604 in 2014), one level IIB hospital (with 3205 deliveries in 2012 and 3075 in 2014) and one level III hospital (with 3878 deliveries in 2012 and 3367 in 2014 were selected randomly for inclusion in the study.

For this study, all the data on nulliparas (groups 1 and 2 according to the TGCS) were collected from the selected hospitals by a single investigator (JK). Where mistakes were found in the records, all the deliveries were checked and reclassified according to the TGCS principles. Socio-demographic and selected personal data (living area, marital status, education and age) were gathered using hospital delivery records and the national database of the Lithuanian Hygiene Institute. Specific delivery-related data were collected from the case notes. Some case notes that were absent, illegible or had missed information directly related to the delivery (i.e. the presence or absence of augmentation, cervical dilatation at the moment when the decision to perform a CS because of dystocia was made etc.) were not included in a specific CS's analysis. Therefore, an imbalance between socio-demographic, personal and delivery-related data might appear.

Outcomes

The primary outcome was the overall CS rate. Secondary outcomes were delivery-related data (indications for CS, cervical dilatation at the moment of oxytocin administration, cervical dilatation at the moment of the decision to perform a CS because of dystocia, and waiting time passed before the decision to perform a CS because of dystocia) and newborn-related outcomes (birth weight, Apgar scores and perinatal mortality). Also, potential risk factors were also assessed – socio-demographic data (living area, education, and marital status), personal data (age, maternal diseases (all diseases that are not related to pregnancy,

i.e. eye, ear, pulmonary, cardiovascular, renal and other pathologies) as well as pregnancy-related conditions (i.e. gestational hypertensive disorders, gestational cholestasis, gestational diabetes etc.).

Based on the analysis of indications for CSs proposed by Robson et al. [13], *a new modified classification* of indications for CSs in nulliparas assigned to group 1 was developed. The main difference was that various conditions (i.e. umbilical cord prolapse after the spontaneous onset of labour, placental abruption etc.) were grouped within a separate group. For the vast majority of such deliveries CS is unavoidable. Therefore, no specific strategies can be created to manage such a delivery vaginally. The other reason for modifying the classification was different management of delivery itself: a different perception of latent and active phases, oxytocine dosage etc. A modified classification included whether variables such as augmentation with or without oxytocin, dilatation of the cervix (complete cervical dilatation (CCD) and incomplete cervical dilatation (< 10 cm) (ICD)), suspected fetal compromise (FC) and other conditions such as placental abruptions, umbilical cord prolapse, and elective CSs with the onset of spontaneous labour. The indications for CS in group 1 were classified as dystocia, FC and others.

Participants

All nulliparous women with a single cephalic, term pregnancy in spontaneous (group 1) or induced labour (group 2A) or an elective CS (group 2B) who gave birth at the selected hospitals during the study period. Nulliparous women without spontaneous labour and falling within groups 2A or 2B formed group 2.

Statistical analysis

The data were analysed using MS Excel and IBM SPSS Statistics 23.0 for Windows. There were 3 groups of hospitals which represented health care facilities providing obstetrical care of different levels. It was estimated that a minimum sample size of 1197 of all deliveries per each stratum would be needed to detect a 5% change in the CS rate with a power of 80% and a significance level of 5%. From these deliveries only nulliparous women falling within groups 1 and 2 according to the TGCS were selected and the outcomes of their deliveries in 2012 and 2014 were compared. The comparison of study groups was conducted using chi-squared test, and if assumptions for it were not met – the Fisher's exact test.

Results

There were 8718 and 8046 deliveries in 2012 and 2014, respectively. Nulliparas accounted for 43% (3746/8718) and 44.6% (3585/8046) of all the deliveries in those years, respectively. The socio-demographic and personal data are compared in Table 2. There were more women living in

Table 2 Socio-demographic and personal data

	2012	2014	p value
Living area			
urban, n (%)	3117 (83.2)	2886 (80.5)	p = 0.003
rural, n (%)	629 (16.8)	699 (19.5)	
Education			
basic, primary and secondary, n (%)	1749 (46.7)	1649 (46.0)	p = 0.552
higher, n (%)	1997 (53.3)	1936 (54.0)	
Marital status			
single, n (%)	1326 (35.4)	1089 (30.4)	p < 0.001
married, n (%)	2420 (64.6)	2496 (69.6)	
Age			
< 20, n (%)	1264 (33.7)	1142 (31.9)	p = 0.198
20–34, n (%)	2270 (60.6)	2224 (62.0)	
≥ 35, n (%)	212 (5.7)	219 (6.1)	
Maternal diseases, n (%)	155 (4.1)	124 (3.5)	p = 0.129

urban areas than in rural ($p = 0.003$) and married vs. single women ($p < 0.001$) in both years. The education, age and number of women with any maternal diseases did not differ between 2012 or 2014 (Table 2).

There were 96.8% (3626/3746) case notes available for analysis in 2012, as compared to 97.7% in 2014 (3502/3585). The CS rate among nulliparas decreased from 23.9% (866/3626) in 2012 to 19.0% (665/3502) in 2014 (p < 0.001) (Table 3).The greatest decrease in absolute contribution to the overall CS rate was recorded in groups 1 ($p = 0.005$) and 2B (p < 0.001) (Table 3).

The greatest contribution to the overall CS rate in group 1 was made by dystocia in both years (Table 4). The majority of operations in this group were performed in patients, who had their labour augmented with oxytocin irrespective the complete cervical dilatation was reached or not (Table 4). The peculiarities of dystocia in group 1 are presented in Table 5. The greatest reduction in the contribution to the overall CS rate

in group 1 was made by operations due to fetal compromise ($p = 0.002$) (Table 4).

The number of CSs in group 2 decreased from 51.8% (440/850) in 2012 to 40.5% (326/804) in 2014. The greatest decrease was seen in group 2B. The vast majority of them were performed because of maternal diseases, post-term pregnancy and fetus related conditions (Table 6).

The study did not reveal any change in perinatal mortality ($p = 0.764$). Among 3746 deliveries in 2012 and 3585 in 2014, it was 3.5 and 3.1 per 1000 deliveries, respectively (Table 7). The Apgar score after 5 min changed in 2014 ($p = 0.003$) mostly because of a decreased number of newborns with the Apgar score ≥ 9 points and an increased number of newborns with the Apgar score of 7–8 points.

Discussion

This study has shown that the implementation of the Robson classification has had a positive impact on the reduction of the CS rate among nulliparas in Lithuania. After the intervention, this rate has decreased by 4.9 pp. The greatest decrease was recorded in group 2B ($p < 0.001$) and group 1 ($p = 0.005$). Moreover, the highest reduction in the CS rate among nulliparas with spontaneous labour was due to the indication "fetal compromise" ($p = 0.002$). Despite the fact that the CS rate decreased, the perinatal morbidity did not change. A statistically significant difference in Apgar score in 5 min can be considered as clinically insignificant – the observed difference was mainly due to large sample size. A reduction of the CS rate after the implementation of the TGCS in clinical practice has been reported in other studies too [13–17]. Scarella et al. reported a 7% reduction (from 32.2 to 25.2%) in CSs among nulliparas who were assigned to group 1 or 2 in one Chilean regional health centre [14]. Despite the fact that this reduction was greater than the one recorded in the present study, it is important to mention that the starting rate in Chile was almost 10% higher, and after the intervention is still 6% higher, than the one recorded in our study. A reduction of more than 20% was reported in a

Table 3 The CS rate in 2012 and 2014

	Number of CS over total number of women in each group		Relative size of groups, %		CS rate in each group, %		p value	Absolute contribution to the overall CS rate, %		p value
	2012	2014	2012	2014	2012	2014		2012	2014	
Group 1	426/2776	340/2698	76.6 2776/3626	77.0 2698/3502	15.3	12.6	p = 0.003	11.7 426/3626	9.7 340/3502	p = 0.005
Group 2	440/850	326/804	23.4 850/3626	23.0 804/3502	51.8	40.5	p < 0.001	12.1 440/3626	9.3 326/3502	p < 0.001
Group 2A	236/646	220/698	17.8 646/3626	19.9 698/3502	36.5	31.5	p = 0.052	6.5 236/3626	6.3 220/3502	p = 0.697
Group 2B	204/204	106/106	5.6 204/3626	3.0 106/3502	100	100	–	5.6 204/3626	3.0 106/3502	p < 0.001
Group 1 and 2	866/3626	666/3502			23.9	19.0	p < 0.001			

Table 4 Indications for CS among women in group 1

Indication	Absolute contribution to the CS rate in group 1, %, 2012	Absolute contribution to the CS rate in group 1, %, 2014	p value	Absolute contribution to the overall CS rate, %, 2012	Absolute contribution to the overall CS rate, %, 2014	p value
FC (without oxytocin)	22.1 94/426	15.9 54/340	$p = 0.032$	2.6 94/3626	1.5 54/3502	$p = 0.002$
Dystocia	70.4 300/426	74.1 252/340	$p = 0.258$	8.3 300/3626	7.2 252/3502	$p = 0.089$
CCD without oxytocin	11.7 50/426	10.0 34/340	$p = 0.447$	1.4 50/3626	1.0 34/3502	$p = 0.11$
CCD with oxytocin	17.6 75/426	20.0 68/340	$p = 0.401$	2.1 75/3626	2.9 68/3502	$p = 0.704$
ICD without oxytocin	7.5 32/426	6.2 21/340	$p = 0.472$	0.9 32/3626	0.6 21/3502	$p = 0.165$
ICD with oxytocin	22.5 96/426	27.9 95/340	$p = 0.085$	2.6 96/3626	2.7 95/3502	$p = 0.865$
FC with oxytocin[a]	11 47/426	10.0 34/340	$p = 0.646$	1.3 47/3626	1.0 34/3502	$p = 0.194$
Others	7.5 32/426	10.0 34/340	$p = 0.222$	0.9 32/3626	1.0 34/3502	p = 0.697
Total				11.7 426/3626	9.7 340/3502	$p = 0.006$

[a]"FC with oxytocin" was attributed to "dystocia" because the reason why oxytocin was administered was dystocia

study from Brazil that was performed at one university hospital [17]. According to the authors of that study, the CS rate in groups 1 and 2 decreased from 34.6 to 13.5% in a 10-month period following the implementation of the Robson classification [17]. This is more than 4 times higher than in our study and could be explained by a very high initial CS rate. Svelato et al. and Blomberg have also reported a reduction in the CS rate after starting to use the TGCS [6, 15]. Yet, the interventions in their studies were multifactorial. They included not only the implementation of the Robson classification, but also the management of labour, interpretation of the cardiotocogram

Table 5 Peculiarities of deliveries when the indication for CS is "dystocia"

	2012	2014	p value
Dystocia: CCD with oxytocin			
Cervical dilatation at the moment of oxytocin administration, cm (mean, SD)	4.69 (2.11)	5.7 (2.21)	0.007
Waiting time passed before making the decision to perform a CS because of dystocia, min (mean, SD)	88.3 (31.55)	87.8 (38.7)	0.933
Dystocia: ICD with oxytocin			
Cervical dilatation at the moment of oxytocin administration, cm (mean, SD)	3.97 (2.16)	4.1 (2.24)	0.68
Cervical dilatation at the moment of the decision to perform a CS because of dystocia, cm (mean, SD)	5.39 (2.53)	5.38 (2.61)	0.991
Waiting time passed before the decision to perform CS because of dystocia, min (mean, SD)	171.3 (125.7)	217.21 (164.47)	0.033

(CTG) etc. [6, 15]. Svelato et al. analysed Robson groups 1–4 in one hospital in Italy. They reported a 6.9 pp. (17.2% to 10.3%) decrease in the CS rate in these groups after the intervention [15]. The target group of Blomberg consisted of nulliparas falling within group 1 according to the TGCS, who delivered in one tertiary level hospital in Sweden [6]. The CS rate in group 1 decreased from 10 to 3% after the study [6]. In addition to this, the CS rate in Robson groups 1 and 2 decreased by 10.5 pp. (from 17.5 to 7%), i.e. twice the decrease reported in our study [6]. It is well known that the CS rates in the Northern European countries are among the lowest [1]. This might be influenced by organizational and cultural differences in the management of deliveries. Despite the fact that the latter two studies describe multifactorial interventions, the impact of the Robson classification cannot be downplayed because the Hawthorne effect might be attributed to it [18]. This effect describes a change in an individual's behaviour after finding out about being observed. It was first noticed when performing experiments in one electricity company [18]. But it is still relevant nowadays and can explain why implementation of the TGCS is enough to work as an audit system and reduce the CS rates [12, 14].

The analysis in this study revealed that the number of CSs decreased the most after the reconsideration of the indications for elective CSs. A major change in the CS rate in group 2B owes to the reduction of the indication "post-term pregnancy". This could be explained by the fact that hospitals could postpone induction of the delivery or elective CS and wait for a spontaneous onset of labour. The other reason for CS is maternal

Table 6 Indications for operations in women with elective CSs

Indication	Absolute contribution to the CS rate in group 2B, %, 2012	Absolute contribution to the CS rate in group 2B, %, 2014	p value	Absolute contribution to the overall CS rate, %, 2012	Absolute contribution to the overall CS rate, %, 2014	p value
Placental and umbilical cord pathology	9.8 20/204	10.4 11/106	$p = 0.873$	0.6 20/3626	0.3 11/3502	$p = 0.129$
Fetus related conditions	16.2 33/204	11.3 12/106	$p = 0.25$	0.9 33/3626	0.3 12/3502	$p = 0.003$
Maternal diseases	48.0 96/204	49.0 52/106	$p = 0.741$	2.7 96/3626	1.5 52/3502	$p < 0.001$
Suspected fetal macrosomia	6.9 14/204	9.4 10/106	$p = 0.424$	0.4 14/3626	0.3 10/3502	$p = 0.465$
Preeclampsia	3.4 7/204	4.7 5/106	$p = 0.575$	0.2 7/3626	0.1 5/3502	$p = 0.603$
Post-term pregnancy	16.7 34/204	15.1 16/106	$p = 0.719$	0.9 34/3626	0.5 16/3502	$p = 0.015$
Total				5.6 204/3626	3.0 106/3502	$p < 0.001$

diseases. Despite the fact the number of women with identifiable maternal diseases did not differ statistically significantly between 2012 and 2014, fewer women were operated because of conditions related to eyes, ears, heart pathologies, previous cervical conisation etc. This means that indications for elective operative deliveries should be stricter in all hospitals and all cases should be discussed in a multi-disciplinary setting in case of uncertainty. The other reason for the reduced number of women in this group might be that some deliveries can be induced rather than ended by an elective CS. The relative size of group 2A increased in 2014, although without statistical significance. On the other hand, the CS rate in this group decreased. This might show that a greater number of induced deliveries were managed successfully.

Table 7 Newborn-related outcomes

Indicator	2012	2014	p value
Newborn weight			
< 3000 g, n (%)	476 (12.7)	429 (12.0)	$p = 0.482$
3000–3999 g, n (%)	2809 (75.0)	2691 (75.1)	
≥ 4000 g, n (%)	461 (12.3)	465 (13.0)	
Apgar score after 5 min			
< 7, n (%)	6 (0.2)	2 (0.1)	$p = 0.003$
7–8, n (%)	141 (3.8)	188 (5.2)	
≥ 9, n (%)	3599 (96.1)	3395 (94.7)	
Perinatal mortality			
antepartum deaths, n	10	7	$p = 0.764$
intrapartum deaths, n	1	0	
not defined, n	–	–	
early neonatal deaths, n	2	4	
perinatal mortality	3.5/1000	3.1/1000	$p = 0.764$

The decrease in the CS rate among nulliparas with spontaneous labour owes mainly to FC managed without oxytocin. This might be explained by two reasons. The first one is that the initial numbers were very high. Our study has revealed that these numbers were more than double the one reported by Robson et al. [12]. The other reason that could explain a significant decrease in CSs in this group is better evaluation of the CTG resulting from the Hawthorne effect. It is possible that changes in the CTG in a woman without oxytocin were attributed to insignificant changes and this was different as it was prior to the intervention phase. It is important to emphasize that newborn-related data and perinatal mortality did not change as our sample size was not calculated to assess these outcome parameters.

The vast majority of operations among nulliparas with spontaneous labour were performed because of dystocia. This outcome correlates with other studies [12]. A more detailed analysis has revealed that operations in this group were mostly performed on women who were treated with oxytocin and irrespective of whether they reached a full dilatation of the cervix or not. A high number of operations in women with full cervical dilatation could be explained by an insufficient waiting time for delivery of the fetus. According to the national guidelines that were developed based on international recommendations, a normal duration of the second stage of delivery in nulliparas is about 2 h [19]. In case of epidural analgesia it is about 3 h [19]. Our study has shown that the mean duration of waiting is approximately 1.5 h. This duration is less than recommended in the national guideline. Therefore, if the number of women in this group increase but the length of second stage is not adhered to national guidance, then an increased number of women will have operative deliveries in the future too.

Strengths and limitations

The strengths of the study are the following: all the data were checked and gathered by the same single study investigator, JK. This have led to an equal classification of all the deliveries; the study represents national data; this study introduces a new classification (based on Robson proposed classification of indications for CSs of intrapartum caesarean sections. This enables us to analyse and compare not only the number of CSs but also the reasons for them.

The limitation of the study is that not all case notes were available for analysis and no maternal outcomes are analysed and discussed.

Conclusions

This two phase study in Lithuania has demonstrated that TGCS can work as an audit intervention that could help to reduce the CS rate without a negative influence on perinatal mortality. This system had the greatest impact on nulliparas for whom an elective CS was planned or those with suspected fetal compromise.

Abbreviations

CCD: Complete cervical dilatation; CS: Caesarean section; CTG: Cardiotocogram; FC: Fetal compromise; ICD: Incomplete cervical dilatation; LSOG: Lithuanian society of obstetricians and gynecologists; TGCS: The 10-group classification system

Authors' contributions

JK, EB and MM were involved in study design, acquisition, analysis and interpretation of data, and drafting of the article. TM and RN were involved in drafting of the article. KS was involved in study data analysis. DRR, AB, MK, KM, GD and DR were involved in critical revision of the article. All authors approved the final version for publication.

Competing interests

The authors declare that they have no competing interests.

Author details

[1]Lithuanian University of Health Sciences, Eiveniu str. 2, 50167 Kaunas, Lithuania. [2]Victoria Hospital, Kirkcaldy, Fife KY2 5AH, Scotland, UK. [3]Vilnius Maternity Hospital, Tyzenhauzu str. 18A, 02106 Vilnius, Lithuania. [4]Vilnius University Hospital Santaros Klinikos, Santariskiu str. 2, 08661 Vilnius, Lithuania.

References

1. World Health Statistics Available from: http://www.who.int/gho/publications/world_health_statistics/en/
2. Medical data of births 2011 Vilnius: institute of hygiene health information Centre; 2012. Availabe from: http://www.hi.lt.
3. Chaillet N, Dumont A. Evidence-based strategies for reducing cesarean section rates: a meta-analysis. Birth. 2007;34(1):53–64.
4. Le Ray C, Blondel B, Prunet C, Khireddine I, Deneux-Tharaux C, Goffinet F. Stabilising the caesarean rate: which target population? BJOG. 2015;122(5):690–9.
5. Hartmann KE, Andrews JC, Jerome RN, Lewis RM, Likis FE, McKoy JN, et al. Strategies to Reduce Cesarean Birth in Low-Risk Women. Rockville (MD): Agency for Healthcare Research and Quality; 2012.
6. Blomberg M. Avoiding the first cesarean section-results of structured organizational and cultural changes. Acta Obstet Gynecol Scand. 2016;95(5):580–6.
7. Boatin AA, Cullinane F, Torloni MR, Betrán AP. Audit and feedback using the Robson classification to reduce caesarean section rates: a systematic review. BJOG. 2018;125(1):36–42.
8. Betran AP, Torloni MR, Zhanh JJ, Gulmezoglu AM. for the WHO working group on caesarean section. WHO statement on caesarean section rates. BJOG. 2016;123:667–70.
9. Robson M. Classification of caesarean sections. Fetal Maternal Med Rev. 2001;12:23–39.
10. Jackson S, Gregory KD. Management of the first stage of labor: potential strategies to lower the cesarean delivery rate. Clin Obstet Gynecol. 2015;58(2):217–26.
11. Robson M, Hartigan L, Murphy M. Methods of achieving and maintaining an appropriate caesarean section rate. Best Pract Res Clin Obstet Gynaecol. 2013;27(2):297–308.
12. Kacerauskiene J, Bartuseviciene E, Railaite DR, Minkauskiene M, Bartusevicius A, Kliucinskas M, et al. Implementation of the Robson classification in clinical practice: Lithuania's experience. BMC Pregnancy Childbirth. 2017;17:432.
13. Robson M, Murphy M, Byrne F. Quality assurance: the 10- group classification system (Robson classification), induction of labor, and caesarean delivery. Int J Gynaecol Obstet. 2015;131(Suppl 1):S23–7.
14. Scarella A, Chamy V, Sepúlveda M, Belizán JM. Medical audit using the ten Group classification system and its impact on the cesarean section rate. EurJ Obstet Gynecol Reprod Biol. 2011;154(2):136–40.
15. Svelato A, Meroni MG, Poli M, Perino A, Spinoso R, Ragusa A. How to reduce caesarean sections in first four Robson's classes. BJOG. 2014;121:91.
16. Piffer S, Pederzini F, Tenaglia F, Paoli A, Nicolodi F, Luewink A. The Robson ten group classification of cesarean section in 7 alpine maternity units in an homogenous area. Eur J Epidemiol. 2012;27:S122–3.
17. Aguiar RAP, Gaspar J, Reis ZSN, Santos MR Jr, Correa MD Jr. Implementation of the Caesarean Births Review using the ten group Robson's classification and its immediate effects on the rate of caesareans, at a university hospital. Poster presented at the international congress Birth: Clinical Challenges in Labor and Delivery. Fortaleza: BJOG; 2015. p. p21.
18. Roethlisberger FJ, Dickson W, Wright H. Management and the worker: an account of a research program conducted by the western electric company, Hawthorne works Chicago. Cambridge: Harvard University Press; 1939.
19. Guidelines and protocols of diagnostics and treatment in obstetrics and neonatology [Internet]. Lithuanian Ministry of Health 2014. Available from: https://sam.lrv.lt/lt/veiklos-sritys/programos-ir-projektai/sveicarijos-paramos-programa/akuserijos-ir-neonatologijos-diagnostikos-ir-gydymo-metodikos/akuserijos-diagnostikos-ir-gydymo-metodikos.

8

Socioeconomic and demographic factors associated with caesarean section delivery in Southern Ghana: evidence from INDEPTH Network member site

Alfred Kwesi Manyeh[1,2]* (iD), Alberta Amu[1,3], David Etsey Akpakli[1,3], John Williams[1,3] and Margarete Gyapong[1,4]

Abstract

Background: In recent years, caesarean section rates continue to evoke worldwide concern because of their steady increase, lack of consensus on the appropriate caesarean section rate and the associated short- and long-term risks. This study sought to identify the rate of caesarean section and associated factors in two districts in rural southern Ghana.

Methods: Pregnancy, birth, and socio-demographic information of 4948 women who gave birth between 2011 and 2013 were obtained from the database of Dodowa Health and Demographic Surveillance System. The rate of C-section was determined and the associations between independent and dependent variables were explored using logistic regression. The analyses were done in STATA 14.2 at 95% confidence interval.

Results: The overall C-section rate for the study period was 6.59%. Women aged 30–34 years were more than twice likely to have C-section compared to those < 20 year (OR: 2.16, 95% CI: 1.20–3.90). However, women aged 34 years and above were more than thrice likely to undergo C-section compared to those < 20 year (OR: 3.73, 95% CI: 1.45–5.17). The odds of having C-section was 65 and 79% higher for participants with Primary and Junior High level schooling respectively (OR: 1.65, 95% CI: 1.08–2.51, OR:1.79, 95%CI: 1.19–2.70). The likelihood of having C-section delivery reduced by 60, 37, and 35% for women with parities 2, 3 and 3+ respectively (OR:0.60, 95% CI: 0.43–0.83, OR: 0.37, 95% CI: 0.25–0.56, OR:0.35, 95% CI: 0.25–0.54). There were increased odds of 36, 52, 83% for women who belong to poorer, middle, and richer wealth quintiles respectively (OR: 1.36, 95%CI: 0.85–2.18, OR: 1.52, 95% CI: 0.97–2.37, OR: 1.83, 95% CI: 1.20–2.80). Participants who belonged to the richest wealth quintile were more than 2 times more likely to have C-section delivery (OR: 2.14, 95%CI: 1.43–3.20). The odds of having C-section delivery reduced by 76% for women from Ningo-Prampram district (OR: 0.76, 95% CI: 0.59.0.96). Women whose household heads have Junior High level and above of education were 45% more likely to have C-section delivery (OR: 1.45, 95% CI: 1.09–1.93).

Conclusion: Age of mother, educational level, parity, household socioeconomic status, district of residence, and level of education of household head are associated with caesarean section delivery.

Keywords: Caesarean section, INDEPTH network, Dodowa, Ghana

* Correspondence: alfredmanyeh4u@gmail.com
[1]Dodowa Health Research Centre, P. O. Box. DD1, Dodowa, Accra, Ghana
[2]Division of Epidemiology and Biostatistics, School of Public Health,
University of the Witwatersrand, Parktown, Johannesburg, South Africa
Full list of author information is available at the end of the article

Background

Accessibility of comprehensive emergency obstetric care (including caesarean section) is crucial to averting the estimated 2.9 million neonatal and 287,000 maternal mortalities that occur worldwide every year [1, 2].

Caesarean section (C-section), is one of the oldest and regularly used surgical procedures in Obstetrics by which fetus is delivered through an abdominal and uterine incision [3–5]. It has been shown that, when C-section is appropriately used, it can improve both infant and maternal health outcomes [6, 7]. According to the World Health Organization (WHO), C-section is a vital treatment in pregnancy [8]. However, the potential risk of C-section may outweigh the benefits when it is used inappropriately [6, 7].

In recent years, the number of C-section deliveries has been increasing in developed and developing countries [9–11]. This increase has however not been clinically justified. This worldwide increase in C-section has become a major public health issue due to potential maternal and perinatal risks, inequality of access and cost involved [12–17]. According to the WHO guidelines, no region is justified for having the rate of C-section more than 10–15% [6, 18]. Despite this WHO guidelines, studies show that the rates of C-sections are high in developing countries [17, 19, 20]. A WHO reports shows that, the global average of C-section rate between 1990 and 2014 increased from 12.4 to 18.6% [21]. While the C-sections rate varies between 12 and 86% across studies done in developed countries [22–25] that of developing countries ranges between 2 and 39% [8, 22, 26–29]. This again shows the cause for concern and hence the need to explore the reasons for the increasing rates in C-section delivery [6, 18].

Although there is no evidence of benefits of C-section to mothers or babies who do not need it [30], however, C-section like any surgery, has complications which may persist for a long period after the current delivery and affect the health of the woman, her child, and future pregnancies. According to literature, the global increase in C-section is associated with uterine rupture such that, women with prior who undergo the procedure are more likely to have uterine rupture in future pregnancies [31–35]. The risk of uterine rupture due to prior C-section are higher in population with limited access to comprehensive obstetric care [17, 36, 37].

Studies have attribute the increase in C-sections to multiple factors ranging from the type of health facility, socio-demographic characteristics to maternal health of women [38–43]. These factors include maternal age [38–40], birth order [44], birth weight [45], place of residence [14], socioeconomic status, maternal educational level [38, 46–48], former C-section [41–43], obstetric complications [49], maternal request [50], and income level [38, 48]. These factors also vary among different populations [16].

The global increase in the rate of the provision of C-section is reflected in Ghana. According to the 2014 Ghana Demographic and Health Survey (GDHS) survey, the C-section rate in Ghana increased from 4.5 to 6.4% between 1990 and 2005 [51]. In 2014, the GDHS reported that 13% of births are delivered by C-section, an increase from 7% in 2008 [52]. Delivery by C-section is highest among births to women aged 35–49 (17%); first-parity births (18%); births for whom women had more than three Antenatal Care (ANC) attendance (15%); deliveries in urban areas (19%) and in the Greater Accra region (23%); births to women with secondary school level and above education (27%), and those with richest socioeconomic status (28%) [52].

Primary C-section usually determines the future obstetric course of any woman [53]. Hence there is a need to assess the rate of C-sections and factors contributing to C-section delivery in the context of Ghana using population based data. The existence of a Health and Demographic Surveillance System provided a unique opportunity to study the factors contributing to C-section delivery at the population level. This is because most studies on C-section used hospital based data which were subject to selection bias. The study of determinants of C-section in a population makes it possible to explore how different elements contribute to the decision to perform a C-section. Therefore, this study aimed to examine the rate of C-section delivery and to explore factors associated with the procedure in two rural districts in Ghana.

Methods

Study area

This study used secondary data from the Dodowa Health and Demographic Surveillance System (DHDSS). The DHDSS site is in the Shai-Osudoku and Ningo-Prampram districts of the Greater Accra Region of Ghana. The two districts together have a total population of 115, 754 people in 380 communities living in 23, 647 households. A detailed description of the DHDSS and its operations can be found elsewhere [54–56]. Health care service delivery in the DHDSS is provided from government hospitals, health centres, clinics, community-based health and planning services (CHPS) compounds/zones, and non-governmental health facilities [54].

Study population

All mothers who were resident in study area and had a delivery between January 1, 2011 to December 31, 2013 were included in the study. Therefore, all mothers who were outside the study area and those who delivered outside the study date were excluded. A total of 4, 948 women were included in the study.

Variables

Dependent variable

The dependent variable is type of delivery and it was dichotomous (coded as 1 if the respondents underwent C-section delivery and 0 if otherwise).

Table 1 Socio-Demographic Characteristics of the study participants

Age group	Frequency[a]	Percentage
< 20	552	11.16
20–24	1151	23.26
25–29	1288	26.03
30–34	1061	21.44
34 +	896	18.11
Mean = 28.01 (SD = 7.06)		
Occupation		
Unemployed	1125	22.74
Farmer	855	17.28
Artisan	608	12.29
Trader	1508	30.48
Civil Servant	84	1.7
Student	669	13.52
Others	99	2
Level of education		
No Education	1333	26.94
Primary	1502	30.36
JHS /Middle school	1691	34.18
SHS and above	422	8.53
Marital status		
Single	1325	27.2
Married	1010	20.73
Separated/Divorced	99	2.03
Cohabiting	2437	50.03
Parity		
Parity 1	1315	26.58
Parity 2	1183	23.91
Parity 3	940	19
Parity 3+	1510	30.52
Timing of ANC visit		
First trimester	2732	55.21
Second trimester	1980	40.02
Third trimester	236	4.77
Type of delivery		
Normal delivery	4621	93.41
C-Section delivery	326	6.59
Child weight at birth		
Low birth weight	232	4.69
Normal birth weight	2760	55.78
Not Weighed	1956	39.53
Delivery place		
Health Facility	3359	67.98
Outside Health Facility	1582	32.02

Table 1 Socio-Demographic Characteristics of the study participants (Continued)

Age group	Frequency[a]	Percentage
Child gender		
Female	2332	47.13
Male	2616	52.87
Household heads education		
No education/Primary	2614	52.83
JHS and above	2334	47.17
Household heads gender		
Female	1893	38.26
Male	3055	61.74
District of residence		
Shai-Osudoku	2165	43.76
Ningo-Prampram	2783	56.24

n = 4948; SD Standard Deviation; [a]due to missing data, the number of participants is may not be 4948 in all categories

Independent variables

From available data, the exposure variables included are maternal age, educational level, marital status, parity, timing of ANC visit, place of delivery, child gender and weight at birth, educational level of household head, district of residence and socio-economic status.

The socio-economic status is calculated using the household's social status, ownership of assets, availability of utilities among others using weights derived through a principal component analysis (PCA) [57]. The socio-economic status is a proxy measure of a household's long term standard of living [54]. The proxies from the PCA were divided into five quintiles; poorest, poorer, middle, richer and richest.

Statistical methods

A descriptive analysis of socio-demographic characteristics of the participants was carried out. The associations between the exposure variables and the outcome of interest were explored in a crude and adjusted ordered logistics regression model. The exposure variables that were significant at $p < 0.05$ in the crude model were entered together into an adjusted model. Stata version 14.2 was used for the analysis and the findings were presented in tables with summary statistics at 95% confidence intervals (CI).

Results

Socio-demographic characteristics

Table 1 presents the socio-demographic characteristics of 4948 study participants. The mean age of the study participants was 28 years (SD = 7.06).

While teenagers (< 20 years) contributed the least proportion of the study participants (11.16%), the 25–29 age group formed the highest proportion (26.03%) followed by the 20–24 and the 30–34 years' groups which accounted for 23.26 and 21.44% respectively.

While 30.48% of the study participants were petty traders, 22.74 and 17.28% were unemployed and farmers respectively. Students formed 13.52% of the study participants. Mothers with Junior high school and primary school level contributed 34.18 and 30.36% respectively.

Participants without formal education accounted for 26.94% of the study's participants. A large proportion of the study participants had their marital status as cohabiting (50.03%) while those married, single, and separated /widowed were 20.73, 27.20, and 2.03% respectively.

Participants with parity 3 or more formed 30.52% of participants while those with parity 1 and 2 were 26.56, and 23.91% respectively.

More than half (55.21%) of the study respondents started ANC visit in the first trimester of gestation. Respondents who initiated ANC attendance in the second and third trimesters formed 40.02 and 4.77% of the sample respectively.

The overall C-section delivery rate for the study period was 6.59%. The C-section rate for Shai-Osoduku District was 7.81% and that of Ningo-Prampram was 5.64%%.

The result of this study shows that 55.78% of the babies were of normal weight. Majority (67.98%) of the study participants delivered in a health facility.

Greater proportion of the babies born (52.87%) were males. More than half (52.83%) of the household heads have no education or primary level of education. As much as 56.24% of the participants were from the Ningo-Prampram district while 43.76% were from Shai-Osoduku district.

Crude and adjusted odds ratio of determinants of C-section delivery

Table 2 presents the crude and adjusted Odds Ratio (OR) at 95% Confidence Interval (CI) of socioeconomic and demographic factors associated with C-section delivery in Dodowa Health and Demographic Surveillance site.

In the crude model, there was a statistically significant association between maternal age and C-section delivery.

The odds of having C-section delivery by women aged 20–24 and 25–29 years is 6 and 43% respectively more likely compared to those aged < 20 years (OR: 1.06, 95% CI: 0.66–1.70, OR: 1.43, 95% CI: 0.91–2.24). Women aged 30–34 and 34+ years were 81 and 74% respectively more likely to have C-section delivery compared to those aged < 20 years (OR; 1.80, 95% CI: 1.15–2.84, OR:1.74, 95% CI: 1.10–2.77). This is statistically significant.

A similar relationship is observed after adjusting other explanatory variables such that, the odds of having C-section went up with increasing maternal age. Women aged 30–34 and 34+ years were more than twice and thrice more likely respectively to have C-section compared to those aged < 20 years (OR:2.16, 95% CI: 1.20–3.90, OR: 3.73, 95% CI: 1.45–5.17). This was statistically significant.

The results further revealed that, the odds of women having C-section delivery went up with increasing level of education in both the crude and adjusted models. In the crude model, odds of women with primary level of formal education having C-section delivery was 75% higher compared to those with no education (OR:1.75, 95% CI: 1.18–2.59). The odds of women with Junior High School (JHS) level of education having C-section delivery as compared to those with no education is almost three times more likely (OR: 2.79, 95% CI: 1.93–4.01). Again, the odds of participants with Senior High level of schooling having C-section delivery was eight times more likely compared to those with no formal education (OR: 7.88, 95% CI: 5.28–11.76).

Holding other variables constant, the odds of having C-section was 65 and 79% higher for participants with Primary and JHS level of schooling respectively compared to those with no education (OR: 1.65, 95%CI: 1.08–2.51, OR:1.79, 95% CI: 1.19–2.70).

In the crude logistics regression model, maternal occupation was statistically significantly associated with C-section. Women who are artisans were more than twice more likely to have C-section compared to those unemployed (OR: 2.37, 95% CI: 1.63–3.44). This was also statistically significant. Women who were civil servants and women who were engaged in other forms of occupation were more than three and two times more likely to undergo C-sections compared with those who were unemployed (OR: 3.56, 95% CI: 1.86–6.83, OR:2.43, 95% CI:1.23–4.81). This is also statistically significant.

Women who were married were 64% more likely to have C-section delivery (OR: 1.64, 95% CI: 1.21–2.22) compared to those who are single. This again was statistically significant. For participants with marital status as separated/divorced and cohabiting, the odds of having a C-section reduced to 96 and 84% respectively compared to those who were single (OR: 0.96, 95% CI: 0.41–2.27, OR:0.84, 95% CI: 0.63–1.11). In the adjusted model, participants who were married had increased odds of 26% of having C-section delivery compared to those who were single (OR: 1.26, 95% CI: 0.85–1.85).

In the crude model, study participants who started ANC visit in the second and third trimesters were 67 and 15% respectively less likely to have a C-section compared with those who started their ANC visit in the first trimester (OR: 0.67, 95% CI: 0.52–0.85, OR: 0.15, 95% CI: 0.05–0.68). After adjusting other explanatory variables, women who started ANC visit in the third trimester were 24% less likely to have C-section compared

Table 2 Crude and adjusted odd ratios of determinates of C-section delivery

Variable	Crude		Adjusted[b]	
	Odd Ratio (95% CI)	P-value	Odd Ratio (95% CI)	P-value
Age group				
< 20	1.00		1.00	
20–24	1.06 (0.66–1.70)	0.825	1.05 (0.64–1.74)	0.839
25–29	1.43 (0.91–2.24)	0.121	1.42 (0.83–2.43)	0.202
30–34	1.81 (1.15–2.84)[a]	0.010	2.16 (1.20–3.90)[a]	0.010
34 +	1.74 (1.10–2.77)[a]	0.019	3.73 (1.45–5.17)[a]	0.002
Level of Education				
No Education	1.00		1.00	
Primary	1.75 (1.18–2.59)[a]	0.006	1.65 (1.08–2.51)[a]	0.019
Junior High school	2.79 (1.93–4.01)[a]	< 0.001	1.79 (1.19–2.70)[a]	0.005
Senior High School and above	7.88 (5.28–11.76)[a]	< 0.001	3.53 (2.17–5.73)[a]	< 0.001
Occupation				
Unemployed	1.00		1.00	
Farmer	1.08 (0.72–1.62)	0.706	1.01 (0.71–1.71)	0.678
Artisan	2.37 (1.63–3.44)[a]	< 0.001	1.48 (0.99–2.20)	0.055
Trader	1.28 (0.91–1.80)	0.159	1.36 (0.95–1.95)	0.095
Civil Servant	3.56 (1.86–6.83)[a]	< 0.001	0.78 (0.38–1.59)	0.496
Student	1.34 (0.89–2.02)	0.159	1.26 (0.77–2.05)	0.363
Others	2.43 (1.23–4.81)[a]	0.011	2.31 (1.10–4.85)[a]	0.026
Marital Status				
Single	1.00		1.00	
Married	1.64 (1.21–2.22)[a]	0.001	1.26 (0.851–1.85)	0.247
Separated/Divorced	0.96 (0.41–2.27)	0.932	1.00 (0.37–2.27)	0.856
Cohabiting	0.84 (0.63–1.11)	0.224	0.94 (0.66–1.32)	0.705
Parity				
Parity 1	1.00		1.00	
Parity 2	0.74 (0.55–0.99)[a]	0.045	0.60 (0.43–0.83)[a]	0.002
Parity 3	0.57 (0.41–0.80)[a]	0.001	0.37 (0.25–0.56)[a]	< 0.001
Parity 3+	0.51 (0.37–0.68)[a]	< 0.001	0.35 (0.23–0.54)[a]	< 0.001
Timing of ANC visit				
First trimester	1.00		1.00	
Second trimester	0.67 (0.52–0.85)[a]	< 0.001	0.81 (0.63–1.05)	0.106
Third trimester	0.15 (0.05–0.47)[a]	< 0.001	0.24 (0.07–0.76)[a]	0.015
Socio Economic Status				
Poorest	1.00		1.00	
Poorer	1.12 (0.71–1.77)	0.627	1.36 (0.85–2.18)	0.205
Middle	1.44 (0.93–2.23)	0.099	1.52 (0.97–2.37)	0.069
Richer	2.15 (1.43–3.23)[a]	< 0.001	1.83 (1.20–2.80)[a]	0.005
Richest	3.84 (2.62–5.63)[a]	< 0.001	2.14 (1.43–3.20)[a]	< 0.001
District of residence				
Shai-Osudoku	1.00		1.00	
Ningo-Prampram	0.71 (0.56–0.88)[a]	0.002	0.76 (0.59–0.96)[a]	0.024

Table 2 Crude and adjusted odd ratios of determinates of C-section delivery *(Continued)*

Variable	Crude		Adjusted[b]	
	Odd Ratio (95% CI)	*P*-value	Odd Ratio (95% CI)	*P*-value
Household heads education				
No education/Primary	1.00		1.00	
Junior High School and above	2.65 (2.08–3.38)[a]	< 0.001	1.45 (1.09–1.93)[a]	0.010
Household heads gender				
Female	1.00		1.00	
Male	1.29 (1.01–1.64)	0.038		
Child weight at birth				
Low birth weight	1.00			
Normal birth weight	0.80 (0.48–1.34)	0.404		
Child Gender				
Female	1.00			
Male	1.12 (0.89–1.41)	0.32		

SD standard deviation, [a]statistical significant, [b]Correct classification rate = 93.41%

to those who initiated their ANC visit in the first trimester of pregnancy. This was statistically significant (OR: 0.24, 95% CI: 0.07–0.76).

The odds of having C-section delivery reduced significantly with increasing parity. There was reduced odds of 74, 57 and 51% of women with parities 2, 3 and 3+ respectively having C-section delivery compared to those with parity 1 (OR: 0.74, 95% CI: 0.55–0.99, OR: 0.57, 95% CI: 0.41–0.80, OR:0.51, 95% CI: 0.37–0.68). In the adjusted model, a similar relationship was observed such that the odds of having C-section delivery reduced with increasing parity. Thus, there was reduced odds of 60, 37, and 35% for women with parities 2, 3 and 3+ respectively compared with those with parity 1(OR:0.60, 95% CI: 0.43–0.83, OR: 0.37, 95% CI: 0.25–0.56, OR:0.35, 95% CI: 0.25–0.54).

The odds of having C-section went up with increasing socioeconomic status. In the crude analysis, participants with middle wealth quintile were 44% more likely to have C-section (OR: 1.44, 95%CI:0.93–2.23) compared to those in the poorest group. Participants who belong to the richer and richest quintiles were more than two times and three times more likely to have C-section delivery compared to those who belong to the poorest group (OR: 2.15, 95% CI: 1.43–3.23, OR: 3.84, 955 CI: 2.62–5.63). Participants' socioeconomic status continued to be increasingly significantly associated with C-section delivery after adjusting other confounding variables in the adjusted model. There were increased odds of 36, 52, 83% for women who belong to poorer, middle, and richer wealth quintiles respectively (OR: 1.36, 95% CI: 0.85–2.18, OR: 1.52, 95% CI: 0.97–2.37, OR: 1.83, 95% CI: 1.20–2.80). Participants who belong to the richest wealth quintile were more than two times more likely to have C-section delivery compared to those who were in the poorest category (OR: 2.14, 95% CI: 1.43–3.20).

The district where participant resides was significantly associated with C-section delivery such that, there was reduced odds of 71 and 76% in the crude and adjusted models respectively for women from Ningo-Prampram district compared to those from Shai-Osudoku district (OR:0.71, 95% CI: 0.56–0.88, OR:0.76, 95% CI: 0.59.0.96).

While there were increased odds of participants giving birth to male babies having C-section delivery (OR: 1.12, 95%CI: 0.89–1.41) compared to those with female babies, there was reduced odds of 80% of having C-section for participants who gave birth to normal weight babies in the crude model (OR: 0.80, 95% CI: 0.48–1.34) compared to those with low birth weight.

There was a statistically significant association between the level of education of household head and C-section such that participants whose household heads have JHS or more education were more than two times more likely to have C-section in the crude model (OR: 2.65, 95% CI: 2.08–3.38) compared to those whose heads had primary/no formal education. In the adjusted model, women whose household heads had JHS and above level of formal education were 45% more likely to have C-section delivery compared to those with primary / no formal education (OR: 1.45, 95% CI: 1.09–1.93).

Discussion

Despite the relevance and worldwide interest in this topic, this is the first study in Ghana to have used population based data at the district level to identify the rate and explore factors associated with C-section delivery. Our analysis of data from 4948 research participants revealed that C-section delivery is associated with maternal age, level of education, occupation, parity and ANC visit. The study also showed that other variables associated with C-section delivery include socioeconomic status, district of residence and level of education of household head.

The overall C-section rate of 7% found by the current study is lower than the national rate of 13% reported in 2014 by GHDS [52]. The current C-section rate is also lower than the WHO recommended rate of 10–15% [6, 18]. It is however similar to the 7.3% reported by Betrán AP et al. for Africa [58] and higher than the 3% estimated for Western Africa [58].

The findings of our study is consistent with the results of previous studies such that factors such as level of education of women, socio-economic status [38, 46–48, 59, 60], maternal occupation status [33], maternal age [38–40, 52, 59, 61], parity [44, 59], place of residence [14], and level of education of household head [60] are associated with C-section delivery.

The findings of our study also confirmed the results of GHDS 2014 which suggested that C-section delivery is associated with advanced maternal age (35–49 years), order of births (parity), ANC visit, maternal level of education, and socioeconomic status [52]. The relationship between advanced maternal age and some adverse pregnancy outcomes and higher risk of medical conditions like hypertension and diabetes as shown by other studies [60, 62] could explain why increasing maternal age was associated with the increased odds of having C-section delivery in our study.

The lower likelihood of C-section delivery among study participants with increasing parity could mean that many women with three caesarean sections do not get pregnant again to avoid further C-section delivery as established by Nilsen C et al. [63]. This could also be due to the fact that once the woman's pelvis has been tested with a previous pregnancy and delivery, subsequent deliveries tend to be less risky until she reaches her fifth delivery (grand-multipara) when the risk increases again as shown in a previous study [64].

The likelihood of mothers in Shai-Osudoku district having C-section delivery as compared to those from Ningo-Prampram district could be explained by the availability of a district hospital in Shai- Osudoku and three other referral hospital in districts that share boundary with Shai-Osudoku district, therefore providing more ready access to C-sections. This finding corroborates results of other studies which suggest that C-section delivery is associated with availability of and access to a medical facility [65–67].

Strengths and limitations

The strengths of this study were its data quality and large sample size. Also, being a community based study with focus on rural communities which are priority for public health interventions was a strength of the study. This notwithstanding, the study had a few limitations.

The secondary data used did not include other important variables on maternal health status, evidence of whether the earlier delivery was by caesarean and fetal characteristics that may influence the risk of C-section. The data used was also not a nationally representative one. This is because the two districts cannot be true representative of 216 districts in Ghana hence the limit in the generalizability of the findings.

Conclusion

The study established that the overall C-section rate in DHDSS site is 6.59%. The findings reinforce the evidence that the odds of having C-section delivery increases with advancing maternal age, level of education and household socioeconomic status. Parity, district of residence, and level of education of household head are other variables that are associated with C-section delivery. To understand other factors influencing C-section delivery and to design an appropriate intervention, we recommend further qualitative research in this area.

Abbreviations
ANC: Antenatal Care; CHPS: Community-based Health Planning and Services; CI: Confidence Intervals; DHDSS: Dodowa Health and Demographic Surveillance System; DHRC: Dodowa Health Research Centre; EOC: Emergency Obstetric Care; GDHS: Ghana Demographic Health Survey; JHS: Junior High school; MDG: Millennium Development Goal; OR: Odd Ratio; PCA: Principal component analysis

Acknowledgments
We want thank the study participants, data collectors, and supervisors involved in the work of the DHDSS. We sincerely thank all staff members of DHRC for their contributions to the HDSS and to this study. We would like to extend our special thanks to Professor Margaret Gyapong for always finding the resources to run the HDSS, for her mentorship and advice to the direction of this paper.

Authors' contributions
AKM conceptualized the paper, participated in the study design, conducted the statistical analysis, and led the writing of the paper. AA and DEA contributed intellectual content and insights and contributed to the writing of the manuscript. JW and MG refined the initial study design and critically reviewed the manuscript. All authors read and approved the manuscript.

Competing interests
The authors declare that they have no competing interests.

Author details

[1]Dodowa Health Research Centre, P. O. Box. DD1, Dodowa, Accra, Ghana. [2]Division of Epidemiology and Biostatistics, School of Public Health, University of the Witwatersrand, Parktown, Johannesburg, South Africa. [3]Ghana Health Service, Accra, Ghana. [4]Centre for Health Policy and Implementation Research, Institute for Health Research, University of Health and Allied Sciences, Volta Region, Ho, Ghana.

References

1. Neuman MAG, Azad K, et al. Prevalence and determinants of caesarean section in private and public health facilities in underserved south Asian communities: cross-sectional analysis of data from Bangladesh, India and Nepal. BMJ Open. 2014;4:e005982.
2. Campbell OM, Graham WJ. Strategies for reducing maternal mortality: getting on with what works. Lancet. 2006;368:1284–99.
3. Joseph PP, Ann MM, Loise JP, Marion S, Rosemary EP. Medical dictionary: a concise and up-to-date guide to medical terms. USA: Houghton Mifflin Company; 1988.
4. Arulkumaran S. Obstetric proceeding: in Dewhurst's textbook of obstetrics and gynecology, 7th ed edn. United States: Edmonds Blackwell publishing; 2007.
5. Kwawukume EY: Caesarean section: Asante and Hittcher printing press limited; 2000.
6. Savage W. The caesarean section epidemic. J Obstet Gynaecol. 2000;20:223–5.
7. Panditrao S. Intra-operative difficulties in repeat cesarean sections. J Obstet Gynecol India. 2008;58(6):507–10.
8. World Health Organization: Monitoring emergency obstetric care: a handbook. 2009.
9. Gomes UA, Silva AA, Bettiol H, Barbieri MA. Risk factors for the increasing caesarean section rate in Southeast Brazil: a comparison of two birth cohorts, 1978-1979 and 1994. Int J Epi. 1999;28:687–94.
10. Leone T, Padmadas SS, Matthews Z. Community factors affecting rising caesarean section rates in developing countries: an analysis of six countries. Soc Sci Med. 2008;67:1236–46.
11. Leung GM, Lam TH, Thach TQ, Wan S, Ho LM. Rates of caesarean birth in Hong Kong: 1987-1999. Birth. 2001;28:166–72.
12. Althabe F, Sosa C, Belizan JM, Gibbons L, Jacquerioz F, Bergel E. Cesarean section rates and maternal and neonatal mortality in low-, medium-, and high-income countries: an ecological study. Birth. 2006;33(6):270–7.
13. Betran AP, Merialdi M, Lauer JA, Bing-Shun W, Thomas J, Van Look P, Wagner M. Rates of caesarean section: analysis of global, regional and national estimates. Paediatr Perinat Epidemiol. 2007;21(2):98–113.
14. Stanton CK, Holtz SA. Levels and trends in caesarean birth in the developing world. Stud Fam Plan. 2006;37(1):41–8.
15. Buekens P, Curtis S, Alayon S. Demographic and health surveys: caesarean section rates in sub-Saharan Africa. BMJ. 2003;326(7381):136.
16. Abebe FE, Gebeyehu AW, Kidane AN, Eyassu GA. Factors leading to cesarean section delivery at Felegehiwot referral hospital, Northwest Ethiopia: a retrospective record review. Reprod Health. 2016;13:6.
17. Villar J, Carroli G, Zavaleta N, Donner A, Wojdyla D, World Health Organization 2005 global survey on maternal and perinatal Health Research Group, et al. Maternal and neonatal individual risks and bene ts associated with caesarean delivery: multicentre prospective study. BMJ. 2007;335:1025.
18. World Health Organization. Appropriate technology for birth. Lancet. 1985;2: 436–7.
19. Souza JP, Gülmezoglu A, Lumbiganon P, Laopaiboon M, Carroli G. WHO global survey on maternal and perinatal Health Research Group, et al. caesarean section without medical indications is associated with an increased risk of adverse short-term maternal outcomes: the 2004-2008 WHO global survey on maternal and perinatal health. BMC Med. 2010;8:71.
20. World Health Organization. Indicator to monitor maternal goals: report of a technical working group. Geneva: World Health Organization; 1994.
21. Betran AP, Ye J, Moller AB, Zhang J, Gumezoglu AM, Torloni MR. The increasing trend in cesarean section rates: global, regional, and national estimates :1990-2014. PLoS One. 2016;11(2):e148343.
22. Adnan A, Abu O, Suleiman H, Abu A. Frequency rate and indications of cesarean sections at Prince Zaid bin Al Hussein Hospital - Jordan. J Med Sci Clin Res. 2012;19(1):82–6.
23. Lauer JA, Betrán AP, Merialdi M, Wojdyla D. Rates of caesarean section: analysis of global, regional and national estimates. Paediatr Perinatal Epidemiol. 2007;28:98–113.
24. Francome C, Savage W. Caesarean section in Britain and the United States 12% or 24%: is either the right rate? Soc Sci Med. 1993;37:1199–218.
25. Thomas J, Paranjothy S. Royal College of Obstetricians and Gynaecologists: clinical effectiveness support unit. The National Sentinel Caesareans section audit report. In. London: RCOG Press; 2001.
26. Shamshad B. Factors leading to increased cesarean section rate. Gomal J Med Sci. 2008;6:1.
27. Belizán J, Althabe F, Barros F, Alexander S. Rates and implications of caesarean sections in Latin America: ecological study. BMJ. 1999;319:1397–400.
28. Lauer J, Betrán A. Decision aids for women with a previous caesarean section: focusing on women's preferences improves decision making. BMJ. 2007;334:1281–2.
29. Najmi R, Rehan N. Prevalence and determinants of caesarean section in a teaching hospital of Pakistan. J Obstet Gynaecol. 2000;20:479–83.
30. Betran AP, Torloni MR, Zhang JJ, Gülmezoglu AM, WHO Working Group on Caesarean Section, Aleem HA, Althabe F, Bergholt T, de Bernis L, Carroli G, Deneux-Tharaux C. WHO Statement on caesarean section rates. BJOG. 2016; 123(5):667–70.
31. Ahmed SM, Daffalla SE. Incidence of uterine rupture in a teaching hospital, Sudan. Saudi Med J. 2001;22:757–61.
32. Eze JN, Ibekwe PC. Uterine rupture at a secondary hospital in Afikpo, Southeast Nigeria. Singap Med J. 2010;51:506–11.
33. Omole-Ohonsi A, Attah R. Risk factors for ruptured uterus in a developing country. Gynecol Obstetric. 2011;21:102. https://doi.org/10.4172/2161-0932. 1000102.
34. Berhe Y, Wall LL. Uterine rupture in resource-poor countries. Obstet Gynecol Surv. 2014;69:695–707.
35. Motomura K, Ganchimeg T, Nagata C, Ota E, Vogel PJ, Betran PA, Torloni RM, Jayaratne K, Jwa CS, Mittal S, et al. Incidence and outcomes of uterine rupture among women with prior caesarean section: WHO multicountry survey on maternal and newborn health. Sci Rep. 2017;7:44093.
36. Lumbiganon P, Laopaiboon M, Gulmezoglu AM, Souza JP, Taneepanichskul S, Ruyan P, et al. Method of delivery and pregnancy outcomes in Asia: the WHO global survey on maternal and perinatal health 2007- 08. Lancet. 2010; 375:490–9.
37. Souza JP, Gulmezoglu A, Lumbiganon P, Laopaiboon M, Carroli G, Fawole B, et al. Caesarean section without medical indications is associated with an increased risk of adverse short-term maternal outcomes: the 2004-2008 WHO global survey on maternal and perinatal health. BMC Med. 2010;8:71.
38. Kun H, FangbiaoT BF, Joanna R, Rachel T, Shenglan T, et al. A mixed-method study of factors associated with differences in caesarean section rates at community level: the case of rural China. Midwifery. 2013;29(8):911–20.
39. Parrish KM, Holt VL, Easterling TR, Connell FA, LoGerfo JP. Effect of changes in maternal age, parity, and birth weight distribution on primary caesarean delivery rates. J Am Medi Asso. 1994;271:443–7.
40. Ecker JL, Chen KT, Cohen AP, Riley LE, Lieberman ES. Increased risk of caesarean delivery with advancing maternal age: indications and associated factors in nulliparous women. Am J Obstet Gynaecol. 2001;185:883–7.
41. Lynch CM, Kearney R, Turner MJ. Maternal morbidity after elective repeat caesarean section after two or more previous procedures. Eur J Obstet Gynaecol Reprod Biol. 2002;4320:1–4.
42. Signorelli C, Cattaruzza MS, Osborn JF. Risk factors for caesarean section in Italy: results of a multicentre study. Public Health. 1995;109:191–9.
43. Spaans WA, Sluijs MB, Van Roosmalen J, Bleker O. Risk factors at caesarean section and failure of subsequent trial of labour. Eur J Obstet Gynaecol Reprod Biol. 2002;100:163–6.
44. Mossialos E, Allin S, Karras K, Davaki K. An investigation of caesarean section in three greek hospitals: the impact of financial incentives and convenience. Eur J Public Health. 2005;15:288–95.
45. Onwude JL, Rao S, Selo-Ojeme DO. Large babies and unplanned caesarean delivery. Eur J Obstet Gynaecol Reprod Biol. 2005;118(1):36–9.

46. Skalkidis Y, Petridou E, Papathoma E, Revinthi K, Tong D, Trichopoulos D. Are operative delivery procedures in Greece sociallyconditioned? IntJ Qual Health Care. 1996;8:159–65.

47. Taffel SM. Cesarean delivery in the United States, 1990. Vital Health Stat 21. 1994;(51):1–24.

48. Tatar M, Gunalp S, Somunoglu S, Demirol A. Women's perceptions of caesarean section: reflections from a Turkish teaching hospital. Soc Sci Med. 2000;50:1227–33.

49. Weiss JL, Malone FD, Emig D, Ball RH, Nyberg DA, Comstock CH, Saade G, Eddleman K, Carter SM, Craigo SD, Carr SR. Obesity, obstetric complications and cesarean delivery rate–a population-based screening study. Am J Obstet Gynecol. 2004;190(4):1091–7.

50. Druzin ML, El-Sayed YY. Caesarean delivery on maternal request: wise use of finite resources? A view from the trenches review article. Semin Perinatol. 2006;30(5):305–8.

51. Tuncalp O, Stanton C, Castro A, Adanu R, Heymann M, et al. Measuring coverage in MNCH: validating Women's self-report of emergency cesarean sections in Ghana and the Dominican Republic. PLoS One. 2013;8(5):e60761.

52. Ghana Statistical Service (GSS), Ghana Health Service (GHS), ICF International. Ghana Demographic and Health Survey 2014. Rockville: GSS, GHS, ICF International; 2015.

53. Hafeez M, Yasin A, Badar N, Pasha MI, Akram N, Gulzar B. Prevalence and indication of caesarean section in a teaching hospital. JIMSA. 2014;27(1):15–6.

54. Manyeh KA, Kukula V, Odonkor G, Ekey RA, Adjei A, Narh-Bana S, Akpakli DE, Gyapong M. Socioeconomic and demographic determinants of birth weight in southern rural Ghana: evidence from Dodowa health and demographic surveillance system. BMC Pregnancy and Childbirth. 2016;16:160.

55. Awini E, Sarpong D, Adjei A, Manyeh AK, Amu A, Akweongo P, Adongo P, Kukula V, Odonkor G, Narh S, Gyapong M. Estimating cause of adult (15+ years) death using InterVA-4 in a rural district of southern Ghana. Glob Health Action. 2014;7(1):25543.

56. Gyapong M, Sarpong D, Awini E, Manyeh KA, Tei D, Odonkor G, Agyepong IA, Mattah P, Wontuo P, Attaa-Pomaa M, et al. Health and demographic surveillance system profile: the Dodowa HDSS. Int J Epidemiol. 2013;42:1686–96.

57. Vyas S, Kumaranayake L. Constructing socio-economic status indices: how to use principal components analysis. Health Policy Plan. 2006;21(6):459–68.

58. Betrán AP, Ye J, Moller A-B, Zhang J, Gülmezoglu AM, Torloni MR. The increasing trend in caesarean section rates: global, regional and National Estimates: 1990-2014. PLoS One. 2016;11(2):e0148343.

59. Janoudi G, Kelly S, Yasseen A, Hamam H, Moretti F, Walker M. Factors associated with increased rates of caesarean section in women of advanced maternal age. J Obstet Gynaecol Can. 2015;37(6):517–26.

60. Zgheib SM, Kacim M, Kostev K. Prevalence of and risk factors associated with cesarean section in Lebanon - A retrospective study based on a sample of 29,270 women. Women Birth. 2017;30(6):e265–e71.

61. Ji H, Jiang H, Yang L, et al. Factors contributing to the rapid rise of caesarean section: a prospective study of primiparous Chinese women in Shanghai. BMJ Open. 2015;5:e008994.

62. Luke B, Brown MB. Elevated risks of pregnancy complications and adverse outcomes with increasing maternal age. Hum Reprod. 2007;22(5):1264–72.

63. Nilsen C, Østbye T, Daltveit KA, Mmbaga TB, Sandøy IF. Trends in and socio-demographic factors associated with caesarean section at a Tanzanian referral hospital, 2000 to 2013. Int J Equity Health. 2014;13:87.

64. Mgaya AH, Massawe SN, Kidanto HL, Mgaya HN. Grand multiparity: is it still a risk in pregnancy? BMC Pregnancy Childbirth. 2013;13:241.

65. Lumbiganon P, Laopaiboon M, Gülmezoglu AM, et al. World health organization global survey on maternal and perinatal Health Research Group. Method of delivery and pregnancy outcomes in Asia: the WHO global survey on maternal and perinatal health 2007–08. Lancet. 2010;375:490–9.

66. Shah A, Fawole B, M'Imunya JM, et al. Cesarean delivery outcomes from the WHO global survey on maternal and perinatal health in Africa. Int J Gynaecol Obstet. 2009;107:191–7.

67. Zhu LP, Qin M, Shi DH, et al. Investigation of cesarean section in Shanghai and effect on maternal and child health. Matern Child Health Care China. 2001;16:763–4.

9

Differences in pregnancy outcomes and obstetric care between asylum seeking and resident women: a cross-sectional study in a German federal state, 2010–2016

Kayvan Bozorgmehr[1*], Louise Biddle[1], Stella Preussler[2], Andreas Mueller[3] and Joachim Szecsenyi[1]

Abstract

Background: Despite large numbers of asylum seekers, there is a lack of evidence on pregnancy outcomes and obstetric care of asylum seeking women in Germany.

Methods: Cross-sectional study (2010–2016) using administrative data of the main referral hospital for pregnant asylum seekers of the reception center of a large federal state in South Germany. Inclusion criteria: women aged 12–50 years, admitted in relation to pregnancy, childbirth or post-partum complications. Outcomes: differences between asylum seekers and residents in the prevalence of high-risk pregnancy conditions, abortive outcomes/stillbirths, peri- and postnatal maternal complications, neonatal complications, and caesarean sections. Analysis: odds ratios (OR) and 95% confidence intervals (CI) obtained by single and multiple logistic regression analysis. Attributable fractions among the exposed (Afe) and among the total population (Afp) were calculated for selected outcomes.

Results: Of 19,864 women admitted in relation to pregnancy, childbirth or post-partum complications, 2.9% (n = 569) were asylum seekers. Adjusted odds for high-risk pregnancy conditions (OR = 0.76, 95%CI: 0.63–0.91, p < 0.0001), caesarean sections (OR = 0.84, 95%CI 0.66–1.07, p = 0.17) and perinatal complications (OR = 0.65, 95%CI: 0.55–0.78, p < 0.0001) were lower; those for abortive outcomes/stillbirths (OR = 1.58, 95%CI: 1.11–2.20, p = 0.01) and postnatal complications (OR = 1.80, 95%CI: 0.93–3.19, p = 0.06) higher among asylum seeking women relative to residents in models adjusted for age, length of admission, and high-risk pregnancy conditions. The Afe for abortive outcomes and stillbirths among asylum seekers was 40.3% (95% CI, 16.3–56.5) and the Afp was 1.8%. The Afe for postnatal complications was 53.1% (95% CI, 7.1–74.0) and the Afp was 3.1%.

Conclusion: Asylum seeking women are at higher risk of abortive outcomes/stillbirths and show a tendency towards higher postnatal complications. This excess risk calls for adequate responses by health care providers and policy makers to improve outpatient postnatal care in reception centers and mitigate adverse birth outcomes among asylum seeking women. Although further research is needed, scaling-up midwivery care, improving outreach by maternity care teams, and routinely identifying and addressing mental illness by psychosocial services could be ways forward to improve outcomes in this population.

Keywords: Migration, Asylum seekers, Health inequality, Pregnancy outcome, Caesarian section, Stillbirth, Reception center, Maternity care, Postnatal care, Social epidemiology

* Correspondence: kayvan.bozorgmehr@med.uni-heidelberg.de
[1]Department of General Practice and Health Services Research, University Hospital Heidelberg, Marsilius Arkaden, INF 130.3, 69120 Heidelberg, Germany
Full list of author information is available at the end of the article

Background

Asylum seeking pregnant women are considered a vulnerable population group with special needs [1]. The Asylum Seekers' Benefits Act (Asylbewerberleistungsgesetz), which regulates legal entitlements to healthcare for asylum seekers in Germany, grants unrestricted access to needed health care for this population [2, 3]. Despite equal legal access to health care, pregnant asylum seekers may face numerous barriers to maternity care as a result of limited availability of specialized services in reception centers as well as geographical and language barriers to accessing regular health services outside reception centers [4, 5]. Adverse living conditions and health system factors of the country of origin, negative experiences and stressors during the peri-migration phase, as well as structural factors related to reception in destination countries may also put asylum seeking pregnant women at high risk of adverse birth outcomes [6–8].

Adverse birth outcomes not only impact the mortality and morbidity of the infant, but can also have detrimental health effects throughout the child's lifecourse, including an increased risk of coronary heart disease, diabetes and hypertension [9]. Thus, adverse birth outcomes may lead not only to an increased utilization of immediate postnatal services [10], but also to increased costs to the healthcare system throughout infancy, childhood, and adulthood [11].

Despite large numbers of asylum seekers, no studies have analyzed maternity care services or maternal outcomes among asylum seeking women in Germany between 1994 and 2014 [12]. Updating the search conducted by the most recent systematic review [12] yielded no additional relevant literature in the German context until 31.12.2017.

We here analyze differences in pregnancy outcomes and obstetric services between asylum seeking women living in a large reception center in Germany and resident women, both delivering in a public hospital between 2010 and 2016. We focus on differences between asylum seekers and residents in the prevalence of (i) high-risk pregnancy conditions, (ii) abortive outcomes and stillbirths, (iii) peri- and postnatal maternal complications, and (iv) neonatal complications. Further, we compare obstetric services provided to asylum seekers and residents with respect to caesarean sections and the timing of hospital admission for labor and delivery.

Methods

Study context and data sources

We used anonymous, administrative data of the largest hospital (Städtisches Klinikum) in the city of Karlsruhe, Germany, to obtain information on pregnancy outcomes and obstetric services provided to resident women and asylum seeking women from the state reception center Karlsruhe between 2010 and 2016.

Until 2015, the state reception center quasi-randomly received about 13% of newly arriving asylum seekers to

Germany based on administrative quota, as it acted as sole reception center for the state of Baden-Württemberg. Further centers were established thereafter in the federal state due to the rising number of asylum seekers. Asylum seekers undergo a mandatory tuberculosis (TB) screening according to §62 of the Asylum Act and remain in the centers until they are transferred to cities in other districts and communities of Baden-Württemberg. In 2015, the maximum duration of stay in the reception centers was prolonged from three to six months, but asylum seekers from so-called "safe" countries of origin remain in the centers throughout the asylum process.

The center provides primary and midwifery care services onsite; specialist outpatient maternity care is provided in private practices. Inpatient specialist services and obstetric care is mainly provided by the public hospital in Karlsruhe. The hospital has a capacity of about 1450 beds and functions as the main tertiary care provider for gynaecological and obstetric services for both resident and asylum seeking women after referral. The only other facility providing obstetric services is a faith-based hospital (with about 530 beds) which is geographically more remote from the reception center facilities.

No standardized medical records exist in the reception center to evaluate antenatal care or determine the total number of pregnant asylum seekers. We hence used data of the mandatory TB screening to approximate the total number of pregnant asylum seekers in the reception center in the period 2010–2016. Pregnant asylum seekers over 15 years old can be identified in the screening data as they undergo a tuberculin skin test or interferon-gamma release assay test, as opposed to the chest radiography administered to non-pregnant individuals.

Inclusion criteria

We included all women admitted to the gynaecological clinic of the public hospital in Karlsruhe between 01.01.2010 and 31.12.2016 due to conditions related to pregnancy, childbirth, or the post-partum period. Women with any of the codes of chapter XV of the German Modification the International Classification of Diseases (ICD-10-GM version 2017) in their primary or secondary diagnoses were considered eligible for inclusion in the analysis. We excluded women above 50 years of age due to low case numbers among asylum seekers ($n = 5$). A unique cost unit was used to reliably identify and distinguish women with asylum seeker status under state-mandate from resident women covered by statutory sickness funds or private insurance companies.

Pregnancy outcomes

We used ICD codes to operationalize high-risk pregnancy conditions (ICD-10-GM O10-O16; O20- O29; and O30-O48), abortive outcomes (ICD-10-GM O00-O08)

and stillbirths (ICD-10-GM Z37.1; Z37.3; Z37.4; Z37.6; and Z37.7), perinatal maternal complications (ICD-10-GM O60-O75), postnatal maternal complications in the post-partum period (ICD-10-GM O85-O92), and neonatal complications (ICD-10-GM P00-P96). Each outcome was coded as binary (1/0) variable.

Obstetric services
We used ICD codes and German operation and procedure (OPS) codes to determine the prevalence of caesarean sections (ICD-10-GM O82; O60.1; O60.2; O60.3 or OPS 5-740; 5-741; 5-742; and 5-749). The timing of hospital admission for labor and delivery was coded as variable with four categories according to weeks of gestation:"≤ 25 weeks" (ICD-10-GM O09.0 - O09.3), "26 - 36 weeks" (ICD-10-GM O09.4 - O09.5), "37 - 41 weeks" (ICD-10-GM O09.6), and "> 41 weeks" (ICD O09.7).

Statistical analysis
We calculated and plotted the prevalence of pregnancy outcomes and caesarian sections per 100,000 women stratified by residence status and age group, as well as the proportion of women admitted to hospital by gestational week. We analyzed differences in pregnancy outcomes and obstetric services between asylum seeking and resident women using single and multiple logistic regression models. All models were adjusted for age, length of admission, and high-risk pregnancy conditions where appropriate. Length of admission was calculated in days using dates of admission and discharge, and the natural logarithm was included in the models. Women's age was categorized in four groups (12-20, 21-30, 31-40, and 41-50) for descriptive purposes, and included as linear variable in the regression analyses. Regression diagnostics were performed by means of standardized residual plots to rule out heteroscedasticity (data not shown). We calculated attributable fractions among the exposed (Afe) to assess the excess rate for selected outcomes among asylum seekers,

as well as the attributable fraction of those outcomes among the total population (Afp). Stata version 15.1 was used for descriptive analysis, single logistic regression, calculation of Afe and Afp, and illustration of results. The function glm of the R-statistical package [13] was used for the multiple logistic regression models.

Results
A total of 42,445 women were admitted to inpatient care of the hospital (2010–2016), of which 2.1% ($n = 870$) were asylum seekers. We excluded 5718 resident women and five asylum seekers aged > 50 years, and 16,562 residents and 296 asylum seekers due to admissions unrelated to pregnancy, childbirth or post-partum complications. The final sample consisted of $N = 19,864$ women of which 2.9% ($n = 569$) were asylum seekers. Data for the timing of hospital admission for labor and delivery was missing for 419 women, 25 of which were asylum seekers; no data was missing for any other variables. The number of asylum seeking women admitted to the hospital during pregnancy, childbirth, or the post-partum period corresponds to 19.3% of all incoming women identified as pregnant ($n = 2944$) in the scope of the mandatory TB screening in the reception center (2010–2016). On average, asylum seeking women were slightly younger than residents and had a shorter length of admission (Table 1).

The prevalence (per 100,000) of high-risk pregnancy conditions was lower among asylum seeking women compared to residents, except for the 41–50 age group (Fig. 1). Asylum seeking women had higher prevalence rates (per 100,000) of abortive outcomes and stillbirths (except for the 41–50 age group) and postnatal complications; and lower prevalence rates (per 100,000) of perinatal complications (except for the 12–20 age group). No case of perinatal complications of the newborn was coded among asylum seekers, so that no further analysis was possible for this outcome. Fewer caesarean sections

Table 1 Age and length of admission by residence status, $N = 19,864$ women admitted to hospital, 2010–2016

	Resident women		Asylum seeking women		Total population	
	n	%	n	%	N	%
Age group						
12–20	602	3.1	88	15.5	690	3.5
21–30	7417	38.4	314	55.2	7731	38.9
31–40	10,460	54.2	154	27.1	10,614	53.4
41–50	816	4.2	13	2.3	829	4.2
Total	19,295	100.0	569	100.0	19,864	100.0
	M (SD)	Min-Max	M (SD)	Min-Max	M (SD)	Min-Max
Age (years)	31.4 (5.4)	15–50	27.1 (6.2)	14–44	31.3 (5.5)	14–50
Length of admission (days)	4.5 (4.6)	1–97	4.0 (3.1)	1–35	4.5 (4.6)	1–97

% column percent, M arithmetic mean, SD standard deviation, Min minimum, Max maximum

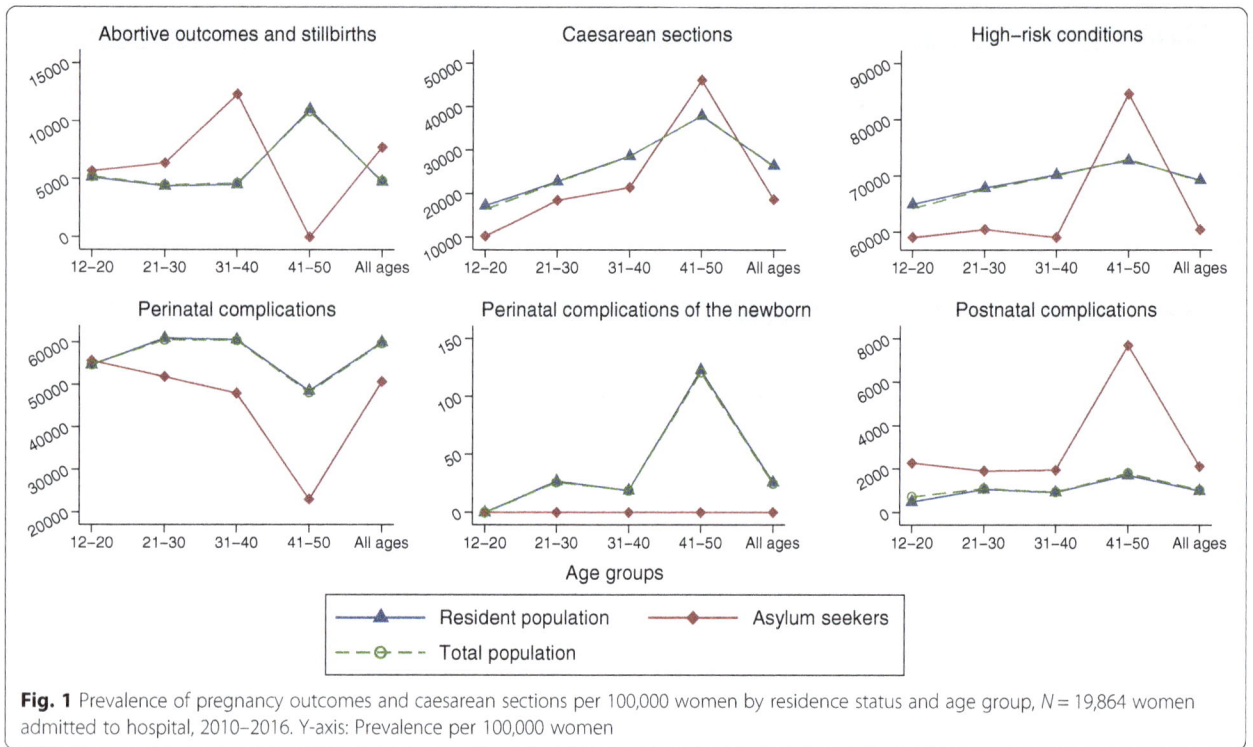

Fig. 1 Prevalence of pregnancy outcomes and caesarean sections per 100,000 women by residence status and age group, $N = 19,864$ women admitted to hospital, 2010–2016. Y-axis: Prevalence per 100,000 women

were conducted per 100,000 women among asylum seekers (except for the 41–50 age group).

The proportion of women admitted to hospital up to 25 weeks of gestation was higher among asylum seekers compared to residents (except for the 41–50

age group), and lower for admissions above 41 weeks of gestation. The pattern of admissions for other categories of gestational week of pregnancy was varied (Fig. 2). The detailed descriptive data is provided in Additional file 1.

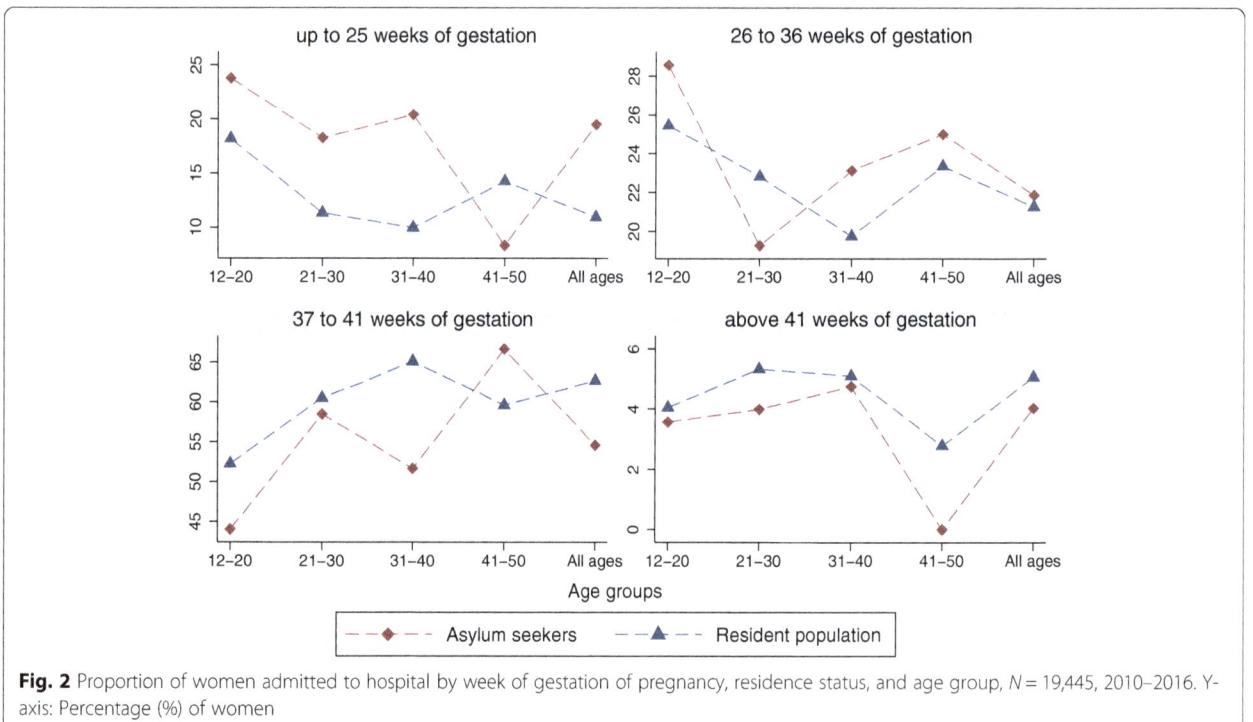

Fig. 2 Proportion of women admitted to hospital by week of gestation of pregnancy, residence status, and age group, $N = 19,445$, 2010–2016. Y-axis: Percentage (%) of women

The unadjusted logistic regression analysis showed higher odds of abortive outcomes and stillbirths, postnatal complications, and admissions up to 25 weeks of gestation among asylum seekers relative to resident women (Table 2).

The excess rate of abortive outcomes and stillbirths among asylum seekers (Afe) was 40.3% (95% confidence interval, CI: 16.3–56.5). These outcomes correspond to 1.8% of abortive outcomes and stillbirths in the total population of women (Afp). For postnatal complications, the excess rate (Afe) among asylum seekers was 53.1% (95% CI: 7.1–74.0) and the Afp was 3.1%.

The unadjusted odds of high-risk pregnancy conditions, perinatal maternal complications, caesarean sections, and admissions during 37 to 41 gestational weeks of pregnancy were significantly ($p < 0.05$) lower among asylum seekers compared to residents (Table 2).

These patterns were confirmed by the multiple regression analysis: the direction of the associations remained stable in the adjusted models, but the strength of the association was slightly reduced (Fig. 3). Differences in caesarean sections and postnatal complications between asylum seeking women and residents were slightly attenuated after full adjustment for age and morbidity variables (Fig. 3). A detailed overview of regression estimates including those of co-variables in the adjusted models is provided in Additional file 2.

Discussion

This is the first study in Germany quantifying differences in pregnancy outcomes and obstetric services between asylum seeking women in a state reception center and resident women. Asylum seeking women were at considerably higher risk for abortive outcomes and stillbirths compared to resident women after full adjustment for age and morbidity-related variables. The excess rate of abortive outcomes and stillbirths among asylum seekers was large. Reducing the rate of adverse outcomes in this group to a level observed among resident women would thus entail high health gains. Several factors across the migration trajectory, ranging from pre- and peri-migration factors to the conditions in the destination country can be associated with the high level of abortions and stillbirths. The lack of adequate health services in the country of origin, perilous migration journeys and near-death experiences, as well as the living conditions in reception centers are experienced as very stressful for asylum seeking women in Germany, affecting their health-related quality of life [14]. Frequent dispersals before reaching the final reception center may also contribute to adverse outcomes and interrupt the continuity of care leading to severe consequences for health and well-being of pregnant women seeking asylum [15, 16]. Furthermore, untreated mental conditions such as depression, anxiety disorders or traumatic stress have adverse consequences for women and their (unborn) children [17]. As shown in a systematic review and meta-analysis in migrant women from low- and middle-income countries, the prevalence of mental illness during pregnancy is very high (e.g. 31.4% for any depressive disorder and 17.3% for major depression) [17]. Adequate and timely identification of mental illness during pregnancy by means of standardized and routinely applied screening interventions, as well as provision of low-threshold psychosocial support based on individual need are thus needed. Such approaches and care provision models, however, do currently not exist in Germany. Integrating routine screening and psychosocial support into maternity care services in reception centers would also be in line with binding EU directives [1] requesting member states to establish process for identifying and addressing

Table 2 Crude odds ratio of pregnancy outcomes and obstetric services for asylum seekers relative to resident women, $N = 19,864$ women admitted to hospital, 2010–2016

	Crude Odds Ratio (Ref.: resident women)	95% CI	p-value
Pregnancy outcome			
High-risk pregnancy	**0.68**	**(0.57–0.81)**	**< 0.0001**
Abortive outcomes/stillbirths	**1.68**	**(1.22–2.30)**	**0.001**
Perinatal complications	**0.69**	**(0.58–0.81)**	**< 0.0001**
Postnatal complications	**2.13**	**(1.18–3.84)**	**0.012**
Obstetric care services			
Caesarean sections	**0.64**	**(0.51–0.79)**	**< 0.0001**
Timing of hospital admission[a]			
Up to 25 weeks of gestation	**1.97**	**(1.59–2.45)**	**< 0.0001**
26–36 weeks of gestation	1.04	(0.84–1.27)	0.736
37–41 weeks of gestation	**0.71**	**(0.60–0.85)**	**< 0.0001**
> 41 weeks of gestation	0.79	(0.51–1.22)	0.283

Ref Reference category, *CI* confidence interval. [a]$N = 19,445$ women ($n = 18,901$ residents and $n = 544$ asylum seekers). Figures in boldface: statistically significant below the 0.05 level

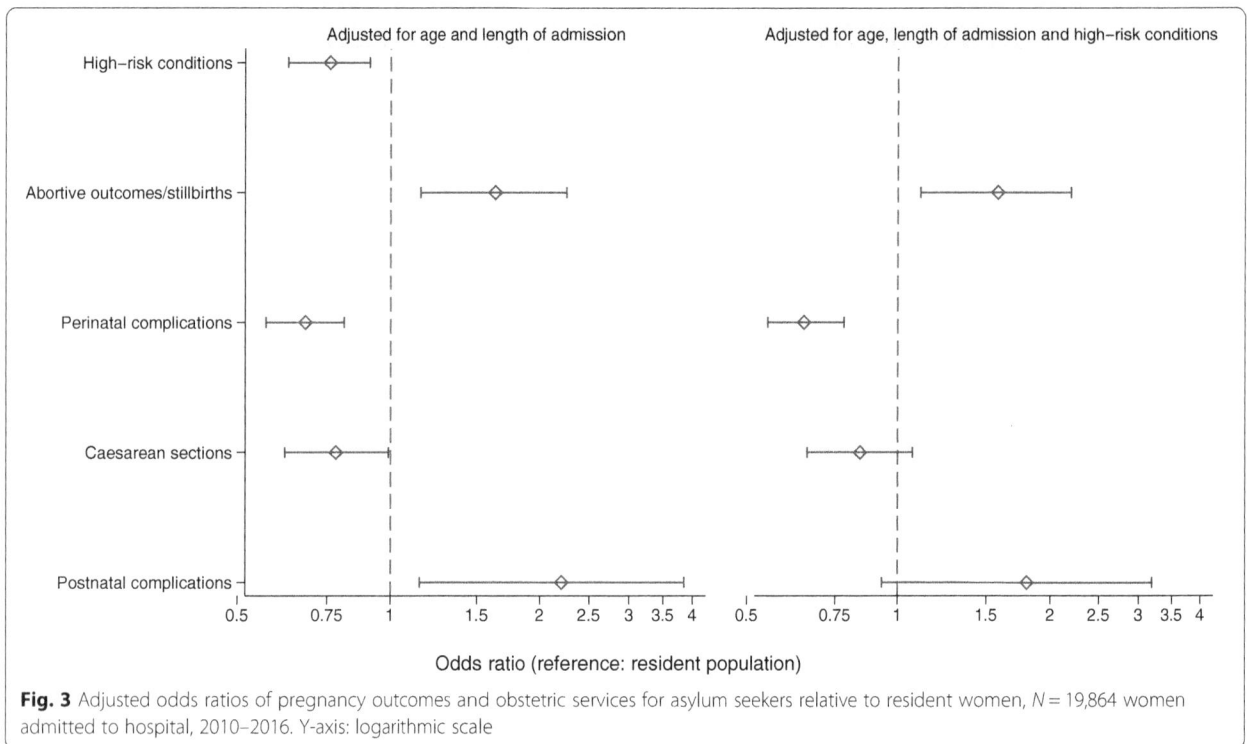

Fig. 3 Adjusted odds ratios of pregnancy outcomes and obstetric services for asylum seekers relative to resident women, N = 19,864 women admitted to hospital, 2010–2016. Y-axis: logarithmic scale

the special needs of vulnerable groups among asylum seekers.

Our study further identified the post-partum period as particularly important to improve maternity care for asylum seeking women: the adjusted odds of admission due to conditions related to the post-partum period was considerably higher compared to residents. We found no indication of delayed referrals using the proxy indicator of gestational weeks of pregnancy to assess differences in timing of hospital admission for labor and delivery. Other adverse outcomes such as perinatal maternal and neonatal complications were lower among asylum seeking women. This could either be related to a higher parity or - in light of the lower odds for high-risk pregnancy conditions - indicate a healthy migrant effect. A health advantage of recent immigrants compared to the native population with comparable socio-demographic characteristics has been observed in several studies [18], also in the context of maternity care and pregnancy outcomes among regular immigrants in Germany [19]. This phenomenon is usually attributed to a self-selection prior to migration, and used to explain why recent immigrants perform better on some health measures despite lower socio-economic status, adverse living conditions, and various barriers to health care [18].

This study has important strengths and limitations. Using administrative hospital data, we reliably identified a group of vulnerable asylum seekers living in reception centers. This allowed us to quantify differences in relevant clinical outcomes related to pregnancy, childbirth, and

post-partum and compare patterns between asylum seeking and resident women over a period of 6 years. We estimate that a large proportion (19.3%) of pregnant asylum seekers were covered by the hospital dataset, but this estimation needs to be interpreted with care. Women becoming pregnant after the health examination while still living in the reception center and pregnant women under 15 years old are not captured using the screening data approach. The unique geographical setting of the public hospital in Karlsruhe as the main referral facility for the reception center minimized - but did not rule out - a referral bias inherent in any study using hospital-based data. The study findings are valid for pregnant asylum seeking women in reception centers, but may not be transferable to asylum seekers who have been transferred to districts and communities. Although the transfer of pregnant asylum seeking women is purely based on administrative criteria, it may not be ruled out that protective factors (e.g. having a more private accommodation) or risk factors (e.g. high number of transfers and discontinuity of care) exert different effects of pregnancy outcomes and access to maternity care.

The use of routine data entailed a lack of relevant socio-demographic parameters (such as country of origin, spoken language, religion or maternal education) and clinical parameters (such as gravidity and parity), so that residual confounding cannot be ruled out. We also lacked information on antenatal care services provided to women, so that the timing of admission is only a crude approximation of the timeliness of outpatient care provision. Better parameters such as early antenatal coverage are needed to monitor equity in access to maternity services [20] for this vulnerable population group. Data on cost of care is theoretically available in the accounts data used here, but the data was not practically available at time of conducting the study. Future research should address this issue and compare morbidity-adjusted differences in cost of care between asylum seekers and residents, making economic evidence available to inform policy and practice and add to the scarce evidence base [10] in this area.

Our findings on elevated risk of stillbirths among asylum seekers are consistent with numerous studies in other countries conducted among general migrant or refugee populations [6–8]. Using the German perinatal data base, Reeske et al. reported an increased risk of stillbirths in migrants (without reference to their residence status) originating from the Middle East and North Africa [21]. A study in Canada reported higher clinical and psychosocial health needs in asylum seeking and refugee women in the postnatal period [22]. The prevalence of caesarean sections (per 100,000) in both residents and asylum seekers was lower than the aggregate national average of 30,700 [23] indicating regional variations. While there is mixed evidence on caesarean section rates among migrants [6–8], a case-control study in London found no significant differences between refugees from Kosovo and residents in the rates of caesarean sections [24]. Overall, cross-country comparisons of such results are very difficult due to differences in societal and health system factors, as well as differences between the underlying migrant populations studied.

The findings of this study have important implications for clinicians and policymakers: pregnant asylum seekers in reception centers are at higher risk of abortive outcomes and stillbirths despite a lower morbidity as measured by high-risk pregnancy conditions. The relative lack of systematic data collection on this population renders such health inequalities invisible. A higher risk of abortive outcomes and stillbirths in asylum seeking women that goes unnoticed by the health system can be regarded as an uncounted toll of forced migration. A wide range of individual circumstances (such as socio-economic status), but also adverse experiences before and during flight [14] can be associated with such negative birth outcomes. However, the post-migration phase is a critical period in which individual risk factors and prior experiences can be mitigated or exacerbated.

Ensuring safe and private accommodation, food security, good access to full antenatal and preventive services, and access to psychosocial and specialized mental health services may help to mitigate negative experiences of the pre- and peri-migration phase. The tendency towards higher risk of postnatal complications in asylum seekers requires improvements in outpatient care in the post-partum period, including better follow-up and continuity of care. Scaling up midwifery care in the post-partum period and strengthening the outreach capacity of maternity care teams may be crucial to achieve this. Maternity care teams, consisting of midwives, social workers, and psychologists implementing care pathways for at-risk women may make big differences in health outcomes for asylum seeking pregnant women [15].

Further research is, however, needed to better understand and explain the reasons for the higher levels of adverse outcomes such as abortions and postnatal complications among asylum seekers. Such research should consider the role of post-migration factors and the relative contribution of pre- and peri-migration factors to adverse birth outcomes among asylum seekers. To this end, prospective studies with expanded geographical reach and better linkage of data from reception centers with data of ante- and perinatal care services are needed.

Conclusions

This study offers first insights into pregnancy outcomes and obstetric care among asylum seeking women using data from a reception center of the third largest federal state in Germany over a period of 7 years. Despite the fact that high-risk pregnancy conditions are lower among asylum seeking compared to resident women, we find substantially higher adjusted odds for postnatal maternal complications and abortive outcomes/stillbirths among asylum seekers. Other adverse outcomes such as perinatal maternal and neonatal complications are lower among asylum seeking women compared to resident women. Measures to improve outpatient postnatal care in reception centers and effectively mitigate adverse birth outcomes among asylum seeking women are needed. Although further research on modifiable post-migration risk factors for such outcomes is needed, scale up of midwifery care in reception centers, improved outreach by maternity care services, and routine identification of mental illness and psychosocial care during pregnancy could be ways forward to improve pregnancy outcomes in this population.

Abbreviations
Afe: Attributable fractions among the exposed; Afp: Attributable fractions among the total population; CI: Confidence interval; ICD-10-GM: German Modification of the International Classification of Disease; OPS: German operation and procedure codes; OR: Odds ratio; TB: tuberculosis

Acknowledgements
We thank Dr. Lorenz Uhlman (IMBI, University Hospital Heidelberg) for statistical advice and Markus Qreini (Dept. for General Practice and Health Services Research) and the Controlling Department of Karlsruhe City Hospital for data management.

Funding
This study was funded by the Federal Ministry of Research and Education (BMBF) in the scope the research project RESPOND (Improving regional health system responses to the challenges of migration though tailored interventions for asylum seekers and refugees); grant number: FKZ 01GY1611.

Authors' contributions
Conceived the study: KB. Study design: KB. Data analysis: SP, KB. Prepared tables and figures: KB. Interpretation of findings: KB, SP, JS, LB, AM. Writing of first and final draft: KB. Revisions for important intellectual content: LB, AM, JS, SP. Guarantor for the study: KB. All authors made important contributions to the study design, participated in drafting the article and revising it critically for important intellectual content, and gave final approval of the version to be submitted.

Competing interests
The authors declare that they have no competing interests.

Author details
[1]Department of General Practice and Health Services Research, University Hospital Heidelberg, Marsilius Arkaden, INF 130.3, 69120 Heidelberg, Germany. [2]Institute for Medical Biometry and Informatics, University Hospital Heidelberg, Heidelberg, Germany. [3]Clinic of Gynaecology, Karlsruhe City Hospital, Karlsruhe, Germany.

References
1. European Parliament, Council of the European Union. Directive 2013/33/EU of the European Parliament and of the Council of 26 June 2013 laying down standards for the reception of applicants for international protection. Offic J Eur Union. 2013;56:96–116.
2. Razum O, Bozorgmehr K. Restricted entitlements and access to health care for refugees and immigrants: the example of Germany. Global Social Policy. 2016;16(3):321–4.
3. Bozorgmehr K, Razum O. Effect of restricting access to health care on health expenditures among asylum-seekers and refugees: a quasi-experimental study in Germany, 1994–2013. PLoS One. 2015;10(7):e0131483.
4. Bozorgmehr K, Nöst S, Thaiss HM, Razum O. Health care provisions for asylum-seekers: a nationwide survey of public health authorities in Germany. Bundesgesundheitsblatt Gesundheitsforschung Gesundheitsschutz. 2016;59(5):545–55.
5. Bradby H, Humphris R, Newall D, Phillimore J. Public health aspects of migrant health: a review of the evidence on health status for refugees and asylum seekers in the European region. Copenhagen: World Health Organization Regional Office for Europe; 2015.
6. Gissler M, Alexander S, MacFarlane A, et al. Stillbirths and infant deaths among migrants in industrialized countries. Acta Obstet Gynecol Scand. 2009;88(2):134–48.
7. Hayes I, Enohumah K, McCaul C. Care of the migrant obstetric population. Int J Obstet Anesth. 2011;20(4):321–9.
8. Andersen A-MN, Gundlund A, Villadsen SF. Stillbirth and congenital anomalies in migrants in Europe. Best Pract Res Clin Obstet Gynaecol. 2016;32:50–9.
9. Osmond C, Barker DJ. Fetal, infant, and childhood growth are predictors of coronary heart disease, diabetes, and hypertension in adult men and women. Environ Health Perspect. 2000;108(Suppl 3):545–53.
10. Mistry H, Heazell AEP, Vincent O, Roberts T. A structured review and exploration of the healthcare costs associated with stillbirth and a subsequent pregnancy in England and Wales. BMC Pregnancy Childbirth. 2013;13(1):236.
11. Petrou S, Khan K. Economic costs associated with moderate and late preterm birth: primary and secondary evidence. Semin Fetal Neonatal Med. 2012;17(3):170–8.
12. Bozorgmehr K, Mohsenpour A, Saure D, et al. Systematic review and evidence mapping of empirical studies on health status and medical care among refugees and asylum seekers in Germany (1990-2014). Bundesgesundheitsblatt Gesundheitsforschung Gesundheitsschutz. 2016; 59(5):599–620.
13. R-CoreTeam. A language and environment for statistical computing. 2016. https://www.R-project.org/.
14. Jesuthasan J, Sönmez E, Abels I, et al. Near-death experiences, attacks by family members, and absence of health care in their home countries affect the quality of life of refugee women in Germany: a multi-region, cross-sectional, gender-sensitive study. BMC Med. 2018;16(1):15.
15. Asif S, Baugh A, Jones NW. The obstetric care of asylum seekers and refugee women in the UK. Obstet Gynaecol. 2015;17(4):223–31.
16. Feldman R. When maternity doesn't matter: dispersing pregnant women seeking asylum. Reprod Health Matters. 2013;21(42):212–7.
17. Fellmeth G, Fazel M, Plugge E. Migration and perinatal mental health in women from low-and middle-income countries: a systematic review and meta-analysis. BJOG. 2017;124(5):742–52.
18. Domnich A, Panatto D, Gasparini R, Amicizia D. The "healthy immigrant" effect: does it exist in Europe today? Ital J Public Health. 2012;9(3).
19. Razum O, Reiss K, Breckenkamp J, et al. Comparing provision and appropriateness of health care between immigrants and non-immigrants in Germany using the example of neuraxial anaesthesia during labour: cross-sectional study. BMJ Open. 2017;7(8):e015913.
20. Razum O, Breckenkamp J, Borde T, David M, Bozorgmehr K. Early antenatal care visit as indicator for health equity monitoring. Lancet Glob Health. 2018;6(1):e35.
21. Reeske A, Kutschmann M, Razum O, Spallek J. Stillbirth differences according to regions of origin: an analysis of the German perinatal database, 2004-2007. BMC Pregnancy Childbirth. 2011;11(1):63.
22. Gagnon AJ, Dougherty G, Wahoush O, et al. International migration to Canada: the post-birth health of mothers and infants by immigration class. Soc Sci Med. 2013;76:197–207.
23. AQUA. German hospital quality report 2012. Goettingen: Institute for Applied Quality Improvement and Research in Health Care; 2014.
24. Yoong W, Wagley A, Fong C, Chukwuma C, Nauta M. Obstetric performance of ethnic Kosovo Albanian asylum seekers in London: a case–control study. J Obstet Gynaecol. 2004;24(5):510–2.

10

Implementation of community based advance distribution of misoprostol in Himachal Pradesh (India): lessons and way forward

Rakesh Parashar[1], Anadi Gupt[2], Devina Bajpayee[3], Anil Gupta[4], Rohan Thakur[5], Ankur Sangwan[6], Anuradha Sharma[7], Deshraj Sharma[7], Sachin Gupta[8], Dinesh Baswal[9], Gunjan Taneja[10] and Rajeev Gera[10*]

Abstract

Background: Postpartum Hemorrhage remains the leading cause of maternal mortality. To prevent PPH, Misoprostol tablet in a dose of 600 micrograms is recommended for use immediately after childbirth in home deliveries wherein the use of oxytocin is difficult. The current article describes an implementation of "community based advance distribution of Misoprostol program" in India which aimed to design an operational framework for implementing this program.

Methods: The intervention was carried out in Janjheli block in Mandi district of the state of Himachal Pradesh which is a mountainous terrain with limited geographical access and reported 90% home deliveries in the year 2014–15. An operational framework to implement program activities was designed which was based on WHO HSS building blocks. Key implementing steps included- Ensuring local ownership through program leadership, forecasting and procurement of 600 mcg misoprostol tablets, training, branding and communication, community engagement and counselling, recording and reporting, monitoring, supportive supervision and feedback mechanisms.

Results: Over the one year of implementation, 512 home deliveries were reported, out of which 89% received the tablets and 84% consumed the tablet within one minute of delivery. No incidence of PPH in tablet consuming mothers was reported. On account of periodic counselling and effective community engagement the intervention also contributed to better tracking of pregnancies till delivery and institutional delivery rates which increased to 93% from 45% and 57% from 11% respectively as compared to the preceding year.

Conclusions: The model has successfully shown the use of single misoprostol tablets of 600 mcg, first time in this program. We also demonstrated a HSS based operational framework, based on which the program is being scaled to additional blocks in Himachal Pradesh as well as to other states of India.

Keywords: Maternal mortality, Misoprostol, Post-partum hemorrhage

* Correspondence: rgera@ipeglobal.com
[10]USAID-VRIDDHI/IPE Global, New Delhi, India
Full list of author information is available at the end of the article

Background

Maternal mortality remains a key concern across the globe with maternal deaths being a core marker of the functioning of the public health care delivery system. Currently 52% of the maternal deaths (in pregnancy, at or soon after childbirth) globally are attributed to the three leading preventable causes of hemorrhage, sepsis and hypertensive disorders [1]. Based on global data from 2003 to 2009, maximum maternal deaths were attributed to hemorrhage and it accounted for more than 27% of maternal deaths in the developing regions and approximately 16% in the developed regions [2]. With a Maternal Mortality Ratio (MMR) of 167 per 100,000 in 2013, India accounts for a substantial number of maternal deaths worldwide [3]. Also, in line with the global scenario hemorrhage accounts for 40% maternal deaths in India with Post-Partum Hemorrhage (PPH) being the major contributor [4].

Recognizing this important fact, the use of Uterotonics immediately after birth has been universally advocated to prevent the occurrence of PPH [5]. Among the available Uterotonics, oxytocin remains the drug of choice with misoprostol identified as the alternate. However a major concern for prevention of PPH is that the administration of oxytocin, requires the assistance of a skilled birth attendant (SBA), and therefore is not available to women experiencing unattended home births, either by choice, lack of access to SBAs [6, 7] or due to gender and wealth disparities [8–10].To address these concerns as regards uterotonic cover, the use of misoprostol for the prevention of PPH by community health care workers and lay health workers is recommended in settings where skilled birth attendants are not present [5]. Various studies have demonstrated misoprostol's effectiveness in preventing PPH, reducing the need for additional interventions and minimizing the need for referrals in a variety of community-based settings [11]. The World Health Organization (WHO) guidelines on "Optimizing health worker roles to improve access to key maternal and newborn health interventions through task shifting" also advocates for the distribution of misoprostol by lay health workers for home births [12]. Multiple programs across the globe have been implemented using misoprostol for prevention of PPH in home births using different approaches [13] and it is now widely recognized that distribution of misoprostol through community health workers (CHWs) for PPH prevention could be a significant step in reducing maternal deaths in low-resource settings [14].

Though the institutional delivery rate in India has improved considerably with the National Family Health Survey (NFHS) 4 data reporting it as 78.9% in 2015–16, an increase of 40.2% as compared to NFHS 3 (2005–06) [15], the country still has geographical pockets with high home delivery rates. As pointed out by global evidence that occurrence of PPH remains high in home deliveries and keeping in perspective the use of misoprostol in home births, the Ministry of Health and Family Welfare (MoHFW) in India undertook the policy decision to permit Accredited Social Health Activists (ASHAs) to undertake advance distribution of misoprostol to pregnant women who are likely to deliver at home to prevent PPH in 2013. Within the Indian context, ASHA is identified as a community health volunteer who creates awareness on health and its social determinants and mobilizes the community towards local health planning and increased utilization and accountability of the existing health services.

This is a marked shift from the initial decision of only allowing Auxiliary Nurse Midwives (ANMs) to administer misoprostol during home deliveries and is supported by global evidence on the effectiveness, feasibility and safety of advance distribution of misoprostol to pregnant women to prevent PPH [13, 14, 16]. Positive results from other low resource setting countries like Bangladesh, Nepal and Zambia which have implemented and scaled up misoprostol for prevention of PPH were also instrumental for Government of India in moving forward with implementing this intervention in the country [17].

Rationale for the intervention

In line with global evidence, MoHFW, advocates for advance community-based distribution of misoprostol to pregnant women on completion of the 8th month of pregnancy by ASHAs in identified high home delivery geographical pockets to women who are likely to deliver at home [4]. The national guidelines put forward criteria to help CHWs to identify women who have a greater chance of delivering at home and hence need to be provided the misoprostol tablets [4]. (Fig. 1):

Though the intervention is an exception to the policy promoting institutional deliveries, it has been enlisted as one of the major interventions within the 5 × 5 matrix developed by Government of India (GOI), which prioritizes high impact interventions across the RMNCH+A spectrum [18].However, so far the uptake of the program has been low with no state in the country having implemented and scaled up the program despite the availability of national guidelines. Two main reasons cited for the intervention not taking off in the country were apprehensions towards offsetting the efforts of promoting institutional deliveries and a leakage of the drug in the system with its possible misuse. In addition, other factors such as dependency of the programme activities on a CHW, drug related adverse events and the operational challenges in implementing the intervention in far off low resource settings requiring strict monitoring and tracking were also cited to be responsible for poor offtake.

- History of one or more home deliveries in the house-hold.
- Families where women customarily deliver at home due to social/religious/cultural/economic reasons.
- Number of ANCs: If the pregnant woman has undertaken less than two ANC visits by the end of the 6th month of the current pregnancy.
- No other care giver at home: Women who do not have anyone at home to take care of her other children/family if she goes to the facility for delivery.
- Choice of the woman/family: Cases where the woman/ her family has indicated that she may/would deliver at home, despite the best counselling and advocacy for institutional delivery by the ANM and ASHAs.
- Women with disabled children, or from families where there is no other support from an adult.
- Women which, due to location of their homes in the following hard to reach areas, are likely to deliver at home:
- Remote villages/hamlets which do not have motorable road connectivity
- Remote villages/hamlets villages on hilltops or in the fields, or in the areas which are cut off from mainland
- Snow bound/waterlogged areas/villages for the period the area/village is cut-off from the mainland for >1 month
- Any other circumstances where the ANM and ASHA are convinced of the probability that the woman might deliver at home.

Fig. 1 Criteria to identify a pregnant woman with likelihood of home delivery (based on GOI guidelines)

To reiterate the importance of the intervention MoHFW reconvened a National Level Workshop in February 2016 for selected states with identified pockets of home deliveries. The workshop brought forward evidences of fractured implementation across the states of Chhattisgarh, Jharkhand and Madhya Pradesh. A need was therefore felt by the national health ministry to identify a framework which could pave the way for effective implementation across the country.

Methods
Aims of the intervention
The current intervention aimed to design and implement an operational framework to implement and scale up the "Community Based Advance Distribution of Misoprostol" program in India.

Objectives
Primary objectives

- To improve uterotonic coverage in the intervention area by advance distribution of misoprostol tablets by community health workers for prevention of PPH in home births
- To test the operational framework for the intervention and understand determinants for success of implementing a community based program in remote, disconnected and a very low resource setting in the Indian context

Secondary objectives

- To understand and report on any other emerging systemic effects of the intervention including an impact on institutional deliveries

Implementation design
The intervention has been designed and implemented based on the WHO Health System Strengthening (HSS) building blocks keeping fidelity with the national framework [4] using existing Antenatal Care (ANC) platforms and CHWs in the public health care delivery system.

The results and achievements have been measured for the following key variables:

- Uterotonic coverage
- Pattern of drug distribution and consumption
- Occurrence of PPH in beneficiaries who consumed the tablet (The operational definition for identification of PPH was used as stated in the national guidelines - a blood loss of more than 500 ml or soaking of an average sized pad in 5 min) [4]
- Drug related adverse events

In addition, the intervention also studied the influence on health system in the intervention geography including tracking of pregnancy outcomes and institutional deliveries through a mix of qualitative and quantitative approaches.

The implementation geography

The state of Himachal Pradesh is a predominantly mountainous state set in the lap of Himalayas in north-west India with an altitude range from 350 m to 6975 m. Climatic conditions vary with heavy snowfall in winter months in higher altitudes making many areas inaccessible [19]. Hence home delivery rates are particularly higher in rural areas in hilly terrain which are geographically difficult to access and have traditionally been pockets of home deliveries. Contextualizing the geographical and climatic conditions the state offers apt conditions to implement the "Advance Community Based Distribution of Misoprostol" program.

It was decided to pilot the implementation in one particular geography with subsequent scale up in other regions of the state. The USAID funded VRIDDHI (Scaling up RMNCH+A Interventions) Project has been providing technical assistance to the state government across the four High Priority Districts (HPDs) of Chamba, Kinnaur, Lahaul-Spiti and Mandi as part of the RMNCH+A strategy in India. Within these districts, high home delivery rates and geographical access were the factors on which the implementation geography was identified. A review of Health Management Information System (HMIS) data for the year 2015–16, identified the community development block of Janjheli in Mandi district with the highest home delivery rates and hence the same was identified for piloting the intervention.

Set at an altitude of 2150 m above sea level in the western Himalayan range, Janjheli has a population of 86,597 (93.73% rural) with two distinct population clusters located at a distance of three to four hours from the district headquarters. The block has difficult terrain with large portions cut off due to snowfall in the winter months. It has 33 public health facilities including one Community Health Center (CHC), 7 Primary Health Centers (PHCs) and 22 Health Sub Centers (HSCs) with only the CHC functioning as a delivery point and providing Basic Emergency Obstetric Services (BEmOC). Access to a Comprehensive Emergency Obstetric Services (CEmOC) center is a major challenge with the nearest one being 3–4 h away from the BEmOC center. The block has a shortage of Medical Officers with 11 medical officers posted at the CHCs and PHCs against a sanctioned strength of 14. Hence the Frontline Health Workers (FLWs) including the 2 health supervisors, 25 Auxiliary Nurse Midwives (ANMs) and 103 Accredited Social Health Activists (ASHAs) form the primary source of health care service delivery beyond CHCs and PHCs.

The implementation began in April 2016 and data from April 2015 – March 2016 was reviewed to assess the Antenatal Care (ANC) and delivery rates. The data review stated that though against an estimated annual cohort of 1700 pregnant women, 1490 women were registered for ANC with 902 (60%) completing three ANC checkups, for the corresponding period only 667 deliveries were reported with 596 (89%) being home deliveries. This is reflective of the Health system not being able to track all registered pregnant women and their delivery outcomes.

Intervention population

Inclusion criteria The beneficiaries of the program were included from all villages of Janjheli block as follows:

- All Pregnant women along with their family members for purpose of counselling (estimated 1400 pregnant women in one year)
- Any visiting pregnant women coming in contact with Front Line Workers (FLWs) during the period of implementation of program

Exclusion criteria-
- Pregnant women and families falling outside administrative area of Janjheli and not visiting Janjheli area during the pregnancy period

The program personnel involved in the implementation included the following -

- All FLWs of the block – 6 health supervisors, 26 health workers /ANMs and 103 ASHAs

All health department officials of the block i.e. Block Medical Officer (BMO), block pharmacist, medical officers (MO) at PHCs in the block.

Operational framework -

Program implementation using the WHO HSS based operational framework [20]– Moving forward on the recommendations from the National Workshop of February 2016, the state of Himachal Pradesh commissioned the program on "Community Based Advance Distribution of Misoprostol tablets to prevent PPH" through the state National Health Mission (NHM). The entire implementation design was developed using the national guidelines. However certain adaptations were undertaken to contextualize the intervention to local needs. This included adaptations for the training material, job-aids, methodology of training and monitoring of the implementation.

The VRIDDHI team worked with the state government and provided technical support for developing the operational framework and its roll-out. Being a government approved program, no ethical clearance was sought prior to initiating the implementation. The state government and the VRIDDHI team undertook meticulous planning prior to the actual roll out of the program.

Key activities undertaken during the implementation phase include the following:

Leadership and governance

A state level steering committee was established under the leadership of the Mission Director (MD), NHM to guide and facilitate the implementation process. The Program Officer (Maternal Health) was the designated nodal officer at the state and district levels while the local level leadership was provided by the block Medical Officer (MO).

Health products - procurement and packaging of tablet

As per GoI guidelines misoprostol is to be administered in the dose strength of 600 mcg to the mother post-delivery for prevention of PPH. However, a major challenge existing in the implementation process was unavailability of the drug in the required strength within the public healthcare system in India. Till date three tablets of 200 mcg were being used for consumption by the beneficiary which made packaging difficult. Availability of only a single vendor manufacturing the 600 mcg tablet further compounded the situation. The state through a major policy change in the procurement process approved single vendor procurement for the 600 mcg drug at the district level. This decision not only facilitated the current program implementation but has positive ramifications on the overall procurement related policies and processes in Himachal Pradesh.

The drug was delivered to the beneficiaries with a guidance leaflet inserted in the drug pack which clearly elaborated key messages regarding the tablet (Fig. 2). In addition to facilitate tracking of distributed, consumed and returned tablets a unique identification number was given to each dose being distributed in the community.

A major initiative was branding of the intervention as "SURAKSHA" which essentially means "Safety" to convey the importance of the drug to the beneficiaries. The drug packets, training and communication tools being used during the implementation phase were branded with the same terminology to convey a homogenous message to all concerned stakeholders.

Human resources - development of training and communication material

Based on the national guidelines due emphasis was given to create a structured and comprehensive training package for the FLWs and communication tools were developed and translated in local language to aid in program service delivery. The national guidelines were adapted into local language and a program booklet containing the program description, roles and responsibilities of service providers was developed for the FLWs. A flip book

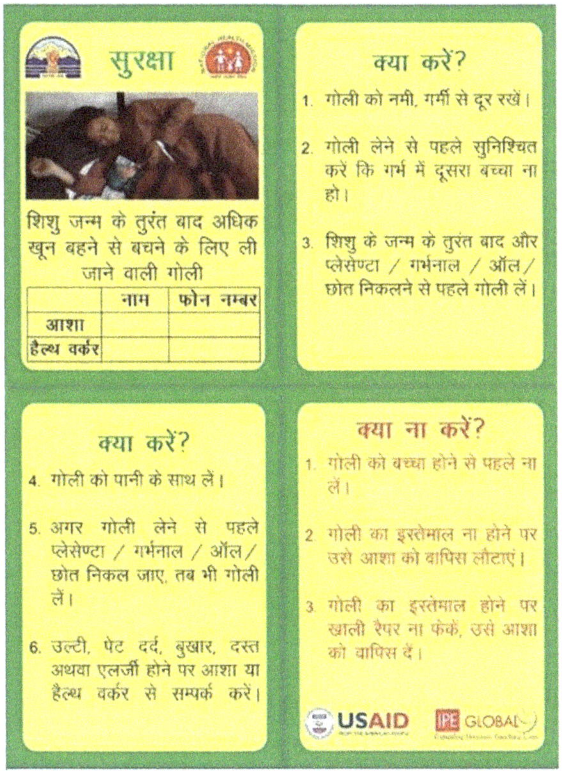

Fig. 2 Pack insert: highlighting Do's and Don'ts for misoprostol use

incorporating all key messages was developed as an Interpersonal Communication and Counselling Tool (IPCC) for the ASHAs for their interaction with expectant mothers (Fig. 3).

The intervention was initiated with a one-day district level orientation on the program guidelines for the district level health officials and program managers in April 2016. This was followed by two block level trainings for the FLWs wherein a total of 100 ASHAs (CHWs), 23 ANMs, block pharmacist and Medical Officer in Charge (MOIC) were trained on the intervention using the program flip book as the training tool. Participatory training methodology was used for the training which provided an opportunity to discuss and deliberate on all issues of the program intervention with the service providers. Key training content included information on the dosage, timing (within a minute of delivery) and route of drug administration and side effects related to the drug. Special impetus was on stressing upon the importance of institutional deliveries which also formed the central theme during the subsequent counselling sessions between the ASHAs and beneficiaries during the drug distribution on completion of the 8th month of pregnancy. In addition, the distribution of tablets to the FLWs was also undertaken during the training, based on the delivery load for the subsequent quarter in the coverage area.

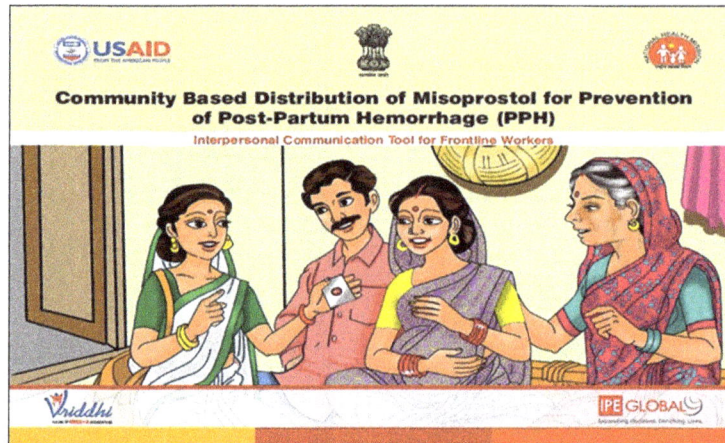

Fig. 3 The Inter-Personal Communication flipbook designed for the intervention

The ANMs of the respective HSCs were involved as field depots to supplement the ASHA with tablets if required.

Health service delivery

Tablet distribution process – To distribute the tablets, AHSAs started visiting the households of pregnant women who had completed their 8th month of pregnancy from the next day of their training. Households were identified from the line list of pregnant women which were made by CHWs for their areas before the trainings.

The distribution work of tablets and related counselling of families was inducted as an additional work for the CHWs in their routine. However, visiting households of potential beneficiaries for reproductive, maternal and child health services was part of exiting routine of the CHWs. This included visiting married couples for family planning services, visiting pregnant women to mobilize them for ante natal checkups and for visiting health facilities for delivering babies, post-delivery follow up care to mother and home-based care for newborn babies. The introduction of 'misoprostol' tablet distribution by CHWs did fit well with the antenatal care support to these PWs and was used as an opportunity to create an additional contact between CHWs and PW or their family members. A detailed, structured counselling process with tablet distribution anchored the message around importance of going to a health institution for delivery. (Fig. 4).

Health information systems

Recording and reporting – The recording formats as available in the national guidelines were adapted and improvised to create a comprehensive recording and reporting mechanism after taking in inputs from involved

- Misoprostol is a safe and effective medicine to prevent bleeding after childbirth
- Misoprostol is not to be consumed before delivery
- Misoprostol is to be consumed within one minute of delivery
- Special care should be taken during the delivery of twin babies, not to take the tablet before both the babies are born
- Misoprostol is to be kept in a safe, dry and cool place, away from children
- Misoprostol is not to be kept under lock and key
- Misoprostol is to be kept in a place where it is easily locatable
- Other elders in the family, and also the *dai*, should be aware of where Misoprostol has been kept
- Once the tablet is consumed the wrapper should be kept carefully and returned to the ASHA
- In case of institutional delivery or any other eventuality, if the tablet is unused, it should be returned to the ASHA
- In case of any problems after delivery and taking the tablet, like – Shivering or chills, continuous bleeding, vomiting etc, a CHW and ANM should be contacted. There contact details are available on the tablet wrapper

Fig. 4 Key messages explained by the ASHAs and ANMs to the pregnant women provided with Misoprostol

stakeholders at all levels. The intervention was initiated with a line listing of current pregnancies in the geography and an Excel based Management Information System (MIS) tool was developed to maintain a database of the beneficiaries as regards consumption of misoprostol tablets and tracking of each drug distributed by collection of unused drug/ wrapper in case of used drug (Additional file 1).

Supportive supervision, monitoring and review mechanisms – A supportive supervision mechanism was institutionalized within the intervention with a structured community monitoring tool developed to facilitate the process. Multiple supportive supervision visits were undertaken primarily by involving the first line supervisors (Lady Health Visitors), block and district level officials and VRIDDHI project team staff. The post-delivery follow up visit served as a method to track the beneficiaries for their pregnancy outcomes, consumption of tablet and any adverse events experienced. Cluster and block level review meetings were held every month to review the progress, identify challenges and refine the intervention. The block level meetings were also used as a platform to assess the tablet usage and distribute tablets to ASHAs as per estimated need.

Health financing

Financial incentives – The distribution of tablet misoprostol at the community level is dependent on ASHA who is a community linked volunteer and incentivized for each service provided. Therefore, a financial incentive structure in line with other health programs has been incorporated for them in the program intervention. The ASHAs were paid a financial incentive of INR 200

for every tablet consumed and INR 100 for return of unused tablet. Moving forward the state has also requested the national ministry for a fixed monthly incentive of INR 300 for submission of monthly reports to the reporting units.

Results

A total of 1265 pregnancy outcomes were reported in Janjheli from 5th May 2016 to 31st May 2017, against 1422 antenatal registrations. Out of this 512 (40%) were reported to be home deliveries, 15 (1%) women delivered on the way to a health facility and 727 (57%) delivered in health facilities, while 11 loss of pregnancy (abortions) were reported. Of the total 1265 deliveries reported, misoprostol was distributed to 979 women who were identified for possible home deliveries. Of the 979 women who were distributed the tablet 511 (52%) had an institutional delivery, 11 (1%) delivered on transit and 457 (47%) had a home delivery. Of the 512 home deliveries reported during the intervention period, the drug was distributed to 457 (89%) women and consumed by 430 beneficiaries thus achieving an uterotonic coverage of 84% for all home deliveries. 55 (11%) women who delivered at home were not distributed the tablet as they were not pre-identified in the home delivery group while 27 (6%) women who were distributed the drug, did not consume the tablet. 6 of these women misplaced the tablets, 7 delivered at their maternal place and did not carry the tablet with them while 11 did not consume it because of apprehensions related to the use (Fig. 5) (Additional file 1).

419 (98%) out of 430 tablets were consumed within 1 min or immediately after delivery of baby while none of the women consumed the tablet before the delivery of the newborn, as reported from the follow up visits of the community health workers.

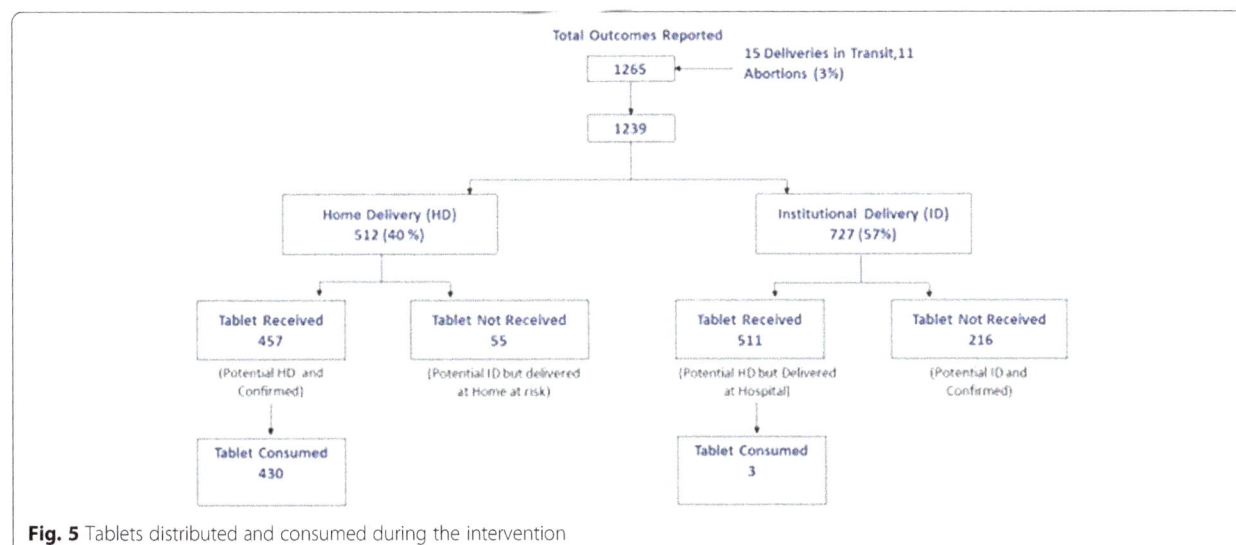

Fig. 5 Tablets distributed and consumed during the intervention

Three women who had institutional deliveries but carried tablets with them consumed the tablet at the health facility itself, while 8 women who delivered on the way while reaching a health facility consumed the tablet. Of the 979 doses distributed, 932 (96%) were successfully tracked either through returned wrappers or unused drugs to the AHSA workers during visits undertaken by them during the Post Natal period. Overall no incidence of PPH was reported among women who consumed misoprostol and only 14 minor adverse events were reported during the intervention period (Table 1). In addition, no maternal death was reported from Janjheli in this period.

An increased involvement of the community with the health system resulted in improved trust between the two. The interaction between the ASHAs and the pregnant women on completion of the 8th month close to the Expected Date of Delivery (EDD) resulted in a five-fold increase in the institutional delivery rates which increased to 57% from just 11% (71 of the 667 reported deliveries) in the preceding year (April 2015 – March 2016). In addition, the interaction also potentiated tracking of pregnancies till delivery. While from April 2015 – March 2016, only 667 (45%) total deliveries were reported against an ANC coverage of 1490, during the intervention period 1265 (89%) pregnancy outcomes were known against 1422 antenatal registrations.

Besides having a direct impact on improving the uterotonic coverage in the home deliveries in the area, the intervention resulted in overall Health System Strengthening (HSS) in Janjheli block. Enhanced capacity of healthcare providers for service delivery, institutionalizing the supportive supervision system, strengthened reporting and effective use of data, improved feedback through regular cluster and block level review meetings and demand generation through community engagement and ownership were key additional learnings from the intervention.

The tangible outcomes of health system improvement as evident from the results of this study were – better

Table 1 Adverse events reported following Misoprostol use

Adverse events reported (N = 430 women who consumed Misoprostol tablet after home based delivery)	Number
Mild Fever	4
Nausea	2
Vomiting	1
Diarrhoea	2
Pain Abdomen	1
Mild tremors	2
Vertigo	1
Temporary Ptosis	1

tracking of pregnancy outcomes and improved institutional delivery rates. The positive effect on various aspects of the health systems in Janjheli block were realized by discussions with the block health functionaries and observations made during the process of implementation. The block health officers recognized that the monthly meetings at block level and cluster level have become more regular and a positive feedback loop during these meetings has become a part of review of other health programs as well. Similarly, the recording and reporting tools used for this intervention are also helping implementation of other programs as they have allowed community health workers to have systematic records of all the pregnant women of their area. The interaction with the community health workers potentiated the fact that the current intervention has built their capacities to communicate with the beneficiary families and also engage them to utilize available health services better. This is also more relevant in the context of Janjheli block, as the community health workers (ASHAs) were commissioned only few months before the intervention and had only gone through an orientation before the trainings for this program were conducted.

There was a positive shift perceived in the antenatal care experience of PW as identified by the CHWs and through follow up interviews by the program supervisors and documentation teams. This could be attributed to an additional antenatal contact at households and a counselling process which allowed enough time to be spent at the households by CHWs. While we did not capture any additional data to look at improved ANC services coverage rate, we interviewed the benefitted family members and CHWs on their experience. Some of the voices which emerged during experience sharing visits are quoted below in Fig. 6.

Discussion

Community based advance distribution of misoprostol tablets for prevention of PPH in home deliveries has been globally recognized as an important intervention contributing to ending preventable maternal deaths [5]. The current intervention has successfully provided a model for effective implementation of the program in India with important implications in reducing incidence of PPH and maternal mortality during home deliveries in the country. Though the country has substantially increased institutional delivery rates, still 6.3 million deliveries are conducted at home. At current national MMR, within this cohort of home deliveries 10,571 maternal deaths are expected with 4228 (40%) being contributed by PPH [4]. Scientific data states that atonic causes contribute to 90% of PPH cases [21–23] and this single intervention reduces deaths due to PPH in home deliveries by 50% [24]. If implemented at 100% coverage the intervention has a potential to possibly avert

"One of the key areas of change because of the Misoprostol program has been the increase in institutional deliveries. The second is improvement in antenatal care. Our FLWs are regularly visiting pregnant women and they have increased the registration of pregnant women in the first trimester of pregnancy, which is very important to provide complete care during pregnancy. Though the percentage of registrations in Janjehli block is lower as compared to other blocks, but the number of registrations in general and registrations in the first trimester have increased during the tenure of the program."
Chief Medical Officer, district Mandi, Himachal Pradesh, India

"Before the intervention, we ourselves did not know clearly about PPH and what its implications are. With this training, our own knowledge base has increased and because if that we can speak with confidence when we go to the community. Even their faith in us has gone up."
An ASHA from Bali Chowki area, district Mandi

"It is an achievement of the Misoprostol program that the number of institutional deliveries has gone up. Our ASHA workers are motivated to visit door-to-door and counsel the pregnant women. The biggest achievement is that women are now aware and ask for Misoprostol on their own."
An ANM from Bali Chowki area, district Mandi

Fig. 6 Experience of Field staff

2114 maternal deaths across the country with more conservative estimates at 70% coverage would avert 1480 maternal deaths across India with an overall reduction in maternal deaths by 3.4–4.8%. Rigorous modelling exercises extrapolated for population estimates in Bangladesh have also demonstrated a reduction of incidence and risk due to death from PPH in home deliveries [25].

The overall uterotonic coverage rate achieved in the current intervention was 84%, which is in line with findings from earlier studies [26–29]. In line with previous studies which have reported minor and transient side effects [26, 30], the current intervention also reported 14 minor, self-limiting side effects (4%) and no PPH case among the 351 women who consumed misoprostol thus strengthening evidence for scale up strategies in India.

The intervention has been able to offset the apprehensions regarding a negative effect on institutional deliveries and drug leakage and misuse. The institutional delivery rate in the area increased five times from 11 to 57% within 6 months of implementation possibly because of an additional contact between the ASHA and the beneficiaries close to the date of delivery and stressing upon the importance of institutional delivery during the counselling sessions. While there is a potential contribution of better tracking of deliveries to the increased proportion of institution-based births, this finding is also in line with three other global interventions which reported an increase in institutional delivery rates during their intervention periods [31–33]. As with the current intervention, the three other programs also appeared to put a high value on counselling of the woman and her family regarding the importance of skilled attendance at birth, the dangers of PPH, and the use of misoprostol

only for the situation where a woman is unable to achieve her plan of a facility-based birth [13].

96% of the distributed drugs were successfully tracked in the intervention with this rate being similar to a study in Ghana in which 98.3% of the doses were successfully tracked and leaks into the system prevented [34]. Giving each tablet a unique identification number and institutionalizing comprehensive operational components of supportive supervision and review meetings were possible reasons for this and again will be defining strategies for scaling up the intervention.

In line with other studies with similar distribution models 98% of the beneficiaries (419 out of 430 home deliveries who received the tablets) consumed the drug within a minute of delivery and as intended no incidence of consumption of the drug was reported prior to delivery, thus underlining the effectiveness of the implementation framework [31, 32, 34].

The current intervention is possibly the first one wherein a single 600 mcg misoprostol has been used instead of the three tablets of 200 mcg each in the public health care system. Though procurement of a single dose 600 mcg tablet was difficult, the state government through pro-active policy level decision making was able to procure the single dose tablet at district level. This not only eased the packaging and distribution of tablet but additionally may have had a positive impact on beneficiary compliance because of ease of consumption of one tablet instead of the usual three, though evidence for the same is currently lacking [35]. Often poor procurement policies limit the success of public health initiatives, but the same was overcome in this program. Taking learnings from the current initiative other states in the country are now procuring the 600 mcg tablet for distribution. Inclusion of the 600 mcg tablet in the country's Essential Drug List (EDL) at all levels of health care will further simplify the process which currently includes only the 100 and 200 mcg tablets for use at tertiary level health facilities [36].

Supply Chain management principles were applied to ensure regular supplies and sufficient stock of tablet Misoprostol. The unique identification number given to each tablet contributed towards effective tracking of the tablet.

Capacity enhancement of the service providers was undertaken through multiple measures during the implementation. A well-designed interactive training package helped improve the understanding and competency of the health workers towards the program while supportive supervision visits and review meetings further potentiated their efforts for effective service delivery. The line listing of pregnant women undertaken at the start of the implementation and the subsequent tracking of beneficiaries helped the service providers have a better understanding of their work area.

Close coordination and team work among the different cadres of health officials and functionaries was demonstrated during the intervention. While the state and district level officials provided clear cut policy level support and guidance, the block MOIC and his team of ANMs, ASHAs, program manager and pharmacist at CHC Janjheli worked closely to ensure smooth and effective service delivery.

Programmatic interpretation and adaptation of the national policy also contributed towards the results. For example, on data review after 4 months of implementation, it was realized that many women having home deliveries were being missed out as they were earlier identified to likely deliver at an institution. Post review the FLWs were advised to ascertain the likelihood of home delivery in PW taking into account the access and time to care and distribute misoprostol to pregnant women who despite all intentions would not be likely to access an institution for delivery. This decision for a more liberal distribution of the drug was taken at the start of winter months with stress on ensuring tracking and collection of unused drug / wrapper and proved pivotal in improving coverage in the later months.

The intervention has again reiterated the importance of active community engagement as a critical contributing factor for the success of any health intervention. Counselling sessions focused at the beneficiary and family members and the contacts between the service providers and the beneficiaries close to the date of delivery not only improved the compliance for institutional deliveries but also improved the trust factor between the two. This aspect of the intervention can definitely help facilitate the implementation of other health programs in the geography.

It is thus imperative that implementation of a community-based program in remote, low resource geographies has to negotiate through challenges of existing program implementation practices. There is a likelihood of unclear program processes clubbed with lack of human resources and their capacities for carrying out these processes. Hence, designing and executing good capacity building measures, carefully curated processes which are co-designed with all involved stakeholders, sustained handholding and problem-solving support, building easy to use data flow processes and relevant mid-course corrections are of high importance.

Limitations of the study –
The current intervention has some limitations in the sense that all the data was reported by the service providers and is subject to bias. However, the tracking of wrappers can be considered as a proxy to the validity of the data. Though the current intervention did not report any incidence of PPH in beneficiaries who consumed misoprostol the relative difficulty in measuring PPH in community based setting can be considered as a limitation. In addition, being a proven intervention with demonstrated effectiveness no baseline and end-line surveys to compare the incidence of PPH was conducted in the intervention area and the entire focus was on optimizing the implementation of the intervention.

Conclusion
Advanced community based distribution of misoprostol has been effective across multiple countries and the current intervention is the first one to demonstrate effectiveness of the program in a field setting in India. The model has successfully demonstrated the implementation of the GOI framework and is now not only being scaled to 11 additional blocks with high home deliveries in the state of Himachal Pradesh, but also to other states of the country. Being a community based intervention, it provides opportunities to build upon other programs targeted at the same geography. Facilitation strategies such as flip book with all key counselling messages, pamphlet with messages on do's & don'ts to beneficiary and documented roles and responsibilities of key stakeholders helped in maintaining implementation fidelity to government programme. The success of this community intervention was also enabled due to constant support and handholding of the FLW delivering the implementation through regular supportive supervision and review by district and state level officials. The intervention also negated the assumption of offsetting the trends of institutional deliveries and in fact contributed to a fivefold increase in hospital based deliveries on account of additional contacts between the service providers and the

beneficiaries which can have huge implications in re-framing of the Ante-Natal Care program in the country.

Key recommendations from the intervention include the use of single 600 mcg tablets instead of the 200 mcg tablets, inclusion of a financial incentive package for the ASHA workers and a more liberal distribution of the tablet to all pregnant women in the intervention geography instead of identifying women with higher chances of home deliveries. Successful scale up of this intervention can contribute towards significant reduction in maternal deaths in the country thereby help achieve the SDG targets.

Abbreviations
ANC: Ante Natal Care; ANMs: Auxiliary Nurse Midwives; ASHAs: Accredited Social Health Activists; BEmOC : Basic Emergency Obstetric Services; BMO: Block Medical Officer; CEmOC : Comprehensive Emergency Obstetric Services; CHC: Community Health Center; CHWs: Community Health Workers; EAG : Empowered Action Group; FLWs : Frontline Health Workers; HMIS: Health Management Information System; HPDs: High Priority Districts; HS : Health Supervisor; HSCs: Health Sub Centers; HSS: Health System Strengthening; MD : Mission Director; MDGs: Millennium Development Goals; MMR: Maternal Mortality Ratio; MO: Medical Officers; MOIC: Medical Officer in Charge; NFHS : National Family Health Survey; PHCs: Primary Health Centers; RMNCH+A: Reproductive Maternal Newborn Child and Adolescent Health; SBA: Skilled Birth Attendant; SDGs: Sustainable Development Goals; SOPs: Standard Operating Procedures; WHO: World Health Organization

Acknowledgements
The authors would like to acknowledge V.S. Sridhar and Sandeep Sharma for designing the Excel based data collation and analysis tool.

Funding
This work was made possible by the support of the American people through the United States Agency for International Development (USAID) and its VRIDDHI – Scaling Up RMNCH+A Interventions Project, implemented by IPE Global Ltd. under the terms of Cooperative Agreement Number AID-386-A-14-00001. USAID has no role in the design of the intervention, data collection, analysis or interpretation. The contents of this paper are the responsibility of IPE Global Ltd. and do not necessarily reflect the views of USAID.

Authors' contribution
RP contributed towards designing the intervention, coordinated the implementation process on ground, undertook data analysis and interpretation and contributed towards writing the methodology, results and discussion section of the manuscript. AG was instrumental in scoping out the intervention, oversaw the implementation of the program in the field and contributed to reviewing and providing inputs to the manuscript. DB1 designed the intervention and the communication package. She also facilitated data analysis and interpretation and reviewed the manuscript. AG facilitated the intervention on ground, oversaw trainings and data collection during the intervention and also analyzed the data and presented the results. RT was involved in the implementation of the intervention and wrote the methodology and description section of the manuscript. AS1 cleaned, managed and analyzed the data, wrote the results section of the manuscript and prepared the Tables. AS2 was instrumental in reviewing the progress of the intervention and provided inputs into the description section of the manuscript. DS facilitated and provided guidance to the implementation process and critically reviewed and provided inputs into the manuscript. SG reviewed and contributed to writing the discussion section of the manuscript. DB2 conceptualized the scope of the intervention and contributed to critically reviewing the manuscript. GT structured the manuscript, drafted the introduction, abstract, methodology and discussions sections. He advised data analysis and coordinated the inputs from all the authors. RG contributed to design and development of the intervention, provided inputs into the data management and analysis sections and also critically reviewed the manuscript. All authors read and approved the final manuscript

Competing interests
The authors declare that they have no competing interests.

Author details
[1]Health Systems, USAID-VRIDDHI/IPE Global, New Delhi, India. [2]Maternal Health, Department of Health and Family Welfare, Government of Himachal Pradesh, Shimla, India. [3]Maternal and Newborn Health, USAID-VRIDDHI/IPE Global, New Delhi, India. [4]USAID-VRIDDHI/IPE Global, Shimla, Himachal Pradesh, India. [5]USAID-VRIDDHI/IPE Global, Mandi, Himachal Pradesh, India. [6]USAID-VRIDDHI/IPE Global, Kinnaur, Himachal Pradesh, India. [7]Department of Health and Family Welfare, Government of Himachal Pradesh, Mandi, Himachal Pradesh, India. [8]Maternal and Child Health, USAID-India, New Delhi, India. [9]Maternal Health, Ministry of Health and Family Welfare, Government of India, New Delhi, India. [10]USAID-VRIDDHI/IPE Global, New Delhi, India.

References
1. Every woman every child. 2015. In: Global Strategy for Women's, Children's, and Adolescents' Health 2016–2030. New York: Every Woman Every Child. Available from: http://www.who.int/life-course/partners/global-strategy/globalstrategyreport2016-2030-lowres.pdf?ua=1.
2. United Nations. The Millennium Development Goals Report. New York; 2015. Available from: http://www.un.org/millenniumgoals/2015_MDG_Report/pdf/MDG%202015%20rev%20(July%201).pdf
3. Office of Registrar General, India. Government of India. Maternal Mortality Ratio Bulletin 2011–13. Available from: http://www.censusindia.gov.in/vital_statistics/mmr_bulletin_2011_13.pdf
4. Ministry of Health and Family Welfare. Operational guidelines and reference manual prevention of post-partum hemorrhage through community based distribution of misoprostol. New Delhi: Ministry of Health and Family Welfare; 2013.
5. World Health Organization. WHO recommendations for the prevention and treatment of postpartum hemorrhage. Geneva: World Health Organization; 2012.
6. Prata N, Passano P, Rowen T, Bell S, Walsh J, Potts M. Where there are (few) skilled attendants. J Health Popul Nutr. 2011;29(2):81–91.
7. Crowe S, Utley M, Costello A, Pagel C. How many births in sub-Saharan Africa and South Asia will not be attended by a skilled birth attendant between 2011 and 2015? BMC Pregnancy Childbirth. 2012;12:4. https://doi.org/10.1186/1471-2393-12-4.
8. Montagu D, Yarney G, Visconti A, Harding A, Yoong J. Where do poor women in developing countries give birth? A multi-country analysis of demographic and health survey data. PLoS One. 2011;6:e17155. https://doi.org/10.1371/journal.pone.0017155.

9. Diaz-Granados N, Pitzul KB, Dorado LM, Wang F, McDermott S, Rondon MB. Monitoring gender equity in health using gender-sensitive indicators: a cross-national study. J Women's Health. 2011;20:145–53. https://doi.org/10.1089/jwh.2010.2057.

10. Payne S. An elusive goal? Gender equity and gender equality in health policy. Gesundheitswen. 2012;74:e19–24.

11. McCormick ML, Sanghvi HCG, Kinzie B, McIntosh N. Averting maternal death and disability: prevention postpartum hemorrhage in low-resource settings. Int J Obstet Gynaecol. 2002;77:267–75. https://doi.org/10.1016/S0020-7292(02)00020-6.

12. WHO. Optimizing health worker roles to improve access to key maternal and newborn health interventions through task shifting. Geneva: WHO; 2012.

13. Smith JM, Gubin R, Holston MM, Fullerton J, Prata N. Misoprostol for postpartum hemorrhage prevention at home birth: an integrative review of global implementation experience to date. BMC Pregnancy Childbirth. 2013; 13:44. https://doi.org/10.1186/1471-2393-13-44.

14. Hundley VA, Avan BI, Sullivan CJ, Graham WJ. Should oral misoprostol be used to prevent postpartum haemorrhage in home-birth settings in low-resource countries? A systematic review of the evidence. Br J Obstet Gynecol. 2013;120(3):277–85. https://doi.org/10.1111/1471-0528.12049.

15. International Institute for Population Sciences (IIPS). National Family Health Survey (NFHS-4), 2015–16. Mumbai: IIPS; 2017. Available from: http://rchiips.org/NFHS/pdf/NFHS4/India.pdf

16. Ejembi CL, Norick P, Starrs A, Thapa K. New global guidance supports community and lay health workers in postpartum hemorrhage prevention. Int J GynecolObstet. 2013;122(3):187–90.

17. Family Care International & Gynuity Health Projects. Reaching women wherever they give birth. Misoprostol for Postpartum Haemorrhage. Stories of success in Bangladesh, Nepal and Zambia; 2012.

18. National Rural Health Mission. Ministry of Health and Family Welfare, Government of India. New Delhi: 5x5 Matrix for High Impact RMNCH+A Interventions; 2013. Available from: https://www.scribd.com/document/334162081/RMNCH-A-5x5-matrix

19. National Disaster Risk Reduction Portal: Himachal Pradesh. Available from: http://lib.icimod.org/record/23446/files/c_attachment_234_2503.pdf

20. Everybody business: strengthening health systems to improve health outcomes: WHO's framework for action. Available from: http://www.who.int/healthsystems/strategy/everybodys_business.pdf

21. Bateman BT, Berman MF, Riley LE, Leffert LR. The epidemiology of postpartum hemorrhage in a large, nationwide sample of deliveries. Anesth Analg. 2010;110(5):1368–73.

22. Carroli G, Cuesta C, Abalos E, Gulmezoglu AM. Epidemiology of postpartum haemorrhage: a systematic review. Best practice & researchClinical obstetrics & gynaecology. 2008;22(6):999–1012.

23. Combs CA, Murphy EL, Laros RK Jr. Factors associated with postpartum hemorrhage with vaginal birth. Obstet Gynecol. 1991;77(1):69–76.

24. Derman RJ, Kodkany BS, Goudar SS, Geller SE, Naik VA, Bellad MB, Patted SS, Patel A, Edlavitch SA, Hartwell T, et al. Oral misoprostol in preventing postpartum haemorrhage in resource-poor communities: a randomised controlled trial. Lancet. 2006;368(9543):1248–53.

25. Prata N, Bell S, Quaiyum M. Modeling maternal mortality in Bangladesh: the role of misoprostol in postpartum hemorrhage prevention. BMC Pregnancy Childbirth. 2014;14(1):78.

26. Smith JM, Baawo SD, Subah M, Sirtor-Gbassie V, Howe CJ, Ishola G, et al. Advance distribution of misoprostol for prevention of postpartum hemorrhage (PPH) at home births in two districts of Liberia. BMC Pregnancy Childbirth. 2014;14:189.

27. Quaiyum A, Gazi R, Hossain S, Wirtz A, Saha NC. Feasibility, acceptability, and Programme effectiveness of misoprostol for prevention of postpartum Haemorrhage in rural Bangladesh: a Quasiexperimental study. International journal of reproductive medicine. 2014;2014(580949):8. https://doi.org/10.1155/2014/580949.

28. Sanghvi H, Wiknjosastro G, Chanpong G, Fishel J, Ahmed S, Zulkarnain M. Prevention of postpartum hemorrhage study. West Java: Jhpiego; 2004.

29. Smith JM, Dimiti A, Dwivedi V, Ochieng I, Dalaka M, Currie S, et al. Advance distribution of misoprostol for the prevention of postpartum hemorrhage in South Sudan. International journal of gynaecology and obstetrics: the official organ of the International Federation of Gynaecology and Obstetrics. 2014;127(2):183–8.

30. Walraven G, Blum J, Dampha Y, et al. Misoprostol in the management of the third stage of labour in the home delivery setting in rural Gambia: a randomised controlled trial. International Journal of Obstetrics and Gynaecology. 2005;112(9):1277–83.

31. Rajbhandari S, Hodgins S, Sanghvi H, McPherson R, Pradhan YV, Baqui AH. Expanding uterotonic protection following childbirth through community-based distribution of misoprostol: operations research study in Nepal. Int J Gynaecol Obstet. 2010;108:282–8. https://doi.org/10.1016/j.ijgo.2009.11.006.

32. Sanghvi H, Ansari N, Prata NJ, Gibson H, Ehsan AT, Smith JM. Prevention of postpartum hemorrhage at home birth in Afghanistan. Int J Gynaecol Obstet. 2010;108:276–81. https://doi.org/10.1016/j.ijgo.2009.12.003.

33. Ministry of Health, Zambia, Venture Strategies Innovations, Bixby Center for Population, Health and Sustainability. Misoprostol Distribution at Antenatal Care Visits for Prevention of Postpartum Hemorrhage: Final Report. Berkely: Venture Strategies Innovation and Bixby Center at University of California; 2010.

34. Geller S, Carnahan L, Akosah E, Asare G, Agyemang R, Dickson R, et al. Community-based distribution of misoprostol to prevent postpartum haemorrhage at home births: results from operations research in rural Ghana. BJOG. 2014;121(3):319–25.

35. Helen JS, Christopher JC, Esther R, Jeffrey R, Geeta S, Kusum T, et al. Programmes for advance distribution of misoprostol to prevent post-partum hemorrhage: a rapid literature review of factors affecting implementation. Health Policy Plan. 2015:1–12 Available from: http://www.academia.edu/25958346/Programmes_for_advance_distribution_of_misoprostol_to_prevent_postpartum_haemorrhage_a_rapid_literature_review_of_factors_affecting_implementation.

36. Ministry of Health and Family Welfare, GOI: National List of Essential Medicines 2015.Available from: http://apps.who.int/medicinedocs/documents/s23088en/s23088en.pdf

11

Missed opportunities in antenatal care for improving the health of pregnant women and newborns in Geita district, Northwest Tanzania

Eveline Thobias Konje[1,2]* [iD], Moke Tito Nyambita Magoma[3], Jennifer Hatfield[2], Susan Kuhn[4], Reginald S. Sauve[2] and Deborah Margret Dewey[2,4,5]

Abstract

Background: Despite the significant benefits of early detection and management of pregnancy related complications during antenatal care (ANC) visits, not all pregnant women in Tanzania initiate ANC in a timely manner. The primary objectives of this research study in rural communities of Geita district, Northwest Tanzania were: 1) to conduct a population-based study that examined the utilization and availability of ANC services; and 2) to explore the challenges faced by women who visited ANC clinics and barriers to utilization of ANC among pregnant women.

Methods: A sequential explanatory mixed method design was utilized. Household surveys that examined antenatal service utilization and availability were conducted in 11 randomly selected wards in Geita district. One thousand, seven hundred and nineteen pregnant women in their 3rd trimester participated in household surveys. It was followed by focus group discussions with community health workers and pregnant women that examined challenges and barriers to ANC.

Results: Of the pregnant women who participated, 86.74% attended an ANC clinic at least once; 3.62% initiated ANC in the first trimester; 13.26% had not initiated ANC when they were interviewed in their 3rd trimester. Of the women who had attended ANC at least once, the majority (82.96%) had been checked for HIV status, less than a half (48.36%) were checked for hemoglobin level, and only a minority had been screened for syphilis (6.51%). Among women offered laboratory testing, the prevalence of HIV was 3.88%, syphilis, 18.57%, and anemia, 54.09%. In terms of other preventive measures, 91.01% received a tetanus toxoid vaccination, 76.32%, antimalarial drugs, 65. 13%, antihelminthic drugs, and 76.12%, iron supplements at least once. Significant challenges identified by women who visited ANC clinics included lack of male partner involvement, informal regulations imposed by health care providers, perceived poor quality of care, and health care system related factors. Socio-cultural beliefs, fear of HIV testing, poverty and distance from health clinics were reported as barriers to early ANC utilization.

Conclusion: Access to effective ANC remains a challenge among women in Geita district. Notably, most women initiated ANC late and early initiation did not guarantee care that could contribute to better pregnancy outcomes.

Keywords: Antenatal care, Missed opportunity, Tanzania, Sequential explanatory mixed method

* Correspondence: etkonje@ucalgary.ca
[1]Department of Biostatistics & Epidemiology, School of Public Health, Catholic University of Health and Allied Sciences, P.O. box 1464 Bugando Area, Mwanza, Tanzania
[2]Department of Community Health Sciences, Cumming School of Medicine, University of Calgary, 3280 Hospital Drive, NW, Calgary, AB, Canada
Full list of author information is available at the end of the article

Background

To reduce preventable maternal and newborn mortality and morbidity, the provision of quality antenatal care (ANC), accessible obstetrics care, and life-saving interventions are essential services [1–5]. In 2015, approximately 303,000 maternal deaths occurred worldwide with sub-Saharan Africa accounting for 66% of all maternal deaths [6]. Although some developing countries have achieved up to a 75% reduction in the maternal mortality ratio (MMR) since 1990, Tanzania has made little progress over the past 25 years [2, 6]. In 1990, the MMR was 529 maternal deaths per 100,000 live births and in 2015/16 it was 545 maternal deaths per 100,000 live births [7]. Most developing countries have achieved a reduction in mortality among under five children; however, the proportion of neonatal deaths and stillborn babies remains unacceptably high [2, 8]. Globally, it was estimated in 2015 that there were 18.4 stillbirths per 1000 births with rural populations accounting for 60% of all stillborn babies [8]. Tanzania ranked ninth in the world among the ten countries with the highest number of stillbirths in 2015 with an estimated 47,000 stillbirths [8]. Most of these stillbirths occurred during labor and delivery and were considered to be due to preventable or manageable health conditions [8, 9].

The sustainable development goal 3.1, emphasizes reducing the MMR to less than 220 per 100, 000 live births for countries with an MMR above the average global level [10]. To end preventable causes of maternal deaths due to pregnancy related complications, scaling up of existing interventions during pregnancy and delivery is crucial [5]. The main causes of maternal deaths are hemorrhage, hypertensive disorder, and infection [11]. Newborn deaths and stillbirths are mainly due to asphyxia, prematurity, and infections [8, 9] and most are preventable with existing evidence-based interventions either directly or indirectly during pregnancy, labor, delivery, and post delivery [1, 3, 5].

Safe motherhood initiative programs recognize the significance of the provision of quality care from preconception to the postnatal period for women and newborn babies. They consist of four pillars, namely, family planning, ANC, clean and safe delivery, and essential obstetric care services [3]. ANC is recognized and emphasized due to its influence on the wellbeing of pregnant women and their unborn babies [1, 3, 5]. In 2002, Tanzania adopted the Focused ANC (FANC) model recommended by the World Health Organisation (WHO). It is still utilized although the WHO introduced a new ANC model in 2016 [1, 12]. The FANC model emphasizes individualized care for all pregnant women as any pregnancy could face complications. It suggests a minimum of 4 visits for uncomplicated pregnancies with the initial visit occurring before 16 weeks gestation, the second visit between 20 and 24 weeks, a third visit between 28 and 32 weeks, and a fourth visit at 36 weeks [13].

Although universal coverage of ANC services is reported globally and at the country level [2, 7, 10, 14], in developing countries, many pregnant women fail to benefit from comprehensive ANC due to factors such as late initiation and the poor quality of ANC services [2, 14–17]. Early initiation during the first trimester and quality ANC over the pregnancy period has been recognized as improving pregnancy outcomes and increasing newborn survival [18, 19]. However, in developing countries, only 25% of pregnant women initiated ANC before 14 weeks gestation and 48% of pregnant women did not complete 4 ANC visits [2, 15]. Several factors have been associated with late initiation including: older age, higher parity/multiparity, lower education level, hidden costs, lack of male support, pregnancy-related cultural beliefs, unplanned pregnancy, and health system related issues such as shortages of supplies and drugs [14, 20–24]. However, most of the studies that have reported on the timing and frequency of ANC utilization were retrospective in nature and included women who had a live birth in the 2–5 years prior to the conduct of the study. The results of these studies could be influenced by survival and recall bias, as the information obtained was from women who survived their pregnancy and were able to provide a self report [14, 20–22, 25, 26]. In addition, these studies were health facility-based, and as a result may suffer from selection bias as attendees were likely to be women with better health care seeking behavior than non-attendees, particularly in rural low income settings, leading to an over estimation of early initiation and utilization of ANC during pregnancy [20, 21, 25].

In Tanzania, early initiation of ANC (i.e., attending antenatal care in the first trimester) is reported to be 24%, and only 51% of women had more than 4 antenatal care visits in 2015/16 [7]. Northwest Tanzania is a region with a low rate of utilization of ANC services despite the existing high fertility rate in this region [7]. The primary objectives of this research study in rural communities of Geita district, Northwest Tanzania were: 1) to conduct a population-based study that examined the utilization and availability of ANC services, and 2) to explore the challenges faced by women who visited ANC clinics and barriers to utilization of ANC among pregnant women.

Methods
Study setting

The study was conducted at Geita district, one of the six districts in Geita region Northwest Tanzania. The district has 35 wards with a district hospital, 5 health centers, and 38 dispensaries. Eleven wards (31%) were randomly selected for inclusion in the study, namely: Lwamgasa, Nyaruyeye, Bukoli, Nyarugusu, Nyakamwaga, Butundwe, Chigunga, Nyamiluluma, Bukondo, Nzera, and Lwenzera. Random selection was accomplished by first alphabetically ordering the wards and numbering them from 1 to 35. Then a random numbers table was used to select eleven wards. Based on the Tanzania Demographic and Health Survey (TDHS) 2015/16, Geita performed poorly on components of ANC and more than a half (52.3%) of pregnant women delivered at home [7].

Study design

This study is part of a large cohort study that is investigating utilization of maternal and child health services, pregnancy outcomes, birth-related complications, and maternal and child mortality and morbidity up to 4 months postpartum. The study utilized a sequential explanatory mixed method approach. This method has two phases. The first phase is characterized by the collection and analysis of quantitative data. The second phase involves the collection and analysis of qualitative data. This method uses the qualitative findings to further explain and interpret the findings of the quantitative data and was selected as it allowed exploring in detail the challenges pregnant women faced when accessing ANC services and the barriers to utilization of ANC services.

Quantitative data collection process

A household survey using a cross sectional design involving pregnant women in the third trimester was conducted between September 2016 and August 2017. Based on 2015 total deliveries for the entire district (36,101), we assumed that approximately 10,000 (28%) pregnant women would be residing in the study area with at least 20% (2000) of them being in their third trimester of pregnancy. The study reached 1805 (90%) of the expected pregnant women in the selected wards, of whom 1719 participated in the survey. Of those who were contacted but not included in our final sample, 81 were not residents of a study area, two had had miscarriages, one woman was in the second trimester of her pregnancy based on her last menstruation period, and two women refused to participate because they were not feeling well.

The household survey consisted of a face-to-face interview. During the conduct of the household survey interview, only pregnant women in their 3rd trimester who voluntarily consented were invited to participate in the study. In the situation that a pregnant woman was not at home during the time the household survey was conducted, that household was re-visited up to three times to see if the woman was interested in participating.

Village leaders, community health workers, and traditional birth attendants assisted in the identification of households with pregnant women. Trained research assistants who were registered nurses, and intern medical doctors conducted the household survey. The research assistants were not health care providers at health facilities in the study areas (they were from college/university and were not employed as health care providers); hence, interview bias was expected to be minimal. The principal investigator (EK) supervised the conduct of the survey.

For the household survey, a structured pretested questionnaire was utilized to capture baseline information including socio-demographic characteristics, gestational age, parity, gravidity, obstetric history, immunization status, intermittent preventive treatement status, deworming status, and the use of iron and folate supplements. The questionnaire also captured information on birth preparedness, an anticipated place for delivery, social support after delivery, money saving for any emergency during pregnancy, and the purchase baby's items, which are included as part of the health education provided through ANC services (seeAdditional file 1). For women who had attended ANC clinics, responses to the household survey questions were crosschecked with their antenatal cards, which are provided to pregnant women who attend ANC clinics. During the household survey, the pregnant women's blood pressure was checked, weight and height were measured, an identification card for follow-up purposes was provided, and counselling regarding the utilization of ANC services was provided. The household surveys were conducted in the homes of the pregnant women unless otherwise specified by the participant. In those rare cases (only four women), the interview was scheduled at a convenient location identified by the participant, usually at their farm or at a friend's house.

Qualitative data collection process

A case study was conducted to explore in depth barriers to utilization of antenatal care services among women in the study area. Women and community health workers from six wards namely Lwenzera, Nzera, Nyarugusu, Bukoli, Lwamgasa, and Bukondo were invited to participate in focus group discussions. Using the results from the analyses of the household survey data, study wards were selected based on the criterion of having a significant number of women who initiated ANC late or who never attended ANC. Community health workers (CHWs) were also invited to participate because of the nature of their work in bridging the community with the health care system. Hence, participants were purposively selected for the focus group discussions (FGDs). FDGs provided the women with a safe environment in which they could present their views and opinions and provided the participants with the opportunity to see that the challenges and barriers that they experienced were similar those of other women. The FGDs also promoted open discussion and sometimes disagreement, and allowed us to observe the group dynamics. Finally, FGDs allowed us to observe whether there was consensus of group members on the challenges faced by women who visited ANC clinics and the barriers to utilization of ANC among pregnant women.

We conducted six FGDs with women who had recently delivered babies, many of whom had not utilized ANC and delivery services. Thirty-five women from the selected wards participated in the FGDs with an average of five to six women in each group. Six focus groups were also conducted with CHWs, one in each of the six wards. On average, five to six CHWs, both male and female participated from each ward making 32 CHWs. A semi-structured interview guide was used to facilitate discussion among participants. The key issues explored were: 1) What do you know about maternal and child health services available to you during pregnancy or to pregnant women? 2) What has been your experience with ANC services in your community? and 3) Why do some pregnant women not utilize the ANC services available in their communities or are late in utilizing these services?

The research team conducted the FDGs in the Swahili language and where necessary in the local language (Sukuma). Members of the research team who were fluent in Sukuma assisted with translation during discussions. None of the research team members involved in conducting the FGDs provided directed medical care to the participants through the local community health centers. Voice recordings were transcribed, translated into English, and back translated into Swahili to ensure content consistency. Field notes were taken by EK and some of the FGDs were supervised by DD. For the purposes of confidentiality, privacy, and friendly environment, FGDs typically occurred at the village leaders' offices or at primary schools. However, in some cases, (two focus groups), they took place at the local health clinic. Each FGD took approximately one hour and thirty minutes.

Data management and analysis

ANC service utilization was the outcome of interest. Three levels were examined, namely no attendance at ANC services, attendance within the first trimester, and attendance in the second or third trimester. Epi-Data version 3.1 software was used for data entry with the double entry system feature to reduce data entry errors. This feature allows double entry of the same questionnaire data by two different clerks. During dataset validation, inconsistencies were resolved by reviewing the original questionnaires and editing accordingly. Cleaned

data were exported and analyzed using STATA version 13 [27]. The 95% confidence intervals and p values reported were based on a 5% level of statistical significance. Chi-squared tests were used to examine associations between categorical variables.

Qualitative data were transcribed and translated into English by two RAs fluent in Swahili and English and cross-checked by EK for discrepancies. Thematic analysis was conducted by EK and reviewed by DD. It involved familiarization with data, identification of the main themes, indexing, charting, mapping, and interpretation. Line by line coding was done manually and identified themes were compared with written field notes for convergence or divergence of ideas. The identified themes were used to gain a deeper understanding of the quantitative results. The data source triangulation was done by having group discussions with community health workers and women in order to confirm the perceived challenges and barriers. The contiguous approach was adapted for data integration at the interpretation and reporting level.

Results

Household survey participant characteristics

Of the 1805 pregnant women visited at their homes, 1719 were eligible for this study. The average age of the participants was 25.7 years (see Table 1). Almost all of the participants (94.71%) were married and the majority of the women reported having a primary school education (68.59%); however, a considerable proportion (23.61%) reported no formal schooling.

Household survey

Antenatal services utilization and availability

Overall, antenatal attendance with at least one visit was 86.74% (1491/1719); however, a considerable proportion of participants 13.26% (228/1719) had not initiated ANC at the time of the household survey. Of the 1491 pregnant women who visited an antenatal clinic at least once, only 3.62% (54/1491; 95% CI 2.67–4.57) initiated ANC at the first trimester while the rest of the participants initiated ANC either in the 2nd or 3rd trimester. Further, although more than three quarters of participants attended antenatal clinics, provision of laboratory and preventive services were not common to all pregnant women. As per the FANC model, pregnant women should receive services related to disease prevention, health promotion, detection and treatment of existing disease, and information on developing a birth preparedness plan. Laboratory testing was limited to 82.96% women for HIV, 48.36% women for hemoglobin level (Hb in g/dL), and 6.51% for syphilis (see Table 2). The prevalence of existing conditions based on the records from antenatal cards was 3.88% for HIV infection,

Table 1 Socio-demographic characteristics of 1719 pregnant women in rural Geita by ANC attendance

Characteristic	Overall		Women attended ANC at least once (N = 1491)		Women not attended ANC (N = 228)	
	Mean(SD)	n (%)	n (%)	Mean (SD)	n (%)	Mean (SD)
Maternal age (in years)	25.73 (6.60)			25.51 (6.52)		27.28 (6.96)
Maternal height (in cm)	155.66 (6.90)			155.77 (6.73)		154.89 (7.92)
Maternal weight (in Kg)	59.49 (8.39)			59.71 (8.38)		57.97 (8.31)
Marital status						
Currently single		91 (5.29)	83 (5.57)		8 (3.51)	
Currently married		1628 (94.71)	1408 (96.43)		220 (96.49)	
Education level						
No formal education		406 (23.61)	347 (23.27)		59 (25.88)	
Primary		1179 (68.59)	1024 (68.68)		155 (67.98)	
Secondary & above		134 (7.80)	120 (8.05)		14 (6.14)	

Table 2 Antenatal care services received and prevalence of screened conditions among 1491 women

Characteristic	Services received at clinics	Prevalence	95% CI
	n (%)	n (%)	
HIV Status			
-Total Screened	1237 (82.96)		
-Tested Positive		48 (3.88)	2.80–4.95
-Tested Negative		1189 (96.12)	
Hemoglobin level			
-Total screened	721 (48.36)		
-Hb level < 10.9 g/dL		390 (54.09)	50.45–57.74
-Hb level > =10.9 g/dL		331 (45.91)	
Syphilis status			
-Total Screened	97 (6.51)		
- Tested Positive		18 (18.57)	10.68–26.43
- Tested Negative		79 (81.43)	
Iron supplements	1135 (76.12)		
Antihelminthic drugs			
- None	520 (34.87)		
- One Dose	475 (31.86)		
- Two Doses	496 (33.27)		
Intermittent preventive treatment			
- None	353 (23.68)		
- One Dose	518 (34.74)		
-Two Doses	620 (41.58)		
Tetanus toxoid vaccine			
- None	134 (8.99)		
- One Dose	229 (15.36)		
-Two or more doses	1128 (75.65)		

54.09% for anemia, and 18.57% for syphilis infection. Regarding preventive measures, 91.01% of participants received a tetanus toxoid vaccination, 76.32%, antimalarial drugs, 65.13%, antihelminthic drugs, and 76.12%, iron supplements at least once.

During the household survey the women were asked about their intentions to deliver at the health facility; plans for transport to the health facility, and saving money for possible emergencies during pregnancy or delivery. They were also asked if they had bought any items for their baby (i.e., basin, clothes, soap), and any social support after the delivery of the baby (i.e., their birth preparedness plan). More than half (54.33%) of the participants indicated that they did not intend to deliver at a health facility. The majority (71.5%) had no plan for transport during labour and 64.39% had not purchased baby items. However, half of the participants had saved money (49.74%) for an emergency during pregnancy or delivery. Significant differences (p value < 0.05) were observed between women who attended ANC clinics at least once and those who did not attend ANC on all components of birth preparedness except social support. ANC clinic attendees were more likely to plan for transport, save money, buy items for their baby, and indicate that they intended to deliver at a health facility compared to those who had not attended an ANC clinic (Table 3).

General characteristics of participants in FGDs

The women who participated in six FGDs (n = 35) were multiparous and had attended ANC clinics at least once in previous pregnancies or the current pregnancy. Of the 32 CHWs who participated in the FGDs, all had at least a year of experience working as a CHW and over half (53%) were male. In terms of the dynamics of the FGDs, the women and the CHWs were very open and forthcoming in their responses to the questions asked by research team members, most women and CHWs contributed to the discussion and participation by all participants was encouraged by the researchers.

Perceived barriers for antenatal care services

This section discusses the perceived barriers that women identified as hindering their utilization of ANC services. It focuses on the issues that women perceived to hinder their utilization of available ANC services. Focus group discussions with women and CHWs were used to identify themes related to perceived barriers to utilization of ANC services in rural Geita district. Women indicated that they do not initiate ANC at all due to the following reasons: poverty, fear of HIV testing, and socio-cultural beliefs (Table 4).

Poverty may influence the health care seeking behavior of pregnant women negatively. Many women have no source of income in the family; therefore, any cost related to health care is a financial burden for the entire family. Fares for transport to ANC clinics, a maternity dress, or other hidden costs can act as a barrier for some women in the rural communities.

Having no income in the family, and [the] health facility being far may lead to women not attending ANC services at all considering the family does not have even a bicycle. Female participant 1

It could be poverty, since nurses here emphasize clean clothes and proper dress such as a maternity dress when a woman wants to attend clinic. If you don't have a maternity dress you may not go. Female participant 5

Participants also identified men's lack of interest and their unwillingness to participate during pregnancy, which resulted in some women not attending ANC clinics. For HIV prevention of mother-to-child transmission, couples are required to go together to the first antenatal visit. This practice aims at providing counselling and HIV testing to both partners. However, some health providers deny ANC services to pregnant women who attended without their male partners. Fear of HIV testing by both female and male partners was also perceived to be a barrier to ANC for couples that were unwilling to participate in HIV testing together.

Table 3 Birth preparedness planning among 1719 pregnant women in rural Geita district

Characteristic		Overall	Women who attended ANC at least once N = 1491	Women who had not attended ANC N = 228	Difference in proportions P value (chi² test)
		n (%)	n (%)	n (%)	
Health facility delivery	Yes	785 (45.67)	730 (48.96)	52 (24.12)	< 0.05
Transport preparation	Yes	490 (28.50)	448 (30.05)	42 (18.42)	< 0.05
Saving money	Yes	855 (49.74)	783 (52.52)	72 (31.58)	< 0.05
Purchase baby items	Yes	574 (33.39)	531 (35.61)	43 (18.86)	< 0.05
Social support	Yes	1438 (83.65)	1254 (84.10)	184 (80.70)	0.20

Some women stay at home throughout their pregnancy period because men are not ready to accompany them to the clinic. It is a "must to go" with your husband on the first visit. Female participant 1

Yes, men not escorting their women is a main problem I can say. When a pregnant woman attends clinic for the first time, the health provider must asks where is your husband, and if you don't have your male partner the possibility of being seen in the clinic is very small and you may end up being scolded. To avoid being harassed, pregnant women may not attend the ANC clinic. Male CHW 1

In the rural settings, parents or in-laws make decisions for couples who live with them. Decisions related to health care seeking may depend upon the attitudes of parents/in-laws towards ANC services and their experiences with the health care system. Men who escort their wives are considered weak in this male dominant society. Participants indicated that parents/in-laws might hinder pregnant women from attending ANC clinics and it becomes a barrier when the couple depends on their parents/in-laws financially.

It is a habit based on parents' experiences. Men do think if my mother did not attend clinic at all or attended only once and gave birth without any problem why bother now. It is common with couples that stay with their parents. If your wife mentions about escorting her to the clinic, your father may say in our times, we did not go with women to their services, why do you want to do it now. This is being weak, your mother did not go and all went well. Then you think no need for my wife to attend clinic. Male CHW 5

Sometimes, a few men may prevent women from attending ANC arguing, do women who miss out ANC face any problems during delivery? But there are those who attended and still experienced complications. So you will stay at home, all will be well. With this response, some women decide not to attend at all. Female participant 6

For those families that stay with their in-laws, since the mother-in-law did not attend clinic, a pregnant woman will find it difficult to attend ANC clinic. Since her mother-in-law will discourage her saying, "We did not go to ANC clinic in those years why do you want to go there?" It becomes more difficult if a man depends on his parent financially. Female CHW 6

Challenges faced by women in visiting ANC clinics

This section highlights the challenges faced by pregnant women who attended an ANC clinic at least once. These challenges included poverty, perceived poor quality of ANC services, and lack of male involvement that hindered pregnant women's timely utilization of ANC services (Table 4).

Participants stated clearly that poverty delayed pregnant women from accessing ANC services in a timely manner. Due to the distance to health facilities and lack of transportation, many pregnant women decided to wait until their third trimester to initiate visits to an ANC clinic. Early ANC initiation meant spending a lot of money on transport, and many women had no source of ongoing income and lacked a bicycle or motorcycle for transport. Factor such as distance may act as both a barrier as well as a challenge to the utilization of ANC services. For some women distance to the ANC clinic could delay their attendance until the third trimester. As a result, they would only make a single visit during their pregnancy for a general check-up.

Due to distance and other issues, instead of visiting to the clinic every month a woman opts to attend only once to avoid the frequency of going to the clinic every month by attending in the last months of the pregnancy from seventh month. Female CHW 1

Sometimes you may feel weak and lazy to walk every month, remember we cannot afford paying for boda boda because we don't have money. Then you decide to wait till you approach the 8th or 9th month so that you have one visit to get an ANC card. Female participant 3

Long distance for some of the villages discourages most of the pregnant women to attend ANC clinics early. Some villages are far away from dispensaries, approximately more than 7 kilometers, making it difficult for pregnant women to walk that long distance. This is worse when the household does not have a bicycle or a motorcycle or money for fare. Even if they know the importance of ANC services, still they may not attend early. Male CHW 1

Women appeared to have some knowledge of the benefits of initiating early ANC services; however, perceived poor quality of ANC services in this community discouraged timely initiation of care. Pregnant women are supposed to receive comprehensive ANC when attending clinics, but in these communities, the absence of health care providers and shortages of supplies and drugs were identified as common challenges.

Most of the services such as antimalarial drugs, iron tablets, mosquito nets are not always available, and laboratory supplies are on and off because our clinics serve a large population, which is not proportional to the available supplies and drugs. Female CHW 1

When you go for ANC they send you back several times because health providers are not there or have gone for seminars. You may go to clinic several times with no luck of receiving any ANC services till you get tired and give up. You may miss the services for several visits because the health providers have gone for seminars or training. Female participant 5

This practice of sending back pregnant women without services has been common in our dispensary and it discourages pregnant women. For example, recently there were no ANC services for the entire week because of the shortage of health providers. There was only one health provider attending only out patients and other emergency care services. Male CHW 6

Lack of male involvement and participation during pregnancy was also a challenge for women who attended ANC clinics in the rural communities. Participants noted that the lack of men's involvement or interest was associated with cultural beliefs, the influence of in-laws, and the environment at the health facilities, which was not male friendly. HIV testing is crucial for both partners; however, and both partners need to agree to HIV testing after proper counselling and health education. In this community, HIV testing was associated with fear by the women as the laboratory test was done in the presence of the male partner. Furthermore, the existing health facilities provided no privacy for the couple during the counselling or the conduct of HIV testing.

Actually, most women in this community go late for antenatal services because of the fear of HIV testing while some men refuse to escort their women for fear of HIV testing. Female participant 4

It is really challenging in this community because of the high rates of HIV infection. The habit of HIV testing among men is not there. Escorting women to the clinic requires men to be ready for HIV testing and results. They think how I can go there when I am not ready to take an HIV test. It is better I just send my wife and I will know if I am safe or not through my wife's HIV result. They believe if a woman is HIV negative they are also negative so there is no need of going there. Male CHW 4

We do not have a friendly environment. For example, with our health facility there is no infrastructure for a reproductive and child health unit. Currently, all patients who come for TB and HIV drugs, out

patients, and pregnant women and under-five children are gathered in one place. There is no privacy and friendly environment for the couple. Male CHW 3

Some cultural beliefs in relation to pregnancy were perceived as causing delays in visiting ANC clinics. For example, in the first trimester, women do not disclose their "invisible" pregnancy to people including health providers for the fear of being witched. In addition, there were misconceptions about use of hematinics as many women thought that iron supplements prolonged the period of pregnancy, tended to exaggerate morning sickness symptoms, and sometimes even cause adverse outcomes. To avoid prolonged use of hematinics, they delay the initiation of ANC care.

We wait for a visible pregnancy for us to start clinic. You cannot start attending clinic with an invisible pregnancy; our fellow women may scold you when we go to fetch water. We do not mention to everyone that you are pregnant. We do this because we fear being witched since you cannot know who your enemy is. Female participant 6

You may visit the household with the aim of identifying a pregnant woman. Nobody in the family would dare to disclose that. To your surprise a few months late, you may meet the same woman with a newborn baby. Misconceptions on haematinics are also a challenge because pregnant women think when you use iron or folate you may experience abortion, fetus progress delay, and annoying side effects. Male CHW 5

Misconception regarding use of iron tablet/syrup exists among women thinking that when you use these drugs you delay the growth of the pregnancy while others complain about the side effects of the drugs such as nausea. So they prefer to visit clinic late to avoid continued use of these drugs. Female CHW 4

How women cope with existing ANC requirements

In these communities, some women circumvent ANC requirements during the first antenatal visit. Since attendance of male partners and HIV testing are mandatory during the first visit, participants reported visiting a clinic away from their ward, and carrying a letter from village leaders confirming that their husband was not present. In addition, some pregnant women paid for men who were willing to escort them and take the HIV test with them, a so-called "husband for hire" Table 4.

Husband for hire do exist in our villages. These are boda boda men. When a woman gets a boda boda to

Table 4 Identified themes and subthemes from FGDs

Key issues	Themes	Sub themes
Perceived barriers to utilization of ANC services	Poverty	• Health facility was far from home and pregnant women feeling tied to walking long distances
		• Women or family not having income to afford transport
		• Having no fare for hiring a bicycle or paying for a boda boda
		• Not having a maternity dress
	Fear of HIV testing	• Pregnant women's fear of HIV testing
		• Male partner fear of HIV testing results
		• Misconception regarding HIV testing
		• Self stigmization arising from HIV results
		• Infidelity among men/risk behaviors in fishing community and mining community
	Socio-cultural beliefs	• Men's refusal to escort women/men feel no need to be involved
		• Normal practices or habits because no history of pregnancy related complications
		• Parental influence especially among those couples who live with their parents
Challenges faced by women when utilizing the ANC services	Lack of male involvement	• Unfriendly male environment
		• Men not willing to escort women
		• Attended ANC clinic but not provided services as male partner did not attend
	Perceived poor quality of care	• Services not available because supplies and/or drugs are out of stock
		• No services available most of the times
		• Long waiting times for services
		• Frequent shortages of health providers
	Informal regulation	• HIV testing is no longer voluntarily
		• Male partner must be there during the first ANC visit
		• Not receiving HIV testing since a man is not with you
Coping strategies for existing ANC requirements	Men for hire	• Husband for hire do exist in our villages
		• Men will not accept escorting their wives
		• Boda boda men are willing to accompany women if they are provided with a little money for escorting you
	Letter from village leaders	• To avoid being scolded and to obtain services you get a letter from village leader to present to the CHWs
		• If your partner refuses to escort you state that he is away
	Health facility	• Attend a health facility that is far away from your home
		• Where health providers do not know you or your husband

take her to the health facility, she also requests if the man is willing to escort her for HIV testing just to pretend being a husband. *Female CHW 6*

Since men will not accept escorting their wives to the antenatal clinic for fear of HIV testing, women decide to go to the village leaders for the letter explaining that the husband for this woman is not present in the village and may be working outside the district. They get a letter because health

providers insist if you come without your husband you will not get any service. *Female CHW 5*

Your husband must be there when you go to the clinic for the first visit. This is a big challenge for women. Therefore, for those who cannot get their husband to escort them [they] may go to a clinic far from this ward because nobody knows their husband there. The boda boda driver usually can pretend to be your husband and you pay him something small. *Female participant 1*

Discussion

Antenatal care is one of the pillars in the Safe Motherhood Initiative for promoting and improving maternal and child health through interventions such as health promotion, treatment of existing diseases, early detection and management of pregnancy-related complications, and disease prevention [3]. Initiating ANC in the first trimester provides opportunities for timely optimal care and treatment of existing conditions [3, 5, 13]. Our findings revealed that the timely attendance at the ANC clinic in the first trimester of pregnancy was low with more than three quarters of participants first attending either in the second or third trimester. This is a significant missed opportunity for improving maternal and child health in Geita district, Northwest Tanzania. The extremely low attendance (3.62%) of women in Geita district, Northwest Tanzania in the first trimester is not consistent with the levels of attendance in Tanzania (24%) and globally (58.6%) [7, 15]. It is important to note that in contrast to previous retrospective studies, this household survey involved pregnant women in their third trimester. Hence, social desirability and recall biases that could have influenced the estimates reported in earlier studies [7, 15] were less likely to bias our results.

We also observed that a considerable proportion of women failed to utilize ANC services fully during their pregnancy due to several reasons including lack of male involvement or lack of men's interest in ANC, perceived poor quality of care, poverty and socio-cultural beliefs. Other studies have documented similar issues that may hinder utilization of ANC [22, 25, 26, 28]. For example, to achieve reduction and elimination of HIV infection through mother to child transmission, male involvement has been observed to increase women's adherence to interventions [29]. In low incomes countries, especially in the rural settings, a shortage of skilled health personnel, lack of drugs and supplies, and long waiting times are common challenges encountered in the health facilities [16, 30–33]. Women in the study area reported similar concerns. Further, ANC requirements such as the male partner being present during the first visit for HIV testing, which is emphasized as one strategy for the prevention of maternal to child transmission (PMTCT) of HIV infection, may lead to unintended consequences as documented in this paper. Although the strategy is intended to promote male involvement for positive pregnancy outcomes, it was reported to impede women from initiating ANC in a timely manner or in some cases women may not initiate ANC. Thus, there is a need to revisit such ANC requirements as they may result in unintended harms to maternal and child health.

While ANC improves and promotes maternal and child health, its effectiveness depends in part on the availability and quality of services provided regardless of the antenatal model implemented in the country [3–5,

19, 34, 35]. However, women in the study setting did not receive all the components of ANC services as per national guidelines. Notably, HIV screening was almost universal but far fewer women were screened for syphilis and anaemia, despite evidence for high rates of syphilis sero-prevalence and anaemia. Low coverage for laboratory services has been mentioned in other studies as a public health challenge in most developing countries [16, 30, 31, 36]. In rural settings, laboratory services for measuring Hb level, syphilis, and HIV infections may not be available in public health facilities due to lack of supplies and limited expertise among health care workers to conduct the tests. Further, in private health facilities, these tests may not be free of charge and many women, particularly in rural districts, may not have the funds to pay for these tests. Strengthening laboratory services in primary care facilities is paramount for quality ANC services and prevention of adverse outcomes such as congenital syphilis, stillbirths, prematurity, low birth weight, and perinatal deaths. Concurrently, early initiation of ANC should be emphasized so that women and their unborn babies will reap the full benefits of ANC.

Normative behaviour and traditional beliefs surrounding pregnancy, labour and delivery must also be addressed, as they appear to shape health-seeking behavior and could negatively affect the well-being of pregnant women and their unborn babies. Importantly, the beliefs that the experience of the mother-in-law applies to her son's wife and that the risk of adverse pregnancy outcomes may not be mitigated by ANC need to be addressed urgently through appropriate channels. In addition, health system factors such as shortages in service providers and important components of ANC (i.e., laboratory tests, vaccines, drugs, supplements), and the demands attached to the prevention of mother to child transmission services such as mandatory partner attendance at ANC initiation, need to be revisited and addressed. ANC clinics are considered "women spaces", and the existing infrastructure does not provide any privacy for couples. Women also live in a cultural atmosphere with norms and gender roles that shape and influence their health care decision-making. In the African context, women and young married couples may lack autonomy on health-related issues. The male dominant social structure gives men autonomy over their female partners on different aspects of life including health care issues. Thus, parents, in-laws, or men in the community influencing or making decisions for young couples or women is common in developing countries like Tanzania. Previous research has documented the existence of male dominated social structures and male partners playing significant decision making roles in developing countries [37, 38].

The integration of the quantitative and qualitative data assisted us in understanding the challenges and barriers that these women experience in attaining timely ANC by shedding light on community and health system related factors that need to be addressed. There is a need to understand how social structures, culture and beliefs could enhance or hinder utilization of health services. The imposed informal regulation on male partner involvement in the initial ANC visit that has been implemented to reduce the prevention of maternal to child transmission (PMTCT) of HIV needs to be re-examined using a participatory approach that emphasizes community involvement and engagement. As observed in this study, "husband for hire" and village leaders' written memos used to navigate the ANC requirements imposed on pregnant women, may fail to achieve their intended purpose. If women are checked for HIV infection with their fake male partners, the goal of promoting safer sex, adherence to PMTCT interventions, and HIV status disclosure between partners will not be realized. Hence, this study highlights the *missed opportunities* associated with early initiation of ANC for promoting health seeking behavior and preventing health conditions that directly or indirectly affect maternal and child health in rural settings in Tanzania.

Study strengths and limitations

The study design accounted for possible biases inherent in previous retrospective studies. In addition, the study was strengthened by triangulation in data collection and the fact that almost all FGD interviews were conducted outside the health facility environment. Finally, a significant strength of this study is that it explored the perspectives of *women who used* ANC services, *women who did not use ANC* services and *health care providers* regarding the challenges and barriers to ANC services in this area of Tanzania. A potential limitation of this study was the use of information/data from the antenatal cards. This could have led to biased estimates of the prevalence of existing conditions such as anemia, syphilis, and HIV. These parameters depend on the quality and completeness of the records of the pregnant women who attended ANC clinics at least once.

Conclusion and recommendations

The study highlights the low attendance of pregnant women at ANC clinics in the first trimester in Geita district, Northwest Tanzania and the limited antenatal services provided to women who utilized ANC services at least once. The goal of improving and promoting maternal and child health through ANC remains elusive in this rural setting. Importantly, not all components of ANC are available to pregnant women even when they initiate ANC early. The critical shortage of human resources, particularly when an ANC provider is invited to attend training away from the health facility further limits women's access to timely ANC services. Based on the findings, in-job training of health providers should be well planned to avoid inconvenience and delays in the provision of care. Improving human resources and timely availability of all essential components of ANC, and a friendly environment for male partners will ensure acceptability and quality services in this and similar rural settings. Further, supportive supervision to health workers during the provision of ANC services and training that specifically focuses on providing services to pregnant women and their partners in an open and sensitive manner needs to be implemented to improve the uptake of ANC services in rural communities. HIV screening for prevention of PMTCT should be conducted voluntarily after provision of health education and counselling and health workers need to ensure that they observe all ethics around ANC services. Finally, community male champions need to be identified. These individuals would take a leading role in exploring and promoting male involvement in maternal and child health services in local communities through family visits, community meetings, and cultural and religious gatherings. Such initiatives are essential for improving the health and outcomes of mothers and newborns.

Abbreviations
ANC: Antenatal care; CHW: Community health worker; FANC: Focused antenatal care; FGD: Focused group discussion; HIV: Human immunodeficiency virus; MMR: Maternal Mortality Ratio; PMTCT: Prevention of mother to child transmission; RCH: Reproductive and Child Health; TDHS: Tanzania Demographic and Health Survey; WHO: World Health Organisation

Acknowledgements
We would like to extend our warm gratitude to the District Medical Officer (DMO-Geita district), the District Reproductive and Child Health coordinator (DRCHço-Geita district), ward leaders, village leaders, community health workers, health providers, and traditional birth attendants who assisted us with this study. Furthermore, we would like to thank all of the women who generously donated their time to participate in this research study. Lastly, thanks to the University of Calgary and the Catholic University of Health and Allied Sciences for their financial support.

Funding
This study received some funding through a grant provided to DD by the Department of Paediatrics, University of Calgary, and a grant provided to EK from the Catholic University of Health and Allied Sciences – CUHAS Bugando, Mwanza, Tanzania (Ph.D. Research Funds). Funding institutions played no role in the study design, data collection, analysis, interpretation of the results, and in writing of the manuscript.

Authors' contributions

ETK conceptualized the idea and MTNM, JH, SK, RS, DMD participated in the design of the study. EK supervised the household survey, DMD supervised focused group discussions, ETK carried out data analysis, wrote the manuscript, and MTNM, JH, SK, RS, and DMD reviewed the manuscript. All authors read and approved the final manuscript.

Competing interests

MM declares that he is an associate editor of the BMC Pregnancy and Childbirth in Low and Middle-Income Countries' series. All other co-authors declare that they have no competing interests.

Author details

[1]Department of Biostatistics & Epidemiology, School of Public Health, Catholic University of Health and Allied Sciences, P.O. box 1464 Bugando Area, Mwanza, Tanzania. [2]Department of Community Health Sciences, Cumming School of Medicine, University of Calgary, 3280 Hospital Drive, NW, Calgary, AB, Canada. [3]Options Tanzania Ltd 76 Ali Hassan, Mwinyi Road, P.O. Box 65350, Dar es Salaam, Tanzania. [4]Department of Paediatrics, University of Calgary, 2888 Shaganappi Tr. NW, Calgary, AB, Canada. [5]Owerko Centre at the Alberta Children's Hospital Research Institute, Cumming School of Medicine, University of Calgary, 2500 University Dr. NW, Calgary, AB, Canada.

References

1. Tunçalp Ö, Pena-Rosas JP, Lawrie T, Bucagu M, Oladapo OT, Portela A, Gülmezoglu AM. WHO recommendations on antenatal care for a positive pregnancy experience - going beyond survival. BJOG. 2017;124:860–2. https://doi.org/10.1111/1471-0528.14599.
2. United Nations Economic Commission for Africa, African Union, African Development Bank, United Nations Development Programme: MDG Report 2015: Assessing progress in Africa toward the millennium development goals. Addis Ababa: The ECA Printing and Publishing Unit; 2015.
3. WHO, editor. Mother baby package: implementing safe motherhood in countries (practical guide), vol. 360. Geneva: WHO. p. 1994.
4. Tunçalp Ö, Were W, MacLennan C, Oladapo OT, Gülmezoglu AM, Bahl R, Daelmans B, Mathai M, Say L, Temmerman M, et al. Quality of care for pregnant women and newborns - the WHO vision. BJOG. 2015;122:1045–9. https://doi.org/10.1111/1471-0528.13451.
5. Bhutta Z, Das J, Bahl R, Lawn J, Salam R, Paul V, Sankar M, Blencowe H, Rizvi A, Chou V, et al. Can available interventions end preventable deaths in mothers, newborn babies, and stillbirths, and at what cost? *Lancet*. 2014; 384(9940):347–70. https://doi.org/10.1016/S0140-6736(1014)60792-60793.
6. WHO, UNICEF, UNFPA, World Bank Group, The United Nations Population Division. Trends in Maternal Mortality: 1990 to 2015. Geneva: World Health Organization; 2015.
7. Ministry of Health, Community Development, Gender, Elderly and Children (MoHCDGEC) [Tanzania Mainland], Ministry of Health (MoH) [Zanzibar], National Bureau of Statistics (NBS): Tanzania Demographic and Health Survey and Malaria Indicator Survey 2015–16. In. Edited by OCGS, ICF. Dar es Salaam, Tanzania and Rockville, Maryland, USA; 2016.
8. Blencowe H, Cousens S, Jassir F, Say L, Chou D, Mathers C, Hogan D, Shiekh S, Qureshi Z, You D, et al. National, regional, and worldwide estimates of stillbirth rates in 2015, with trends from 2000: a systematic analysis. Lancet Glob Health. 2016;4:e98–108. https://doi.org/10.1016/s2214-1109x(1015)00275–00272.
9. McClure EM, Goldenberg RL. Stillbirth in Developing Countries: A review of causes, risk factors and prevention strategies. J Matern Fetal Neonatal Med. 2009;22(3):183–90. https://doi.org/10.1080/14767050802559129.
10. WHO: Health in 2015: From MDGs, Millennium Development Goals to SDGs, Sustainable Development Goals. 2015. http://www.who.int/iris/handle/10665/200009. (Accessed 9 May 2017).
11. Say L, Chou D, Gemmill A, Tunçalp Ö, Moller A, Daniels J, Gülmezoglu AM, Temmerman M, Alkema L. Global causes of maternal death: a WHO systematic analysis. Lancet Glob Health. 2014;2:e323–33. https://doi.org/10.1016/s2214-1109x(1014)70227-x.
12. WHO. Antenatal Care Randomized Trial. Manual for the implementation of the new model. Geneva: Department of Reproductive Health and Research, Family and Community Medicine, World Health Organization; 2002.
13. Maternal Health Task Force. Focuses antenatal Care in Tanzania: delivering individualized, targeted, high-quality care. Harvard: HARVARD, School of Public Health, Department of Global Health and Population; 2002.
14. Yaya S, Bishwajit G, Ekholuenetale M, Shah V, Kadio B, Udenigwe O. Timing and adequate attendance of antenatal care visits among women in Ethiopia. PLoS One. 2017;12(9):e0184934.
15. Ann-Beth M, Petzold M, Chou D, Say L. Early antenatal care visit: a systematic analysis of regional and global levels and trends of coverage from 1990 t0 2013. Lancet Glob Health. 2017;5:e977–83.
16. Kanyangarara M, Munoa M, Walker N. Quality of antenatal care services provision in health facilities across sub-Saharan Africa: Evidence from nationally representative health facility assessments. J Glob Health. 2017;7(2). https://doi.org/10.7189/jogh.7107.021101.
17. Conrad P, Schmid G, Tientrebeogo J, Moses A, Kirenga S, Neuhann F, Muller O, Sarker M. Compliance with focused antenatal care services: Do health workers in rural Burkina Faso, Uganda and Tanzania perform all ANC procedures? Trop Med Int Health. 2012;17(3):300–7. https://doi.org/10.1111/j.1365.3156.2011.02923.x.
18. Hawkes SJ, Gomez GB, Broutet N. Early antenatal care: does it make a difference to outcomes of pregnancy associated with syphilis? A systematic review and meta-analysis. PLoS One. 2013;8(2). https://doi.org/10.1371/journal.pone.0056713.
19. Arunda M, Emmelin A, Asamoah BO. Effectiveness of antenatal care services in reducing neonatal mortality in Kenya: Analysis of national survey data. Glob Health Action. 2017;10. https://doi.org/10.1080/16549716.16542017.11328796.
20. Gross K, Alba S, Glass TR, Schellenberg JA, Obrist B. Timing of antenatal care for adolescent and adult pregnant women in South-Eastern Tanzania. BMC Pregnancy Childbirth. 2012;12(16). https://doi.org/10.1186/1471-2393-1112-1116.
21. Exavery A, Kant'e AM, Hingora A, Mabaruku G, Pemba S, Phillips JF. How mistimed and unwanted pregnancies affect timing of antenatal care initiation in three districts in Tanzania. BMC Pregnancy Childbirth. 2013; 13(35). https://doi.org/10.1186/1471-2393-13-35 .
22. Gupta S, Yamada G, Mpembeni R, Frumence G, Callaghan-Koru JA, Stevenson R, Brandes N, Baqui AH. Factors associated with four and more antenatal care visits and its decline among pregnant women in Tanzania between 1999 and 2010. PLoS One. 2014;9(7):e101893. https://doi.org/10.1371/journal.pone.0101893.
23. Magadi MA, Madise NJ, Rodrigues RN. Frequency and timing of antenatal care in Kenya: explaining the variations between women of different communities. Soc Sci Med. 2000;51:551–61.
24. Ndidi EP, Oseremen IG. Reasons given by pregnant women for late initiation of antenatal care in the Niger Delta, Nigeria. Ghana Med J. 2010;44(2).
25. Simkhada B, van Teijlingen ER, Porter M, Simkhada P. Factors affecting the utilization of antenatal care in developing countries: systematic review of the literature. J Adv Nurs. 2008;61(3):244–60. https://doi.org/10.1111/j.1365-2648.2007.04532.x.
26. Finlayson K, Downe S. Why do women not use antenatal services in low and middle income countries? A meta-synthesis of qualitative studies. PLoS Med. 2013;10(1):e1001373p.

27. StataCorp. Stata Statistical Software: Release 13. College Station: StataCorp LP; 2013.

28. Hagen JP, Rulisa S, Pe'rez-Escamilla R. Barriers and solutions for timely initiation of antenatal care in Kigali Rwanda: Health facility professionals' perspective. Midwifery. 2013;30:96–102. https://doi.org/10.1016/j.midw.2013.1001.1016.

29. Aluisio A, Richardson BA, Bosire R, John-Stewart G, Mbori-Ngacha D, Farquhar C. Male antenatal attendance and HIV testing are associated with decreased infant HIV infection and increased HIV-free survival. J Acquir Immune Defic Syndr. 2011;56(1):76–82. https://doi.org/10.1097/QAI.1090b1013e3181fdb1094c1094.

30. Gross K, Schellenberg JA, Kessy F, Pfeiffer C, Obrist B. Antenatal care in practice: An exploratory study in antenatal care clinics in the Kilombero Valley, South-Eastern Tanzania. BMC Pregnancy Childbirth. 2011, 36;11. https://doi.org/10.1186/1471-2393-11-36.

31. Nyamtema AS, Jong AB, Urassa DP, Hagen JP, Roosmalen J. The quality of antenatal care in rural Tanzania: What is behind the number of visits? BMC Pregnancy Childbirth. 2012;12(70). https://doi.org/10.1186/1471-2393-12-70.

32. Mahiti GR, Mkoka DA, Kiwara AD, Mbekenga CK, Hurtig A, Goicolea I. Women's perceptions of antenatal, delivery, and postpartum services in rural Tanzania. Glob Health Action. 2015;8. https://doi.org/10.3402/gha.v3408.28567.

33. Mrisho M, Obrist B, Schellenberg JA, Haws RA, Mushi AK, Mshinda H, Tanner M, Schellenberg D. The use of antenatal and postnatal care: perspectives and experiences of women and health care providers in rural southern Tanzania. BMC Pregnancy Childbirth. 2009;9(10). https://doi.org/10.1186/1471-2393-1189-1110.

34. McDonagh M: Is antenatal care effective in reducing maternal morbidity and mortality? Health Policy Plan 1996, 11(1):1–15.

35. Bergsjø P. What is the evidence for the role of antenatal care strategies in the reduction of maternal mortality and morbidity? Stud HSO   P. 2001:35–54.

36. Baker U, Okuga M, Waiswa P, Manzi F, Peterson S, Hanson C, Group TEs. Bottlenecks in the implementation of essential screening tests in antenatal care: Syphilis, HIV, and anemia testing in rural Tanzania and Uganda. Int J Gynecol Obstet. 2015;130:S43–50. https://doi.org/10.1016/j.ijgo.2015.1004.1017.

37. Paruzzolo S, Mehra R, Kes A, Ashbaugh C. Targeting poverty and gender inequality to improve maternal health. Washington DC: International Center for Research on Women; 2010.

38. Adjiwanou V, LeGrand T. Gender inequality and the use of maternal healthcare services in rural sub-Saharan Africa. Health Place. 2014;29:67–78. https://doi.org/10.1016/j.healthplace.2014.1006.1001.

12

First do no harm - interventions during labor and maternal satisfaction: a descriptive cross-sectional study

Kıymet Yeşilçiçek Çalik[1]*, Özlem Karabulutlu[2] and Canan Yavuz[3]

Abstract

Background: Interventions can be lifesaving when properly implemented but can also put the lives of both mother and child at risk by disrupting normal physiological childbirth when used indiscriminately without indications. Therefore, this study was performed to investigate the effect of frequent interventions during labor on maternal satisfaction and to provide evidence-based recommendations for labor management decisions.

Methods: The study was performed in descriptive design in a state hospital in Kars, Turkey with 351 pregnant women who were recruited from the delivery ward. The data were collected using three questionnaires: a survey form containing sociodemographic and obstetric characteristics, the Scale for Measuring Maternal Satisfaction in Vaginal Birth, and an intervention observation form.

Results: The average satisfaction scores of the mothers giving birth in our study were found to be low, at 139.59 ± 29.02 (≥ 150.5 = high satisfaction level, < 150.5 = low satisfaction level). The percentages of the interventions that were carried out were as follows: 80.6%, enema; 22.2%, perineal shaving; 70.7%, induction; 95.4%, continuous EFM; 92.3%, listening to fetal heart sounds; 72.9%, vaginal examination (two-hourly); 31.9%, amniotomy; 31.3%, medication for pain control; 74.9%, intravenous fluids; 80.3%, restricting food/liquid intake; 54.7%, palpation of contractions on the fundus; 35.0%, restriction of movement; 99.1%, vaginal irrigation with chlorhexidine; 85.5%, using a "hands on" method; 68.9%, episiotomy; 74.6%, closed glottis pushing; 43.3%, fundal pressure; 55.3%, delayed umbilical cord clamping; 86.0%, delayed skin-to-skin contact; 60.1%, controlled cord traction; 68.9%, postpartum hemorrhage control; and 27.6%, uterine massage. The satisfaction levels of those who experienced the interventions of induction, EFM, restriction of movement, two-hourly vaginal examinations, intravenous fluid, fundal pressure, episiotomy, palpation of contractions on the fundus, closed glottis pushing, delayed umbilical cord clamping, delayed skin-to-skin contact, fluid/food restriction, and of those who were not provided pharmacological pain control were found to be lower ($p < 0.05$).

Conclusion: Medical interventions carried out at high rates had a negative impact on women's childbirth experience. Therefore, a proper assessment in the light of medical evidence should be made before deciding that it is absolutely necessary to intervene in the birthing process and the interdisciplinary team should ensure that intrapartum caregivers will "first do no harm."

Keywords: Interventions during labor, Birth, Maternal satisfaction, Turkey

* Correspondence: omrumyesilcicek@hotmail.com; kyesilcicek@ktu.edu.tr
[1]Obstetrics and Gynaecology Nursing Department, Karadeniz Technical University, Faculty of HealthScience, University District, Farabi Street, Ortahisar, Trabzon, Turkey
Full list of author information is available at the end of the article

Background

"A natural birth that takes place of its own accord without interventions of any sort is a complicated process in itself, but also equally fine-tuned and balanced, prone to having its optimal properties eliminated with each intervention. Therefore, the only intervention asked of those supervising childbirth should be to respect this awe-inspiring phenomenon and adhere to medicine's first fundamental principle which reads 'Pimum non nocere' [1]." Indiscriminately resorting to medical intervention where it is not needed violates the principle of respect for medical physiology and the fundamental medical principle of "PRIMUM NON NOCERE."

Advances in medical technologies have undeniably provided significant benefits in terms of maternal and infant health, especially in high-risk pregnancies and premature births. In recent years in some countries, however, almost all pregnant mothers undergo interventions (enema, perineal shaving, liquid and food intake restrictions, routine IV fluid infusion, continuous EFM (electronic fetal monitoring), routine amniotomy, frequent vaginal examinations, use of vaginal antiseptic agents) without proper assessment of whether it is really needed [2–7]. For example, studies conducted in countries in Latin America, the Caribbean, Canada, Spain, China, South Africa and Turkey indicate that unnecessary medical interventions are common during normal labor [2–7]. It is known that unnecessary interventions undertaken without indication disrupt the natural progression of labor, causing complications to the fetus and the mother (ketosis, dehydration, prolonged labor, interventional delivery, postpartum hemorrhage, hypoglycemia, hyponatremia, cost increase, restriction of options for subsequent births, negative and unhappy childbirth experiences, feelings of failure and guilt, longer hospitalization periods, etc.) [8, 9]. For example, in many hospitals, obstetric interventions such as eating and drinking restrictions, IV fluid infusion, continuous EFM, induction, enema and episiotomy are routinely performed on all women without a specific medical justification [3, 4, 6, 8–11]. In fact, recent evidence-based studies indicate that routine interventions during low-risk births have failed to make births safer for either the mother or the baby, and that some medical practices disrupt the natural course of birth, creating unwanted complications during labor. Furthermore, such interventions tend to cause women to be dissatisfied with the childbirth experience, causing them to seek alternative methods for their next child's birth [1, 2, 8]. Care must therefore be taken to maximize the use of preventive measures during the normal delivery process to minimize the need for interventions [8]. The World Health Organization (WHO) envisions a world in which all pregnant women and their babies are provided quality care during pregnancy, birth and the postnatal period. In order to reduce maternal and infant morbidity and mortality, every pregnant woman needs competent care with evidence-based practices during birth in a supportive environment. Quality care includes efficient clinical and nonclinical interventions, a health staff with optimum competence, and a strong health infrastructure to obtain better health outcomes and ensure the positive experience of women and healthcare providers. Moreover, quality of care is considered a key component of the right to health and the route to equity and dignity for women and children. In order to achieve this, healthcare needs to be safe, effective, timely, efficient, equitable, and people-centered [12]. To achieve this, midwives/nurses/physicians should be trained to feel more confident with practices that facilitate normal childbirth, encouraged to more carefully assess the potential consequences and risks that come with each intervention, and to resort to interventions only when the situation calls for it, while mothers should also be educated to raise their awareness so that they can actively participate in the decision-making process with regard to how the child should be delivered. Women should be properly informed before any intervention is made and their approval should be sought [8, 10].

We believe that with an evidence-based approach to childbirth, useless treatment methods and unnecessary practices will be abandoned, women's expectations will gain more weight leading to higher levels of maternal satisfaction, and costs will be reduced. The aim of this study is to examine the use of routine interventions in labor and maternal satisfaction at birth. In addition, the results of this study will contribute to the current literature on childbirth, filling a significant gap of knowledge regarding the frequency of routine interventions implemented during labor and the impact of such practices on maternal satisfaction.

Methods

This descriptive study was conducted at the Turkish Ministry of Health, Kars Harakani Regional Training and Research Hospital over the period May 13–December 1, 2015. The study's target population comprised all women who fulfilled the study criteria and who experienced spontaneous vaginal childbirth. The study sample included 351 women aged between 19 and 45 who gave birth normally and at term, had healthy fetuses, no chronic diseases, who did not experience complications during pregnancy, childbirth and the postpartum period, and who were admitted to the delivery ward in the latent stage of labor.

Using the sample selection formula for a known universe size, the sample size was calculated as an optimum 347 with a 95% confidence interval, a 5% margin of error, 5% significance, and 50% prevalence (due to the lack of prior knowledge). The study was completed with 351 participants. A year prior to the study, the number of women who gave birth by normal labor at the hospital was 3470.

Questionnaires, observation forms, and the Scale for Measuring Maternal Satisfaction in Vaginal Birth (SMMSVB) were used to collect the study data. After an examination of the related literature, some sociodemographic and obstetric characteristics of the women were included in the questionnaire, while the observation form contained a list of practices performed in the first, second, third and the early postpartum stages of labor [2–9, 11].

Two methods were used for collecting the study data. In the first stage, all interventions carried out during the period from the latent to the early postpartum stage, starting with the admission of the expecting mother to the delivery ward, were duly observed by the investigator and recorded in the observation form. The data collected through observations were corroborated by entries from records kept by the delivery staff. At this stage, all women who came to the delivery room in spontaneous labor were randomly selected using the simple random sampling technique and recorded as participants in the study by the researcher. In the second stage of data collection, an evaluation was made of the women's satisfaction with the birth. The researcher administered the satisfaction scale to the participants immediately before their discharge (between the 20th–24th hours) via a face-to-face interview in the postpartum room.

Written and verbal informed consent was received from the pregnant women (regardless of their socio-demographic-obstetric characteristics)) admitted for delivery (in the delivery room in the first admissions stage) were provided with information about the study and informed that observations would be made at any time throughout the stages of the delivery. Because the relevant ethics research unit of the hospital demands both written and verbal consent for such studies (a descriptive, cross-sectional and observational study). Prior to the implementation of the data collection instruments and before the observations, the pregnant women were explained the purpose of the study in compliance with the principle of "Informed Consent," their willful participation in the study was ensured in line with the principle of "Respect for Autonomy," and they were assured that the information obtained about them would be kept confidential in accordance with the principle of "Confidentiality and the Protection of Privacy." İnstitution approval (No: 82134845/730.08.03) was obtained from the the Kars Harakani Regional Training and Research Hospital, Turkey. İnstitution consent was preferred in our context without violating the ethical principles and it was approved by the committee.

Scale for Measuring Maternal Satisfaction in Vaginal Birth (SMMSVB):

Developed by Güngör and Beji and with its validity and reliability confirmed, this scale is a 5-point Likert-type instrument consisting of 43 items and 10 sub-dimensions. Thirteen items are reversely scored. The reversely scored items are converted first to calculate the scale score. The sum of the points of all the items on the scale yields the "total scale score" after the reversely scored items have been converted. The total raw score ranges from 43 to 215. A higher score on the scale indicates a higher level of maternal satisfaction in terms of the care received at the hospital for normal delivery. The cut-off score of the scale was 150.5 (≥150.5 = high maternal satisfaction level, < 150.5 = low maternal satisfaction level) [11].

Data analysis

Data from the study were evaluated using the SPSS 21.0 statistical package program. Nonparametric tests were used in the data analysis as it was seen that the scale scores had no normal distribution ($p < 0.05$) when the scale's normality distribution was examined (Kolmogorov - Smirnov). The Mann Whitney U test and other descriptive statistical methods [(frequency, percentage, median, interquartile range (IQR)] were also employed. The results were evaluated at a 95% confidence interval.

Results

Of the surveyed women, 57.8% were between the ages 20–29, 40.7% had a maximum elementary level education, 90% were unemployed, 44.2% lived in rural areas, 69.5% were in the middle household income bracket, 84.3% had social security, 54.7% lived in extended families, 64.9% were multiparous, 87.5% had planned their pregnancies and 56.1% had received antenatal education (Table 1).

The level of maternal satisfaction among the women in our study was 139.59 ± 29.02, which is low (cut-off scale score 150.5). The birth satisfaction of the women was evaluated according to the interventions they experienced during the three stages of birth (In **the first stage of labor:** perineal shaving, enema, induction, continuous EFM, palpation of contractions on the fundus, listening to fetal heartbeat via doppler/fetoscopy, movement restrictions, two-hourly vaginal examinations, amniotomy, analgesic medication for pain control, intravenous fluids, and nutrition/liquid intake restriction; **in the second stage of labor,** episiotomy, pushing techniques, fundal pressure, vacuum/forceps, vaginal irrigation with chlorhexidine, perineum protection using the "hands-on" method, early clamping of the umbilical cord, early skin-to-skin contact; and **in the third stage of labor,** removal of the placenta with controlled cord

Table 1 Socio-demographic and obstetric characteristics of the women

Characteristics		Number	Percent
Age	15–19	39	11.1
	20–29	203	57.8
	30 and up	109	31.1
Education level	Primary school and below	143	40.7
	Secondary school	95	27.1
	High school	60	17.1
	College and university	53	15.1
Employment status	Yes	35	10.0
	No	316	90.0
Place of residence	Village	155	44.2
	District	73	20.8
	Province	123	35.0
Household income	Low	75	21.4
	Medium	244	69.5
	High	32	9.1
Health coverage	Yes	296	84.3
	No	55	15.7
Family structure	Extented	159	45.3
	Nuclear	192	54.7
Number of pregnancies	1	123	35.0
	2	92	26.2
	3	66	18.8
	4 and up	70	19.9
Unwilling pregnancy	Yes	307	87.5
	No	44	12.5
Receiving prenatal education	Yes	197	56.1
	No	154	43.9

traction, bleeding control in the early postpartum period, uterine massage).

In the first stage of labor, the women underwent the following procedures: 22.2%, perineal shaving; 80.6%, enema; 70.7%, oxytocin induction (elective: 67.3%); 95.4%, continuous EFM; 54.7%, palpation of contractions on the fundus; 92.3%, listening to fetal heartbeat with Doppler/fetoscopy; 35.0%, movement restrictions; 72.9%, two-hourly vaginal examinations; 31.9%, amniotomy; 31.3%, analgesic medication for pain contros; 74.9%, intravenous fluids; and 80.3%, nutrition/liquid intake restriction (Table 2).

Accordingly, in the second stage of labor, the following procedures were carried out: 68.9%, episiotomy, 74.6%, pushing techniques (closed glottis); 43.3%, fundal pressure; 1.4%, vacuum/forceps; 99.1%, vaginal irrigation with chlorhexidine; 85.5%, perineum protection with the "hands-on" method; 55.3%; early clamping of the umbilical cord; and 86.0% did not engage in skin-to-skin contact in the early stage (Table 2).

In the third stage of labor, the placenta was removed with controlled cord traction in 60.1% of the women, 68.9% underwent bleeding control in the early postpartum period, and 27.6% were applied uterine massage (Table 2).

In the median (IQR) analysis, according to the cut-off score of the maternal satisfaction scale (cut-off scale score 150.5: ≥150.5 = high maternal satisfaction level, < 150.5 = low maternal satisfaction level), women who underwent the following interventions had lower scores of maternal satisfaction when compared to the women who did not: women who were induced ($p = 0.005$ < 0.05), who experienced continuous EFM ($p = 0.021 < 0.05$), palpation of contractions on the fundus ($p = 0.024 < 0.05$), whose fetus' heartbeat was listened to through the abdomen ($p = 0.021 < 0.05$), women who experienced restricted mobility ($p = 0.000 < 0.05$), received two-hourly vaginal examinations ($p = 0.001 < 0.05$), were not administered analgesic medication ($p = 0.007 < 0.05$), were administered

Table 2 The distribution of the median scores obtained from SMMSVB according to the interventions at normal birth

Interventions in labor		Total scores of maternal satisfaction assessment scale at normal birth		
		N (%)	Median (IQR)	p*
In the first stage of labor				
Perineal shaving	Yes	78 (22.2)	127.5 (101.7–143)	0.158
	No	273 (77.8)	120 (100–150)	
Enema	Yes	283 (80.6)	123 (100–150)	0.607
	No	68 (19.4)	116 (105–150)	
Oxytocin induction	Yes	248 (70.7)	106 (94.2–138)	0.005
	No	103 (29.3)	116 (100–153)	
Continuous Electronic Fetal Monitoring	Yes	335 (95.4)	117 (100–146)	0.021
	No	16 (4.6)	158.5 (123–183.7)	
Palpation of contractions	Yes	192 (54.7)	121 (88.2–142)	0.024
	No	159 (45.3)	146 (110–182)	
Fetal heart sound with Doppler /fetoscopy	Yes	324 (92.3)	108 (98–140)	0.021
	No	27 (7.7)	146 (105–157)	
Restricted movement	Yes	123 (35.0)	126 (88–156)	0.000
	No	228 (65.0)	134 (107–168.7)	
Vaginal examinations (two hourly)	Yes	256 (72.9)	122.5 (97–145.7)	0.001
	No	95 (27.1)	143 (102–181)	
Amniotomy	Yes	112 (31.9)	122.5 (98–158.7)	0.001
	No	239 (68.1)	132 (100–159)	
Administration of analgesics	Yes	110 (31.3)	138 (113.2–179.7)	0.007
	No	241 (68.7)	126 (100–151.5)	
Intravenous fluids	Yes	263 (74.9)	114 (98–143)	0.034
	No	88 (25.1)	132 (109–157)	
Restriction of liquids/nutrition	Yes	282 (63.0)	121.5 (100–145)	0.014
	No	69 (37.0)	145 (105.5–168)	
In the second stage of labor				
Chlorhexidine vaginal irrigation	Yes	344 (98.0)	126 (102–159)	0.877
	No	7 (2.0)	113 (95–143)	
Pushing techniques	"Open" Glottis	89 (25.4)	134 (107–157)	0.000
	"Closed" glottis	262 (74.6)	119 (100–144)	
Fundal pressure	Yes	152 (43.3)	121 (98–150)	0.007
	No	199 (56.7)	134 (108–157)	
Episiotomy	Yes	242 (68.9)	109 (99–145.2)	0.004
	No	109 (31.1)	136 (117–165)	
Manual protection of perineum	Hands off	51 (14.5)	126 (100–153)	0.519
	Hands on	300 (85.5)	122 (101–150)	
Vacuum / Forceps application	Yes	5 (1.4)	116 (95–135)	0.155
	No	346 (98.6)	126 (102–151)	
Time of umbilical cord clamping	Early	194 (55.3)	133 (108–168)	0.039
	Delay	157 (44.7)	114 (100.5–150)	
Skin-to-skin	Yes	49 (14.0)	147 (108.5–180)	0.000
	No	302 (86.0)	126 (102.7–152)	

Table 2 The distribution of the median scores obtained from SMMSVB according to the interventions at normal birth *(Continued)*

Interventions in labor		Total scores of maternal satisfaction assessment scale at normal birth		
		N (%)	Median (IQR)	p*
In the third stage of labor				
Removal techniques of the placenta	With controlled cord traction	211 (60.1)	119 (100–150)	0.002
	Spontaneously	140 (39.9)	131 (106.2–164)	
Control of bleeding in early postpartum period	Yes	242 (68.9)	124 (101–153)	0.730
	No	109 (31.1)	126 (101–144)	
Uterine massage	Yes	97 (27.6)	117 (100.5–152)	0.243
	No	254 (72.4)	127 (102–150)	

*Mann Whitney U test

intravenous fluids infusion ($p = 0.034 < 0.05$), were subjected to restricted liquid/nutrition intake ($p = 0.014 < 0.05$), made to push using the closed glottis technique ($p = 0.000 < 0.05$), who underwent the application of fundal pressure ($p = 0.007 < 0.05$), had an episiotomy ($p = 0.004 < 0.05$), delayed umbilical cord clamping ($p = 0.039 < 0.05$), had the placenta removed with controlled cord traction ($p = 0.002 < 0.05$). Women who underwent amniotomy were found to have higher levels of satisfaction ($p = 0.000 < 0.05$) (Table 2).

Discussion

"First know what is normal. Expect what is normal and do not intervene when the state is normal! If a pathological condition develops, choose the correct intervention to bring the mother and baby back to normal state and apply it. Every intervention has a powerful impact and sometimes that impact may lead to the development of further pathologies, moving the situation further away from normality. Extra caution and care is advised when choosing which intervention to apply!" [1, 13].

There have been important changes in the management of birth over the last 30 years. One trend is toward more natural childbirth, emphasizing the human emotional aspects of labor and delivery and seeing the mother as an active participant in the birth process rather than a baby-producing machine [2]. In addition to paying attention to the wellbeing of mother and child, an attempt is made to decrease unnecessary interventions at birth, protect mothers' choices during the process, and reduce the cost of care [2, 4]. In Turkey, however, it has been reported that routine interventions, especially those used to accelerate the birth, are over-utilized [11, 14]. In the present study, two out of every three women were administered an enema, underwent elective induction, continuous EFM, had the fetus' heart sounds listened to with Doppler/fetoscopy, experienced frequent vaginal examinations, had restrictions in intravenous fluids and nutrients and other intrapartum interventions in the first stage of labor. Almost one out of every three women experienced perineal shaving, palpation of contractions on the fundus, movement

restrictions, amniotomy, and the administration of analgesics for pain control. These women however did not display satisfaction with these interventions. Similarly, 92.7% of the women in another study in Chile experienced medically augmented labor (artificial rupture of the membranes, continuous fetal monitoring, no oral hydration, while almost all received intravenous hydration, oxytocin, epidural analgesia, episiotomy, and most delivered in the lithotomy position). One-third of the women reported dissatisfaction with the care they received [4]. However, international organizations and evidence-based studies suggest that there is no need to restrict water and nutrient intake during labor at non-risk births [15, 16], no routine perineal shaving [17, 18], and enema should be applied at birth [19], delivery pain should be relieved [20, 21], intravenous fluids are not beneficial or harmful at birth [22, 23], women should be encouraged to take the position they are most comfortable during the birth, they should be allowed to move freely and their upright positions should be supported [24], vaginal examinations at 4-h intervals in the first stage of labor are adequate [25] and induction without indication and early amniotomy should not be applied as they would cause serious complications [26–29]. However in this study, surprisingly, 31.9% of the women who participated in the study and received amniotomy were found to be satisfied with the practice. It is thought that women's satisfaction with this practice has to do with midwives/nurses telling women they are performing amniotomy "to speed up the child's delivery."

In the present study, one reason for continuous EFM or frequent monitoring of the fetal heart beat with Doppler/fetoscopy may be tied to the fact that in Turkey gynecologists and obstetricians are the group, after general practitioners, that receive the greatest number of complaints of malpractice and therefore this group of specialists prefers to apply this practice to avoid complaints and paying costly compensation amounts [30]. Evidence-based studies, ACOG and NICE suggest that continuous EFM not be used in low-risk pregnancies and even that intermittent auscultation is a "convenient and safe alternative" [31–33]. In fact, palpation of contractions on the fundus is not a common practice that is used by midwives/nurses in normal birth management because of the widespread use of continuous EFM. However, those who are new to the profession and student midwives/nurses perform it to hone their skills and gain experience.

In this study, a large majority of the women in the 2nd stage of labor underwent an episiotomy, performed Valsalva pushing, received fundal pressure, vaginal irrigation with chlorhexidine, were offered perineal protection with a "hands on" technique, had the umbilical cord clamped early and were not exposed to skin-to-skin contact at an early stage. These interventions proved to have a negative impact on the women's maternal satisfaction. However, evidence-based studies and available data do not provide any convincing evidence to support intrapartum vaginal irrigation with chlorhexidine to reduce the risk of maternal and neonatal infection [34] and the ideal clinical practice is to support spontaneous pushing and to encourage women to choose their own pushing techniques [35], intact perineal ratios are high and anal sphincter tears are frequently seen in women under fundal pressure [36], using limited episiotomy (mediolateral) when needed, reporting that routine episiotomy does not prevent pelvic floor injury [37–39], the perineum should not be touched during the second stage of birth until crowning [40], and umbilical cord be clamped not too soon (approximately at minutes 1–3, after the cord pulse stops) in terms of achieving positive neonatal outcomes, and that the maternal-infant relationship should be started as early as possible [41–43].

In this study, more than half of the women in the 3rd stage of labor had the placenta removed with controlled cord traction, bleeding control was achieved in the early postpartum period, and one-third were administered uterine massage. It was however found that women who experienced the removal of the placenta by controlled cord traction displayed a low level of maternal satisfaction. Evidence based studies, the routine performed of controlled umbilical cord traction by experienced health professionals using uterotonics, such as oxytocin [44, 45], and postpartum uterine massage performed every 10 min for a duration of 60 min reduced blood loss and the need for additional uterotonics, reducing the number of women experiencing more than 500 ml of blood loss by 50% [46, 47]. It is assumed that women are not satisfied with the practice because of the pain and sensitivity created by the pressure on the fundus during controlled cord traction.

Birth and maternal satisfaction in this period, which is seen as a very important experience in a woman's life, is of the utmost importance in terms of the woman's own health, the baby's health and a positive family relationship [48]. Giving birth safely by receiving adequate and effective medical assistance is the principal expectation of a woman [47]. For this reason, unless there is a serious problem, most women do not want medical interventions that are performed to accelerate or facilitate the birth such as oxytocin, induction, enema, amniotomy, vacuum, fundal pressure, etc. [14]. It is therefore thought that interventions at birth affect childbirth satisfaction. However, findings in this study showed that despite recommendations provided by WHO in 1985 and further confirmed in 2015 by the most important related international associations, obstetric procedures are still over-utilized [12, 44]. Such interventions and restrictions cause women to have limited mobility, restricting their freedom of movement, making them feel less comfortable and experiencing more pain and anxiety because of not being able to direct their attention to other things other than lessening the impact of contractions. These procedures disrupt the hormonal balance of birth, protract the labor process, wear down the mother, cause the baby distress, increase the likelihood of an interventional birth, turn childbirth into a distressing experience, and reduce maternal satisfaction. The literature also supports the theory that obstetric intervention is linked with reduced birth satisfaction [6, 11, 14, 49]. Although maternal satisfaction is influenced by many factors, the prevailing view is that having a sense of control over the process, labor pain, personal support, expectations about childbirth, and medical interventions play a key role in maternal satisfaction [50]. It is especially having that sense of control over the birth process that determines maternal satisfaction levels. However, administering medications and excessive routine interventions cause women to lose all sense of control over the process, resulting in maternal dissatisfaction and postpartum complications [51]. The study conducted in accordance with the current literature found that the average satisfaction score for women who underwent routine interventions was 139.59 ± 29.02, which is low. That is to say, the women were not satisfied with induction, EFM, palpation of contractions on the fundus, movement restrictions, frequent vaginal examinations, lack of labor pain relief interventions, IV fluid infusions, fundal pressure, episiotomy, delayed cord clamping, removal of the placenta with controlled cord traction, and delayed skin-to-skin contact. Similarly, Binfa et al. [3] reported that although the majority of perceptions of wellbeing during labor was adequate or optimum, it is concerning that almost 1 out of every 4 mothers reported their general wellbeing as poor. It is remarkable that in Brazil, where unnecessary interventions are less applied, women have a higher and optimum level of birth satisfaction. The findings from this study are aligned with many of the categories of mistreatment identified in a systematic review of the global literature on mistreatment of women during labor and childbirth [52]. Chalmers and Dzakpasu [53] reported that among women having vaginal births, fewer interventions during labour was significantly associated with higher overall satisfaction with the labour and birth experience (ranging from 75% of women having no interventions to 46.4% having eight or more interventions rating their experiences as 'very postive'). The WHO affirms that disrespectful treatment violates the rights of women and also infringes on their health, bodily integrity, right to life and freedom from discrimination. In this context, instead of traditional care services focusing on morbidity and mortality, efforts to provide women in participatory models of antenatal care are recommended to promote women-centered care in accordance with the WHO guidelines. This approach requires respect and familiarity for the childbearing woman and her family's psychological, social, and cultural needs. Therefore, the focus and evaluation of care must be centered on emotional, social, and cultural aspects, rather than solely on the physical dimension [12, 33].

Limitations

Several limitations of this study should be noted. First, the present findings are based on a cross-sectional survey. Second, the fact that the results are representative only for the institutions in a province of Turkey where the study was conducted was accepted as the limitation of the study. Third, iIn this study almost every woman was intervened at least once, so each intervention was compared with the general satisfaction status. Finally, further multivariate analyses are needed, and planned, to explore whether the observations emerging from this analysis of independent "Interventions during labor and maternal satisfaction" variables are robust or influenced by more complex associations in the data.

Conclusion

Unnecessary interventions without medical indications spoil the physiology of birth. A birth where physiology is spoiled is traumatic for the mother, hazardous for the baby and exhausting for the physician/midwife/nurse. Our study results show that interventions not supported by evidence-based studies (such as continuous EFM, enema, induction, frequent vaginal examinations, food/ liquid restrictions, the closed glottis pushing technique, episiotomy, movement restrictions, manual preservation of the perineum, early clamping of the umbilical cord, delayed skin-to-skin contact) were routinely performed at the discretion of the medical staff and that the women were not happy with this. The women were not properly informed about the procedures performed on them and their approval was not sought. Using clinically proven practices at all stages of labor instead of traditional practices and methods based on personal experiences will ensure standardization of the care provided and increase maternal satisfaction. Accordingly, health professionals should be encouraged to participate in on-the-job training programs and follow up on current trends in medical care. Additionally, qualitative aspects, such as the satisfaction of the woman and her family with the productive process, must also be assessed and the health professionals (midwife/nurse and physician) must also use appropriate precautions to ensure that interventions do not impose unnecessary risks for the women. Unintended consequences of intrapartum interventions make it imperative that educators cooperate with nurses, midwives, and physicians to promote natural processes for childbirth and advocate for policies that focus on ensuring informed consent and alternative options.

Abbreviations

EFM: Electronic fetal monitoring; FHR: Fetal Heart Rate; FIGO: International Gynecology and Obstetrics Federation; HIV: Human Immunodeficiency Virus; ICM: International Midwives Confederation; ICSI: Institute for Clinical Systems Improvement; IV: Intravenous; NICE: National Institute of Health and Clinical Excellence / UK; RCM: The Royal Collage of Midwifes; SMMSVB: Scale for Measuring Maternal Satisfaction in Vaginal Birth; WHO: World Health Organization

Acknowledgements

The authors are grateful to the women who participated in study.

Authors' contributions

Involved in the development of the proposal: KYÇ, ÖK. Participated in data collection: ÖK., CY. Participated in analysis: KYÇ. Prepared the draft: KYÇ, ÖK. Revised drafts of the paper: KYÇ, ÖK. All authors contributed to drafting and finalizing the manuscript. All authors read and approved the final manuscript.

Authors' information

KYÇ: Asst. Prof., Head of the Department of Midwifery, Karadeniz Technical University, Faculty of Health Sciences, Department of Obstetrics and Gynecology Nursing, Trabzon / Turkey.
ÖK: Asst. Prof. Kafkas University, Kars School of Health Midwifery, Kars, Turkey.
CY: Midwife, Tekirdağ Community Health Center, Tekirdağ, Turkey.

Competing interests

The authors declare that they have no competing interests.

Author details
[1]Obstetrics and Gynaecology Nursing Department, Karadeniz Technical University, Faculty of HealthScience, University District, Farabi Street, Ortahisar, Trabzon, Turkey. [2]Department of Midwifery, Kafkas University, Faculty of Health Sciences, Kars, Turkey. [3]Midwife, Tekirdağ Community Health Center, Tekirdağ, Turkey.

References
1. Kloosterman G. Programma Rotterdam, de Doelen. 2015. www.tropenopleiding.nl/.../Programma-Doelencongres.pdf. Accessed 22 June 2017.
2. Chen CY, Wang KG. Are routine interventions necessary in normal birth? Taiwan J Obstet Gyne. 2006. https://doi.org/10.1016/S1028-4559(09)60247-3.
3. Binfa L, Pantoja L, Ortiz J, Cavada G, Schindler P, Burgos RY, et al. Midwifery practice and maternity services: A multisite descriptive study in Latin America and the Caribbean. Midwifery. 2016. https://doi.org/10.1016/j.midw.2016.07.010.
4. Binfa L, Pantoja L, Ortiz J, Gurovich M, Cavada G, Foster J. Assessment of the implementation of the model of integrated and humanised midwifery health services in Chile. Midwifery. 2016. https://doi.org/10.1016/j. midw.2016.01.018.
5. Yıldırım G, Beji NK. Effects of pushing techniques in birth on mother and fetus: a randomized study. Birth. 2008. https://doi.org/10.1111/j.1523-536X.2007.00208.x.
6. Chalmers B, Kaczorowski J, Levitt C, Dzakpasu S, O'Brien B, Lee L. Use of routine interventions in vaginal labor and birth: findings from the maternity experiences survey. Birth. 2009. https://doi.org/10.1111/j.1523-536X.2008.00291.
7. Xu Q, Simit H, Liang H, Garner P. Evidence-informed obstetric practice during normal birth in China: trends and influences in four hospital. BMC Health Serv Res. 2006. https://doi.org/10.1186/1472-6963-6-29.
8. Jansen L, Gibson M, Bowles BC, Leach J. First do no harm: interventions during childbirth. J Perinat Educ. 2013. https://doi.org/10.1891/1058-1243.22.2.83.
9. Rossen J, Økland I, Nilsen OB, Eggebø TM. Is there an increase of postpartum hemorrhage, and is severe hemorrhage associated with more frequent use of obstetric interventions? Acta Obstet Gyn Sca. 2010. https://doi.org/10.3109/00016349.2010.514324.
10. Lothian JA. Safe, healthy birth: What every pregnant woman needs to know. J Perinat Educ. 2009. https://doi.org/10.1624/105812409X461225.
11. Gungor I, Kizilkaya BN. Development and psychometric testing of the scales for measuring maternal satisfaction in normal and caesarean birth. Midwifery. 2012. https://doi.org/10.1016/j.midw.2011.03.009.
12. Tunçalp Ö, Were WM, MacLennan C, Oladapo OT, Gülmezoglu AM, Bahl R, et al. Quality of care for pregnant women and newborns—the WHO vision. BJOG. 2015. https://doi.org/10.1111/1471-0528.13451.
13. Ozer S. What is birth? 2015. https://hthayat.haberturk.com/yazarlar/semra-ozer/1030140-dogum-nedir. Accessed 22 June 2017.
14. Özcan Ş, Aslan E. Determination of maternal satisfaction at normal and cesarean birth. F N Hem Derg. 2015. https://doi.org/10.17672/fnhd.88951.
15. ACOG The American Congress of Obstetricians and Gynecologists. Oral intake during labor. Committee Opinion. The ACOG register; 2009. https://www.acog.org/...and.../Oral-Intake-During-Labor. Accessed 29 Apr 2017.
16. Singata M, Tranmer J, Gyte GML. Restricting oral fluid and food intake during labour. Cochrane Database Syst Rev, Issue 8. Art. No.: CD003930. 2013; doi: https://doi.org/10.1002/14651858.CD003930.pub3.
17. Kovavisarach E, Jirasettasiri P. Randomised controlled trial of perineal shaving versus hair cutting in parturients on admission in labor. J Med Assoc Thail. 2005;88(9):1167–71.
18. Basevi V, Lavender T. Routine perineal shaving on admission in labor. Cochrane Database Syst Rev, Issue 11. Art. No.: CD001236.2014; doi: https://doi.org/10.1002/14651858.CD001236.pub2.
19. Reveiz L, Gaitán HG, Cuervo LG. Enemas during labor. Cochrane Database Syst Rev, Issue 7. Art. No.: CD000330. 2013; doi: https://doi.org/10.1002/14651858.CD000330.pub4.
20. Jones L, Othman M, Dowswell T, Alfirevic Z, Gates S, Newburn M. et al. Pain management for women in labour: an overview of systematic reviews.

21. Hodnett ED, Gates S, Hofmeyr GJ, Sakala C, Weston J. Continuous support for women during childbirth. Cochrane Database Syst Rev, Issue 2. Art. No.: CD003766.2011; doi: https://doi.org/10.1002/14651858.CD003766.pub3.
22. ICS Institute for Clinical Systems Improvement. Health Care Guideline. The ICSI register. https://www.icsi.org/ (2006). Accessed 15 May 2017.
23. Dawood F, Dowswell T, Quenby S. Intravenous fluids for reducing the duration of labour in low risk nulliparous women. Cochrane Database Syst Rev, Issue 6. Art. No.: CD007715. 2013; doi: https://doi.org/10.1002/14651858.CD007715.pub2.
24. Lawrence A, Lewis L, Hofmeyr GJ, Styles C. Maternal positions and mobility during first stage labour. Cochrane Database Syst Rev, Issue 10. Art. No.: CD003934. 2013; doi: https://doi.org/10.1002/14651858.CD003934.pub4.
25. Downe S, Gyte GML, Dahlen HG, Singata M. Routine vaginal examinations for assessing progress of labour to improve outcomes for women and babies at term. Cochrane Database Syst Rev, Issue 7. Art. No.: CD010088. 2013; doi: https://doi.org/10.1002/14651858.CD010088.pub2.
26. Gülmezoglu AM, Crowther CA, Middleton P, Heatley E. Induction of labour for improving birth outcomes for women at or beyond term. Cochrane Database of Syst Rev, Issue 6. Art. No.: CD004945. 2012; doi: https://doi.org/10.1002/14651858.CD004945.pub3.
27. WHO World Health Organization. Recommendations for augmentation of labour. The WHO register. www.who.int/.../publications/.../augmentation-labour/en/(2015). Accessed 29 June 2017.
28. Kokanalı MK, Kokanalı D, Güzel Al, Topçu HO, Cavkaytar S, Doğanay M. Analysis of factors that influence the outcomes of labor induction with intravenous synthetic oxytocin infusion in term pregnancy with favourable bishop score. Cukurova Med J. 2015;40(2):317–25.
29. Smyth RMD, Alldred SK, Markham C. Amniotomy for shortening spontaneous labour. Cochrane Database Syst Rev, Issue 1. Art. No.: CD006167. 2013; doi: https://doi.org/10.1002/14651858.CD006167.pub3.
30. T.C. Istanbul Medical Chamber. The Istanbul Medical Chamber Register. www.istabip.org.tr/ (2016). Accessed 27 June 2017.
31. ACOG The American Congress of Obstetricians and Gynecologists. Obstetric Care Consensus Series. The ACOG register. https://www.acog.org/Resources-And-Publications/Obstetric-Care-Consensus-Series-List (2016). Accessed 20 Apr 2017.
32. Devane D, Lalor JG, Daly S, McGuire W, Smith V. Cardiotocography versus intermittent auscultation of fetal heart on admission to labour ward for assessment of fetal wellbeing. Cochrane Database Syst Rev, Issue 2. Art. No.: CD005122. 2012; doi: https://doi.org/10.1002/14651858.CD005122.pub4.
33. NICE Natioanal Institue for Health and Care Excellence intrapartum care: Intrapartum care for healthy women and babies. Clinical guideline. The NICE register. https://www.nice.org.uk/guidance/cg190 (2016). Accessed 15 Apr 2017.
34. Lumbiganon P, Thinkhamrop J, Thinkhamrop B, Tolosa JE. Vaginal chlorhexidine during labour for preventing maternal and neonatal infections (excluding Group B Streptococcal and HIV). Cochrane Database Syst Rev. Issue 10. Art. No.: CD004070. 2014; doi:https://doi.org/10.1002/14651858.CD004070.pub2.
35. Prins M, Boxem J, Lucas C, Hutton E. Effect of spontaneous pushing versus valsalva pushing in the second stage of labor on mother and fetus: a systematic review of randomized trials. BJOG-Int Obstet Gy. 2011. https://doi.org/10.1111/j.1471-0528.2011.02910.x.
36. Verheijen EC, Raven JH, Hofmeyr GJ. Fundal pressure during the second stage of labour. Cochrane Database Syst Rev, Issue 4. Art. No.: CD006067. 2009; doi: https://doi.org/10.1002/14651858.CD006067.pub2.
37. Karaahmet AY, Yazıcı S. The current stage of episiotomy. HSP. 2017; doi: https://doi.org/10.17681/hsp.270072.
38. FIGO Management of the second stage of labor. The FIGO register. www.figo.org › Our Work › FIGO Committees (2012). Accessed 20 Mar 2017.
39. Carroli G, Mignini L. Episiotomy for vaginal birth. Cochrane Database Syst Rev, Issue 1. Art. No.: CD000081. 2009; doi: https://doi.org/10.1002/14651858.CD000081.pub2.
40. Aasheim V, Nilsen ABV, Lukasse M, Reinar LM. Perineal techniques during the second stage of labor for reducing perineal trauma. Cochrane Database Syst Rev, Issue 12. Art. No.: CD006672. 2011; doi: https://doi.org/10.1002/14651858.CD006672.pub2.
41. WHO World Health Organization. Recommendations for the prevention and treatment of postpartum hemorrhage. The WHO register. http://www.who.int/reproductivehealth/publications/maternal_perinatal_health/9789241548502/en/ (2012). Accessed 29 May 2017.

42. Moore ER, Anderson GC, Bergman N, Dowswell T. Early skin-to-skin contact for mothers and their healthy newborn infants. Cochrane Database Syst Rev, Issue 10. Art. No.: CD003519. 2012; doi:https://doi.org/10.1002/14651858.CD003519.pub3.

43. McDonald SJ, Middleton P, Dowswell T, Morris PS. Effect of timing of umbilical cord clamping of term infants on maternal and neonatal outcomes. Cochrane Database Syst Rev, Issue 7. Art. No.: CD004074. 2013; doi: https://doi.org/10.1002/14651858.CD004074.pub3.

44. WHO World Health Organization. Managing complications in pregnancy and childbirth: A guide for midwives and doctors. The WHO register. whqlibdoc.who.int/publications/2007/9241545879_eng.pdf (2000). Accessed 29 June 2017.

45. Hofmeyr GJ, Mshweshwe NT, Gülmezoglu AM. Controlled cord traction for the third stage of labour. Cochrane Database Syst Rev, Issue 1. Art. No.: CD008020. 2015; doi: https://doi.org/10.1002/14651858.CD008020.pub2.

46. Hofmeyr GJ, Abdel-Aleem H, Abdel-Aleem MA. Uterine massage for preventing postpartum hemorrhage. Cochrane Database of Syst Rev, Issue 7. Art. No.: CD006431. 2013; doi: https://doi.org/10.1002/14651858.CD006431.pub3.

47. ICM Essential competencies for basic midwifery practice. The ICM register. international midwives.org. Education Core Documents (2013). http://internationalmidwives.org/what-we-do/education-coredocuments/essential-competencies-basic-midwifery-practice/. Accessed 13 June 2017.

48. Waldenström U, Hildingsson I, Rubertsson C, Radestad I. A negative birth experience: prevalence and risk factors in a national sample. Birth. 2004. https://doi.org/10.1111/j.0730-7659.2004.0270.x.

49. Hollins Martin CJ, Martin CR. A survey of women's birth experiences in Scotland using the Birth Satisfaction Scale (BSS). Eur J Pers Cent Healthc. 2015. https://doi.org/10.5750/ejpch.v3i4.1019.

50. Christiaens W, Bracke P. Assessment of social psychological determinants of satisfaction with childbirth in a cross-national perspective. BMC Pregnancy Childb. 2007; doi.org/10.1186/1471-2393-7-26.

51. Srivastava A, Avan BI, Rajbangshi P, Bhattacharyya S. Determinants of women's satisfaction with maternal health care: a review of literature from developing countries. BMC Pregnancy Childb. 2015; doi.org/10.1186/s12884-015-0525-0.

52. Bohren MA, Hunter EC, Munthe-Kaas HM, Souza JP, Vogel JP, Gulmezoglu AM. Facilitators and barriers to facility-based delivery in low- and middle-income countries: a qualitative evidence synthesis. Reprod Health. 2014. https://doi.org/10.1186/1742-4755-11-71.

53. Chalmers BE, Dzakpasu S. Interventions in labour and birth and satisfaction with care: the Canadian maternity experiences survey findings. Journal of Reproductive and Infant Psychology.2015. https://doi.org/10.1080/02646838.2015.1042964 .

13

Maternal mortality in the Gaza strip: a look at causes and solutions

Bettina Böttcher[1][*] [iD], Nasser Abu-El-Noor[2], Belal Aldabbour[1], Fadel Naim Naim[1] and Yousef Aljeesh[2]

Abstract

Background: Maternal mortality is an important health indicator for the overall health of a population. This study assessed the causes and contributing factors to maternal mortality that occurred in the Gaza-Strip between July 2014 and June 2015.

Methods: This is a retrospective study that used both quantitative and qualitative data. The data were collected from available medical records, investigation reports, death certificates, and field interviews with healthcare professionals as well as families.

Results: A total of 18 maternal mortalities occurred in Gaza between 1st July 2014 and June 30th 2015. Age at time of death ranged from 18 to 44 years, with 44.4% occurring before the age of 35 years. About 22.2% were primiparous, while 55.6% were grand multiparous women. The most common causes of death were sepsis, postpartum haemorrhage, and pulmonary embolism.

The most striking deficiency was very poor medical documentation which was observed in 17 cases (94%). In addition, poor communication between doctors and women and their families or among healthcare teams was noticed in nine cases (50%). These were repeatedly described by families during interviews. Further aspects surfacing in many interviews were distrust by families towards clinicians and poor understanding of health conditions by women. Other factors included socioeconomic conditions, poor antenatal attendance and the impact of the 2014 war.

Low morale among medical staff was expressed by most interviewed clinicians, as well as the fear of being blamed by families and management in case of adverse events. Substandard care and lack of appropriate supervision were also found in some cases.

Conclusions: This study revealed deficiencies in maternity care, some of which were linked to the socioeconomic situation and the 2014 war. Others show poor implementation of clinical guidelines and lack of professional skills in communication and teamwork. Specialised training should be offered for clinicians in order to improve these aspects. However, the most striking deficiency was the extremely poor documentation, reflecting a lack of awareness among clinicians regarding its importance. Local policymakers should focus on systematic application of quality improvement strategies in order to achieve greater patient safety and further reductions in the maternal mortality rate.

Keywords: Gaza-strip, Maternal mortality, Quality improvement, Medical documentation, Patient safety, Clinical audit, Palestine

* Correspondence: Bettina.bottcher@yahoo.co.uk
[1]Faculty of Medicine, Islamic University of Gaza, P. O. Box 108, Gaza strip, Gaza, Palestine
Full list of author information is available at the end of the article

Background

Maternal mortality is an important health indicator, widely acknowledged as a general indicator of the overall health of a population, the status of women in a society, and the functioning of the healthcare system. Maternal mortality is defined as death of a woman during pregnancy or within 42 days after childbirth, spontaneous abortion or termination of pregnancy, but excluding deaths from incidental or accidental causes [1]. In the year 2000, the United Nations set ten Millennium goals to be reached by 2015. Among these was Millennium Goal Number five: "To reduce maternal mortality by three quarters from 1990 to 2015" [2]. Many Middle Eastern countries are believed to have reached this goal. However, this was not achieved globally and conflicts in the Region have made it more difficult to reach this goal at a regional level [3].

According to the Palestinian Ministry of Health (MoH), the Maternal Mortality Rate (MMR) in the Gaza-Strip was 30/100,000 live births in 2014, and 25 in 2015 [4, 5], which differed from that in the West Bank with 20/100, 000 in 2014 [4]. On the other hand, MMR was 7 in Israel, 58 in Jordan and 33 in Egypt [3, 5, 6]. The Gaza-Strip suffers from several severe social and economic challenges due to a blockade that has been imposed on Gaza since 2006, which might have an impact on health indicators including maternal mortality [7]. This may explain the obvious difference in the MMR between the Gaza-Strip and the West Bank (the two parts of Palestine). Moreover, Abdo et al. suggested that recurring conflicts affecting the Gaza-Strip also contributed to differing maternal mortality rates [8].

This study aimed to identify causes of maternal mortality in the Gaza-Strip that occurred between 1st July 2014 and 30th June 2015. Furthermore, this study sought to explore the relationship between MMR and socioeconomic status as well as the relationship between MMR and access to healthcare facilities during the war that took place in July and August 2014. Finally, it was intended to identify ways of improving the quality of maternal health services and reduce MMR in the Gaza-Strip to achieve the WHO goal of reduction in MMR by two-thirds [2].

Methods

A descriptive, retrospective design that included a mixed (triangulation) approach of quantitative and qualitative data collection was used in this study. The use of both quantitative and qualitative approaches strengthens the design and reduces any weaknesses in either approach [9, 10]. It also provides richer and more in-depth data that will reduce bias of using a single method [11, 12].

The study population included all women who died during pregnancy or within 42 days post-delivery or abortion that occurred between 1st July 2014 and 30th June 2015 in the Gaza-Strip. A central register of maternal deaths exists in the Gaza-Strip and is kept by the Palestinian Ministry of Health. Identification and registration of these cases is mandatory for all hospitals. During the study period, 18 maternal deaths, that met the definition of maternal mortality, had been registered and were included in this study [1]. Pregnant women who died due to accidents were excluded from the study, as they do not meet the WHO definition of maternal mortality [1]. The available clinical notes, investigation reports and death certificates for the 18 women were reviewed. Data collection sheets, developed by the research team, were completed for each case. The sheet covered five main domains which included: socioeconomic status, past medical history, obstetrical history, received antenatal care, and the index pregnancy.

Interviews were conducted with the families of the deceased women. When possible, home visits were made to meet these families. In 14 cases the husbands were interviewed, while four of the interviews involved other family members in addition to the husband, and in two cases only relatives without the husband of the deceased were interviewed. The research team could not interview the family members of two women; one family refused any contact with the research team and for the other family, contact information could not be found. In seven cases, for the convenience of family members, the interviews were made by phone. Besides that, the research team members interviewed 12 medical clinicians who had been involved in caring for the deceased women. In total, three medical directors were interviewed, eight consultants, including four obstetricians, two intensive care physicians, one cardiologist and one microbiologist, as well as one primary care manager. Interviews with clinicians lasted between 20 to 90 min, while interviews with family members took more time, ranging from 45 to 100 min.

During the data collection process, several obstacles and challenges had to be overcome. Firstly, finding the medical case notes for the deceased women; only 12 case notes could be located. In the remaining cases, notes were not available, mostly due to poor contact with the health services or care providers during the war in July and August of 2014. Similarly, contact information for women were not recorded systematically in the notes. Contact phone numbers were found to be scribbled at odd places in the case notes, but were completely missing in eight cases. Therefore, contact details were obtained informally in these cases, by asking people who knew the families of the deceased women.

Ethical considerations

Ethical approval for this study was obtained from the Human Resources Department of the Palestinian

Ministry of Health (MoH), which is the body in Gaza to issue ethical and administrative approvals for studies involving patients and their families. Further approval to conduct the study was obtained from the administrative bodies of the governmental and one private hospitals, that had provided care for the deceased women. Before conducting the interviews with family members or healthcare providers, the aims of the study were explained to the participants, and a formal consent to participate in this study was obtained. Prior to data collection and after obtaining ethical approval from the Human Resources Department, verbal consent was obtained from participants who preferred to be interviewed over the phone, while written consent was taken from those interviewed face-to-face. Participants were informed that they had the right to refuse participation in the study or to withdraw at any time without being penalized. The collected data were kept under high confidentiality and anonymity as each case was assigned a code number. The women's confidentiality was preserved throughout the study.

Data analysis

Data analysis was done with the help of EXCEL (Microsoft Inc.) and mainly in terms of descriptive statistics with means, standard deviations and percentages. For qualitative data analysis, the researchers read the transcripts of the interviews independently. Transcripts were reviewed several times by each researcher in order to gain an increased understanding of the study phenomenon at multiple levels if possible [12]. While reading the transcripts, each researcher coded data and organized the participants' sentences and paragraphs of the interviews with similar properties into different themes and subthemes [11]. After each researcher finished his/her analysis, the research team met in person and discussed patterns relating to a core category. During the meeting, data were coded using constant comparison among themes from each researcher until a consensus was reached on the common core themes of the study. From these themes, the main categories of

contributing factors were identified and quantified as listed in Table 1. The manuscripts and coding of the data was read by several experts to ensure rigor of the study and avoid bias [13, 14].

Results

Characteristics of deceased women

The age of the 18 women, who died during the study period, ranged from 18 to 44 years, with a mean age of 33.5 ± 7.1 years. From these, four women (22%) were primiparous, while ten (55%) were grand multiparous women (para five and more). The majority of deaths occurred during the antepartum period (10 cases; 55%) followed by the postpartum period (seven cases; 38.9%). Only one death occurred intrapartum. Eight women (44%) had been identified as high risk pregnancies due to a variety of reasons including previous Caesarean section, pregnancy-induced hypertension (complicated by gestational diabetes mellitus), epilepsy, poorly-controlled bronchial asthma, deep vein thrombosis during a previous pregnancy and one had an aortic stenosis.

Causes and frequency of mortalities over time

The most frequent causes for mortality were found to be pulmonary embolism (PE), infection/septicemia, and post-partum hemorrhage (PPH) (Fig. 1). Four women (22.2%) died during the war in July and August 2014 (Fig. 2). A further two peaks were noted in October 2014, following the war, when five women (27.8%) died and then again in January 2015 with another four (22.2%) deaths, indicating exposure to cold weather due to poor home insulation as a possible factor, confirmed by home visits to families whose relative died of uncontrolled asthma.

Contributing factors to mortalities

From the collected data, including the interviews, several recurring themes could be identified as contributing factors to these deaths, which were mainly poor documentation (including patient notes, progress reports, operation and birth records as well as investigation results), poor

Table 1 Contributing Factors to Poor Outcome and Aspects of Care

Contributory Factor	Total Number	Percentage of Total
Substandard care and poor documentation	17	94.4%
Poor communication	9	50%
Impact of war	4	22.2%
Poor educational achievements of patients	3	16.7%
Socioeconomic factors and cultural beliefs	5	27.8%
Poor understanding of illness/ self-neglect	4	22.2%
Access difficulties	2	11.1%
Irregular/ late antenatal care attendance	5	27.8%

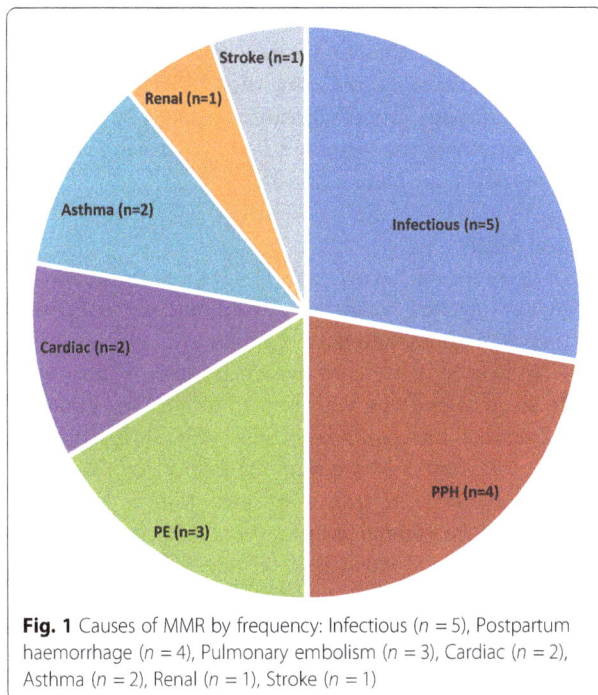

Fig. 1 Causes of MMR by frequency: Infectious (*n* = 5), Postpartum haemorrhage (*n* = 4), Pulmonary embolism (*n* = 3), Cardiac (*n* = 2), Asthma (*n* = 2), Renal (*n* = 1), Stroke (*n* = 1)

communication within teams and between healthcare professionals and women and their families, socioeconomic factors as well as irregular, late or no antenatal care attendance (Table 1). Furthermore, direct impact of the war as well as self-neglect contributed to some maternal deaths. Poor educational achievements were evident in three women (which included one woman who had not benefitted from the most basic schooling and two who had only completed four years of education) (Table 1).

Substandard care and poor documentation

Evidence of substandard care was found in the care of 10 women (55.6%). In all of these, documentation was significantly substandard, compounding the poor care. In particular, no attention was being paid to recording

timings of events or the given medications in any of the medical case notes. Essential details, such as estimated blood loss in cases of haemorrhage or intraoperative complications in case of Caesarean sections, were also consistently missing in the notes. The condition of two women (11.1%), deteriorated slowly overnight, which was not recognised by healthcare providers. Lack of supervision was evident in the care of some women, as in the case of one woman who suffered from severe dyspnoea, a serious sign in a young adult, which was not recognised to have been caused by irritation of the diaphragm. As a consequence, the hypovolaemia from the massive intra-abdominal haemorrhage had been overseen by the resident doctor. Senior obstetric help and support were not called, despite ongoing symptoms.

Poor communication

Poor communication was evident in the care of nine women (50%) and included a lack of safety netting, inappropriate reassurance of women and their families, even if the women's conditions were critical, poor skills at breaking bad news and avoiding to see families following poor outcomes. One husband said: "*They did a CT scan* (computed tomography) *and blood tests and the doctor told us that everything was 100% good and we went home.*" However, his wife had a severe and ongoing headache and died within 48 h due to meningitis, after staying at home and re-presenting very late to the hospital. At the time of discharge, she had been completely reassured that everything was OK and had not been instructed to return in case of ongoing or worsening symptoms, illustrating the close connection between poor communication and substandard care. In another case, the husband reported that he asked a doctor about the condition of his wife, who had been admitted to the intensive care unit (ICU), and was told that: "*She is fine. Everything is good.*" But his wife died within one hour after this reassurance was given to him. Another husband illustrated his experience in the following words:

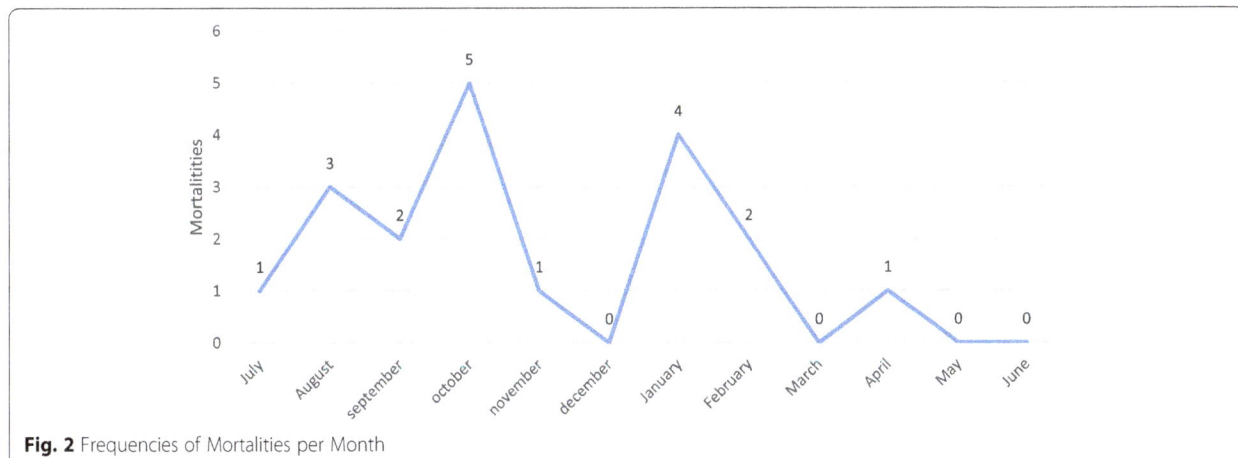

Fig. 2 Frequencies of Mortalities per Month

"My wife was unconscious on that day. Her condition was getting worse and worse every day... the ICU doctors did not give us accurate information about her condition. Even when they discovered that she had kidney failure, they told me that she will need kidney dialysis only one time and her kidney will come back to work."

The transfer process of two women between hospitals within the Gaza-Strip was impeded by poor communication between healthcare professionals, leading to an extreme delay in care provided to the women, probably contributing to their death. This was described by one husband as follows: *"In the last week of her pregnancy, we went to Hospital B, but they referred us to Hospital A. When we arrived there, they refused to receive us. So, we went back to Hospital B, who sent us back to [Hospital A] (a more specialized hospital), who refused to receive my wife again. This happened four times in the midst of the war."* Further factors contributing to this delay included a lack of agreed referral protocols for the transfer of patients and a situation of extreme stress also for medical personnel during the war. A formal referral and transfer policy has since been agreed and implemented. One director said: *"These were difficult conditions and lack of agreement on the transfer process contributed to the delays during the war. We have since come together and agreed on a transfer policy".*

Poor communication between healthcare professionals and its impact on the care delivered to women was also described by physicians. One physician recounted the care of a patient with severe aortic stenosis, where obstetricians and cardiologists could not establish effective multidisciplinary care. The woman was cared for on the cardiac care unit for a large part of her pregnancy. The physician related: *"The obstetric team did not visit her regularly, but only when they were called to see the woman. No care arrangements were made by obstetric and cardiac teams together."*

Impact of war

The clinical care of four women (22.2%) was directly impacted by the ongoing war in July and August 2014, mainly with limitations of safe transportation to access care or impact of smoke from explosions, as one husband reported: *"They (the doctors) told me that the difficulty of breathing was due to the smoke from the explosions of rockets."* Another two families found that certain stressors had an effect on patients even after hostilities had ceased. At least seven families (38.9%) were displaced during the war and found shelter either in a mosque, a school or with relatives. However, only six deaths (33.3%) occurred during or in the first month following the war (Fig. 2).

Socioeconomic factors

Socioeconomic factors were immediate contributors to the poor outcome in the care of five women (27.8%). Two women with bronchial asthma died in January, the coldest month of the year, and lived in inadequate, very cold and poorly insulated, housing (Fig. 2).

Cultural beliefs

Social pressure for having male children contributed to a pregnancy against medical advice and a concealed pregnancy without antenatal care in two women, who were known to have cardiovascular disease, one with aortic stenosis and one with hypertension. One husband expressed his unawareness of his wife's pregnancy as follows: *"She had told me that she had a coil. But after her death, I learned from her sister that it had been removed as she wanted another son."* The family of the woman with aortic stenosis described that she had met another woman *"with a heart problem like hers,"* who had had three children and believed this was also possible for her. She already had one daughter and had been strongly advised against a further pregnancy, but her maternal aunt said: *"She believed she could have more children as the other woman she had met and she wanted a son."*

Distrust in physicians

Eight of the interviewed families (44.4%) expressed a high degree of disappointment and the view that their relatives had been treated negligently. In five cases (28%), this view was very strong. To express his distrust in physicians, one husband described them as *"licensed killers"*. In all of these cases, there were evident communication shortfalls between medical staff and families. Eight cases (44.4%) reported a lack of information given to them or 'inappropriate reassurance', meaning that husbands had been reassured that everything was OK regarding the condition of their wives until shortly before their deaths.

Low morale among clinicians

When talking to clinicians, low morale was found in most cases. This was largely due to high workloads and pressures that were rewarded with only small salaries, which were not received regularly. Employees in the Palestinian Ministry of Health receive only 50% of their monthly salary every 40 days for the last few years, including the study period. Furthermore, doctors perceived a lack of support from managers and the MoH in case of adverse events. On the contrary, the health officials and managers were perceived by clinicians to seek individuals to blame and discipline for such events. As a result, clinicians avoided involvement in difficult cases, as in the case of a 20-year old woman with aortic stenosis. She had been warned against pregnancy and was told that this might endanger her life. In spite of that, she decided to get pregnant. However, she did not receive any antenatal care until she was in the second trimester when she had already developed dyspnoea. Although she was advised to terminate her pregnancy, at this stage, obstetricians avoided undertaking such a procedure, for fear of her death occurring in the process and being blamed for it. One obstetrician described this problem and said: *"If she died on the table, the doctors would be blamed by families and managers."* This led to care being delivered reactively rather than proactively. Clinicians described being trapped in a culture of blame. One obstetrician described the team, who investigated maternal mortalities, as *"policemen"* who search for faults.

Discussion

The causes of maternal death that were found in this study were close to the causes reported in a previous study (5). No major changes occurred in the frequency of PE and PPH as a cause of maternal death. However, an increase was noted in the percentage of women who died due to infectious causes, bronchial asthma and renal disease. On the other hand, a decrease occurred in the percentage of women dying due to cardiovascular diseases (Table 2). Hypertension was only implicated as a contributory factor to death in one case. This is probably an expression of the excellent routine antenatal care available to women across the Gaza-Strip free of charge, which was described in one study as high quality care [15].

Determination of causes of maternal death was done without postmortem examination in all cases. In one case an evident discrepancy was noted between the 'official' cause of death 'postpartum haemorrhage' and the one supported by interviews with clinicians, who suspected 'pulmonary embolism'. This difference in opinion between attending obstetricians and investigators, which

could not be resolved, demonstrates the poor communication and lack of teamwork among clinicians, managers and investigation teams. Rather than focusing on learning points and improvements as well as system failures, adverse event investigators from the MoH were perceived by clinicians to be more concerned about pointing out wrongful acts and blame rather than investigating system failures.

The lack of interest in investigating and confirming causes of maternal death, once they had occurred, was evident. For example, in two cases of sepsis, samples had been obtained for investigation (one sample from a pleural infusion as well as blood cultures), but laboratory results were not followed up or documented in the notes. It appeared that clinicians felt that documentation was not necessary and did not feel the obligation to follow up on them after the woman had died.

In the Gaza-Strip, antenatal care is provided by governmental as well as UNRWA (United Nations Relief and Works Agency) clinics to all women free of charge and meets the basic care needs of all pregnant women [15]. In total, 95.3% of women in Gaza were reported to have taken advantage of this in 2015 [5]. However, ultrasound examinations are not routinely available, so women have to seek these in the private sector; a service that not all women can afford. In this study, 22.2% of the mortalities did not take advantage of regular antenatal care and this is a large proportion compared to the < 5% of women in the general population of Gaza, who are reported to have < 4 antenatal visits [5, 7].

The vast majority of women in the Gaza-Strip give birth in governmental hospitals, which was also the case in this sample. Only one woman in this sample had delivered in a private hospital, where she suffered a PPH and was transferred instantly to the local governmental hospital. Postnatal care is reported to reach 91.8% of women in the Gaza-Strip, attending a healthcare institution for a postnatal care visit within two days after childbirth [16].

A broad lack of trust by patients in the healthcare system of Gaza became evident, reinforced by families of deceased women feeling excluded by healthcare teams. Inappropriate reassurance by the medical teams, as well as avoidance of seeing the family shortly following their relative's death, revealed a lack of skills by clinicians in breaking bad news. Yet, the lack of effective communication has been shown to be an obstacle to providing appropriate healthcare and safeguarding patient safety [17–19]. Effective communication between teams, amongst healthcare professionals and between healthcare professionals and their patients is essential in the transfer of information (handover), getting a clear picture of the problem, referral between hospitals, follow up and safety netting. To this effect, including the

Table 2 Frequency of Causes of Death in Percent in 2008/09 and 2014/15

Cause of Death	2008/09(16) N = 11 (2008) N = 18 (2009) N = 30 (total – 2 years)	2014/15 Current study N = 18 (1 year)
Pulmonary Embolism	20.0%	16.7%
Postpartum Haemorrhage	16.7%	22.2%
Infectious Causes	16.7%	27.8%
Cardiovascular Disease	30.0%	16.7%
Bronchial Asthma	0	11.1%
Renal Disease	0	5.6%
Others	16.7%	0

patient as part of the team is essential for obtaining information and decision making [18, 20, 21]. In this study, one or all of these aspects were missing or insufficient in 66% of the cases.

The extremely poor standard of documentation shown in this study has proven another obstacle in providing safe maternity care. Unfortunately, this has been shown to be a widespread problem in the Gaza-Strip [22, 23]. Meticulous, contemporaneous and accurate documentation is the backbone of evaluation and quality improvement in any healthcare system [24]. This study shows evidence of significantly substandard documentation even in the most severe and moribund cases. However, documentation is essential for patient care and safety as well as for effective clinical audit. The lack of simple measures of documentation, such as the use of early warning scores, contributed to maternal mortality in this study and underline documentation to be clinicians' duty and not a choice [25, 26].

The development of a culture of openness, encouraging clinical audit and transparency, is not optional when improving the healthcare system. Clinicians often voiced fears of transparency in adverse events, suggesting that this would lead to less trust by patients in local clinicians, which has also been identified in other studies [27]. Clinical audit allows the identification of weaknesses and facilitates improvements. As such it is the cornerstone of quality improvement processes in healthcare and mandatory for ensuring patient safety [28, 29]. Contrary to current local opinion, it would increase trust in the healthcare system [30].

The impact of the 2014 war, as well as socioeconomic factors, were great and affected about 50% of women. Subtler and more difficult to measure is the influence of the blockade, which has been imposed on the Gaza-Strip since 2006. It has led not only to shortages and to varying availability of drugs, disposables, and medical equipment, but it also caused difficulties or impossibilities for healthcare professionals from Gaza to join international conferences and advanced medical training, contributing to increasing isolation of healthcare professionals in the Gaza-Strip [31]. Due to these factors, professionals in Gaza do not partake easily in global developments and advances in medicine and practice. This might be one factor contributing to the fact that clinical audit and quality improvement initiatives have largely been absent in Gaza and no significance is currently attached to adequate documentation in medical notes. The healthcare system seems to have 'missed out' on these important developments, despite access to the internet. Currently, local initiatives and debates are gathering speed, promoting clinical audit as well as local quality improvement initiatives to benefit the healthcare system across the Gaza-Strip. This has been supported by non-governmental organisations, local universities, visiting teams of clinicians, as well as, most recently official support by the Palestinian MoH and also the Palestinian Medical Council. These interventions have brought the process of continuous quality improvement in healthcare into focus, but have yet to reach all clinicians.

Conclusion

Multiple factors were identified to be contributing to maternal mortality in the Gaza-Strip. In order to reduce MMR, in an attempt to meet the WHO goal, further measures, such as improvement of documentation, clinical audit activity and development of skills in communication are all relatively inexpensive interventions, which are within the reach of the healthcare system in the Gaza-Strip. It is due to local leadership to pick up this baton and realise greater patient safety and reduction in MMR by more systematically applying quality improvement strategies.

Abbreviations
ICU: Intensive Care Unit; MMR: Maternal Mortality Rate; MoH: Palestinian Ministry of Health; NGO: Non-Governmental Organisation; PE: Pulmonary Embolism; PPH: Postpartum Haemorrhage; UNFPA: United Nations Population Fund; UNRWA: United Nations Relief and Works Agency; WHO: World Health Organisation

Acknowledgements
Dr. Abdelrazaaq Al Kurd for critical reading of the study and plentiful good advice.
Osama Abueita from the UNFPA for his trust and ongoing support in completion of this study.
Aiman Momani MD, PhD for his contribution to editing the final draft.

Funding
Limited funding for this study was provided by the United Nations Population Fund (UNFPA), Palestine. This did not include publication fees. The UNFPA played no role in the design of the study, collection, analysis, and interpretation of data. The UNFPA also played no role in writing the manuscript.

Authors' contributions
BB, NAEN, BA designed the study, collected the data, analysed and interpreted the data and drafted the manuscript. FN and YA contributed to the design of the study. All authors read and approved the final manuscript.

Competing interests
The authors declare that they have no competing interests.

Author details
[1]Faculty of Medicine, Islamic University of Gaza, P. O. Box 108, Gaza strip, Gaza, Palestine. [2]Faculty of Nursing, Islamic University of Gaza, P. O. Box 108, Gaza Strip, Gaza, Palestine.

References

1. Say L, Chou D, Gemmill A, Tunçalp Ö, Moller A-B, Daniels J, et al. Global causes of maternal death: a WHO systematic analysis. Lancet Glob Health. 2014;2(6):e323–e33.
2. United Nations. Millennium Development Goals Report 2015 New York 2015 [updated 6 July 2015]. Available from: http://www.un.org/en/development/desa/publications/mdg-report-2015.html. Accessed 3 Apr 2017.
3. World Health Organization. State of inequality: Reproductive, maternal, newborn and child health 2015 [updated 2015]. Available from: http://www.who.int/gender-equity-rights/knowledge/state-of-inequality/en/. Accessed 10 Jun 2017.
4. Awwad J. Ministry of Health. State of Palestine. The health conditions of the population of occupied Palestine. Report submitted to the Sixty-ninth World Health Assembly of the. World Health Organization (Geneva, 23–28 May 2016). Available from: https://who.int/gb/ebwha/pdf_files/WHA69A69_INF6-en.pdf Accessed 3 Apr 2017.
5. Palestinian Central Bureau of Statistics. Palestinian Multiple Indicator Cluster Survey 2014 Nablus, Palestine 2015 [updated 2015]. Available from: http://www.pcbs.gov.ps/post.aspx?lang=en&ItemID=1377. Accessed 10 Jun 2017.
6. World Health Organization, United Nations Childrens Fund, United Nations Population Fund (UNFPA), The World Bank, United Nations Population Division. Trends in Maternal Mortality: 1990 to 2013. Estimates by WHO, UNICEF, UNFPA, The World Bank and the United Nations Population Division 2014 [updated May 2014]. Available from: http://www.who.int/reproductivehealth/publications/monitoring/maternal-mortality-2013/en/. Accessed 3 Apr 2017.
7. Abdul Rahim HF, Wick L, Halileh S, Hassan-Bitar S, Chekir H, Watt G, et al. Maternal and child health in the occupied Palestinian territory. Lancet. 2009; 373(9667):967–77.
8. Abdo S, Jarrar K, El-Nakhal S, Ramlawi A, Hijaz T, Saman K, et al. Report on Maternal Mortality in Palestine 2012. Available from: http://www.unfpa.ps/resources/file/publications/Maternal%20Mortality%20Report%20-%20English.pdf. Accessed 3 Apr 2017.
9. Patton MQ. Qualitative interviewing. Qual Res Eval methods. 2002;3:344–7.
10. Punch KF. Introduction to social research: quantitative and qualitative approaches. Sage; 2013.
11. Neuman WL. Social research methods: quantitative and qualitative approaches. Boston: Allyn and bacon, 2005.
12. Creswell JW. Research design: qualitative, quantitative, and mixed methods approaches: sage publications; 2013.
13. Cohen DJ, Crabtree BF. Evaluative criteria for qualitative research in health care: controversies and recommendations. The Annals of Family Medicine. 2008;6(4):331–9.
14. Polit DF, Beck CT. Nursing research: principles and methods. Philadelphia: Lippincott Williams & Wilkins; 2004.
15. Abu-El-Noor NI, El-Shokry M, Fareed M, Abu-Sultan N, Saleh K, Alkasseh AS. Quality of antenatal Care in Governmental Primary Health Care Centers in the Gaza strip as perceived by nurses and midwives: an indication for policy change. IUG J Nat Stud. 2018;26(2):38–4816.
16. Press Release on the Occasion of International Health Day 07/04/2015 [Internet]. 2015 [cited 25/8/2017]. Available from: http://www.pcbs.gov.ps/post.aspx?lang=en&ItemID=1367.
17. Tongue JR, Epps HR, Forese LL. Communication skills for patient-centered care. J Bone Joint Surg Am. 2005;87(3):652–8.
18. Almond S, Mant D, Thompson M. Diagnostic safety-netting. Br J Gen Pract. 2009;59(568):872–4.
19. Maguire P, Pitceathly C. Key communication skills and how to acquire them. BMJ. 2002;325(7366):697–700.
20. Ha JF, Longnecker N. Doctor-patient communication: a review. Ochsner J. 2010;10(1):38–43.
21. Neighbour R. The inner consultation: how to develop an effective and intuitive consulting style. London: Radcliffe publishing; 2005.
22. Abukhalil M, Bottcher B, Mehjez O, Alankah L, Abuyusuf M, Hasan S. Medical records of emergency caesarean sections in the Gaza strip: a clinical audit. Lancet. 2018;391:S26.
23. El-Shami M, Alaloul E, Dabbour R, Alkhatib M, Abdelghafour T, Böttcher B. An evidence-based study: evaluating the Management of Acute Heart Failure in the Gaza-strip hospitals. J Card Fail. 2017;23(8):112.
24. Gutheil TG. Fundamentals of medical record documentation. Psychiatry (Edgmont). 2004;1(3):26.
25. Prytherch DR, Smith GB, Schmidt PE, Featherstone PI. ViEWS—towards a national early warning score for detecting adult inpatient deterioration. Resuscitation. 2010;81(8):932–7.
26. Cuthbertson BH, Boroujerdi M, McKie L, Aucott L, Prescott G. Can physiological variables and early warning scoring systems allow early recognition of the deteriorating surgical patient? Crit Care Med. 2007; 35(2):402–9.
27. Zimmo M, Laine K, Hassan SJ, Fosse E, Lieng M, Ali-Masri H, et al. Differences in rates and odds for emergency caesarean section in six Palestinian hospitals: a population-based birth cohort study. BMJ Open. 2018;8(3):e019509.
28. Reason J. Beyond the organisational accident: the need for "error wisdom" on the frontline. Qual Saf Health Care. 2004;13(suppl 2):ii28–33.
29. Tantrige PM. Clinical audits must improve to benefit patients, providers, and doctors. BMJ Career. 2014;349:g4534.
30. Wachter RM. The end of the beginning: patient safety five years after 'to err is human'. Health Aff. 2004;23:W4.
31. United Nations Office for the Cooperation of Humanitarean Affairs. 2016 [cited 2017 3rd Apr]. Available from: https://www.ochaopt.org/content/gaza-crossings-operations-status-monthly-update-june-2016. Accessed 10 Jun 2017.

14

Association between fluid management and dilutional coagulopathy in severe postpartum haemorrhage: a nationwide retrospective cohort study

Ada Gillissen[1,2,3], Thomas van den Akker[3,4], Camila Caram-Deelder[1,2], Dacia D C A Henriquez[1,2,3], Kitty W M Bloemenkamp[5], Jos J M van Roosmalen[3,6], Jeroen Eikenboom[7], Johanna G van der Bom[1,2*] and on behalf of the TeMpOH-1 study group

Abstract

Background: The view that 2 l of crystalloid and 1.5 l of colloid can be infused while awaiting compatible blood for patients with major postpartum haemorrhage is based on expert opinion documents. We describe real-world changes in levels of coagulation parameters after the administration of different volumes of clear fluids to women suffering from major postpartum haemorrhage.

Methods: We performed a nationwide retrospective cohort study in the Netherlands among 1038 women experiencing severe postpartum haemorrhage who had received at least four units of red cells or fresh frozen plasma or platelets in addition to red cells. The volume of clear fluids administered before the time of blood sampling was classified into three fluid administration strategies, based on the RCOG guideline: < 2 L, 2–3.5 L and > 3.5 L. Outcomes included haemoglobin, haematocrit, platelet count, fibrinogen, aPTT and PT levels.

Results: Haemoglobin, haematocrit, platelet count, fibrinogen and aPTT were associated with volumes of clear fluids, which was most pronounced early during the course of postpartum haemorrhage. During the earliest phases of postpartum haemorrhage median haemoglobin level was 10.1 g/dl (IQR 8.5–11.6) among the women who received < 2 L clear fluids and 8.1 g/dl (IQR 7.1–8.4) among women who received > 3.5 L of clear fluids; similarly median platelet counts were 181×10^9/litre (IQR 131–239) and 89×10^9/litre (IQR 84–135), aPTT 29 s (IQR 27–33) and 38 s (IQR 35–55) and fibrinogen 3.9 g/L (IQR 2.5–5.2) and 1.6 g/L (IQR 1.3–2.1).

Conclusions: In this large cohort of women with severe postpartum haemorrhage, administration of larger volumes of clear fluids was associated with more severe deterioration of coagulation parameters corresponding to dilution. Our findings provide thus far the best available evidence to support expert opinion-based guidelines recommending restrictive fluid resuscitation in women experiencing postpartum haemorrhage.

Keywords: Coagulation parameters, Dilutional coagulopathy, Fluid management, Postpartum haemorrhage

* Correspondence: j.g.vanderbom@lumc.nl; J.G.van_der_Bom@lumc.nl
[1]Center for Clinical Transfusion Research, Sanquin Research, Plesmanlaan 1a –
5th floor, 2333, BZ, Leiden, The Netherlands
[2]Department of Clinical Epidemiology, Leiden University Medical Center,
Albinusdreef 2, 2333, ZA, Leiden, The Netherlands
Full list of author information is available at the end of the article

Background

Postpartum haemorrhage continues to be a leading cause of maternal health problems worldwide [1]. Depending on the primary cause of haemorrhage, acquired coagulopathy may develop during the course of postpartum haemorrhage and aggravate bleeding [2]. Rapid intravenous infusion of clear (crystalloid and colloid) fluids is generally applied during on-going haemorrhage to establish haemodynamic stability, restore adequate intravascular volume and improve oxygen carrying capacity and oxygen tissue delivery [3]. When given in large volumes, clear fluids initiate dilution of clotting factors resulting in impairment of coagulation and coagulopathy [4–6]. On top of that, rapid consumption of fibrinogen, clotting factors and platelets as a result of persistent blood loss, aggravates coagulopathy [5]. The use of colloid fluids has proven to negatively influence coagulation capacity and endothelial function [7, 8]. These findings have led to less aggressive fluid management in patients with traumatic haemorrhagic shock [9].

International guidelines on management of women with severe postpartum haemorrhage elucidate the lack of quantitative evidence on the effect of different fluid management strategies on parameters of coagulopathy. For instance, the RCOG green-top guideline advises to follow the expert opinion-based recommendation to administer up to 3.5 l of warmed clear fluids, starting with 2 l of warmed isotonic crystalloids until blood products are available in case of persistent postpartum blood loss exceeding 1000 ml [10]. The experts formed their opinions based on experiments in laboratories, animals, healthy volunteers, and observations from trauma patients. However, findings from these studies may not apply to pregnant women, since pregnancy induces haemodynamic and haematologic changes that protect them against haemorrhage during birth. Maternal blood volume increases between 1.2 and 1.6 l above non-pregnant values, creating a hypervolemic state during pregnancy [4]. To enable evidence-based recommendations on fluid management strategies in women with major postpartum haemorrhage, more insight is needed on the changes of coagulation parameters after administration of different volumes of fluids [4]. To the best of our knowledge no previous studies have been conducted into different fluid management strategies and their possible effect on coagulation parameters in women experiencing postpartum haemorrhage.

The aim of this study was to describe the association between administration of different volumes of clear fluids and levels of coagulation parameters in women experiencing postpartum haemorrhage.

Methods

Design and study population

We studied volumes of clear fluids and results of coagulation parameter measurements during postpartum haemorrhage in a cohort of women who had been included in a nationwide retrospective cohort study in 61 hospitals in the Netherlands, the TeMpOH-1 (Transfusion strategies in women during Major Obstetric Haemorrhage) study. Included in the TeMpOH-1 study were women who received at least four units of red cells or any transfusion of fresh frozen plasma (FFP) and/or platelets in addition to red cells because of *obstetric haemorrhage* defined as ≥1000 mL blood loss during pregnancy, childbirth or puerperium between January 1st, 2011 and January 1st, 2013. For the present analyses, we selected women from the TeMpOH-1 cohort who met criteria for *primary postpartum haemorrhage*: any amount of blood loss exceeding 1000 mL within the first 24 h after childbirth. Women with no coagulation parameters measured during active postpartum haemorrhage and women with missing data on volumes and timing of clear fluids were excluded. In case transfusion of blood products occurred before onset of clear fluid administration, patients were also excluded. The Ethical Committee of Leiden University Medical Centre (P12.273) and the institutional review boards of all participating hospitals approved of the study. The study was registered in the Netherlands Trial Register (NTR4079). Details regarding study design have been reported elsewhere [11]. The need to obtain informed consent was waived by the ethics committee because of the retrospective design. Women 18 years of age and older who met the inclusion criteria were selected.

Data collection

To identify all consecutive women who had been transfused with the aforementioned amount of blood products because of postpartum haemorrhage in the participating hospitals, data from the hospitals' blood transfusion services were merged with data from birth registers of contributing hospitals. Qualified medical students and research nurses collected routine data from the medical records with regard to (obstetric) history and course of the current pregnancy, as well as data pertaining to characteristics of participating women, mode of birth, primary cause of haemorrhage, placentation, characteristics of shock (defined as systolic blood pressure < 90 mmHg or heartrate > 120 bpm), surgical and haemostatic interventions to stop bleeding and coagulation parameters. Results of all measurements of haemoglobin level (Hb, g/dl), haematocrit (Ht, fraction), platelet count ($\times 10^9$/litre), activated partial thromboplastin time (aPTT, seconds), prothrombin time (PT, seconds) and fibrinogen (g/L) levels from the first measurement of blood loss onwards were documented; this included parameters drawn from cases before they had bled a total volume of 1000 mL. Outliers of levels of coagulation parameters were verified in the medical records. In addition, detailed information on crystalloid and colloid fluids administered during the course of postpartum haemorrhage was collected: total volume and type of clear fluids given, as well as timing information with regard to onset and end of infusion. Information on timing and volume of repetitive blood loss measurements was also retrieved from the medical files. In most cases blood loss was measured by weighing soaked gauzes during and after birth and by use of a collector bag and suction system in the operating theatre.

Severe acute maternal morbidity and maternal mortality

The composite endpoint severe acute maternal morbidity and mortality comprised emergency peripartum hysterectomy, ligation of the uterine arteries, B-Lynch suture (in the Netherlands only used as emergency procedure), arterial embolization or admission into an intensive care unit.

Statistical analyses

The aim was to describe values of measured laboratory parameters according to increasing "volume of blood loss" and "volume of clear fluids administered" during the course of severe postpartum haemorrhage. In order to have an estimate of the "volume of blood loss" and of "volume of clear fluids administered" for all blood samples (and their respective laboratory results) we used linear interpolation of the actual measurement of "volume of blood loss" and "volume of clear fluids administered" before and after each blood sample. The volume of blood loss at the time of blood sampling was categorised in 8 groups: 0–1.0 L, 1.0–1.5 L, 1.5–2.0 L, 2.0–2.5 L, 2.5–3.0 L, 3.0–3.5 L, 3.5–4.0 L and > 4.0 L. Coagulation parameters were allocated to the category representing the volume of blood loss at sampling. In case of multiple laboratory measurements per patient within one blood loss category, the mean of the values was used in the analyses, calculating a patient just once per category. Subsequently, within these blood loss categories, the volume of clear fluids administered at the time of blood sampling was calculated and classified into three fluid administration strategies: < 2.0 L, 2.0–3.5 L and > 3.5 L. These three administration strategies were based on the RCOG green-top guideline, which recommends to administer up to 3.5 l of warmed clear fluids, starting with 2 l of warmed isotonic crystalloids if blood is not available [10]. Since blood sampling during postpartum haemorrhage was not performed at predefined time points and samples were obtained on request of the physician on call during postpartum haemorrhage, patients could have different frequencies and panels of coagulation parameters. Reference ranges of aPTT varied somewhat for the 61 participating hospitals as a result of use of different types of reagents. Therefore, an aPTT

ratio was calculated by dividing the aPTT level of cases by the mean of the hospital specific reference range.

Results

Patient characteristics

A total of 1038 women with severe postpartum haemorrhage had at least one valid measurement of coagulation parameters sampled during active bleeding in addition to data on volume and timing of clear fluids administered (Fig. 1). Baseline characteristics are reported in Table 1. Women were on average 31 years of age, gave birth at a median gestational age of 39.7 weeks and 25% delivered by caesarean section. Uterine atony was the primary cause of bleeding in 66% of the cases and 34% of women developed a composite endpoint of severe acute maternal morbidity or mortality. The median total volume of blood loss among all 1038 women with postpartum haemorrhage was 3.0 L (interquartile range 2.5–4.0). In our cohort, women in the lowest fluid categories showed fewer signs of shock and were administered fewer blood products when compared to women in the other fluid categories for all coagulation parameters (*data presented in table adjacent to* Fig. 3).

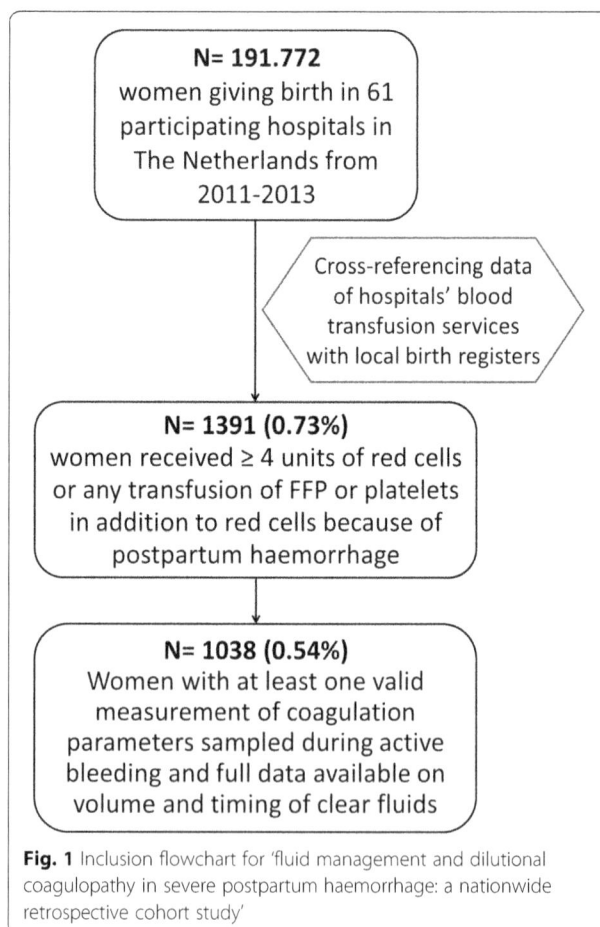

Fig. 1 Inclusion flowchart for 'fluid management and dilutional coagulopathy in severe postpartum haemorrhage: a nationwide retrospective cohort study'

Table 1 Clinical characteristics of the cohort of 1038 women with ongoing postpartum haemorrhage included in this analysis

Patients	$n = 1038$
Maternal characteristics	
Age (years)	31.0 (28.0–35.0)[a]
BMI (kg/m^2)	23.2 (21.0–26.3)
Ethnicity Caucasian	747 (72%)[b]
Nulliparity	534 (51%)
Gestational age	39.7 (38.1–40.7)
Mode of birth	
Caesarean section	254 (24%)
Vaginal	780 (75%)
Comorbidity	
Pre-eclampsia/ HELLP	104 (10%)
Anti-coagulant use	6 (0.6%)
Transfer to hospital	
No transfer (birth in hospital)	753 (73%)
Transfer to hospital during labour	157 (15%)
Postpartum transfer (birth at home)	128 (12%)
Primary cause of bleeding	
Uterine atony	684 (66%)
Retained placenta	168 (16%)
Pathological ingrowth of placenta	89 (9%)
Surgical bleeding and abruption/ coagulopathy	97(9%)
Placentation	
Abnormal localisation placenta	65 (6%)
Pathological ingrowth placenta	97 (9%)
Composite endpoint severe maternal morbidity and mortality	355 (34%)
Embolisation	124 (12%)
Hysterectomy	57 (5%)
Emergency B-Lynch	27 (3%)
Ligation arteries	7 (0.7%)
ICU admission	295 (28%)
Maternal mortality	6 (0.6%)
Haemostatic Interventions	
Fibrinogen administered	98 (9%)
Tranexamic acid administered	473 (46%)
Recombinant FVIIa administered	29 (3%)
Bleeding characteristics	
Bleeding rate (ml/min) [c]	2.4 (1.3–4.8)
Shock	927 (89%)
Total volume blood loss (L)	3.0 (2.5–4.0)
Total volume of clear fluids (L)	3.0 (2.0–4.0)
Total units of blood products (n)	6.0 (4.0–8.0)

[a]Values are presented as median with (interquartile range), [b]percentage, [c] maximum

Volume expansion and volume of blood loss

Figure 2 presents volumes of blood loss and volumes of infused fluids. Among women who had one or more laboratory parameters measured during the first phases of postpartum haemorrhage ($n = 245$ for 0 to 1 L; $n = 306$ for 1 to 1.5 L; and $n = 351$ for 1.5 to 2 L) the mean volume of replacement therapy (clear fluids and blood products) administered was less or equal the total volume of blood loss. During the next phases of postpartum haemorrhage (blood loss between 2 and 2.5 L) the mean volume of replacement therapy (clear fluids and blood products) was higher than the volume of blood loss. This "overload" enlarged with increasing blood loss volumes, reaching 32% more volume replacement compared to blood loss in the phase in which the women had lost 3.5-4 L (5.3 L infused /4 L lost). For all categories of blood loss, mean volume of clear fluids administered did not exceed and in most cases was similar to the maximum blood loss. With increasing blood loss, the proportion of blood products (versus clear fluids) administered showed a gradual increase, from 118/1178 mL (10%) at 1000-1500 mL blood loss to 1605/5279 mL (30%) after blood loss up to 4000 mL.

Laboratory parameters after different volumes of clear fluids in the course of postpartum haemorrhage

Figure 3 presents results of laboratory tests according to received volumes of clear fluids (0 to 2 L, 2 to 3.5 L or more than 3.5 L) during the first two litres of postpartum haemorrhage. From 1031 women a total of 2714 haemoglobin measurements were available. Administration of higher volumes of clear fluids was associated with lower haemoglobin and haematocrit levels and this was most pronounced in the earlier phases of postpartum haemorrhage (Fig. 3 and Additional file 1: Table S1 and Additional file 2: Figure S2). For example, when the women had lost less than 1.0 L of blood, the median haemoglobin level was 10.1 g/dl (IQR 8.5–11.6) if they had received < 2.0 L of clear fluids, whereas after receiving 2.0–3.5 L clear fluids median haemoglobin was 8.4 g/dl (IQR 8.4–9.7).

Platelet counts of 804 women decreased over the three increasing fluid administration categories. In samples drawn in the earliest phase of postpartum haemorrhage (0-1 L blood loss), median platelet counts were 181 (IQR 131–239), 154 (IQR 99–205) and 89×10^9/litre (IQR 84–135) in the three categories of increasing volumes of fluids administered. A similar pattern was observed in consecutive blood loss categories.

Fibrinogen measurements of 438 women were available for analyses. Administering higher volumes of clear fluids was associated with a decreasing level of fibrinogen in measurements in the early phases of postpartum haemorrhage (up to 2 L of blood loss). The largest

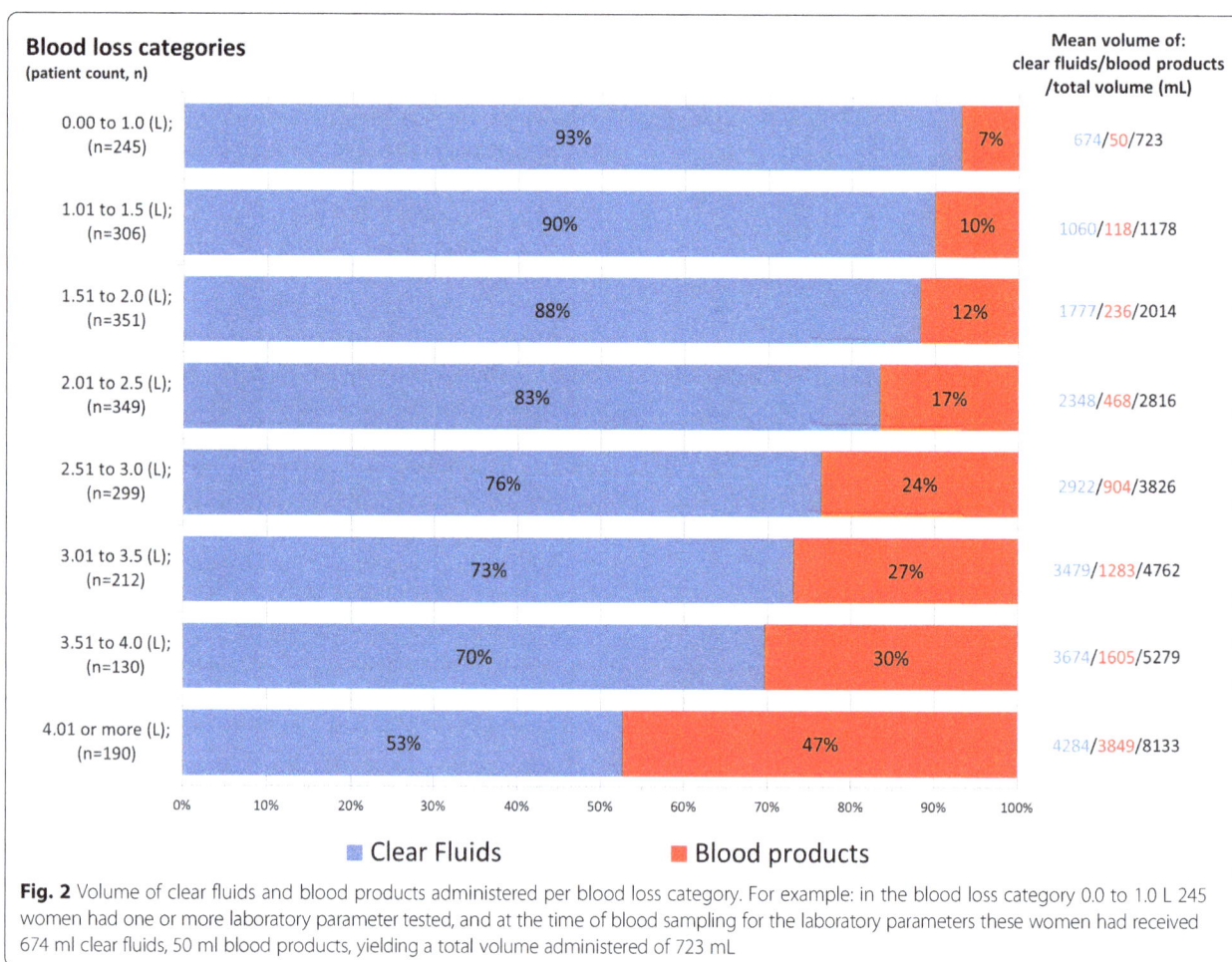

Fig. 2 Volume of clear fluids and blood products administered per blood loss category. For example: in the blood loss category 0.0 to 1.0 L 245 women had one or more laboratory parameter tested, and at the time of blood sampling for the laboratory parameters these women had received 674 ml clear fluids, 50 ml blood products, yielding a total volume administered of 723 mL

change was displayed for measurements performed in the earliest phase of postpartum haemorrhage (blood loss 0-1000 mL): 3.9 g/L (IQR 2.5–5.2), 2.6 g/L (IQR 1.6–3.7), 1.6 g/L (IQR 1.3–2.1) over the three fluid management categories.

PT and aPTT were longer after administration of larger volumes of clear fluids. For both, the largest difference was observed between measurements in the most restrictive fluids category (< 2 L) and the most liberal category (> 3.5 L). In samples drawn between 0 and 1 L blood loss, PT was 13 (IQR 11–15) and 17 s (IQR 12–19) and aPTT 29 (IQR 27–33) and 38 s (IQR 35–55) in lowest and highest fluid administration categories respectively. Levels of PT and aPTT of women administered 2–3.5 L of fluids were similar to blood samples of women who were administered less than 2 L of fluids. Results of the aPTT ratio showed similar results (Additional file 3: Figure S3).

Discussion

This nationwide retrospective multicentre cohort study describes coagulation parameters after administering different volumes of resuscitation fluids in 1038 women

with ongoing severe postpartum haemorrhage. The administration of larger volumes of clear fluids was associated with deterioration of levels of haemoglobin, haematocrit, platelet count, fibrinogen, aPTT and PT which was most pronounced during the earlier phases of postpartum haemorrhage.

Strengths and limitations of our study

A strength of the study is that we included a large cohort of women who had suffered severe postpartum haemorrhage and who had been treated with different volume replacement strategies. Women in our study were categorised based on similar volumes of blood loss at time of blood sampling, thereby making them comparable on a clinical level during the course of haemorrhage. Volume replacement had been carefully documented in the medical files in all the participating hospitals ensuring correct classification of women according to the different replacement strategies. Both these strengths allow for reliable description of abnormalities in coagulation in relation to volume replacement therapy.

We stratified our findings according to volume of blood loss. Volume of blood loss was measured in most cases by

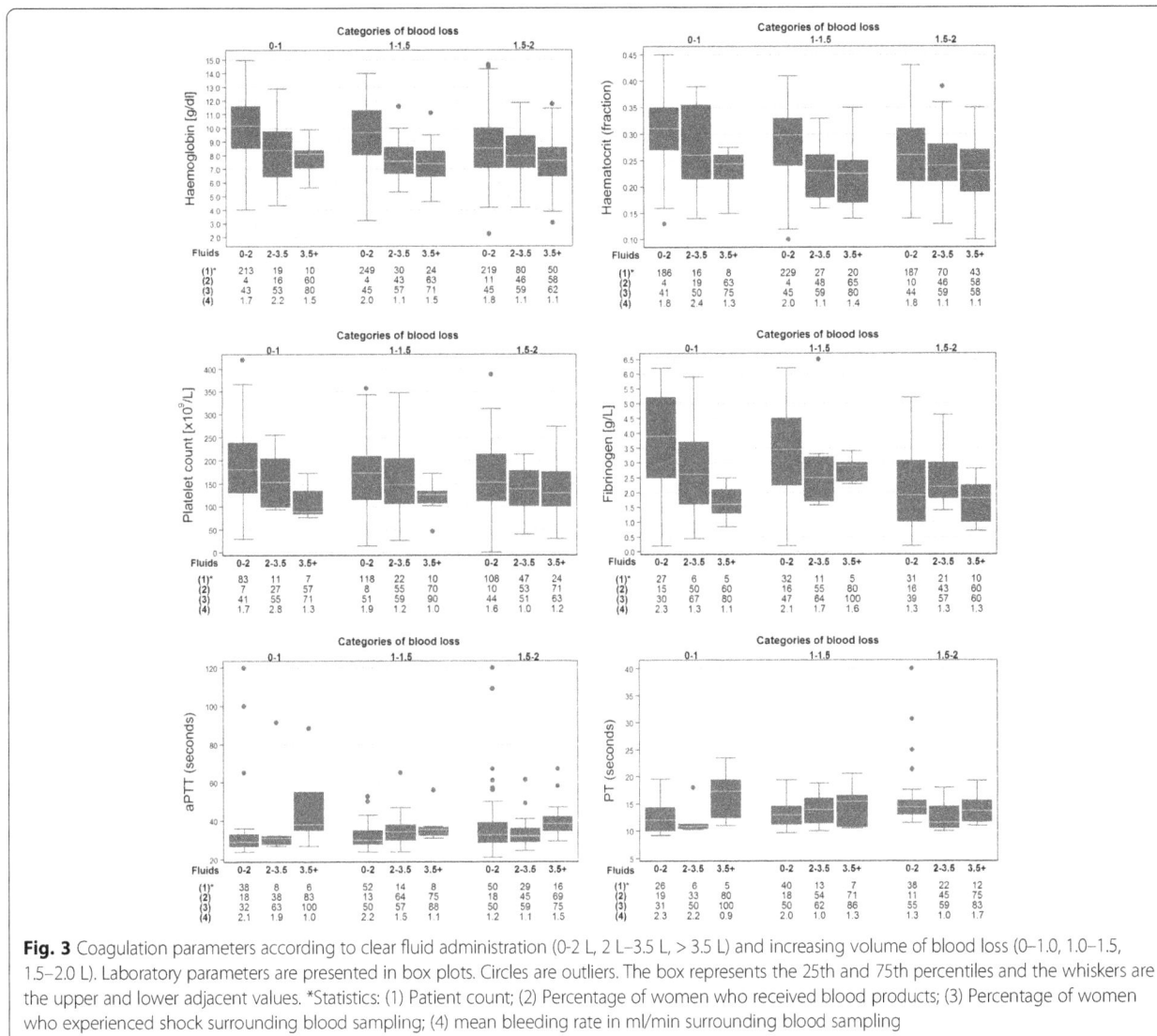

Fig. 3 Coagulation parameters according to clear fluid administration (0-2 L, 2 L–3.5 L, > 3.5 L) and increasing volume of blood loss (0–1.0, 1.0–1.5, 1.5–2.0 L). Laboratory parameters are presented in box plots. Circles are outliers. The box represents the 25th and 75th percentiles and the whiskers are the upper and lower adjacent values. *Statistics: (1) Patient count; (2) Percentage of women who received blood products; (3) Percentage of women who experienced shock surrounding blood sampling; (4) mean bleeding rate in ml/min surrounding blood sampling

Haemoglobin [g/dl] — Categories of blood loss

	0-1			1-1.5			1.5-2		
Fluids	0-2	2-3.5	3.5+	0-2	2-3.5	3.5+	0-2	2-3.5	3.5+
(1)*	213	19	10	249	30	24	219	80	50
(2)	4	16	60	4	43	63	11	48	58
(3)	43	53	80	45	57	71	45	59	62
(4)	1.7	2.2	1.5	2.0	1.1	1.5	1.8	1.1	1.1

Haematocrit (fraction) — Categories of blood loss

	0-1			1-1.5			1.5-2		
Fluids	0-2	2-3.5	3.5+	0-2	2-3.5	3.5+	0-2	2-3.5	3.5+
(1)*	186	16	8	229	27	20	187	70	43
(2)	4	19	63	4	48	65	10	46	58
(3)	41	50	75	45	59	80	44	59	58
(4)	1.8	2.4	1.3	2.0	1.1	1.4	1.8	1.1	1.1

Platelet count [×10⁹/L] — Categories of blood loss

	0-1			1-1.5			1.5-2		
Fluids	0-2	2-3.5	3.5+	0-2	2-3.5	3.5+	0-2	2-3.5	3.5+
(1)*	83	11	7	118	22	10	108	47	24
(2)	7	27	57	8	55	70	10	53	71
(3)	41	55	71	51	59	90	44	51	63
(4)	1.7	2.8	1.3	1.9	1.2	1.0	1.6	1.0	1.2

Fibrinogen [g/L] — Categories of blood loss

	0-1			1-1.5			1.5-2		
Fluids	0-2	2-3.5	3.5+	0-2	2-3.5	3.5+	0-2	2-3.5	3.5+
(1)*	27	6	5	32	11	5	31	21	10
(2)	15	50	60	16	55	80	16	43	60
(3)	30	67	80	47	64	100	39	57	60
(4)	2.3	1.3	1.1	2.1	1.7	1.6	1.3	1.3	1.3

aPTT (seconds) — Categories of blood loss

	0-1			1-1.5			1.5-2		
Fluids	0-2	2-3.5	3.5+	0-2	2-3.5	3.5+	0-2	2-3.5	3.5+
(1)*	38	8	6	52	14	8	50	29	16
(2)	18	38	83	13	64	75	18	45	69
(3)	32	63	100	50	57	88	50	59	75
(4)	2.1	1.9	1.0	2.2	1.5	1.1	1.2	1.1	1.5

PT (seconds) — Categories of blood loss

	0-1			1-1.5			1.5-2		
Fluids	0-2	2-3.5	3.5+	0-2	2-3.5	3.5+	0-2	2-3.5	3.5+
(1)*	26	6	5	40	13	7	38	22	12
(2)	19	33	80	18	54	71	11	45	75
(3)	31	50	100	50	62	86	55	59	83
(4)	2.2	2.2	0.9	2.0	1.0	1.3	1.1	1.0	1.7

weighing soaked gauzes during and after birth and by use of a collector bag and suction system in the operating theatre, in addition to visual estimation. Thus, there may be misclassification of volume of blood loss in both directions, over- and underestimation and it is therefore difficult to know whether and how our findings are affected by this misclassification. Our findings are also affected by the fact that inherently more blood samples are drawn from women with more severe bleeding. This may have led to overestimation of the number of women with abnormal laboratory test results. Because of the design of the study we did not have influence on the number and specific panels of coagulation samples requested. Therefore, our results show different selections of women in all blood loss categories that we present. Although it is tempting to infer that high volumes of clear fluids are causally related to the observed dilution our study does not allow such inference. There are many other factors that may have influenced coagulation parameters such as the primary cause of haemorrhage, bleeding and treatment characteristics and the presence of comorbidities. This descriptive study does not allow for disentanglement of the separate effects of these joint risk factors. We excluded 353 women because they had no valid lab measurement available during active bleeding or data were missing on volume or timing of clear fluids administered. To be certain their exclusion did not induce a systemic error to our data resulting from selection bias, we compared these women on the most relevant Table 1 items: mode of birth, nulliparity, primary cause of haemorrhage, the composite endpoint of severe maternal morbidity and mortality, bleeding rate at sampling, presence of shock and total volume of blood loss. No differences were observed compared to the women that were included in the study, ruling out the presence of a systemic error influencing the results.

Comparison with other studies

To the best of our knowledge no previous studies have described the association between different fluid management strategies and coagulation parameters during the various phases of severe postpartum haemorrhage. Yet, our findings corroborate results of previous studies into the effect of dilution on coagulation parameters. An in vitro study evaluating the effect of haemodilution on coagulation factors found that PT and aPTT were significantly prolonged after 60% and 80% dilution [12]. Another in vitro study investigated the effect of haemodilution on the course of global coagulation tests and clotting factors. Levels of dilution-dependent coagulation factors and aPTT were found to decrease in an almost linear manner. Critically low activities for coagulation factors and a critically low level of fibrinogen were measured at dilutions of between 60 and 75% [13]. An in vivo study reported coagulation parameters in hypotensive patients with penetrating torso injuries who were treated with immediate versus delayed fluid resuscitation. Patients in the immediate fluid administration group showed worse levels of haemoglobin, platelet count, PT and APTT compared to patients in the delayed fluid administration group [14]. No previous studies were found that examined the change in coagulation parameters as a result of different fluid management strategies in women experiencing postpartum haemorrhage.

Clinical implications

In our cohort of women experiencing postpartum haemorrhage, we displayed changes occurring on coagulation parameter level after administering different volumes of fluids. Administration of larger volumes of clear fluids was associated with more severe worsening of levels of haemoglobin, haematocrit, platelet count, fibrinogen, aPTT and PT which was most pronounced during the earlier phases of postpartum haemorrhage. Our findings provide quantitative evidence to reinforce expert opinion-based guidelines recommending restrictive fluid resuscitation strategies in case of postpartum haemorrhage;

Conclusions

In this nationwide retrospective cohort study in 1038 women on the change in coagulation parameters with increasing volumes administered during the course of postpartum haemorrhage necessitating blood transfusion, the administration of large volumes of clear fluids was associated with changes in coagulation parameters corresponding to dilutional coagulopathy. Our findings provide thus far the best available evidence to support expert opinion-based guidelines recommending restrictive fluid resuscitation in women experiencing postpartum haemorrhage.

Abbreviations

aPTT: Activated Partial Thromboplastin Time; Hb: Haemoglobin; Ht: Haematocrit; IQR: Interquartile range; PT: prothrombin time; RCOG: Royal College of Obstetricians and Gynaecologists

Acknowledgements

We would like to thank all 61 participating hospitals and the Dutch Consortium for Healthcare Evaluation and Research in Obstetrics and Gynaecology - NVOG Consortium 2.0, medical students R.M. Loeff, R.J. van Goeverden, B. Eijlers, A. Hillebrand, S.E. Spelmink, T.J. Beunder, V. Harskamp, M. Wind, M.D. Koning, R.A. Cramer, A. Veenstra, S.M. Smith and E.E. Ensing, datamanagers C.J. van Brussel-de Groot and O. Zouitni, research nurses C. Kolster-Bijdevaate, M.S. Bourgonje-Verhart, C.E. Bleeker-Taborh, E. Roos-van Milligen and A. de Graaf for their contributions to the TeMpOH-1 study. Also we would like to thank Professor J.C.M Meijers for critically reading and providing feedback on the manuscript.
TeMpOH-1 study group.
H.J. Adriaanse (PhD), Gelre Hospital, Medical Laboratory Head; E.S.A. van den Akker (MD, PhD), Onze Lieve Vrouwe Hospital, Obstetrician; M.I. Baas (MD, PhD), Hospital Rivierenland Tiel, Obstetrician; C.M.C. Bank (MSc), Admiraal de Ruyter Hospital, Medical Laboratory Head; E. van Beek (MD, PhD), St. Antonius Hospital, Obstetrician; B.A. de Boer (PhD), Atalmedial, Medical Laboratory Head; K. de Boer (MD, PhD), Rijnstate Hospital, Obstetrician; D.M.R. van der Borden (MD, PhD), Regional Hospital Koningin Beatrix, Obstetrician; H.A. Bremer (MD, PhD), Reinier de Graaf Hospital, Obstetrician; J.T.J. Brons (MD, PhD), Medical Centre Twente, Obstetrician; J.M. Burggraaf (MD, PhD), Scheper Hospital, Obstetrician; H. Ceelie (PhD), Vlietland Hospital, Medical Laboratory Head; H. Chon (PhD), Tergooi Hospital, Medical Laboratory Heads; J.L.M. Cikot (MD, PhD), Van Weel-Bethesda Hospital, Obstetrician; F.M.C. Delemarre (MD, PhD), Elkerliek Hospital, Obstetrician; J.H.C. Diris (PhD), Bernhoven Hospital, Medical Laboratory Head; M. Doesburg–van Kleffens (PhD), Maas Hospital Pantein, Medical Laboratory Head; I.M.A. van Dooren (MD, PhD), St. Jans Hospital, Obstetrician; J.L.P. van Duijnhoven (PhD), Elkerliek Hospital, Medical Laboratory Head; F.M. van Dunné (MD PhD), Medical Centre Haaglanden, Obstetrician; J.J. Duvekot (MD, PhD), Erasmus Medical Centre, Obstetrician; P. Engbers (PhD), Bethesda Hospital, Medical Laboratory Head; M.J.W. van Etten–van Hulst (MD, PhD), Fransiscus Hospital, Obstetrician; H. Feitsma (MD, PhD), Haga Hospital, Obstetrician; M.A. Fouraux (PhD), Ikazia Hospital, Medical Laboratory Head; M.T.M. Franssen (MD, PhD), University Medical Centre Groningen, Obstetrician; M.A.M. Frasa (PhD), Groene Hart Hospital, Medical Laboratory Head; A.J. van Gammeren (PhD), Amphia Hospital, Medical Laboratory Head; N. van Gemund (MD, PhD), Sint Fransiscus Hospital, Obstetrician; F. van der Graaf (PhD), Máxima Medical Centre, Medical Laboratory Head; Prof. C.J.M. de Groot (MD, PhD), VU Medical Centre, Obstetrician; C.M. Hackeng (PhD), St. Antonius Hospital, Medical Laboratory Head; D.P. van der Ham (MD, PhD), Martini Hospital, Obstetrician; M.J.C.P. Hanssen (MD, PhD), Bethesda Hospital, Obstetrician; T.H.M. Hasaart (MD, PhD), Catharina Hospital, Obstetrician; H.A. Hendriks (MSc) Sint Lucas Andreas Hospital, Medical Laboratory Head; Y.M.C. Henskens (PhD), Maastricht University Medical Centre, Medical Laboratory Head; B.B.J. Hermsen (MD, PhD), Sint Lucas Andreas Hospital, Obstetrician; S. Hogenboom (PhD), Flevo Hospital, Medical Laboratory Head; A. Hooker (MD, PhD), Zaans Medical Centre, Obstetrician; F. Hudig (PhD), Haga Hospital, Medical Laboratory Head; A.M.G. Huijssoon (MD, PhD), Vlietland Hospital, Obstetrician; A.J.M. Huisjes (MD, PhD), Gelre Hospital, Obstetrician; N. Jonker (PhD), Wilhelmina Hospital, Medical Laboratory Head; P.J. Kabel (PhD), St. Elisabeth Hospital, Medical Laboratory Head; C. van Kampen (PhD), Gelderse Vallei Hospital, Medical Laboratory Head; M.H. de Keijzer (PhD), Rivierenland Tiel Hospital, Medical Laboratory Head; D.H. van de Kerkhof (PhD), Catharina Hospital, Medical Laboratory Head; J.F.W. Keuren (PhD), Zuwe Hofpoort Hospital, Medical Laboratory Head; J.F.W. Keuren (PhD), Groene Hart Hospital, Medical Laboratory Head; G. Kleiverda (MD, PhD), Flevo Hospital, Obstetrician; J.H. Klinkspoor (PhD), Amsterdam Medical Centre, Medical Laboratory Head; S.G.A. Koehorst (PhD), Slingeland Hospital, Medical Laboratory Head; M. Kok (MD, PhD), Amsterdam Medical Centre, Obstetrician; R.D. Kok (MD, PhD), Bernhoven Hospital, Obstetrician; J.B. de Kok (PhD), Deventer Hospital, Medical Laboratory Head; A. Koops (MD, PhD), Wilhelmina Hospital, Obstetrician; W. Kortlandt (PhD),

Diakonessen Hospital, Medical Laboratory Head; J. Langenveld (MD, PhD), Atrium Medical Centre, Obstetrician; M.P.G. Leers (PhD), Atrium Medical Centre, Medical Laboratory Head; A. Leyte (PhD), Onze Lieve Vrouwe Gasthuis, Medical Laboratory Head; A. de Mare (PhD), Medlon, Medical Laboratory Head; G.D.M. Martens (MD, PhD), Zuwe Hofpoort Hospital, Obstetrician; J.H. Meekers, University Medical Centre Groningen, Employee laboratory; C.A. van Meir (MD, PhD), Groene Hart Hospital, Obstetrician; G.C.H Metz (MD, PhD), Ikazia Hospital, Obstetrician; E.C.H.J. Michielse (PhD), St. Jans Hospital, Medical Laboratory Head; L.J. Mostert (PhD), Van Weel-Bethesda Hospital, Medical Laboratory Head; S.W.H. Nij Bijvank (MD, PhD), Isala clinics, Obstetrician; E. Oostenveld (MD, PhD), Tjongerschans Hospital, Obstetrician; N. Osmanovic (PhD), Zaans Medical Centre, Medical Laboratory Head; M.A. Oudijk (MD, PhD), University Medical Centre Utrecht, Obstetrician; C. Pagano Mirani–Oostdijk (PhD), Fransiscus Hospital, Medical Laboratory Head; E.C.M. van Pampus (PhD), University Medical Centre St. Radboud, Medical Laboratory Head; D.N.M. Papatsonis (MD, PhD), Amphia Hospital, Obstetrician; R.H.M. Peters (MD), Tjongerschans Hospital, Medical Laboratory Head; G.A.E. Ponjee (PhD), Medical Centre Haaglanden, Medical Laboratory Head; M. Pontesilli (MD, PhD student), Medical Centre Alkmaar, Fertility doctor; M.M. Porath (MD, PhD), Máxima Medical Centre, Obstetrician; M.S. Post (MD, PhD), Medical Centre Leeuwarden, Obstetrician; J.G.J. Pouwels (PhD), Scheper Hospital, Medical Laboratory Head; L. Prinzen (PhD), Sint Fransiscus Hospital, Medical Laboratory Head; J.M.T. Roelofsen (MD, PhD), Lange Land Hospital, Obstetrician; J.J.M. Rondeel (PhD), Isala clinics, Medical Laboratory Head; P.C.M. van der Salm (MD, PhD), Meander Medical Centre, Obstetrician; H.C.J. Scheepers (MD, PhD), Maastricht University Medical Centre, Obstetrician; D.H. Schippers (MD, PhD), Canisius-Wilhelmina Hospital, Obstetrician; N.W.E. Schuitemaker (MD, PhD), Diakonessen Hospital, Obstetrician; J.M. Sikkema (MD, PhD), Hospital group Twente, Obstetrician; J. Slomp (PhD), Medical Spectre Twente, Medical Laboratory Head; J.W. Smit (PhD), Martini Hospital, Medical Laboratory Head; Y.S. Snuif–de Lange (MD, PhD), Admiraal de Ruyter Hospital, Obstetrician; J.W.J. van der Stappen (PhD), Canisius-Wilhelmina Hospital, Medical Laboratory Head; P. Steures (MD, PhD), St. Elisabeth Hospital, Obstetrician; G.H.M. Tax (MD, PhD), Reinier de Graaf Hospital, Medical Laboratory Head; M. Treskes (PhD), Tergooi Hospital, Medical Laboratory Heads; H.J.L.M. Ulenkate (PhD), Zorgsaam Zeeuws-Vlaanderen Hospital, Medical Laboratory Head; G.A. van Unnik (MD, PhD), Diaconessen Hospital, Obstetrician; B.S. van der Veen (PhD), Medical Centre Leeuwarden, Medical Laboratory Head; T.E.M. Verhagen (MD, PhD), Slingeland Hospital, Obstetrician; J. Versendaal (MD), Maasstad Hospital, Obstetrician; B. Visschers (MD, PhD), Zorgsaam Zeeuws-Vlaanderen Hospital, Obstetrician; O. Visser (MD, PhD), VU Medical Centre, Hematologist; H. Visser (MD, PhD), Tergooi Hospital Obstetrician; K.M.K. de Vooght (PhD), University Medical Centre Utrecht, Medical Laboratory Head; M.J. de Vries (MD, PhD), Rijnland Hospital, Obstetrician; H. de Waard (PhD), Rijnstate Hospital, Medical Laboratory Head; F. Weerkamp (PhD), Maasstad Hospital, Medical Laboratory Head; M.J.N. Weinans (MD, PhD), Gelderse Vallei Hospital, Obstetrician; H. de Wet (MD, PhD), Refaja Hospital Stadskanaal, Obstetrician; M. van Wijnen (PhD), Meander Medical Centre, Medical Laboratory Head; W.J. van Wijngaarden (MD, PhD), Bronovo Hospital, Obstetrician; A.C. de Wit (MD, PhD), Maas Hospital Pantein, Obstetrician; M.D. Woiski (MD, PhD), University Medical Centre St. Radboud, Obstetrician.

Funding
Sanquin, Grant PPOC 11–032. Sanquin did not have any role in the conduction of the TeMpOH-1 study. Also, Sanquin was not involved in any analyses or scientific writing involving this manuscript.

Authors' contributions
Contribution: AG, TA, DH, JB designed the research and AG wrote the original draft of the paper. AG, CC, and DH were responsible for data curation. CC and AG analysed results and made the figures and Tables. AG, DH, JR, JE, KB, JB were involved in conceptualization and methodology. All co-authors reviewed and edited the paper and gave final approval. JB and TA had supervision over the project. All authors read and approved the final manuscript.

Competing interests
One of the co-authors of this manuscript, Jos J. M. van Roosmalen is a member of the editorial board (Section Editor) of BMC pregnancy and childbirth.

Author details
[1]Center for Clinical Transfusion Research, Sanquin Research, Plesmanlaan 1a – 5th floor, 2333, BZ, Leiden, The Netherlands. [2]Department of Clinical Epidemiology, Leiden University Medical Center, Albinusdreef 2, 2333, ZA, Leiden, The Netherlands. [3]Department of Obstetrics, Leiden University Medical Center, Albinusdreef 2, 2333, ZA, Leiden, The Netherlands. [4]National Perinatal Epidemiology Unit, University of Oxford, University of Oxford, Old Road Campus, Oxford OX3 7LF, UK. [5]Department of Obstetrics, Birth Centre Wilhelmina's Children Hospital, University Medical Center Utrecht, Lundlaan 6, 3584, EA, Utrecht, The Netherlands. [6]Athena Institute, VU University Amsterdam, De Boelelaan 1105, 1081, HV, Amsterdam, The Netherlands. [7]Department of Internal Medicine, Division of Thrombosis and Haemostasis, Leiden University Medical Center, Leiden, the Netherlands.

References
1. Say L, Chou D, Gemmill A, Tuncalp O, Moller AB, Daniels J, Gulmezoglu AM, Temmerman M, Alkema L. Global causes of maternal death: a WHO systematic analysis. Lancet Glob Health. 2014;2(6):e323–33.
2. Collis RE, Collins PW. Haemostatic management of obstetric haemorrhage. Anaesthesia. 2015;70(Suppl 1):78–86 e27–78.
3. Ruth D, Kennedy BB. Acute volume resuscitation following obstetric hemorrhage. J Perinatal Neonatal Nurs. 2011;25(3):253–60.
4. Bonnet MP, Basso O. Prohemostatic interventions in obstetric hemorrhage. Semin Thromb Hemost. 2012;38(3):259–64.
5. Schorn MN, Phillippi JC. Volume replacement following severe postpartum hemorrhage. J Midwifery Women's Health. 2014;59(3):336–43.
6. Cotton BA, Guy JS, Morris JA Jr, Abumrad NN. The cellular, metabolic, and systemic consequences of aggressive fluid resuscitation strategies. Shock (Augusta, Ga). 2006;26(2):115–21.
7. Fenger-Eriksen C. Acquired fibrinogen deficiency caused by artificial colloid plasma expanders. Wien Klin Wochenschr. 2010;122(Suppl 5):S21–2.
8. Fenger-Eriksen C, Moore GW, Rangarajan S, Ingerslev J, Sorensen B. Fibrinogen estimates are influenced by methods of measurement and hemodilution with colloid plasma expanders. Transfusion. 2010;50(12):2571–6.
9. Chang R, Holcomb JB. Optimal fluid therapy for traumatic hemorrhagic shock. Crit Care Clin. 2017;33(1):15–36.
10. Mavrides EAS, Chandraharan E, Collins P, Green L, Hunt BJ, Riris S, Thomson AJ, On behalf of the Royal College of Obstetricians and Gynaecologists. Prevention and Management of Postpartum Haemorrhage: green-top guideline no. 52. BJOG. 2017;124(5):e106–49.
11. Gillissen A, Henriquez D, van den Akker T, Caram-Deelder C, Wind M, Zwart JJ, van Roosmalen J, Eikenboom J, Bloemenkamp KWM, van der Bom JG. The effect of tranexamic acid on blood loss and maternal outcome in the treatment of persistent postpartum hemorrhage: a nationwide retrospective cohort study. PLoS One. 2017;12(11):e0187555.

12. Darlington DN, Delgado AV, Kheirabadi BS, Fedyk CG, Scherer MR, Pusateri AE, Wade CE, Cap AP, Holcomb JB, Dubick MA. Effect of hemodilution on coagulation and recombinant factor VIIa efficacy in human blood in vitro. J Trauma. 2011;71(5):1152–63.

13. Weiss G, Lison S, Spannagl M, Heindl B. Expressiveness of global coagulation parameters in dilutional coagulopathy. Br J Anaesth. 2010;105(4):429–36.

14. Bickell WH, Wall MJ Jr, Pepe PE, Martin RR, Ginger VF, Allen MK, Mattox KL. Immediate versus delayed fluid resuscitation for hypotensive patients with penetrating torso injuries. N Engl J Med. 1994;331(17):1105–9.

15

The effect of Ramadan fasting during pregnancy on perinatal outcomes: a systematic review and meta-analysis

Jocelyn D. Glazier[1], Dexter J. L. Hayes[1], Sabiha Hussain[1], Stephen W. D'Souza[1], Joanne Whitcombe[2], Alexander E. P. Heazell[1] and Nick Ashton[3]* (iD)

Abstract

Background: Although exempt, many pregnant Muslim women partake in the daily fast during daylight hours during the month of Ramadan. In other contexts an impoverished diet during pregnancy impacts on birth weight. The aim of this systematic review was to determine whether Ramadan fasting by pregnant women affects perinatal outcomes. Primary outcomes investigated were perinatal mortality, preterm birth and small for gestational age (SGA) infants. Secondary outcomes investigated were stillbirth, neonatal death, maternal death, hypertensive disorders of pregnancy, gestational diabetes, congenital abnormalities, serious neonatal morbidity, birth weight, preterm birth and placental weight.

Methods: Systematic review and meta-analysis of observational studies and randomised controlled trials was conducted in EMBASE, MEDLINE, CINAHL, Web of Science, Google Scholar, the Health Management Information Consortium and Applied Social Sciences Index and Abstracts. Studies from any year were eligible. Studies reporting predefined perinatal outcomes in pregnancies exposed to Ramadan fasting were included. Cohort studies with no comparator group or that considered fasting outside pregnancy were excluded, as were studies assuming fasting practice based solely upon family name. Quality of included studies was assessed using the ROBINS-I tool for assessing risk of bias in non-randomised studies. Analyses were performed in STATA.

Results: From 375 records, 22 studies of 31,374 pregnancies were included, of which 18,920 pregnancies were exposed to Ramadan fasting. Birth weight was reported in 21 studies and was not affected by maternal fasting (standardised mean difference [SMD] 0.03, 95% CI 0.00 to 0.05). Placental weight was significantly lower in fasting mothers (SMD -0.94, 95% CI -0.97 to -0.90), although this observation was dominated by a single large study. No data were presented for perinatal mortality. Ramadan fasting had no effect on preterm delivery (odds ratio 0.99, 95% CI 0.72 to 1.37) based on 5600 pregnancies (1193 exposed to Ramadan fasting).

Conclusions: Ramadan fasting does not adversely affect birth weight although there is insufficient evidence regarding potential effects on other perinatal outcomes. Further studies are needed to accurately determine whether Ramadan fasting is associated with adverse maternal or neonatal outcome.

Keywords: Birth weight, Fasting, Placenta, Pregnancy, Ramadan

* Correspondence: nick.ashton@manchester.ac.uk
[3]Division of Cardiovascular Sciences, Faculty of Biology, Medicine and Health, University of Manchester, 3rd Floor Core Technology Facility, 46 Grafton Street, Manchester M13 9NT, UK
Full list of author information is available at the end of the article

Background

During the month of Ramadan, healthy adult Muslims abstain from eating and drinking from sunrise until sunset. This represents a form of intermittent fasting where both the quantity and quality of food eaten are altered [1]. Although pregnant Muslim women are exempt from fasting, evidence suggests that up to 90% partake in Ramadan fasting for at least part of the month [2, 3], being keen to share the cultural experience with their families. The estimate of 230 million Muslim women of childbearing age worldwide [4], with a fertility rate averaging 3.1 children per woman [4], leads to the potential for up to 535 million babies in each generation to be exposed *in utero* over Ramadan to a repeated cyclical pattern of maternal intermittent fasting.

Exposure to a restricted or sub-optimal diet during pregnancy affects fetal development and has life-long health impacts on the offspring [5]. Low birth weight and altered neonatal growth trajectories are associated with an increased risk of cardiovascular disease, diabetes [5], obesity [6] and impaired cognitive function [7]. Preterm delivery and reduced birth weight are more prevalent in women who eat less frequently while pregnant [8], suggesting that pregnant women who fast during Ramadan may be more likely to give birth to premature or underweight babies.

Although the impact of Ramadan fasting during pregnancy on the health of the child has been investigated [9–13], individual studies show conflicting results and sample sizes are often too small to allow evaluation of serious, but infrequent, outcomes. Furthermore, the timing of exposure to maternal fasting during Ramadan may affect the outcome [14], yet the trimester of fetal exposure to fasting is generally poorly defined in studies. Although fasting could arise at any pregnancy stage, occurrence early in the first trimester seems most likely as the mother may be unaware that she is already pregnant. Fasting during the first trimester has been reported to be associated with reduced birth weight [15], whereas placental weight, another predictor of health outcomes in offspring [16], is reportedly lower if the mother fasted during the second or third trimester [17].

Muslim women may seek advice from health practitioners regarding the safety of Ramadan fasting; however the current information available to pregnant women is contradictory [18] and clear guidance is lacking. Therefore, available evidence regarding associations between Ramadan fasting and pregnancy outcomes needs to be evaluated.

The aim of this systematic review and meta-analysis was to determine the effects of maternal intermittent fasting during Ramadan on a range of pregnancy outcomes.

Methods

The systematic review and meta-analysis is reported in accordance with PRISMA guidelines [19]; the review protocol was registered with the International Prospective Register of Systematic Reviews (PROSPERO) on 8 July 2016 (CRD42016041949).

Eligibility criteria, information sources, search strategy

Searches were carried out in EMBASE, MEDLINE, CINAHL, Web of Science, Google Scholar, the Health Management Information Consortium (HMIC) and Applied Social Sciences Index and Abstracts. In order to reduce publication bias, searches were also carried out in the Centre for Reviews and Dissemination databases, ProQuest and EThOS to uncover any relevant unpublished studies and grey literature. Reference lists of eligible studies were checked for other potentially eligible studies for inclusion. The search was not limited by dates but was limited to English-only publications. All searches were updated on 11 April 2018. See Additional file 1 for the EMBASE search strategy. Searches were performed by JW, SH and DH.

We included observational studies which reported either primary or secondary outcomes in pregnancies that were exposed to intermittent fasting during Ramadan compared to unexposed pregnancies. Randomised controlled trials or cluster randomised controlled trials were also eligible. Cohort studies with no comparator group (which only reported an outcome of interest in women who fasted during pregnancy) were excluded. If studies assumed fasting practice based solely upon ethnic group or family name then they were excluded as this was deemed to be unreliable. Studies were not excluded based on their geographical location or the timing of fasting with regard to trimester of pregnancy.

Studies were included if they reported a relevant pregnancy outcome in women who intermittently fasted during their pregnancy. The exposure of interest was intermittent fasting during the month of Ramadan during any stage of pregnancy. Studies looking at fasting during any other time period (prior to conception, postnatal period) were excluded.

Primary outcomes for this study were: perinatal mortality (the death of a baby before birth or during the first week of life), preterm birth (before 37 weeks of pregnancy) and small for gestational age (SGA) infants (as defined by each study or below the tenth centile for gestational age). Secondary outcomes were: stillbirth (the death of a baby before birth after 20 weeks' gestation), neonatal death (the death of a baby during the first 28 days of life), maternal death (the death of the mother during pregnancy or the first 6 weeks postnatally), hypertensive disorders of pregnancy, gestational diabetes, congenital abnormalities (structural abnormalities of the fetus), serious neonatal morbidity, birth weight (continuous variable), low birth weight (< 2500 g), very low birth weight (< 1500 g), extremely preterm birth (< 28 weeks gestation) and placental weight (continuous variable).

Data extraction

After removal of duplicates, all citations were screened for relevance using the full citation, abstract and indexing terms. Relevant studies were assessed for eligibility by two out of four reviewers (SH, DH, JG and SDS) according to the pre-specified inclusion and exclusion criteria, and where possible full manuscripts were obtained. Final decisions were made by two reviewers independently and a third (AH or NA) consulted to resolve any issues where necessary. Where data were missing or incomplete, attempts were made to contact the authors for clarification.

Assessment of risk of bias

Included studies were assessed using the Risk Of Bias In Non-randomised Studies – of Interventions (ROBINS-I) tool [20], which categorises risk of bias as low, moderate, serious, critical and unclear, and the risk of bias category for each study was reported; if a study's risk of bias was categorised as serious, critical or unclear, the effect of removing this study was tested and the relevant outcome(s) reported.

Data synthesis

Meta-analysis was performed in STATA (Version 14) [21] using the *metan* [22] and *metabias* [23] commands. Random effects meta-analysis was used in anticipation of heterogeneity due to differences in study design.

For continuous variables (birth weight and placental weight), standardised mean differences (SMD) (Hedges' g) with 95% confidence intervals were calculated. For binary variables (low birth weight and preterm delivery), odds ratios and 95% confidence intervals were calculated. The I^2 statistic was calculated; this is derived from Cochran's chi-squared statistic Q and is used to describe the percentage of between-study variation that is attributable to variability in the true exposure effect [24]. An I^2 value of 0–30% was classified as low, 31–60% as moderate, 61–90% substantial and 91–100% considerable [25]. Funnel plots were created to test for small-study effects.

Where studies presented continuous data grouped by trimester in which fasting took place, length of fasting or stratified by other measures (e.g. fetal sex), then averages were taken to obtain overall means and standard deviations. Where outcome data were available by fasting trimester then data were stratified by trimester and the effect of this was investigated.

Results

Study selection

The search strategy identified 375 records (Fig. 1). After duplicates were removed 118 papers were screened on the basis of their titles and abstracts. Forty papers were

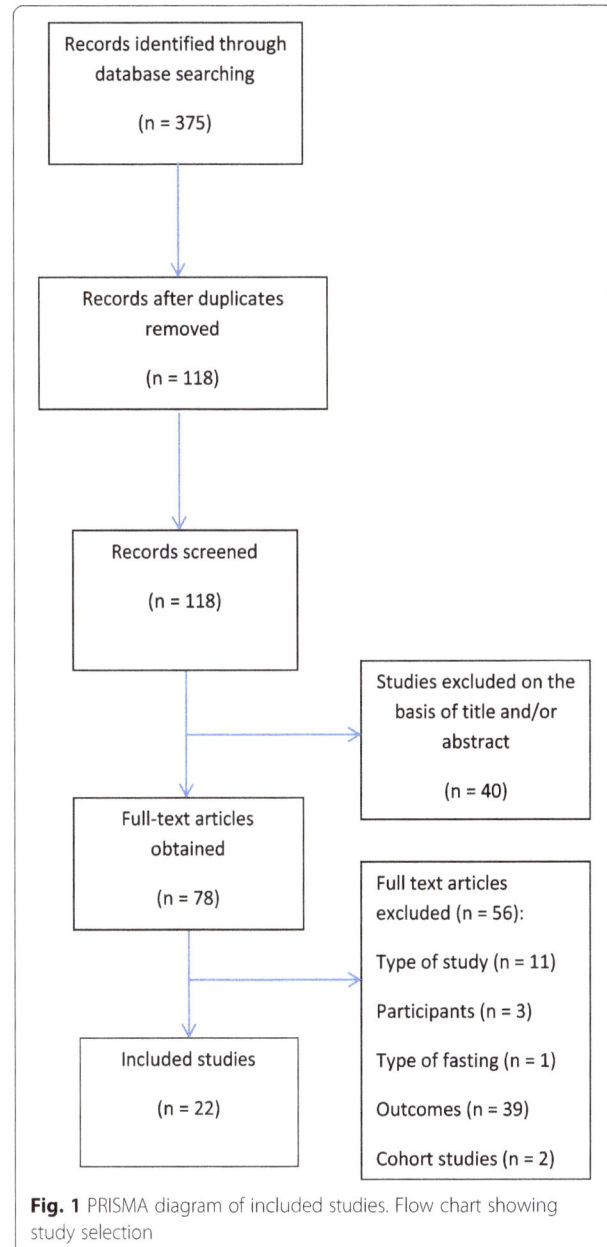

Fig. 1 PRISMA diagram of included studies. Flow chart showing study selection

excluded on this basis, resulting in 78 papers to be evaluated using their full text. After exclusions, 22 studies of 31,374 pregnancies were included in the final analysis.

Study characteristics

Seven studies reported data for at least one of the co-primary outcomes (perinatal mortality, SGA infants and preterm birth) and all but one study [9] reported data on at least one secondary outcome (Table 1). Six studies were judged to be at moderate risk of bias; the other 16 were determined to be at low risk (Table 2). Heterogeneity for outcomes ranged from 0 to 98.5%.

Table 1 Characteristics of included studies

Authors	Year	Location and study period	Total pregnancies	Cases	Controls	Primary outcomes	Secondary outcomes	Trimester of fasting	Length and duration of fasting (days and average hours/day)	Risk of bias (ROBINS-I)
Alwasel	2011	Saudi Arabia, August 2000–April 2009	17,626	13,220	4406	–	BW, PW	1st, 2nd, 3rd	n/a	Moderate
Arab	2001	Iran, 1999	4343	3086	1257	SGA	BW, LBW	n/a	1 to 20+ days n/a	Moderate
Awwad	2012	Lebanon, September 2008	402	201	201	PTB	BW, LBW	1st, 2nd, 3rd	22 +/– 9 days n/a	Low
Azizi	2004	Iran, April–September 2001	191	98	93	–	BW	3rd	28 +/– 2 days 13 h20 min	Low
Bayoglu Tekin	2016	Turkey, June–July 2014	48	23	25	–	BW	3rd	18.2 +/– 2 days 17.24 h	Low
Daley	2017	United Kingdom, March 2007 – December 2010	5156	479	4677	PTB	BW, LBW	1st	n/a	Moderate
Hefni	1993	Egypt, 1991	322	167	155	–	BW, SB	3rd	n/a >10 h	Low
Hizli	2012	Turkey, August–September 2010	110	56	54	–	BW	3rd	12.9 +/– 2.5 days 15.3 h (12–19)	Low
Karateke	2016	Turkey, June–July 2014	240	120	120	–	BW, LBW	1st, 2nd, 3rd	n/a n/a	Low
Kavehmanesh	2004	Iran, January–September 2000	539	284	255	PTB	BW	n/a	24 +/– 9 days 13 h	Low
Makvandi	2013	Iran, 2013	300	150	150	–	BW, LBW	3rd	16.6+/–13.2 days n/a	Low
Malhotra	1989	United Kingdom, April–May 1987	22	11	11	SGA	BW, CA, NND, PW	3rd	n/a 7 h	Moderate
Naderi	2004	Iran, November 2001	101	51	50	–	BW	n/a	20+ days n/a	Low
Ozturk	2011	Turkey, September 2008	72	42	30	PTB	–	2nd	10+ days Approximately 12 h	Low
Petherick	2014	United Kingdom, October–December 2010	300	128	172	PTB	BW, GD, Hyp, LBW	1st, 2nd, 3rd	1–29 days Up to 18 h	Moderate
Rezk	2016	Egypt, June–July 2015	450	210	240	–	BW	3rd	30 days 12-16 h	Low
Sakar	2016	Turkey, August–October 2013	338	168	170	–	BW, PW	3rd	25.17 +/– 5.44 days n/a	Low
Sarafraz	2014	Iran, 2008	293	200	93	–	BW	1st, 2nd, 3rd	1 to 20+ days n/a	Low
Savitri	2018	Indonesia, July 2012 – July 2014	139	110	29	–	BW	1st, 2nd, 3rd	1–30 days n/a	Moderate
Seckin	2014	Turkey, July–August 2013	169	82	87	–	BW	3rd	23 +/– 3.6 days 18.7 h (17–20)	Low
Shahgheibi	2005	Iran, (dates unknown)	163	63	100	–	BW, LBW	3rd	10 to 20+ days n/a	Low
Ziaee	2010	Iran, October 2004	189	123	66	–	BW, LBW	1st, 2nd, 3rd	1 to 20+ days 13 h	Low

Primary outcomes: *SGA* small for gestational age, *PTB* preterm birth. Secondary outcomes; *BW* birth weight, *CA* congenital abnormalities, *GD* gestational diabetes, *Hyp* hypertension, *LBW* low birth weight, *NND* neonatal death, *PW* placental weight, *SB* stillbirth

Table 2 Risk of bias of included studies

Author	Year	Bias domain						
		Bias due to confounding	Bias in selection of participants into the study	Bias in classification of exposure	Bias due to missing data	Bias in measurement of outcomes	Bias in selection of the reported result	Overall
Alwasel	2011	**Low/Moderate**	Low	**Serious**	Low	Low	Low	**Moderate**
Arab	2001	Low	Low	Low	**Serious**	Low	Low	**Moderate**
Awwad	2012	**Moderate**	Low	Low	Low	Low	Low	**Low**
Azizi	2014	Low	Low	Low	**Moderate**	Low	Low	**Low**
Bayoglu Tekin	2016	Low	Low	Low	Low	Low	Low	**Low**
Daley	2018	**Moderate**	Low	**Moderate**	**Moderate**	Low	Low	**Moderate**
Hefni	1993	**Low/Moderate**	Low	Low	Low	Low	**Low/Moderate**	**Low**
Hizli	2012	Low	Low	Low	Low	Low	Low	**Low**
Karateke	2016	**Moderate**	Low	Low	Low	Low	Low	**Low**
Kavehmanesh	2004	**Low/Moderate**	Low	Low	Low	**Low/Moderate**	Low	**Low**
Malhotra	1989	**Moderate**	Low	Low	**Low/Moderate**	Low	Low	**Moderate**
Makvandi	2013	**Moderate**	Low	Low	Low	Low	Low	**Low**
Naderi	2004	**Moderate**	Low	Low	Low	Low	Low	**Low**
Ozturk	2011	**Moderate**	Low	Low	Low	**Low/Moderate**	Low	**Low**
Petherick	2014	**Moderate/Serious**	Low	**Moderate**	Low	Low	Low	**Moderate**
Rezk	2016	Low	Low	Low	Low	Low	Low	**Low**
Sakar	2016	Low	Low	Low	Low	Low	Low	**Low**
Sarafraz	2013	Low	Low	Low	Low	Low	Low	**Low**
Savitri	2018	Low	**Serious**	Low	Low	Low	Low	**Moderate**
Seckin	2014	Low	Low	Low	Low	Low	Low	**Low**
Shahgheibi	2005	**Low/Moderate**	Low	Low	Low	Low	Low	**Low**
Ziaee	2010	Low	Low	Low	Low	Low	Low	**Low**

Studies found to have a moderate or greater risk of bias in one or more domains are highlighted in bold

Synthesis of results

No studies presented data regarding perinatal mortality, and only two [10, 11] had data for SGA infants so meta-analysis was not performed. There was no significant effect of Ramadan fasting on the frequency of preterm delivery (OR 0.99, 95% CI 0.72 to 1.37) (Fig. 2); data were available on 5600 pregnancies from five studies [9, 10, 12, 13, 26] of which 1193 were exposed to Ramadan fasting. One study defined preterm delivery as < 38 weeks gestation so these data were not included [27]. Another study excluded preterm deliveries from the cohort [28].

All but one study [9] examined birth weight as a continuous variable; data were available on 31,441 pregnancies, of which 19,030 were exposed to fasting. There was no significant effect of maternal Ramadan fasting on birth weight (SMD 0.03, 95% CI 0.00 to 0.05) (Fig. 3). Three studies [29–31] presented mean results stratified by trimester in which fasting occurred, and an additional ten studies [11, 27, 32–39] were of third trimester exposure allowing a comparison to be performed; however no individual trimester showed a significant effect of fasting on birth weight and there was no difference between trimester groups ($p = 0.99$).

Eight studies [10, 13, 26, 30, 31, 35, 39, 40] investigated the effects of maternal fasting on low birth weight (LBW); there were 11,080 births from these studies, of which 4344 were from mothers who fasted. Fasting did not significantly affect the proportion of LBW babies (OR 1.05, 95% CI 0.87 to 1.26) (Fig. 4). Three of these studies [30, 31, 40] stratified their data by trimester ($n = 2411$ first trimester fasting, $n = 2571$ second trimester, $n = 2356$ third trimester); there was no significant difference in the effect (I^2 0.0% $p = 0.57$).

Three studies comprising 17,986 pregnancies measured placental weight as an outcome [11, 29, 37]. Placental weight was significantly lower in fasting mothers (SMD -0.94, 95% CI -0.97 to – 0.90) (Fig. 5).

Two authors were contacted for information. One responded [33], providing clarification on study outcomes. No information was provided regarding discrepancies between numbers in tables and text in another paper [40]; data from the text were used as these were consistent with data reported in the abstract.

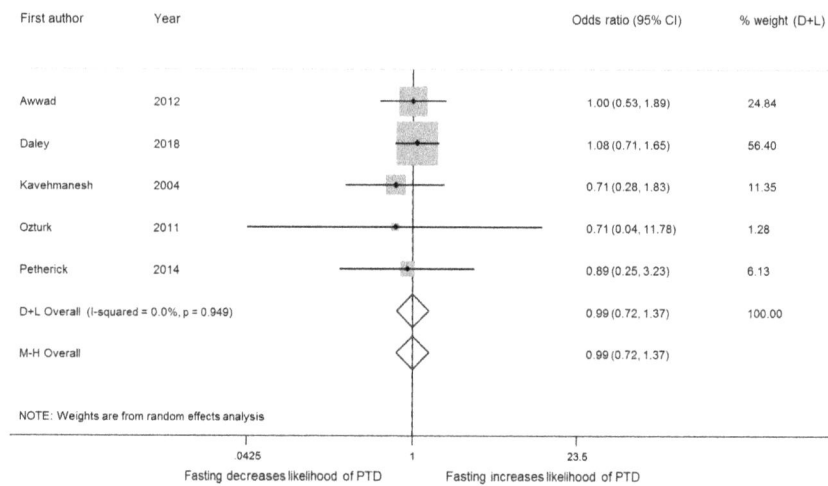

Fig. 2 Effect of fasting on the likelihood of preterm delivery. Forest plot showing the effect of maternal fasting on preterm delivery

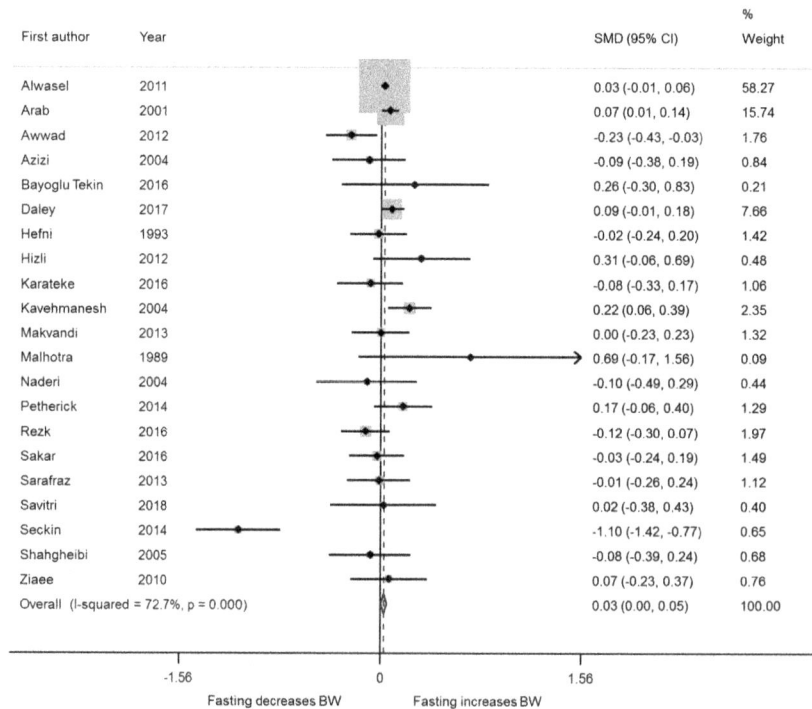

Fig. 3 Effect of fasting on birth weight. Forest plot showing the effect of maternal fasting on birth weight as a continuous variable

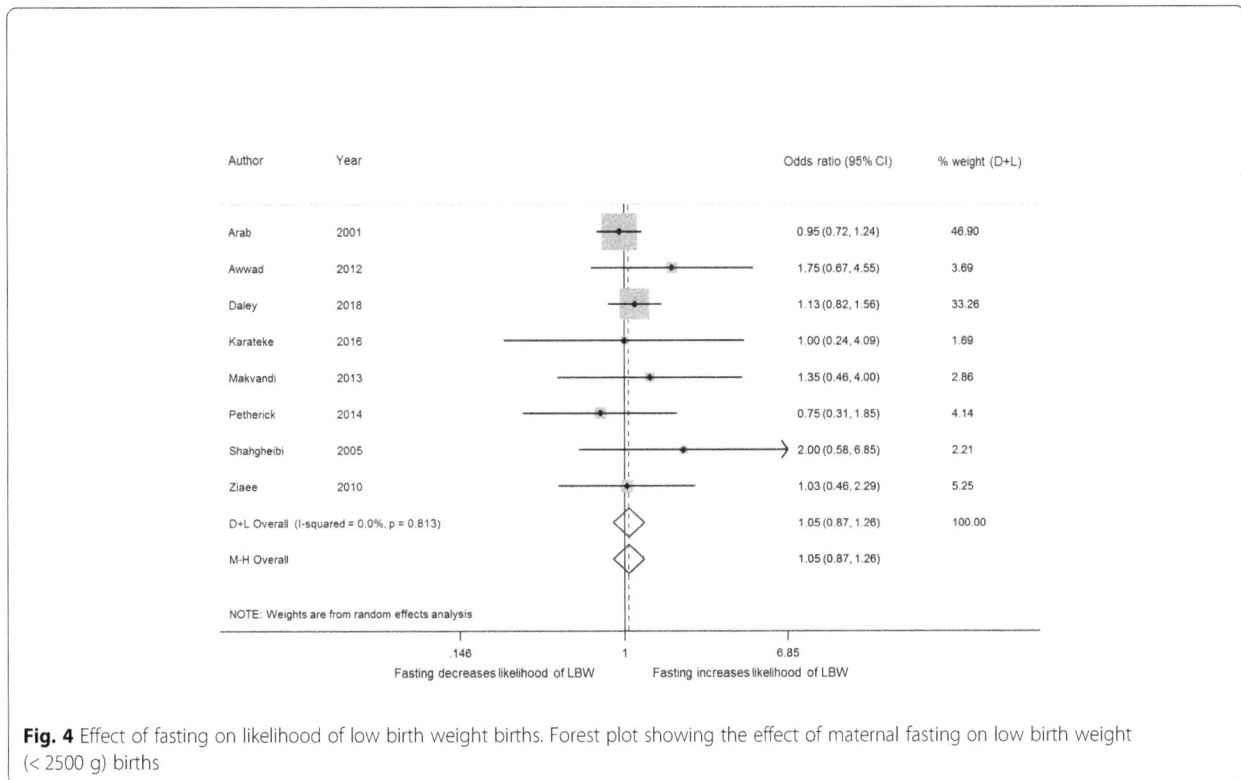

Fig. 4 Effect of fasting on likelihood of low birth weight births. Forest plot showing the effect of maternal fasting on low birth weight (< 2500 g) births

Risk of bias of included studies

Egger's test gave a value of $p = 0.082$ indicating that there was no significant influence of small study effects on our results (Fig. 6). No studies were assessed as having a high risk of bias so the analyses presented include all results. However, of the 31,441 pregnancies where birth weight was measured as an outcome, 17,626 were from one study [29]. A sensitivity analysis was performed to determine how much of an effect this study had on the overall result; without this study a SMD of 0.03 (95% CI -0.01 to 0.07) was obtained, still demonstrating no significant effect of fasting on birth weight.

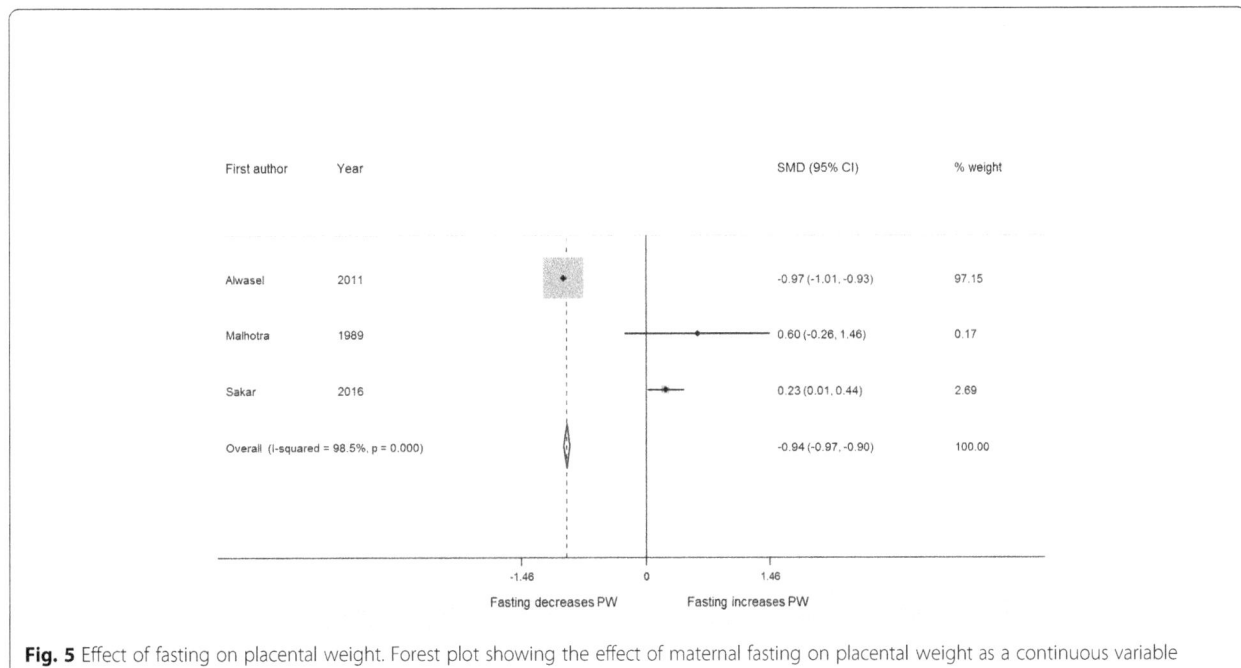

Fig. 5 Effect of fasting on placental weight. Forest plot showing the effect of maternal fasting on placental weight as a continuous variable

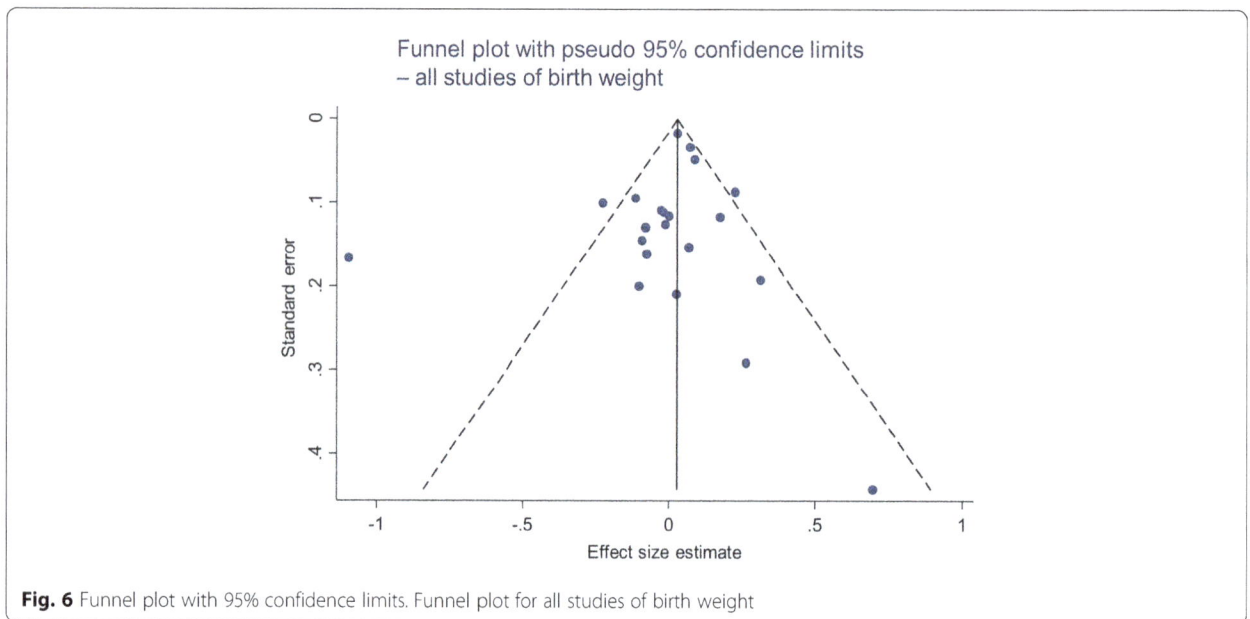

Fig. 6 Funnel plot with 95% confidence limits. Funnel plot for all studies of birth weight

Discussion

Of our co-primary outcomes, only preterm birth had sufficient studies for meta-analysis which found no significant effect of Ramadan fasting. Data were available for some secondary outcomes: birth weight, placental weight and low birth weight; only placental weight was reduced by Ramadan fasting. However, this result was dominated by one study [29], which comprised 17,626 of 17,986 births for this outcome; one of the other two studies found a significant increase in placental weight [37]. There were insufficient data to perform meta-analysis for other outcomes, including: congenital abnormalities, gestational diabetes, hypertension, stillbirth and neonatal death. Stillbirth and neonatal death are arguably the most serious of these outcomes, yet due to the relatively small number of studies and their comparatively low incidences this study was underpowered to detect a difference. The paucity of data indicates a need for further large scale studies which report data on these rare but serious outcomes.

Strengths and limitations

This study was strengthened in that it was carried out in accordance with a prospective protocol with pre-specified eligibility criteria and primary outcomes. This is the first meta-analysis to examine the effects of Ramadan fasting and provides a dataset that can be updated as the number of studies grows. It has also highlighted the current lack of data and identified research gaps to be addressed. This study was limited by the fact that due to resources only English language papers were included. Furthermore, other potential effects of Ramadan fasting may not have been included in our outcome measures. Other studies have shown effects of Ramadan fasting on fetal movement

[41], maternal glucose levels [42] and various fetal growth indices [43]. Furthermore, our review did not examine whether fasting in the periconceptional period was associated with pregnancy outcome. As enduring effects of fasting and maternal undernutrition in this period have been shown in animal models [44, 45], this hypothesis merits further exploration.

The studies reviewed suggest that pregnant women who are well nourished may have nutritional reserves to support fetal adaptations during Ramadan fasting. However, longitudinal information on fetal growth was not available; the only feasible measure recorded was birth weight. Therefore, it remains to be established whether Ramadan fasting alters fetal growth patterns. Furthermore, there is little known about postnatal growth or growth and development in infancy and childhood.

Our literature search also identified papers that reported data on co-primary or secondary outcomes but presented the data in ways that could not be incorporated; Salleh [46] used linear regression to examine the effects of Ramadan fasting on birth weight and Boskabadi et al. [47] also looked at birth weight but presented data as medians and interquartile ranges; there was no control group in the study. One of our included studies [9] contained usable data for preterm delivery; however birth weight data were presented as medians and IQRs. Neither of these studies found differences between the control and fasting groups. Other studies were excluded because study groups were not sufficiently clear: Almond and Mazumder [48] acknowledged that not all women in their 'fasting' group fasted and that a large number of non-Muslims may also have been included. Cross et al. [49] defined maternal Muslim status (and assumed fasting status) based on the first three letters of maternal surnames.

Data showed significant heterogeneity for some outcomes. This variation may not relate to trimester of fasting, as when data were stratified by trimester there were no significant differences in the observed effect, although this may also represent a type 2 error as this meta-analysis may not have sufficient statistical power to detect such a difference. Only three studies presented usable data stratified by trimester of fasting for birth weight [29–31], of which one [31] found an association between trimester and mean neonatal weight. Alwasel et al. [29] showed significant associations in the second and third trimesters but not the first. Savitri et al. [28] performed regression analysis to investigate the effect of fasting trimester and found no significance, although they state that there was a trend towards lower birth weight with fasting, particularly in the second and third trimester. It may be that fasting later in pregnancy, when fetal growth is exponential, would be more likely to impact birth weight; further human studies are needed.

We were not able to investigate potential effects of Ramadan fasting length (in days) and duration (hours/day) due to limitations in available data. Duration of fasting was not documented by all studies and data were recorded in different ways; some studies stated the average number of fasting hours per day [9, 12, 32–34, 36] while others gave the upper [13] or lower [27] limits. In total, 16 included studies recorded the average number of fasting days (Table 1), but few papers stratified by number of days fasting so meta-regression could not be performed. However, only one paper that divided data by number of fasting days [40] found a significant difference in outcome: that birth weight following more than 20 days of fasting was significantly greater than that after fasting for 1–9 days. Makki [50] found no relationship between the number of fasting days and incidence of low birth weight. However, this paper could not be included in our analysis as there was no comparator group.

Another potential source of heterogeneity was geographical location of study. The majority of studies were from Asia and the Middle East (8 from Iran [12, 31, 32, 35, 39, 40, 51, 52], 6 from Turkey [9, 30, 33, 34, 37, 38], 2 from Egypt [27, 36], 1 from Indonesia [28], 1 from Saudi Arabia [29] and 1 from Lebanon [10]). Three included studies [11, 13, 26] were from the UK. Geographical location may alter the number of hours of fasting, and thus the physiological challenge on the developing fetus, as the timing of the daily fast is determined by sunrise and sunset.

Risk of bias is unlikely to account for the observed heterogeneity as overall risk of bias of the included studies was low, with only six studies [11, 13, 26, 28, 29, 40] judged to be at moderate risk of bias. The majority of bias was due to uncertainty of the trimester affected by fasting. Three studies were judged to be at serious risk of bias for individual domains: one paper was due to missing data [40], another for selection of participants [28], and the other due to classification of exposure [29]. Therefore, subgroup analysis for risk of bias was not conducted.

Conclusions

This meta-analysis did not find any significant associations between Ramadan fasting and pregnancy outcome. Although studies were drawn from a large literature base, only a relatively small number met the inclusion criteria for analysis, limiting the breadth of robust conclusions. Until more definitive data are available, clinicians and other pregnancy healthcare providers cannot make firm recommendations that Ramadan fasting has no adverse consequences for mother or infant. Further observational studies of the effects of Ramadan fasting are required. Even if individual studies are not sufficiently large to determine differences in rare outcomes such as stillbirth or neonatal death, these should still be reported to facilitate subsequent meta-analysis. Additional studies are also needed to explore the origin of the considerable heterogeneity in observations; these should determine the effects of fasting in the periconceptional period, in different trimesters of pregnancy and whether geographical location, time of year and consequent duration of fasting alters the effect. Thus, well-designed studies investigating Ramadan fasting during pregnancy are needed to investigate the full impacts on maternal and fetal health, as well as to give potential fasting mothers an informed choice whilst addressing an issue that could have enduring public health consequences [53].

Abbreviations
CI: Confidence interval; CINAHL: Cumulative Index of Nursing and Allied Health Literature; EMBASE: Excerpta Medica database; ETHOS: E thesis online service; HMIC: Healthcare Management Information Consortium; LBW: Low birth weight; MEDLINE: National Library of Medicine journal citation database; OR: Odds ratio; PROSPERO: International prospective register of systematic reviews; ROBINS-I: Risk of bias in non-randomised studies - of interventions; SGA: Small for gestational age; SMD: Standardised mean difference

Authors' contributions
JDG, SH, SDS, DJLH, AEPH and NA contributed to the study concept and design. AEPH and DJLH wrote the protocol. SH and JW developed the search strategy. SH, SDS, DJLH and NA acquired the data for the study. DJLH and AEPH analysed and interpreted the data. JDG, NA, DJLH and AEPH developed the first draft of the manuscript and JDG, SH, SDS, DJLH, AEPH and NA revised all drafts and approved the final version. All authors read and approved the final manuscript.

Competing interests

The authors declare that they have no competing interests

Author details

[1]Maternal and Fetal Health Research Centre, Division of Developmental Biology and Medicine, Faculty of Biology, Medicine and Health, University of Manchester, 5th Floor (Research), St Mary's Hospital, Oxford Road, Manchester M13 9WL, UK. [2]Trust Library, Central Manchester University Hospitals NHS Foundation Trust, Education South, Oxford Road, Manchester M13 9WL, UK. [3]Division of Cardiovascular Sciences, Faculty of Biology, Medicine and Health, University of Manchester, 3rd Floor Core Technology Facility, 46 Grafton Street, Manchester M13 9NT, UK.

References

1. Arab M. Ketonuria and serum glucose of fasting pregnant women at the end of a day in Ramadan. Acta Med Iran. 2004;42:209–12.
2. Baynouna Al Ketbi LM, Niglekerke NJ, Zein Al Deen SM, Mirghani H. Diet restriction in Ramadan and the effect of fasting on glucose levels in pregnancy. BMC Res Notes. 2014;7:392.
3. Prentice AM, Prentice A, Lamb WH, Lunn PG, Austin S. Metabolic consequences of fasting during Ramadan in pregnant and lactating women. Hum Nutr Clin Nutr. 1983;37:283–94.
4. Pew Research Center. Religion & Public Life Project: Muslim population by country. 2011. http://www.pewforum.org/2011/01/27/table-muslim-population-by-country/. Accessed 19 Dec 2014.
5. Barker DJ, Thornburg KL. The obstetric origins of health for a lifetime. Clin Obstet Gynecol. 2013;56:511–9.
6. Martin CL, Siega-Riz AM, Sotres-Alvarez D, Robinson WR, Daniels JL, Perrin EM, et al. Maternal dietary patterns during pregnancy are associated with child growth in the first 3 years of life. J Nutr. 2016;146:2281–8.
7. Sorensen HT, Sabroe S, Olsen J, Rothman KJ, Gillman MW, Fischer P. Birth weight and cognitive function in young adult life: historical cohort study. BMJ. 1997;315:401–3.
8. Siega-Riz AM, Herrmann TS, Savitz DA, Thorp JM. Frequency of eating during pregnancy and its effect on preterm delivery. Am J Epidemiol. 2001; 153:647–52.
9. Ozturk E, Balat O, Ugur MG, Yazicioglu C, Pence S, Erel O, et al. Effect of Ramadan fasting on maternal oxidative stress during the second trimester: a preliminary study. J Obstet Gynaecol Res. 2011;37:729–33.
10. Awwad J, Usta IM, Succar J, Musallam KM, Ghazeeri G, Nassar AH. The effect of maternal fasting during Ramadan on preterm delivery: a prospective cohort study. BJOG. 2012;119:1379–86.
11. Malhotra A, Scott PH, Scott J, Gee H, Wharton BA. Metabolic changes in Asian Muslim pregnant mothers observing the Ramadan fast in Britain. Br J Nutr. 1989;61:663–72.
12. Kavehmanesh Z, Abolghasemi H. Maternal Ramadan fasting and neonatal health. J Perinatol. 2004;24:748–50.
13. Petherick ES, Tuffnell D, Wright J. Experiences and outcomes of maternal Ramadan fasting during pregnancy: results from a sub-cohort of the born in Bradford birth cohort study. BMC Pregnancy Childbirth. 2014;14:335.
14. Roseboom TJ, van der Meulen JH, Ravelli AC, Osmond C, Barker DJ, Bleker OP. Effects of prenatal exposure to the Dutch famine on adult disease in later life: an overview. Mol Cell Endocrinol. 2001;185:93–8.
15. Savitri AI, Yadegari N, Bakker J, van Ewijk RJ, Grobbee DE, Painter RC, et al. Ramadan fasting and newborn's birth weight in pregnant Muslim women in the Netherlands. Br J Nutr. 2014;112:1503–9.
16. Thornburg KL, O'Tierney PF, Louey S. Review: the placenta is a programming agent for cardiovascular disease. Placenta. 2010;31:S54–9.
17. Alwasel SH, Abotalib Z, Aljarallah JS, Osmond C, Alkharaz SM, Alhazza IM, et al. Changes in placental size during Ramadan. Placenta. 2010;31:607–10.
18. British Nutrition Foundation. Ramadan and Pregnanacy. April 2015. https://www.nutrition.org.uk/healthyliving/nutritionforpregnancy/ramadanpregnancy.html. Accessed 17 Oct 2018.
19. Moher D, Liberati A, Tetzlaff J, Altman DG, Group P. Preferred reporting items for systematic reviews and meta-analyses: the PRISMA statement. PLoS Med. 2009;6:e1000097.
20. Sterne JA, Hernán MA, Reeves BC, Savović J, Berkman ND, Viswanathan M, et al. ROBINS-I: a tool for assessing risk of bias in non-randomised studies of interventions. BMJ. 2016;355:i4919.
21. StataCorp. STATA Statistical Software, release 14. College Station: StataCorp LP; 2015.
22. Harris R, Bradburn M, Deeks J, Harbord R, Altman D, Sterne J. Metan: fixed- and random-effects meta-analysis. Stata J. 2008;8:3.
23. Sterne JA, Harbord RM. Funnel plots in meta-analysis. Stata J. 2004;4:127–41.
24. Higgins J, Thompson SG, Deeks JJ, Altman DG. Measuring inconsistency in meta-analyses. BMJ. 2003;327:557–60.
25. Deeks JJ, Higgins J, Altman DG. Analysing data and undertaking meta-analyses. Cochrane Handb Syst Rev Interv. 2008:243–96.
26. Daley A, Pallan M, Clifford S, Jolly K, Bryant M, Adab P, et al. Are babies conceived during Ramadan born smaller and sooner than babies conceived at other times of the year? A born in Bradford cohort study. J Epidemiol Community Health. 2017;71:722–8.
27. Hefni M, Fikry S, Abdelkhalik M. Fasting in Ramadan and preterm labour. Saudi Med J. 1993;14:130–2.
28. Savitri AI, Amelia D, Painter RC, Baharuddin M, Roseboom TJ, Grobbee DE, et al. Ramadan during pregnancy and birth weight of newborns. J Nutr Sci. 2018;7:1–9.
29. Alwasel S, Abotalib Z, Aljarallah J, Osmond C, Alkharaz S, Alhazza I, et al. Secular increase in placental weight in Saudi Arabia. Placenta. 2011;32:391–4.
30. Karateke A, Kaplanoglu M, Avci F, Kurt RK, Baloglu A. The effect of Ramadan fasting on fetal development. Pak J Med Sci. 2015;31:1295–9.
31. Ziaee V, Kihanidoost Z, Younesian M, Akhavirad M-B, Bateni F, Kazemianfar Z, et al. The effect of Ramadan fasting on outcome of pregnancy. Iran J Pediatr. 2010;20:181–6.
32. Azizi F, Sadeghipour H, Siahkolah B, Rezaei-Ghaleh N. Intellectual development of children born of mothers who fasted in Ramadan during pregnancy. Int J Vit Nutr Res. 2004;74:374–80.
33. Bayoglu Tekin Y, Guvendag Guven ES, Mete Ural U, Yazici ZA, Kirbas A, Kir Sahin F. Evaluation of the effects of fasting associated dehydration on maternal NGAL levels and fetal renal artery Doppler parameters. J Matern Fetal Neonatal Med. 2016;29:629–32.
34. Hızlı D, Yılmaz SS, Onaran Y, Kafalı H, Danışman N, L M. Impact of maternal fasting during Ramadan on fetal Doppler parameters, maternal lipid levels and neonatal outcomes. J Matern Fetal Neonatal Med. 2012;25:975–7.
35. Makvandi S, Nematy M, Karimi L. Effects of Ramadan fasting on neonatal anthropometric measurements in the third trimester of pregnancy. J Fasting Health. 2013;1:53–7.
36. Rezk MA-A, Sayyed T, Abo-Elnasr M, Shawky M, Badr H. Impact of maternal fasting on fetal well-being parameters and fetal–neonatal outcome: a case–control study. J Matern Fetal Neonatal Med. 2016;29:2834–8.
37. Sakar M, Balsak D, Verit F, Zebitay A, Buyuk A, Akay E, et al. The effect of Ramadan fasting and maternal hypoalbuminaemia on neonatal anthropometric parameters and placental weight. J Obstet Gynaecol. 2016;36:483–6.
38. Seckin KD, Yeral MI, Karslı MF, Gultekin IB. Effect of maternal fasting for religious beliefs on fetal sonographic findings and neonatal outcomes. Int J Gynecol Obstet. 2014;126:123–5.
39. Shahgheibi S, Ghadery E, Pauladi A. Effects of fasting during the third trimester of pregnancy on neonatal growth indices. Ann Alquds Med. 2005;1:58–62.
40. Arab M, Nasrollahi S. Interrelation of Ramadan fasting and birth weight. Med J Islamic Academy of Sci. 2001;14:91–5.
41. Mirghani H, Weerasinghe D, Ezimokhai M, Smith J. The effect of maternal fasting on the fetal biophysical profile. Int J Gynecol Obstet. 2003;81:17–21.

The effect of Ramadan fasting during pregnancy on perinatal outcomes: a systematic review...

151

42. Mirghani HM, Salem M, Weerasinghe SD. Effect of maternal fasting on uterine arterial blood flow. J Obstet Gynaecol Res. 2007;33:151–4.

43. Sakar MN, Gultekin H, Demir B, Bakir VL, Balsak D, Vuruskan E, et al. Ramadan fasting and pregnancy: implications for fetal development in summer season. J Perinat Med. 2015;43:319–23.

44. Rumball CWH, Harding JE, Oliver MH, Bloomfield FH. Effects of twin pregnancy and periconceptional undernutrition on maternal metabolism, fetal growth and glucose–insulin axis function in ovine pregnancy. J Physiol. 2008;586:1399–411.

45. Watkins AJ, Lucas ES, Wilkins A, Cagampang FRA, Fleming TP. Maternal periconceptional and gestational low protein diet affects mouse offspring growth, cardiovascular and adipose phenotype at 1 year of age. PLoS One. 2011;6:e28745.

46. Salleh H. Ramadan fasting among pregnant women in Muar district, Malaysia and its association to health outcomes. Malays J Reprod Health. 1989;7:69–83.

47. Boskabadi H, Mehdizadeh A, Alboumiri Z. Effect of the number of Ramadan fasting days on maternal and neonatal outcomes. J Fasting Health. 2014;2: 84–9.

48. Almond D, Mazumder BA. Health capital and the prenatal environment: the effect of Ramadan observance during pregnancy. Am Econ J Appl Econ. 2011;3:56–85.

49. Cross J, Eminson J, Wharton B. Ramadan and birth weight at full term in Asian Moslem pregnant women in Birmingham. Arch Dis Child. 1990;65: 1053–6.

50. Makki AM. Impact of Ramadan fasting on birth weight in 4 hospitals in Sana'a city, Yemen. Saudi Med J. 2002;23:1419–20.

51. Naderi T, Kamyabi Z. Determination of fundal height increase in fasting and non-fasting pregnant women during Ramadan. Saudi Med J. 2004;25:809–10.

52. Sarafraz N, Kafaei Atrian M, Abbaszadeh F, Bagheri A. Effect of Ramadan fasting during pregnancy on neonatal birth weight. J Fasting Health. 2014;2: 37–40.

53. Susser E, Ananth CV. Is prenatal fasting during Ramadan related to adult health outcomes? A novel and important question for epidemiology. Am J Epidemiol. 2013;177:737–40.

16

Women's perception of support and control during childbirth in The Gambia, a quantitative study on dignified facility-based intrapartum care

Saffie Colley[1] ⓘ, Chien-Huei Kao[2*], Meeiling Gau[2] and Su-Fen Cheng[3]

Abstract

Background: In The Gambia, a woman faces 1 in 24-lifetime risk of maternal death due to pregnancy and childbirth, yet, only 57% of deliveries are conducted by skilled birth attendants. However, poor provider attitude has been identified as one of the contributing factors hampering the efforts of the government in improving access to skilled care during childbirth. This study, therefore, explored women's perception of support and control during childbirth in The Gambia.

Methods: A descriptive cross-sectional study was employed. A convenience sampling method was used to select participants in two regions in The Gambia. A sample size of 200 women who met the eligibility criteria was recruited after informed consent. The demographic-obstetric information sheet and the Support and Control in Birth scale (SCIB) were used to collect data. Data analysis was done using SPSS software version 23.0.

Results: Women's perceptions of support and control were low. External control 1.85 (SD ± 0.43) recorded the least perception compared to internal control 2.41 (SD ± 0.65) and perception of support 2.52 (SD ± 0.61). Participants reported the lowest perceptions in pain control, involvement in decision making, information sharing and the utilization of different position during birth. Women's age ($p < .001$) and mode of delivery ($p = .01$), significantly predicted women's perception of internal control. Educational status ($p = .02$), mode of delivery ($p = .04$), place of delivery ($p < .001$) and perception of support ($p < .001$) significantly predicted women's perception of external control, whilst birth plan ($p = .001$), mode of delivery ($p = .04$), and perception of external control ($p < .001$) significantly predicted women's perception of support.

Conclusion: This study concluded that an environment that promotes women feeling a sense of control and support during childbirth should be created in order to ensure a dignified intrapartum care in The Gambia. This can be achieved through effective training of skilled birth attendants on non-pharmacological pain management, effective communication with clients and promoting women's participation in decision-making regarding their care throughout the process of childbirth.

Keywords: Perception, Control, Support, Childbirth, Women

* Correspondence: chienhuei@ntunhs.edu.tw
[2]Graduate Institute of Nurse-Midwifery National Taipei University and Health Sciences, 365 Ming-Te Road, Taipei 112, Taiwan
Full list of author information is available at the end of the article

Background

In The Gambia, a woman faces 1 in 24-lifetime risk of maternal death due to pregnancy and childbirth, yet, only 57% of deliveries are conducted by skilled birth attendants [1]. Ensuring universal access to reproductive health service is the aim of all health systems in developing countries including The Gambia, in an effort to reduce maternal morbidity and mortality so as to meet the Sustainable Development Goals by 2030. One of the strategies in achieving this aim is the promotion of skilled care before, during and after childbirth [2]. However, poor provider attitude has been identified as one of the contributing factors hampering the efforts of The Gambian government in improving access to skilled birth care [3]. Addressing the key obstacles to the utilization of skilled care and creating an environment that supports women's needs during childbirth is, therefore, crucial [4].

Childbirth is a stressful experience for women worldwide, therefore, it is of paramount importance for caregivers to be supportive and create an atmosphere that allows women to gain autonomy over the process of childbirth to ensure positive dignified birth experience [2, 5]. Ensuring client satisfaction, promoting clients participation in decision making about their care, and providing a respectful and nondiscriminatory health care are among The Gambia national health policy guiding principles, to improving access to quality healthcare delivery [6]. Supportive care from providers and care that help women to obtain their level of control enhances dignity during childbirth [7], promote women's participation in decision-making regarding their care [8], reduce obstetric interventions during birth [9, 10], and promote positive decisions concerning the utilization of maternity health services in future pregnancies [11]. Women's loss of control and lack of supportive care are forms of mistreatment during childbirth and may have an effect on decisions about the utilization of intrapartum care services in the future [11].

Studies on factors influencing the utilization of maternal healthcare services in The Gambia mainly focused on economic and sociocultural factors [12, 13]. Little attention is given to understanding women's view about intrapartum care services that recognize their needs. This study, therefore, seeks to assess women's perception of support and control during childbirth in The Gambia. The findings will help midwives to have a better understanding of women's needs during intrapartum care to enhance effective dignified maternity care. The findings will also help to address the challenges faced by developing countries of moving towards dignified childbirth.

The aim of this study was to explore women's perception of support and control during childbirth in The Gambia and to identify related factors influencing perceptions of support and control during childbirth. The findings will not only help to improve obstetric care in The Gambia but, will contribute to the global body of knowledge related to dignified maternity care.

Methods

Setting and sample

A quantitative, cross-sectional descriptive approach was employed. Due to the limited time available and the lack of funding to conduct this study, convenience sampling was used to select the study areas and recruit participants, between August 2016 and September 2016, at three major health centers in Western and Lower River Regions in The Gambia. Western Region is located in the western part of The Gambia, with nearly 75% of the total population [14] and the highest number of deliveries (approximately 27,200 per year) [15]. Lower River Region which is in the southern part of the country has a population of 82,361 [14] and a number of about 2000 deliveries annually [15].

Based on the two stated objectives to this paper; (1) to assess women's perception of support and control during childbirth; (2) to identify related factors influencing perceptions of support and control during childbirth, the researchers calculated a sample size that will achieve both the descriptive and inferential statistics needed to analyze the data. The researchers used a 95% confidence level, an estimated number of deliveries of 29,200 per year in Western and Lower River Regions [14, 15], an estimated confidence interval of 10% from a previous study on a similar population [16] and a 10% non-response rate. The minimum sample size required for the descriptive statistics was 165 participants. The G-power 3.1.9.2 was used to calculate the sample size for the inferential statistics using an F test, a linear multiple regression with fixed model and R^2 increase, effect size of 0.2, alpha of 0.05, a power (1-β err prob) of 0.95, 9 predictors (all tested), and a 10% non-response rate. A minimum sample size of 140 participants was required. However, we recruited 200 participants in this study to ensure that all statistical analysis for the two research objectives required were achieved.

The predictors used in this study included the independent variables (demographic and obstetric characteristics of participants). The operational definitions of these predictors are clearly stated in the research instrument section in this paper.

Eligibility criteria for participants

Women between the ages of 18 and 35 years, with no medical or obstetric complication during pregnancy, were eligible to participate. They were also eligible if admitted for at least 3 h in a public major health facility in Western and Lower River Regions prior to delivery. Women with multiple pregnancies and those who delivered before arrival at the health facility were excluded.

Data collection process and instruments

Ethics approval was obtained from The Gambia government and Medical Research Council ethics committee, reference number R016005. A demographic-obstetric questionnaire (Additional file 1) and the Support and Control in Birth (SCIB) scale (Additional file 2) were used to obtain participants' information. The structured demographic-obstetric questionnaire was developed by the researcher based on evidence. That is, the variables that were included in the questionnaire such as age, education, place of delivery, marital status, parity, number of antenatal attendance and birth plan were selected based on similar studies [17–22]. Participants in this study were classified as either married or single. The married participant was classified as being in monogamous or polygamous families, and those not married were single, cohabiting, or widowed. Age of participants ranges from 18 to 35 years, participants ages were grouped as 24 years and below and 25 years and above. This age cut-off was based on a previous study by Aitken and colleagues [23]. Educated participants were those with primary education or above, and those uneducated have no formal education. The parity of participants' ranges from 1 to 4, primiparous were participants who have given birth for the first time and multiparous were those having given birth two or more times. Birth planning is one of the components of antenatal care in The Gambia and in this study, a participant who had a birth plan is one who was educated on a birth preparedness plan and complication readiness in one or more antenatal visits during pregnancy. Participants ethnicities in this study are those found in The Gambia [14].

The Support and Control in Birth (SCIB) scale was developed by Ford et al. [22]. It is a 33-item scale with three subscales, namely; internal control, external control, and support. Internal control subscale assessed participants' ability to control oneself during childbirth including events such as pain, emotion, behavior, physical functioning and thoughts through their own efforts. The external control subscale assessed participants' control over events being controlled by external forces such as pain relief (comfort measures or analgesic), information, environment, decisions and procedures, and birth outcome. The support subscale assessed coaching, coping techniques, staff attitude, empathy, understanding and reassurance, encouragement, listening to women's wishes, informational support, and physical support for pain relief.

The SCIB scale is a 5-point Likert scale with responses ranging from completely agree to completely disagree, the middle number (3) representing neither agree nor disagree. The 5-point response scale ranges from 1 to 5, with high scores indicating more support or control, low scores indicating less support or control, and a score of 3 indicating an average support or control. Negative items in the scale were reversed scored. The scale has an overall Cronbach's alpha coefficient of 0.95, internal subscale (0.86), external subscale (0.93) and the support subscale (0.93) [22]. It was tested by Ford et al. (2009) and the psychometric properties were compared well with other published scale of the same field, notably, the Labour Agentry Scale [22]. Similarly, the scale was used by Inci, Gokce, and Tanhan (2015), to develop and validate a Turkish version of the SCIB scale, which was concluded to be reliable and valid with an internal consistency coefficient of 0.86 [24]. All the variables explained in the subscales are incorporated in the health system of the Gambia as per WHO standard. However, as a result of the difference in demography and culture, the SCIB scale was adapted and it was pretested to ensure consistency. The Cronbach's alpha for the total scale was 0.78, internal control subscale was 0.78, external control subscale was 0.75 and support subscale was 0.81. The Cronbach's alpha in this study is lower compared to a study conducted in the United Kingdom, to measure maternal perception of support and control during childbirth [22]. The inter-items correlation indicated an increase in the Cronbach's Alpha if items such as "I was overcome by the pain" and "I gained control by working with my body" in the internal control subscale and "I could get up and move around as much as I wanted" in the external control subscale, were deleted. There was no irrelevant item in the support subscale. Cultural beliefs and demography of participants may be responsible for the difference in the Cronbach's Alpha of the two studies.

In each health facility, participants admitted more than 3 h post- delivery in the postnatal ward for observation, and who met the eligibility criteria and signed the consent form, were invited to participate. As a result of the low literacy rate among women in The Gambia, the questionnaires were administered to the eligible participants that were in the ward at the time of data collection and are willing to participate using the face-to-face interview.

Data processing and analysis

SPSS statistical software version 23.0 was used to analyze the data. Frequency distributions, mean and standard deviation were used to analyze participants' demographic-obstetric characteristics and perceptions of support and control during childbirth. As a result of the non-normal data, non-parametric tests such as Mann-Whitney U test, Kruskal-Wallis H test and Spearman's *rho* correlation were used to compare difference in participants' demographic-obstetric characteristics and perceptions of support and control during childbirth, and relationship between perceptions of support and control during childbirth. Linear multiple regression was used to analyze participants' demographic-obstetric characteristics predicting perceptions of support and control during childbirth.

Results
Demographic and obstetric characteristics of study participants

In this study, there was a 100% response rate and no missing data. Most (55%, $n = 110$) of the participants had no formal education, were married (97%, $n = 194$), and of Mandinka ethnicity (40.0%, $n = 80$). The mean age of the participants was 25. 8 (SD ± 5.09), and about three quarters (74%, $n = 148$) were multiparous. More than half (50.5%, $n = 101$) of the participants had less than four antenatal visits, reported having a birth plan (55.5%, $n = 111$) and had a normal vaginal delivery (95.5%, $n = 191$). In terms of place of delivery, majority of participants delivered in Western Two Health Region (37.5%, $n = 75$). Table 1 shows the demographic and obstetric characteristics of participants.

Women's perception of support and control during childbirth
Perception of internal control

The mean score for internal control was 2.41 (SD ± 0.65), indicating a low perception. The three lowest mean scores in this subscale included; "I was able to control my reactions to the pain" 2.03 (± 1.00); "I was mentally calm" 2.07 (SD ± 1.17); and "the pain was too great for me to gain control over it" 2.09 (SD ±1.08). Items with the highest scores were "I was overcome by the pain" 3.76 (SD ± 0.97); and "I gained control by working with my body" 3.29 (SD ± 1.19).

Perception of external control

External control, 1.85 (SD ± 0.43) equally revealed a low perception. Of the 11 items, the three lowest scores were observed in, "I could decide when I received information" 1.48 (SD ± 0.56); "I could influence which procedures were carried" 1.54 (SD ± 0.61); and "I had control over what information I was given" 1.56 (SD ± 0.63). The only item with a high mean score was observed in "I could get up and move around as much as I wanted" 3.59 (SD ± 1.32).

Perception of support

The overall mean score for support was 2.52 (SD ± 0.62), revealing a moderately low perception and the items such as "the staff helped me to try different positions" 1.45 (SD ± 0.89); "I was given time to ask questions" 2.01 (SD ± 1.24); and "the staff stopped doing something if I asked them to stop" 2.18 (SD ± 1.03), showed the lowest mean scores. Items with high scores were "the staff realized the pain I was in" 3.45 (SD ± 1.17); the staff encouraged me not to fight what my body was doing" 3.20 (SD ± 1.15); and "the staff helped me find energy to continue when I wanted to give up" 2.98 (SD ± 1.29). Table 2

Table 1 Demographic-obstetric Characteristic of Participants ($N = 200$)

Variables	n (%)	Mean ± SD	Range
Age		25.82 ± 5.09	18–35 Yrs.
Less than 25 yrs	83 (41.5)		
25 yrs. or more	117 (58.5)		
Education			
No formal education	110 (55.0)		
Primary education and above	90 (45.0)		
Marital status			
Married (monogamy or polygamy)	194 (97.0)		
Not married (single, cohabiting, widowed)	6 (3.0)		
Ethnicity			
Jola	18 (9.0)		
Fula	47 (23.5)		
Wollof	32 (16.0)		
Mandinka	80 (40.0)		
Others	23 (11.5)		
Parity			1–4
Nullipara (1)	52 (26.0)		
Multipara (≥ 2)	148 (74.0)		
No. of antenatal visits			
Less than 4	101 (50.5)		
4 or more	99 (49.5)		
Place of delivery			
Western one health region	70 (35.0)		
Western two health region	75 (37.5)		
Lower river health region	55 (27.5)		
Birth plan			
No	89 (44.5)		
Yes	111 (55.5)		
Mode of Delivery			
Vaginal delivery	191 (95.5)		
Assisted vacuum delivery	3 (1.5)		
Caesarean section	6 (3.0)		

shows women's perception of maternal support and control during childbirth.

The difference in demographic-obstetric characteristics and Women's perception support and control during childbirth
Perception of internal control

Higher levels in perception of internal control was significantly associated with participants aged 25 years and older ($rho = .20$; $p = .004$), and vaginal delivery (median $= 2.20$, $U = 374.0$, $p = .004$).

Table 2 Women's Perception of Support and Control during Childbirth (N = 200) [22]

Variables	Mean ± SD	Ranking	
		Lowest	Highest
Internal control	2.41 ± 0.65		
1.The pain was too great for me to gain control over it*	2.09 ± 1.08	3	
2.I was overcome by the pain	3.76 ± 0.97		1
3.I was able to control my reactions to the pain	2.03 ± 1.00	1	
4.I was mentally calm	2.07 ± 1.17	2	
5.I was in control of my emotions	2.22 ± 1.21		
6.I felt my body was on a mission that I could not control*	2.16 ± 1.18		
7.Negative feelings overwhelmed me*	2.16 ± 1.21		
8.I gained control by working with my body	3.29 ± 1.19		2
9.I could control the sounds I was making	2.15 ± 1.14		
10.I behaved in a way, not myself*	2.18 ± 1.13		
External control	1.85 ± 0.43		
1. I had control over when procedures happened	1.57 ± 0.64		
2.I could influence which procedures were carried	1.54 ± 0.61	2	
3.I decided whether procedures were carried out or not	1.61 ± 0.73		
4.People in the room took control*	1.94 ± 0.80		
5.I had control over the decisions that were carried out or not	1.75 ± 0.84		
6.I could get up and move around as much as I wanted	3.59 ± 1.32		1
7.People coming in and out of the room was beyond my control*	1.92 ± 1.12		
8.I chose whether I was given information or not	1.54 ± 0.68	3	
9.I could decide when I received information	1.48 ± 0.56	1	
10.I had control over what information I was given	1.56 ± 0.63		
11. I felt I had control over the way my baby was finally born	1.90 ± 0.70		
Support	2.52 ± 0.62		
1. The staff helped me find the energy to continue when I wanted to give up.	2.98 ± 1.29		3
2. The staff seemed to know instinctively what I wanted or needed	2.68 ± 1.15		
3. The staff went out of their way to try a new way to try to keep me comfortable.	2.73 ± 1.16		
4. The staff encouraged me to try new ways of coping (such as breathing techniques).	2.42 ± 1.10		
5. The staff realized the pain I was in	3.45 ± 1.17		1
6. The staff encouraged me not to fight what my body was doing	3.20 ± 1.15		2
7. I felt like the staff had their own agenda*	2.40 ± 1.05		
8. I felt like the staff tried to move things along for their own convenience*	2.48 ± 1.13		
9. I was given time to ask questions	2.01 ± 1.24	2	
10. The staff helped me to try different positions	1.45 ± 0.89	1	
11. The staff stopped doing something if I asked them to stop	2.18 ± 1.03	3	
12. The staff dismissed things I said to them	2.26 ± 1.13		

* Items = Reversed scored
Ford, Ayers & Wright (2009); Measurement of Maternal Perceptions of Support and Control in Birth (SCIB)

Perception of external control

Higher levels in perception of external control was significantly associated with participants aged 25 years and older (rho = .17; p = .02), vaginal delivery (median = 1.91, U = 419.0, p = <.001), and higher parity (median = 1.91, U = 2661.0, p = .001); and a low level in perception of external control significantly associated with women who delivered in Western Region (median = 1.73, U = 2721.0, p = .001), and those who had primary or higher education (median = 1.73, U = 3647.0, p = .001).

Perception of support

There was a statistically significant higher level in perception of support among married women (median = 2.58, $U = 310$, $p = .05$), women who had a vaginal delivery (median = 2.58, $U = 326.50$, $p = .002$), participants aged 25 years and older ($rho = .18$, $p = .01$), higher parity (median = 2.58, $U = 2960.50$, $p = .01$) and those who had a birth plan (median = 2.67, $U = 3649.0$, $p = .001$). 2.58). (Additional file 3: Table S3), shows the difference in demographic-obstetric factors and women's perception of maternal support and control during childbirth.

Predictors of Women's perception of support and control during childbirth

Perception of internal control

Mode of delivery ($p = .01$) and age ($p < .001$) were significant predictors for women's perception of internal control during childbirth, $F_{(3,196)} = 6.74$, $p < .001$, and 8% of the variance in perception of internal control was explained by the model. Women with aged 25 years and older and those who had a vaginal delivery were more likely to have a higher level in the perception of internal control during childbirth.

Perception of external control

Women's perception of external control was significantly predicted by mode of delivery ($p = .04$), place of delivery ($p < .001$), educational status ($p = .02$) and perception of support ($p < .001$), ($F_{(6, 182)} = 10.12$; $p < .001$), indicating that 27% of the variance in perception of external control was explained by the model. Women who had a vaginal delivery were more likely to have a higher level in the perception of external control. Perception of external control was more likely to be high as the perception of support increased during childbirth, and women who had primary or higher education, and those who delivered in Western Region were less likely to have higher levels in the perception of external control during childbirth.

Perception of support

Birth plan ($p = .001$), mode of delivery ($p = .04$), and perception external control ($p < .001$) significantly predicted women's perception of support, $F_{(7, 192)} = 8.75$; $p < .001$, and 25% of variance in perception of support was explained by the model. Women who had a vaginal delivery, those who had a birth plan, and those with a higher level in the perception of external control had a high perception of support during childbirth. (Additional file 4: Table S4), shows related factors predicting women's perception of support and control during childbirth.

Discussion

The purpose of this study was to explore women's perception of support and control during childbirth in the Gambia. According to Ford et al. (2009), perception of control is on two folds namely; internal control which measured women's experience of labour in terms of thoughts, emotions, behaviours, pain and physical functioning during labour and delivery. External control assessed women's control over events controlled by external forces such as access to information, the birth environment, decision making and procedures, and birth outcomes. Perception of support assessed women's perception of supportive care from skilled birth attendants, including staff attitude, encouragement, coaching, empathy, listening and providing information [22]. The findings, therefore, help to answer the following research questions.

What is the women's perception of support and control during childbirth in the Gambia?

As evident in this study, the overall perceptions of control and support were low. Among the three subscales, external control 1.85 (SD ± 0.43) recorded the least perception, which implies that women had the lowest perceived control over external factors such as accessing information and decision making during childbirth. The finding is in line with a similar study conducted in the United Kingdom, which revealed a lower level of perception in external control than the perception of internal control among women during childbirth [22]. Internal control is when women trust in their capability to control events through their own efforts [20] and their experience of labor in terms of their thoughts, emotions, behaviors, pain and physical functioning during labor and delivery [22]. Therefore, this finding could be related to participants' belief in culture, because childbirth in The Gambia is viewed as a transition to adulthood and an experience to showcase womanhood [25], therefore, women are expected to endure labor pains and behave positively during the process.

Factors with the lowest perception of internal control included "the inability to control reactions to pain", "being mentally calm during labor" and "the pain being too great to gain control". This finding supports Green and Baston [17] in which labor pain was regarded as the factor influencing poor control during childbirth. Severe pain during childbirth increases the production of adrenaline, which may interfere with the progress of labor. Therefore, non-pharmacological pain management such as massage, which is the only intrapartum pain management intervention available in The Gambia, should be provided to women.

External factors such as "deciding when they receive information", "inability to influence which procedures were carried out" and "inability to gain control over what information was given to them" had the lowest scores. This implies that women had less autonomy as regards to information sharing and involvement in decision-making during childbirth, and this is a form of mistreatment and loss of dignity [11]. Women's involvement in decision making, makes them feel dignified and respected during labor. [17]. Effective communication which is both woman-initiated and provider-initiated is a main element of gaining external control [8].

Though women's perception of support was low, it was higher than the perception of both internal and external control in this study. This corroborates with the findings of a similar study conducted in the United Kingdom [22]. One of the factors with the lowest perception of support included "women not helped to try different positions during birth". Empowering and encouraging women to change positions during the first and second stage of labour is an integral part of quality intrapartum care [26]. Maternal positioning as preferred by women during birth act as a coping mechanism for pain and promote comfort [26], and utilizing positions such as the upright position during the second stage of labor, minimizes obstetric complications and interventions, shorten the duration of labor and reduces the feeling of pain [27]. In The Gambia, the supine/lithotomy position is the most widely used position during the second stage of labor in the health facilities across the country, this is also evident in Malawi [28]. Lack of knowledge and competence in conducting deliveries using positions other than the supine position could be one of the reasons for women not helped to try different positions in this study. Positioning during delivery is not captured in The Gambia Maternity Care Guideline and Service Delivery Standards [29], therefore, it should be incorporated, and training on the use of different positions during delivery should be provided to skilled birth attendants (midwives), to improve competence. The skills should also be incorporated in all the midwifery curricula in The Gambia.

Women not given the time to ask questions was also one of the factors with the lowest perception of support. This implies that the interaction between skilled birth attendants and women was poor. Effective client-centered communication by healthcare providers during childbirth is regarded as an enhancer for respectful and dignified childbirth [30]. The Reproductive and Child Health Unit and the midwifery institutions in The Gambia should put more emphasis on improving the interpersonal skills of skilled birth attendants to enhance effective maternity care.

Women's inability to stop skilled birth attendants in doing something to them they don't like is a form of non-consent care, which is a violation of women's right and an intentional act of disrespect and abuse during childbirth [30, 31]. Therefore, women should be empowered to make their own decisions about the care provided, which must be respected as it is crucial in promoting control during childbirth.

What are the related factors influencing women's perception of support and control during childbirth in the Gambia?

Women with aged 25 years and older were more likely to have an increase in perception of internal control. The finding agrees with Weisman et al. [20], in which the perception of internal control was negatively associated with younger maternal age. In the same vein, women who had a normal vaginal delivery were more likely to have a higher level in the perception of internal control and perception of external control as compared to those who had instrumental delivery. This finding is consistent with the findings of Ford et al. and Bertucci et al. [22, 32], which stated that birth interventions such as instrumental deliveries may influence the perception of control among women during childbirth.

Education is one of the social determinants of health, and research has shown that the higher the patients' level of education, the higher the expectation of care provided [33]. In this study, higher levels of education were associated with a decrease in perception of external control, which shows that educated women had a lower expectation about the care received and this may be due to their ability to express their wishes. Due to the low literacy rate among women compared to their male counterparts in The Gambia [34], this study supports the need for the government to step up efforts in promoting female education.

Women who delivered in Western Region were less likely to have a higher level in the perception of external control. Though the reason for this finding is not clear, the high number of deliveries [15] and the low provider-client ratio [35] in health facilities may be responsible. However, further research is needed to understand this phenomenon.

Perception of support was positively associated with the perception of external control. Supportive care from health care providers is an important factor that promotes control during childbirth [8]. Therefore, supportive care from skilled birth attendants should be provided to women in order to enhance external control during childbirth.

Regarding the perception of support, the findings further demonstrated that mode of delivery, the perception of external control and birth plan were the significant predictors. Women who had a birth plan and those who had a vaginal delivery were more likely to have higher levels in the perception of support. Effective implementation of the birth preparedness and complication readiness strategies should be strengthened in antenatal care services across the country, as the birth plan has been identified as a factor that enhances the feeling of support during childbirth [8]. Individualized care in which care is provided based on women's needs should be strengthened to improve quality care.

The study revealed a positive association between perception of external control and perception support. Therefore, for women to feel supported, external factors that affect women's autonomy during childbirth such as poor client-provider communication and women's inability to make decisions about their own care should be eliminated.

The study findings therein will enhance the formulation and implementation of effective tailor-made dignified intrapartum care policies that will have a positive impact on women's experience of childbirth, so as to improve the utilization of facility-based intrapartum care service in The Gambia.

Concerning the limitations of this study, a convenience sampling was the method employed in selecting participants in this study. This sampling method is liable to selection bias. The three health facilities identified for the study may differ in the implementation of intrapartum care protocols, and this may have an impact on the results of this study.

Conclusion

Ensuring universal access to reproductive health for all women is one of the components of the Sustainable Development Goals, and is the fundamental desired goal for countries worldwide. Therefore, The Gambia as a developing country with high maternal and infant mortality rates needs to double up attempts to improving the utilization of reproductive health services nationwide. It is therefore critical for The Gambia and other developing countries facing the challenges of moving towards dignified birth, to create an environment within all maternity units that will provide supportive care and promote feelings of control during childbirth, so as to enhance positive decisions about the utilization of maternity care services in future pregnancies.

This study indicated that participants had the lowest perception in pain control, involvement in decision making regarding the care provided, information sharing and utilising different position during birth. Age, mode of delivery, educational status, place of delivery and birth plan significantly predicted participants' perceptions of support and control during childbirth.

From these findings, it is clear that there is a need for the Reproductive and Child Health Unit (RCH) and the Nurses and Midwives Council of The Gambia to strengthen efforts in ensuring that women are given the right support and control during childbirth. This can be achieved through effective supervision and training of skilled birth attendants on non-pharmacological pain management, effective client-provider communication during the intrapartum period, and promote women's involvement in decision making. The findings also support the need for all midwifery curricula to incorporate the training of skilled birth attendants (midwives) on the use of different positions to conduct deliveries, as they are equally important in promoting women feeling a sense of control and support during childbirth.

Abbreviations
GBOS: Gambia Bureau of Statistics; ICPD: International Conference on Population and Development; MOHSW: Ministry of Health and Social Welfare; RCH: Reproductive and Child Health; SCIB: Support and Control in Birth Scale; TBA: Traditional Birth Attendants; UNDP: United Nation Development Programme; WHO: World Health Organisation

Authors contributions
SC planned the current study, did data collection, analyzed and interpreted the findings, did the first draft of the writing and also the final document. C-H. K, M. G, and S-F. C acted as second reviewers. All authors read and approved the final document.

Competing interests
The authors declared that they have no competing interest.

Author details
[1]Ministry of Health & Social Welfare, West Africa, Banjul, The Gambia. [2]Graduate Institute of Nurse-Midwifery National Taipei University and Health Sciences, 365 Ming-Te Road, Taipei 112, Taiwan. [3]Graduate Institute of Nursing, National Taipei University and Health Sciences, 365 Ming-Te Road, Taipei 112, Taiwan.

References
1. WHO. Trends in maternal mortality: 1990 to 2015: estimates by WHO, UNICEF, UNFPA, World Bank Group and the United Nations Population Division. Geneva: World Health Organization. 2015.
2. WHO. Maternal mortality [https://apps.www.who.int/mediacentre/factsheets/fs348/en/index.html].
3. Cham M, Sundby J, Vangen S. Maternal mortality in the rural Gambia, a qualitative study on access to emergency obstetric care. Reprod Health. 2005;2(1):3.

4.   WHO. WHO statement on the prevention and elimination of disrespect and abuse durig facility-based childbirth [http://apps.who.int/iris/bitstream/handle/10665/134588/WHO_RHR_14.23_eng.pdf?sequence=1].

5.   WHO: Respectful Maternity Care Charter [https://www.whiteribbonalliance.org/wp-content/uploads/2017/11/Final_RMC_Charter.pdf].

6.   MOHSW. National health policy. MOHSW: The Republic of The Gambia; 2012-2020.

7.   Matthews R, Callister LC. Childbearing Women's perceptions of nursing care that promotes dignity. J Obstet Gynecol Neonatal Nurs. 2005;33(4):498–507.

8.   Fair CD, Morrison T. I felt part of the decision-making process': a qualitative study on techniques used to enhance maternal control during labor and delivery. International Journal of Childbirth Education. 2011;26(3):21–5.

9.   Kashanian M, Javadi F, Haghighi MM. Effect of continuous support during labor on duration of labor and rate of cesarean delivery. Int J Gynecol Obstet. 2010;109(3):198–200.

10. Hodnett ED, Gates S, Hofmeyr GJ, Sakala C. Continuous support for women during childbirth. Cochrane Libr. 2013.

11. Bohren MA, Vogel JP, Hunter EC, Lutsiv O, Makh SK, Souza JP, Aguiar C, Saraiva Coneglian F, Diniz ALA, Tunçalp Ö, et al. The mistreatment of women during childbirth in health facilities globally: a mixed-methods systematic review. PLoS Med. 2015;12(6):e1001847.

12. Lowe M, Chen D-R, Huang S-L. Social and cultural factors affecting maternal health in rural Gambia: an exploratory qualitative study. PLoS One. 2016; 11(9):e0163653.

13. Jammeh A, Sundby J, Vangen S. Barriers to Emergency Obstetric Care Services in Perinatal Deaths in Rural Gambia: A Qualitative In-Depth Interview Study, vol. 2011; 2011.

14. GBOs. The Gambia 2013 Population and Housing Census Preliminary Results. The Gambia: GBOS. Banjul; 2013.

15. Sowe MMMKN, Bah A, Jallow F. Service statistics report 2014. The Gambia: MOHSW; 2015. p. 13.

16. Anya SE, Hydara A, Jaiteh LE. Antenatal care in the Gambia: missed opportunity for information, education and communication. BMC Pregnancy Childbirth. 2008;8(1):9.

17. Green JM, Baston HA. Feeling in control during labor: concepts, correlates, and consequences. Birth. 2003;30(4):235–47.

18. Kuo S, Lin K, Hsu C, Yang C, Chang M, Tsao C, Lin L. Evaluation of the effects of a birth plan on Taiwanese women's childbirth experiences, control and expectations fulfilment: a randomised controlled trial. Int J Nurs Stud. 2010;47(7):806–14.

19. Cheung W, Ip W, Chan D. Maternal anxiety and feelings of control during labour: a study of Chinese first-time pregnant women. Midwifery. 2007;23(2): 123–30.

20. Weisman CS, Hillemeier MM, Chase GA, Misra DP, Chuang CH, Parrott R, Dyer A. Women's perceived control of their birth outcomes in the Central Pennsylvania Women's health study. implications for the use of preconception care Womens Health Issues. 2008;18(1):17–25.

21. Morhason-Bello IO, Adedokun BO, Ojengbede OA, Olayemi O, Oladokun A, Fabamwo AO. Assessment of the effect of psychosocial support during childbirth in Ibadan, south-West Nigeria: a randomised controlled trial. Austrailian and New Zealand Journal Obstetric and Gynaecology. 2009;49(2): 145–50.

22. Ford E, Ayers S, Wright DB. Measurement of maternal perceptions of support and control in birth (SCIB). Journal of Women's Health (15409996). 2009;18(2):245–52.

23. Aitken Z, Hewitt B, Keogh L, LaMontagne AD, Bentley R, Kavanagh AM. Young maternal age at first birth and mental health later in life: does the association vary by birth cohort? Soc Sci Med. 2016;157:9–17.

24. Inci F, Gokce Isbir G, Tanhan F. The Turkish version of perceived support and control in birth scale. J Psychosom Obstet Gynecol. 2015;36(3):103–13.

25. Sawyer A, Ayers S, Smith H, Sidibeh L, Nyan O, Dale J. Women's experiences of pregnancy, childbirth, and the postnatal period in the Gambia: a qualitative study. Br J Health Psychol. 2011;16(3):528–41.

26. Simkin P, Ancheta R: The labor progress handbook, early interventions to prevent and treat dystocia, 3rd edn. West Sussex: Wiley-Blackwell; 2011.

27. Valiani M, Rezaie M, Shahshahan Z. Comparative study on the influence of three delivery positions on pain intensity during the second stage of labor. Iranian Journal Nursing and Midwifery Research. 2016;21(4):372–8.

28. Zileni BD, Glover P, Jones M, Teoh K-K, Zileni CW, Muller A. Malawi women's knowledge and use of labour and birthing positions: a cross-sectional descriptive survey. Women & Birth. 2017;30(1):e1–8.

29. RCH. The Gambia National Maternity Care Guidelines and Service Delivery Standards. The Gambia: MOHSW. Banjul; 2010.

30. Ratcliffe HL, Sando D, Willey Lyatuu G, Emil F, Mwanyika-Sando M, Chalamilla G, Langer A, McDonald KP. Mitigating disrespect and abuse during childbirth in Tanzania: an exploratory study of the effects of two facility-based interventions in a large public hospital. Reprod Health. 2016;13:1–13.

31. Bowser DHK. Exploring evidence for disrespect and abuse in facility-based childbirth. Report of a landscape analysis. Washington. In: DC: USAID; 2010.

32. Bertucci V, Boffo M, Mannarini S, Serena A, Saccardi C, Cosmi E, Andrisani A, Ambrosini G. Assessing the perception of the childbirth experience in Italian women: a contribution to the adaptation of the childbirth perception questionnaire. Midwifery. 2012;28(2):265–74.

33. Köberich S, Feuchtinger J, Farin E. Factors influencing hospitalized patients' perception of individualized nursing care: a cross-sectional study. BMC Nurs. 2016;15(1):14.

34. Women's Bureau. Gender and women empowerment policy. The Gambia: Women's bureau; 2010-2020.

35. Annual Services Statistics Report. MOHSW; 2012.

17

Using a composite adherence tool to assess ART response and risk factors of poor adherence in pregnant and breastfeeding HIV-positive Cameroonian women at 6 and 12 months after initiating option B+

Pascal N. Atanga[1,2,3]* , Harrison T. Ndetan[4,5], Peter N. Fon[2], Henry D. Meriki[7,8], Tih P. Muffih[1], Eric A. Achidi[6], Michael Hoelscher[3,9,10] and Arne Kroidl[9,10]

Abstract

Background: Antiretroviral therapy (ART) adherence in preventing HIV mother-to-child transmission in association with virological suppression and risk factors of low adherence in the Cameroon's Option B+ programme are poorly understood. We used a composite adherence score (CAS) to determine adherence and risk factors of poor adherence in association with virological treatment response in HIV-positive pregnant and breastfeeding women who remained in care at 6 and 12 months after initiating ART.

Methods: We prospectively enrolled 268 women after ART initiation between October 2013 and December 2015 from five facilities within the Kumba health district. Adherence at 6 and 12 months were measured using a CAS comprising of a 6-month medication refill record review, a four-item self-reported questionnaires and a 30-day visual analogue scale. Adherence was defined as the sum scores of the three measures and classified as high, moderate and low. Measured adherence levels were compared to virological suppression rates at month 12 and risk factors of poor adherence were determined.

Results: At 6 and 12 months, 217 (81.0%) and 185 (69.0%) women were available for adherence evaluation. Respectively. Of those, 128 (59.0%) and 68 (31.4%) had high or moderate adherence as per the CAS tool at month 6, and 116 (62.7%) and 48 (24.9%) at month 12, respectively. Viral loads were assessed in 165 women at months 12, and 92.7% had viral suppression (< 1000 copies/mL). Viral suppression was seen in 100% of women with high, 89.5% with moderate, and 52.9% with low adherence using the CAS tool. Virological treatment failure was significantly associated with low adherence [OR 7.6, (95%CI, 1.8–30.8)]. Risk factors for low adherence were younger age [aOR 3.8, (95%CI, 1.4–10.6)], primary as compared to higher levels of education [aOR 2.7, (95%CI, 1.4–5.2)] and employment in the informal sector compared to unemployment [aOR 1.9, (95%CI,1.0–3.6)].

(Continued on next page)

* Correspondence: abonkwechinje@gmail.com
[1]Cameroon Baptist Convention Health Service (CBCHS), P. O. Box 152, Tiko, Health Services Complex, Mutengene, South West Region, Cameroon
[2]Department of Public Health and Hygiene, Faculty of Health Sciences, University of Buea, P.O. Box 63, Buea, Cameroon
Full list of author information is available at the end of the article

(Continued from previous page)

Conclusions: During the first year of Option B+ implementation in Cameroon our novel CAS adherence tool was feasible, and useful to discriminate ART adherence levels which correlated with viral suppression. Younger age, less educated and informal sector employed women may need more attention for optimal adherence to reduce the risk of virological failure.

Keywords: Option B + , Adherence, Viral load, Risk factors, Cameroon

Background

Adherence to antiretroviral therapy (ART) for HIV infection is essential for plasma viral load suppression. This is key to treatment success as it reduces both morbidity and mortality but most importantly improves the quality of life and reduces drug resistance development [1–3]. Non-adherence is the most important factor that leads to viral resistance [4]. As test and treat is being adopted worldwide including Option B+ procedures for newly diagnosed HIV-positive pregnant and breastfeeding women, additional adherence and retention support are needed as most of the patients initiating ART present with asymptomatic HIV infection [5, 6]. Since the introduction of Option B+ in Malawi in 2011, ART uptake has significantly improved for this target group but there are still concerns that women with asymptomatic HIV infection may not be adequately retained or poorly adhere to treatment [7–9]. Recent studies since the introduction of Option B+ have focused on retention in care [8, 10, 11] and very little data is available assessing patients' adherence to ART. Evidence also shows that retention, which is often used as a surrogate for adherence, may fail to account for the pattern of clinic attendance and drug taking behaviour [12]. The few studies evaluating adherence to Option B + used a single adherence measure such as self-report or pharmacy refill which both have been shown to overestimate adherence [13, 14]. Overestimated adherence could result in patient misclassification and lead to inaccurate targeting of adherence-improving interventions or delays in addressing adherence problems. Self-reported adherence is subjective and its reliability drops overtime as patients get acquainted with the assessment tool used [15]. Pharmacy refills and pill counts on their part, though objective and not easily affected by recall and social desirability biases, may result in 'pill-dumping', thus overestimating adherence [16, 17]. Viral load (VL) suppression data can provide additional information to improve adherence assessment conducted using any subjective measure, though it could also be affected by pre-treatment HIV drug resistance [18]. To optimise the Option B+ programme and reduce the risk of treatment failure, timely and adequate assessment of adherence in HIV-positive pregnant and breastfeeding women with a simple but robust tool is critical in resource limited settings where second line medication options are limited and third line regimens are virtually non-existent or are still very expensive [2, 5]. Sub-optimal adherence needs to be identified and addressed

early prior to treatment failure and the development of viral drug resistance. This is possible only if we understand the risk factors of poor adherence and those enablers of proper medication taking behaviour. These factors have been studied in other settings but are poorly understood in Cameroon [19, 20]. In order to meet the UNAIDS 90–90-90 objective by 2020 [21], treatment programmes should not only focus on HIV testing, ART initiation and retention in care, but also on adherence to lifelong ART which is key to reaching the 3rd 90. However, notwithstanding the importance of near perfect adherence on viral suppression, recent research findings are showing that newer ART regimens may only require moderate adherence levels to achieve viral suppression [22–24].

In our previous analysis of this cohort of pregnant or breastfeeding women, we observed good uptake of HIV testing and counselling, ART and retention in care, which however, declined over time. We analysed treatment discontinuation taking into account women lost to follow up, transferred out to other ART clinics, intentionally stopped medication or died. Discontinuation from Option B+ was highest at small sites with a high staff turnover [8]. Based on those findings, we now specifically evaluated information on women who remained in care with respect to ART adherence in association with viral suppression using a multiple method tool. We further investigated risk factors associated with poor adherence alongside enablers of proper drug taking behaviour.

Methods

Study design and settings

This prospective cohort study was carried out between October, 2013 and December 2015 at five health facilities located within the Kumba Health District, South West Region, Cameroon, which all provide integrated maternal, neonatal, child health and prevention of mother to child transmission (PMTCT) services. These sites were among the ten facilities that piloted Option B + in the region from October, 2013. They receive well over 90% of all pregnant women seeking antenatal care (ANC) in the health district, and also had their staff trained in Option B+ procedures and task shifting as part of the pilot project. Task shifting allows midwives and nurses to prescribe ART and follow-up the mother baby pair [25].

Study participants, procedures, outcomes and definitions

The study participants and procedures were previously described [8]. For the current analysis, which focused on adherence using a composite adherence score and viral suppression, we included women who remained in care at six and twelve months after ART initiation. In brief, ART was offered as a once daily regimen with a fixed dose combination of tenofovir, lamivudine and efavirenz regardless of clinical or immunological status in accordance with WHO and national guidelines [5, 26]. ART follow-up cards were opened for each ART initiating client from which information on age, date and timing of ART initiation, previous ART history, WHO staging, CD4 T-cell counts, level of education, profession, religious affiliation, and marital status was documented. Adherence and VL information were completed on subsequent follow-up visits when available. ART visits were scheduled monthly in a way that provided at least 4 days buffer supply of medications. Visits were managed at ANC or infant welfare clinics (IWC) post-delivery by trained nurses or midwives. During each refill visit, women received routine information and support on adherence, and every 6 months each women underwent a comprehensive adherence assessment. Data extraction and interviews were conducted by nurses and midwives who were trained as study staff. VL testing was performed 12 months after ART initiation when VL became routine for patient monitoring using the Real Time HIV-1 m2000™ System (Abbott Laboratories, Illinois, USA). VL samples were not collected if either the woman missed her clinic visit on the day of sample collection or had multimonth refills during a previous visit. Virological suppression was defined as any value < 1000 copies/mL on a single measurement according to WHO and national guidelines [4, 26]. Women with low replicating viraemia (40 and 999 copies/mL) were subjected to re-enforced adherence counselling, those with suspected virological treatment failure (VL ≥1000 copies/mL) also received re-enforced adherence support and repeated VL testing within 3 months if adherence was judged satisfactory. During re-enforced adherence, individual adherence challenges were identified by psychosocial support staffs who then worked with individual clients until viral load retesting after adherence was judged satisfactory.

The primary study outcome was ART adherence at six and twelve months after Option B+ initiation using a validated multi-method tool adapted from South Africa [27]. We included medication refill record review (ARV pick-up appointments) as ARVs in Cameroon are sourced and distributed by a sole body through approved ARV treatment centres and Option B+ sites free of charge. Adherence was assessed using a six monthly medication refill record review, a four-item self-reported adherence questionnaire, and a thirty days visual analogue scale (VAS).

Medication refill records for each woman over the past 6 months were reviewed by the study staff to track the total number of refills effected using the patient ART cohort register. A face-to-face interview was then administered, prefaced by a normalizing language in order to reduce social desirability bias [28, 29]. The interviewer then administered the four closed ended questions formulated such that the right answer was a no to reduce the "white coat effect" [27]. The four questions used to evaluate self-reported adherence were (i) *"Do you sometimes find it difficult to remember to take your medicine?"*; (ii) *"When you feel better, do you sometimes stop taking your medicine?"*; (iii) *"Thinking back over the past 4 days, have you missed any of your doses?"*; and (iv) *"Sometimes if you feel worse when you take the medicine, do you stop taking it?"* [27]. Two additional questions were administered to probe for reasons of missing doses and enhancers of drug taking behaviour as follows; (i) *"What causes you to miss some doses of your drug?"*, and (ii) *"What helps you remember to take your drugs?"* Women were finally asked to estimate adherence on a linear VAS, (Fig. 1), which included a score ranging from zero (no adherence) to ten (optimal adherence) over the last 30 days [30, 31].

Adherence was scored separately for each adherence measure with a score on 3 indicating high, 2 moderate and 1 low adherence (Table 1). Overall adherence was estimated by creating a composite adherence score (CAS), which included the sum of the scores from each of the three measures and classified adherence as high, moderate or low. To avoid overweighting, once adherence was scored as poor on pharmacy refill the CAS was low irrespective of the scores on the questionnaire and the VAS.

Secondary outcomes included risk factors of poor adherence, reasons for missing medications, reminders commonly used to enhance adherence, and the correlation between different adherence tools and the CAS. In

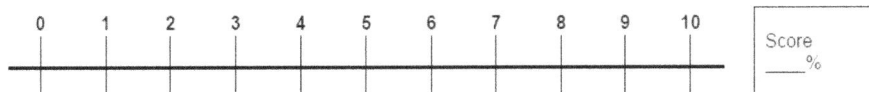

Fig. 1 Visual Analogue Scale (VAS)

Table 1 Interpretation of the single adherence measures and the composite adherence score (CAS)

Single adherence tool*	Medication refill	Had 6 refills (3)	Missed 1 refill (2)					Missed 2 or more refills (1)			
	Self-report questionnaire	No to all 4 questions (3)	Yes to 1 question (2)					Yes to 2 or more questions (1)			
	VAS	90% or more (3)	80% to less than 90% (2)					Less than 80% (1)			
Composite adherence tool	Medication refill score	3	3	3	3	3	2	3	2	2	1
	Self-report questionnaire score	3	3	3	2	2	2	1	2	1	1
	VAS score	3	2	1	2	1	2	1	1	1	1
	CAS	9	8	7	7	6	6	5	5	4	3
	Overall adherence	High	Moderate					Low			

CAS composite adherence score, VAS visual analogue scale; Single adherence scores: 3 = high adherence, 2 = moderate adherence, 1 = low adherence;

assessing the risk factors associated with poor adherence, all women who had discontinued treatment at or before 12 months after ART initiation were considered as the worst case of adherence and were included into the low adherence category.

Statistical analysis

Data were collected on study specific case report forms, entered into an Excel spread sheet and corrected for inconsistency before extraction for analysis. Descriptive statistics were used to examine the baseline socio-demographic, laboratory and clinical characteristics of the study participants at ART initiation. Binary logistic regression was used to assess the association between adherence scores by different adherence tools and viral suppression, as well as to assess the risk factors for poor adherence. Unadjusted odd ratios (OR) and 95% confidence intervals (CI) were reported. For risk factor, variables with significant or marginal association ($p < 0.100$) and those previously reported to be associated with poor adherence were included into the multivariate analyses reporting the adjusted odd ratios (aOR) for poor adherence. An alpha level of < 0.05 was set to define significance. Spearman correlation was used to compare the performance of the different adherence measures with each other and with the CAS. Data were analysed using the IBM Statistical Package for Social Sciences (version 21, IBM SPSS Inc., Chicago IL, USA).

Results
Baseline characteristics of the study participants
Of the 268 women starting Option B+, 253 (94.4%) initiated ART prior to labour/delivery and 15 (5.6%) during breastfeeding. Patients' baseline socio-demographic, HIV status, clinical and laboratory characteristics are provided in Table 2. In brief, the median age at ART initiation was 27 (IQR 24–31) years, a minimum of primary level of education was attained in 263 (98.1%) and 105 (39.2%) were unemployed. At ART initiation the median CD4+ T-cell count was 376 cells/mL, (IQR 244–544.8), 234 (87.3%) were ART naïve, whereas 4 (1.5%) had been exposed to ARV during previous pregnancies. In

addition, 30 (11.2%) women already received Option A during their current pregnancy and were switched to Option B+ triple regimens.

Adherence measurements and the performance of the different tools
After six and twelve months 217 (81.0%) and 185 (69.0%) of women were still available for adherence analysis, respectively. Adherence levels determined by CAS for women retained in care at months 6 and 12 were high in 128 (59.0%) and 116 (62.7%) cases, moderate in 68 (31.4%) and 48 (24.9%), and low in 21 (9.6%) and 23 (12.4%), respectively (Table 3).

Differences within adherence estimates were further assessed by comparing correlation coefficients at each adherence time-point (Table 4). All adherence measures were correlated with each other. Significant correlation with the CAS by Spearman correlation were seen for all comparisons ($p < 0.001$), ranging from 0.36 to 0.83. However, the highest linear correlation was observed between the VAS and CAS which remained consistent both at 6 and 12 months with a Spearman correlation of 0.83.

Adherence and virological suppression
Of the 185 women assessed for adherence at months 12, VL was performed in 165 (90.7%) women. Of those 139 (84.2%) had undetectable VL < 40 copies/mL, 14 (8.5%) low level replication between 40 and 999 copies/mL, and 12 (7.3%) evidence for virological treatment failure ≥ 1000 copies/mL. Viral suppression < 1000 copies/mL was positively associated with high adherence as estimated by CAS in 100%, with moderate adherence in 89.5% and low adherence in 52.9% (Table 5). All adherence measures showed statistically significant differences between high adherence when compared with low adherence and virological suppression. In bivariate regression analysis there was a strong positive association between virological failure and low adherence for all adherence tools. Using the CAS, all clients who reported high adherence were virologically suppressed and moderate adherence showed statistically significant difference

Table 2 Baseline socio-demographic, clinical and laboratory characteristics of women who started triple ART for PMTCT Option B+ in Kumba Health District, South West Region, Cameroon between October 2013 and December 2014

Variables	Description	N = 268
Age, years	Median (IQR)	27 (24–31)
Age groups, years	15–24	76 (28.4)
	25–34	156 (58.2)
	35 and above	36 (13.4)
Educational Level	None	5 (1.9)
	Completed primary	147 (54.8)
	Completed secondary and above	116 (43.3)
Marital Status	Single	60 (22.4)
	Married	171 (63.8)
	Others (divorced, widow)	37 (13.8)
Religious affiliation	Catholic	59 (22.0)
	Presbyterian	88 (32.8)
	Baptist	16 (6.0)
	Pentecostals	100 (37.3)
	Muslim	5 (1.9)
Occupation	Unemployed	105 (39.2)
	Employed (formal public sector)	14 (5.2)
	Employed (informal sector) or others	149 (55.6)
HIV status	Known HIV positive, not on ART	34 (12.7)
	New HIV diagnosis	234 (87.3)
ART status	ART naive	234 (87.3)
	Not on ART, but previously exposed	4 (1.5)
	Currently on Option A	30 (11.2)
Timing of ART initiation	After delivery	15 (5.6)
	Prior to labour /delivery	253 (94.4)
CD4 cell count at ART initiation, cells/µL	Median (IQR)	376 (244–544.8)
CD4 cell count groups	> 350 cells/µL	153 (57.1)
	≤350 cells/µL	115 (42.9)
WHO stage	WHO stage 1	226 (84.3)
	WHO stage 2	35 (13.1)
	WHO stage 3	7 (2.6)
	WHO stage 4	0 (0)

Data are in numbers and percentages [n (%)] or for continuous variables in median and Interquartile range (IQR)

Table 3 Antiretroviral treatment adherence as assessed by different measures (pharmacy refill, self-reported questionnaire, and Visual Analogue Scale) and the composite adherence score at month 6 and 12 after ART initiation

Adherence variable	Adherence score	Adherence month 6 N = 217	Adherence month 12 N = 185
Pharmacy refill	High	183 (84.3)	150 (81.1)
	Moderate	17 (7.8)	12 (6.5)
	Low	17 (7.8)	23 (12.4)
Self-reported questionnaire	High	159 (69.1)	143 (77.3)
	Moderate	43 (19.8)	31 (16.8)
	Low	15 (6.9)	11 (5.9)
Visual Analogue Scale (VAS)	High	150 (69.1)	135 (73.0)
	Moderate	39 (18.0)	25 (13.5)
	Low	28 (12.9)	25 (13.5)
Composite adherence score (CAS)	High	128 (59.0)	116 (62.7)
	Moderate	68 (31.4)	46 (24.9)
	Low	21 (9.6)	23 (12.4)

Data are in numbers and percentages [n (%)]

with virological suppression when compared to low adherence [OR 7.6, (95%CI, 1.8–30.8)] .

Risk factors associated with low adherence

In both bivariate and multivariate regression analyses adjusted for socio-demographics and other HIV and laboratory characteristics, low adherence was statistically significant with younger as compared to older ages [aOR 3.8, (95%CI, 1.4–10.6)], completed primary compared to completed secondary education and above [aOR 2.7, (95%CI, 1.4–5.2)] and employment in the informal sector when compared to unemployment [aOR 1.9, (95%C, 1.0–3.6)] (Table 6).

Religious affiliation, marital status, initial CD4 T-cell count at ART initiation, WHO stage and timing of ART initiation were not associated with low adherence.

Reasons for missed medication doses and factors that helped to remind medication taking

During adherence assessment at month 12, 121 women gave reasons why doses were missed. Frequently cited reasons were forgetfulness by 43 (35.5%), travel away from home by 21 (24.0%) and lack of transport to the clinic by 28 (23.1%) women. Side effects, stigmatization, distracted by the baby, being away for work and being involved in church or other social activities were less frequently cited. Asking about factors that helped to remind medications taking, 172 women provided one or more responses. The most frequently cited were the use of cell phone by 64 (37.2%) women, 63 (36.6%) indicated that drug taking had become a routine in their life so it

Table 4 Correlation coefficient between each two adherence measures and between each adherence measure and the CAS at 6 and 12 months (Spearman correlation)

| | Timing of adherence evaluation | | | | | | | |
| | 6 month | | | | 12 month | | | |
Adherence Tool	Pharmacy refill	Self-report	VAS	CAS	Pharmacy refill	Self-report	VAS	CAS
Pharmacy refill	1.00	0.42	0.52	0.62	1.00	0.36	0.66	0.72
Self-report	–	1.00	0.53	0.77	–	1.00	0.49	0.71
VAS	–	–	1.00	0.83	–	–	1.00	0.83

occurs more as an instinct, and 22 (12.8%) mentioned the use of alarm clocks. Among the less frequently cited, 14 (8.1%) declared being reminded by their husbands, 4 (2.3%) relied on a television series and 4 (2.3%) had their drugs by their bedside. Two additional tables show the clients responses to these two questions in more details [see Additional file 1; Tables 1 and 2].

Discussion

Using a composite adherence score (CAS) we determined adherence in association with viral suppression and risk factors of poor adherence in a cohort of HIV-positive pregnant and breastfeeding women who remained in care at 6 and 12 months after initiating ART as part of Option B+. The study demonstrated that of those women who remained in care after Option B+ initiation, 59.0 and 31.4% were either highly or moderately adhering to their treatment as per our CAS tool at

6 month, and 62.7 and 24.9% at month 12, respectively. The predictive accuracy of the CAS tool was reflected by virological suppression rates, which were 100% in women who scored high, 89.5% who scored moderate, and 52.9% who scored low with the CAS tool at month 12. Low CAS adherence as compared to moderate adherence was significantly associated with virological failure (OR 7.6, $p = 0.005$). In our cohort, moderate to high adherence scores by the CAS tool were sufficient to reach more than 90% of viral suppression (< 1000 copies/mL) as defined by the UNAIDS targets, thus 90.8% of women at 6 months and 87.6% at 12 months were considered with good adherence to reach durable treatment response. Our adherence levels were comparable with findings of earlier reports of good adherence with Option B+ from Eastern Africa [13, 32], but slightly higher than adherence reported for the same target group from an Option A study [33]. Adequate adherence

Table 5 Association between adherence scores by different adherence tools and virological suppression in pregnant and breastfeeding women at 12 months after ART initiation

Adherence variable	Participants who received VL assessments N = 165	VL ≥ 1000 copies/mL N = 12 (7.3)	VL < 1000 copies/mL N = 153 (92.7)	[a]OR (95%CI)	P-value
Pharmacy refill					
Low adherence	17 (10.3)	6/17 (35.3)	11/17 (64.7)	14.4 (3.8–54.8)	0.0001
Moderate adherence	11 (6.7)	1/11 (9.1)	10/11 (90.9)	2.6 (0.3–24.8)	0.395
High adherence	137 (83.0)	5/137 (3.6)	132/137 (96.4)	1	
Self-report					
Low adherence	7 (4.2)	4/7 (57.1)	3/7 (42.9)	21.2 (4.0–111.2)	0.0003
Moderate adherence	25 (15.2)	2/25 (8.0)	23/25 (92.0)	1.4 (0.3–6.9)	0.695
High adherence	133 (80.6)	6/133 (4.5)	127/133 (95.5)	1	
VAS					
Low adherence	18 (10.9)	9/18 (50.0)	9/18 (50.0)	124.0 (14.1–1090.4)	< 0.0001
Moderate adherence	22 (13.3)	2/22 (9.1)	20/22 (90.9)	12.4 (1.1–143.0)	0.06
High adherence	125 (75.8)	1/125 (0.8)	124/125 (99.2)	1	
CAS					
Low adherence	17 (10.3)	8/17 (47.1)	9/17 (52.9)	7.6 (1.8–30.8)	0.005
Moderate adherence	38 (23.0)	4/38 (10.5)	34/38 (89.5)	1	
High adherence	110 (66.7)	0 (0.0)	110/110 (100)	–	

Data are in numbers and percentages [n (%)].[a]binary logistic regression, OR (crude odd ratio)

Table 6 Risk factors for low adherence using the composite adherence score (CAS) at 12 months following Option B+ initiation with adjusted odd ratios (aOR) for 5 health facilities in Kumba health district

Variables	Low adherence N = 85	Moderate or high adherence N = 162	Bivariate analysis[a]		Multivariate analysis[b]	
			OR (95% CI)	P-value	aOR (95% CI)	P-value
Age (years)						
15–24	29 (42.0)	40 (58.0)	2.4 (0.9,5.9)	0.07	3.8 (1.4, 10.6)	0.01
25–34	48 (33.3)	96 (66.7)	1.6 (0.7,3.9)	0.27	1.9 (0.8,4.6)	0.18
35 and above	8 (23.5)	26 (76.5)	1		1	
Educational Level						
None	1(20.0)	4 (80.0)	0.8 (0.1,7.8)	0.87	1.3 (0.1,15.2)	0.81
Completed primary	59 (44.0)	75 (56.0)	2.6 (1.5,4.6)	0.001	2.7 (1.4,5.2)	0.001
Completed secondary and above	25 (23.1)	83 (76.9)	1		1	
Occupation						
Unemployed	23 (24.2)	72 (58.8)	1		1	
Employed formal sector	5 (38.5)	8 (61.5)	2.0 (0.6,6.6)	0.28	3.9 (1.0,14.8)	0.055
Employed informal sector	57 (41.0)	82 (59.0)	2.2 (1.2,3.9)	0.01	1.9 (1.0,3.6)	0.05
Religious affiliation						
Catholic	20 (36.4)	35 (63.6)	1		1	
Protestants (Presbyterians/Baptist)	26 (28.3)	66 (71.7)	0.7 (0.3,1.4)	0.31	0.6 (0.3,1.4)	0.24
Pentecostals	39 (41.1)	56 (58.9)	1.2 (0.6,2.4)	0.57	1.1 (0.5,2.3)	0.88
Muslim	0 (0.0)	5 (100.0)	–		–	
CD4 at initiation						
$\leq$ 350 cells/µL	41 (38.7)	65 (61.3)	1.4 (0.8,2.4)	0.22	1.4 (0.8,2.3)	0.23
> 350 cells/µL	44 (31.2)	97 (68.8)	1		1	

Data are in numbers and percentages [n (%)],[a]binary logistic regression, OR (crude odd ratio), aOR (adjusted odd ratio)]. [b]adjusted for age, level of education, occupation, religious afiliation, WHO staging and CD4 count at ART initiation

assessment is important to better understand and optimise the success of the Option B+ programme.

A key strength of this study was the use of a CAS to assess adherence in this population. To our knowledge this is the first study to measure adherence to ART in the context of Option B+ using a CAS. We found a high level of correlation between all single adherence measures (pharmacy refill, self-reported adherence, and VAS) and the CAS which were also all associated with the 12 months viral suppression indicating the validity of each of the measures. It has been argued that the use of a CAS to measure adherence may be cumbersome in routine clinical settings [34]. Our observed close correspondence between the VAS and the CAS suggests that a single and less cumbersome tool like the VAS could be more conveniently used in clinical settings, and this observation was also reported in other older studies [30, 31, 35]. Furthermore, in a recent review of adherence and retention beyond Option B+ the authors' claimed that the paucity of literature on adherence in this population was due to the lack of adherence measure systematically used in routine care [36]. This thus justifies the importance of a simple tool like the VAS for routine adherence assessment at the point of care. Among clients with virologic failure who reported a high adherence, 50% came from self-reported adherence indicating its high vulnerability to social desirability and recall biases [29]. Despite its mediocre performance as an adherence assessment tool in predicting virologic failure, we would still argue that self-reported questionnaires remains useful in providing additional information necessary to provide adequate adherence support to clients with adherence challenges.

Viral suppression rates in women who remained in care at 12 months in our study (92.7%) outreached the UNAIDS 2020 target [21], suggesting that viral suppression is achievable both in pregnancy and/or breastfeeding. However, 8.5% of our women had low replicating viraemia between 40 and 999 copies/mL, and given the low genetic resistance barrier of non-nucleotide reverse transcriptase inhibitor containing regimens, close monitoring is required to promptly identify treatment failure and switch clients to a second line therapy.

Risk factors for low adherence to ART were younger age, low level of education and employment in the informal sector. Younger age and low level of education had been reported as predictors of lost to follow-up and treatment discontinuation [8, 20]. Older women with more experience and better self-care skills/abilities may be more responsible towards their health compared to younger women [20]. Employees in the informal sector have their own unique work challenges and stresses, which can adversely affect their ability to concentrate on health and medication adherence. A South African study showed that conflict with work commitment and the difficulty of disclosing ones HIV status to an employer affected ARV adherence in women on Option B+ [37]. Potential strategies to mitigate these challenges include flexible clinics opening hours like evenings or weekends when most workers are free and do not need employer's permission or a day off just to attend clinic.

Like other studies from sub-Saharan Africa, most participants in this study cited forgetfulness, being away from home and lack of transport to the health facility as possible reasons for missing doses [32, 38, 39]. Our study participants also indicated that reminder aids like cell phones, alarm clocks and reminder from family members helped improved their adherence. A good proportion of the respondents (36.6%) claimed that medication taking had become a routine for them so they needed no reminders. Of these, 88.2% had viral suppression showing that they had in fact adapted this routinely. This claim for those not virally suppressed may just covey their good intentions to continue taking their medication or methodological problems such as social desirability concerns. Recent studies have shown that the use of cell phones short message reminders can greatly improve adherence [40–42]. The role of family members like husbands and sisters to remind clients take their medication could improve adherence [13, 33].

Limitations

The main limitation in this study was that adherence and virological suppression might had been overestimated as assessment was limited to women who retained in treatment, and may therefore not be representative of all HIV-positive women engaged in the Cameroon's Option B + programme. Despite the fact that we prefaced with a normalising language, the self-reported questionnaires and VAS may still had been prone to recall and social desirability biases. The small sample size also limited further analyses. Despite these limitations, our findings had shown that the VAS and the CAS both reliably predicted virological response in a clinical context thus could be used to assess adherence especially in resource limited settings where VL access may be limited. We therefore, believe that the study findings are useful to inform implementation of PMTCT Option B+ and to a certain extent the Test and Treat strategy in Cameroon and other comparable settings.

Conclusions

During the first year of the Option B+ implementation in Cameroon we used a novel adherence tool, which effectively provided an adherence score that correlated well with viral suppression. However, younger, less educated and informal sector employed pregnant and breastfeeding women may need more attention for optimal adherence to help reduce the risk of virological failure.

Abbreviations

ANC: Antenatal care; aOR: Adjusted odds ratio; ART: Antiretroviral therapy; ARV: Antiretroviral; CAS: Composite adherence score; CBCHS: Cameroon Baptist Convention Health Service; CD4: Cluster of differentiation 4; CI: Confidence interval; CIH: Centre for International Health; DZIF: German Centre for Infection Research; HIV: Human Immunodeficiency Virus; HIV/AIDS: Human Immunodeficiency Virus/Acquired Immunodeficiency Syndrome; IWC: Infant welfare clinic; LMU: University of Munich; OR: Crude odds ratio; PEPFAR: President's emergency plan for AIDS relief; PMTCT: Prevention of Mother-To-Child Transmission; UNAIDS: Joint United Nations Programme on HIV/AIDS; VAS: Visual analogue scale; VL: Viral load; WHO: World Health Organization

Acknowledgements

The authors would like to thank all the study participants, the study staff and all site staff of the participating health units. We sincerely appreciate the efforts of Dr. Atashili Julius who significantly contributed to the conception and data collection but the cold hands of death did not permit him to see the final product of this work. We also thank late Dr. Aguh Valentine F. a gynaecologist obstetrician at the mother and child reference hospital, Douala, Cameroon for reviewing the manuscript. Our special thanks also go to the staff and administration of the Emerging Disease laboratory of the University of Buea for providing us with the necessary laboratory assistance and space for the storage of our samples. We are equally very grateful to the Cameroon Baptist Convention Health Services who secured the funds from PEPFAR through CDC-Cameroon for the pilot project within which this study was conducted.

Funding

The data for this study was collected from routine patient information with permission from the ministry of public health in an on-going pilot project fully funded by PEPFAR. Neither the pilot project funder nor the implementing partner had any role in the study design, data collection and analysis, preparation of the manuscript, or the decision to publish.

Authors' contributions

PN conceived and designed the study, took overall responsibility for implementing the study and led the manuscript writing. PN, AK, MH, EA, HN and HM contributed in developing the study concept and design. PA, HN, EA, HM, AK, NP and TM participated in the data collection, sample collection and analysis and the statistical analyses. PA, EA, AK and NP developed the manuscript structure and wrote the original draft. PN, HN, NP, EA, HM, MH, AK and TM reviewed the manuscript critically for intellectual content and provided guidance and editorial support. All authors have read and approved the final version of the submitted manuscript.

Competing interest
The authors declare no competing interest.

Author details
[1]Cameroon Baptist Convention Health Service (CBCHS), P. O. Box 152, Tiko, Health Services Complex, Mutengene, South West Region, Cameroon. [2]Department of Public Health and Hygiene, Faculty of Health Sciences, University of Buea, P.O. Box 63, Buea, Cameroon. [3]Centre for International Health (CIH), University of Munich (LMU), Munich, Germany. [4]Department of Epidemiology and Biostatistics, University Texas Health Northeast, School of Community and Rural Health, Tyler, USA. [5]Department of Biostatistics and Epidemiology, School of Public Health, University of North Texas Health Science Center, Fort Worth, TX, USA. [6]Faculty of Science, University of Buea, P.O. Box 63, Buea, Cameroon. [7]Department of Microbiology and Parasitology, Faculty of Sciences, University of Buea, P.O. Box 63, Buea, Cameroon. [8]Laboratory Department, Regional Hospital Buea, Buea, Cameroon. [9]Division of Infectious Diseases and Tropical Medicine, Medical Centre of the University of Munich (LMU), Munich, Germany. [10]German Centre for Infection Research (DZIF), Partner Site Munich, Munich, Germany.

References
1. Mills EJ, et al. Adherence to antiretroviral therapy in sub-Saharan Africa and North America: a meta-analysis. Jama. 2006;296(6):679–90.
2. Bangsberg DR, Preventing HIV. Antiretroviral resistance through better monitoring of treatment adherence. J Infect Dis. 2008;197(Supplement_3): S272–8.
3. Ngarina M, et al. Virologic and immunologic failure, drug resistance and mortality during the first 24 months postpartum among HIV-infected women initiated on antiretroviral therapy for life in the Mitra plus study, Dar Es Salaam, Tanzania. BMC Infect Dis. 2015;15:175.
4. WHO. Consolidated guidelines on the use of antiretroviral drugs for treating and preventing HIV infection: summary of key features and recommendations. June. 2013:2013.
5. WHO, Consolidated guidelines on the use of antiretroviral drugs for treating and preventing hiv infection: Recommendations for a Public Health approach. 2016.
6. Takow SE, et al. Time for option B+? Prevalence and characteristics of HIV infection among attendees of 2 antenatal clinics in Buea, Cameroon. Journal of the International Association of Providers of AIDS Care. 2013; 14(1):77–81.
7. CDC. Impact of an innovative approach to prevent mother-to-child transmission of HIV--Malawi, July 2011–September 2012. MMWR Morb Mortal Wkly Rep. 2013, 62(8):148.
8. Atanga PN, et al. Retention in care and reasons for discontinuation of lifelong antiretroviral therapy in a cohort of Cameroonian pregnant and breastfeeding HIV-positive women initiating 'option B+'in the south west region. Tropical Med Int Health. 2016;22(2):161–70.
9. Coutsoudis A, et al. Is option B+ the best choice?: forum. Southern Afr J HIV Med. 2013;14(1):8–10.
10. Haas AD, et al. Retention in care during the first 3 years of antiretroviral therapy for women in Malawi's option B+ programme: an observational cohort study. Lancet HIV. 2016;3(4):e175–82.
11. Tenthani L, et al. Retention in care under universal antiretroviral therapy for HIV-infected pregnant and breastfeeding women ('Option B+') in Malawi. AIDS (London, England). 2014;28(4):589–98.
12. Rollins NC, et al. Defining and analyzing retention-in-care among pregnant and breastfeeding HIV-infected women: unpacking the data to interpret and improve PMTCT outcomes. J Acquir Immune Defic Syndr. 2014;67: S150–6.
13. Ebuy H, Yebyo H, Alemayehu M. Adherence level to and predictors of option B+ PMTCT program in Tigray, northern Ethiopia. Int J Infect Dis. 2015;33:123–9.
14. Haas AD, et al. Adherence to antiretroviral therapy during and after pregnancy: cohort study on women receiving care in Malawi's option B+ program. Clin Infect Dis. 2016;63(9):1227–35.
15. Nieuwkerk PT, Oort FJ. Self-reported adherence to antiretroviral therapy for HIV-1 infection and virologic treatment response: a meta-analysis. J Acquir Immune Defic Syndr. 2005;38(4):445–8.
16. Kitahata MM, et al. Pharmacy-based assessment of adherence to HAART predicts virologic and immunologic treatment response and clinical progression to AIDS and death. Int J STD AIDS. 2004;15(12):803–10.
17. Berg KM, Arnsten JH. Practical and conceptual challenges in measuring antiretroviral adherence. J Acquir Immune Defic Syndr. 2006;43(Suppl 1):S79.
18. Fokam J, et al. Short communication: population-based surveillance of HIV-1 drug resistance in Cameroonian adults initiating antiretroviral therapy according to the World Health Organization guidelines. AIDS Res Hum Retrovir. 2016;32(4):329–33.
19. Mitiku I, et al. Factors associated with loss to follow-up among women in option B+ PMTCT programme in Northeast Ethiopia: a retrospective cohort study. J Int AIDS Soc. 2016;19(1):20662.
20. Tweya H, et al. Understanding factors, outcomes and reasons for loss to follow-up among women in option B+ PMTCT programme in Lilongwe, Malawi. Tropical Med Int Health. 2014;19(11):1360–6.
21. UNAIDS. 90-90-90: an ambitious treatment target to help end the AIDS epidemic. Geneva: UNAIDS; 2014.
22. Parienti J-J, et al. Not all missed doses are the same: sustained NNRTI treatment interruptions predict HIV rebound at low-to-moderate adherence levels. PLoS One. 2008;3(7):e2783.
23. Kobin AB, Sheth NU. Levels of adherence required for virologic suppression among newer antiretroviral medications. Ann Pharmacother. 2011;45(3):372–9.
24. Bezabhe WM, et al. Adherence to antiretroviral therapy and virologic failure: a meta-analysis. Medicine. 2016;95(15).
25. MOPH. National Guidelines on Taskshifting for the Management of HIV/AIDS. Yaounde: Cameroon Ministry of Public Health; 2016.
26. CNLS, Directives nationales des prevention et de prise en charge du VIH au Cameroon. National Guidelines, 2015.
27. Steel, G., J. Nwokike, and M.P. Joshi, Development of a multi-method tool to measure ART adherence in resource-constrained settings: the South Africa experience. RPM Plus, 2007.
28. Vinten G. Taking the threat out of threatening questions. J R Soc Promot Heal. 1998;118(1):10–4.
29. Wagner G, Miller LG. Is the influence of social desirability on patients' self-reported adherence overrated? J Acquir Immune Defic Syndr. 2004; 35(2):203–4.
30. Walsh JC, Mandalia S, Gazzard BG. Responses to a 1 month self-report on adherence to antiretroviral therapy are consistent with electronic data and virological treatment outcome. Aids. 2002;16(2):269–77.
31. Giordano TP, et al. Measuring adherence to antiretroviral therapy in a diverse population using a visual analogue scale. HIV Clin Trials. 2004;5:74–9.
32. Ayuo P, et al. Frequency and factors associated with adherence to and completion of combination antiretroviral therapy for prevention of mother to child transmission in western Kenya. J Int AIDS Soc. 2013;16(1):17994.

33. Igwegbe A, Ugboaja J, Nwajiaku L. Prevalence and determinants of non-adherence to antiretroviral therapy among HIV-positive pregnant women in Nnewi, Nigeria. Int J Med Med Sci. 2010;2(8):238–45.

34. Simoni JM, et al. Self-report measures of antiretroviral therapy adherence: a review with recommendations for HIV research and clinical management. AIDS Behav. 2006;10(3):227–45.

35. Oyugi JH, et al. Multiple validated measures of adherence indicate high levels of adherence to generic HIV antiretroviral therapy in a resource-limited setting. J Acquir Immune Defic Syndr. 2004;36(5):1100–2.

36. Myer L, et al. Beyond "option B+": understanding antiretroviral therapy (ART) adherence, retention in care and engagement in ART Services among pregnant and postpartum women initiating therapy in sub-Saharan Africa. J Acquir Immune Defic Syndr. 2017;75:S115–22.

37. Clouse K, et al. "What they wanted was to give birth; nothing else": barriers to retention in option B+ HIV care among postpartum women in South Africa. J Acquir Immune Defic Syndr. 2014;67(1):e12–8.

38. Shubber Z, et al. Patient-reported barriers to adherence to antiretroviral therapy: a systematic review and meta-analysis. PLoS Med. 2016;13(11): e1002183.

39. Kim MH, et al. Why did I stop? Barriers and facilitators to uptake and adherence to ART in option B+ HIV care in Lilongwe, Malawi. PLoS One. 2016;11(2):e0149527.

40. Fenerty SD, et al. The effect of reminder systems on patients' adherence to treatment. Patient Prefer Adherence. 2012;6:127–35.

41. Hardy H, et al. Randomized controlled trial of a personalized cellular phone reminder system to enhance adherence to antiretroviral therapy. AIDS Patient Care STDs. 2011;25(3):153–61.

42. Mbuagbaw L, Bonono-Momnougui RC, Thabane L. Considerations in using text messages to improve adherence to highly active antiretroviral therapy: a qualitative study among clients in Yaounde, Cameroon. HIV/AIDS (Auckl). 2012;4:45.

18

First trimester medication use in pregnancy in Cameroon: a multi-hospital survey

Aminkeng Zawuo Leke[1,3]* ⓘ, Helen Dolk[2], Maria Loane[2], Karen Casson[2], Nkwati Michel Maboh[1], Susan Etta Maeya[1], Lerry Dibo Ndumbe[1], Pauline Bessem Nyenti[1], Obale Armstrong[1] and Derick Etiendem[1]

Abstract

Background: There is a paucity of epidemiological data on medication use in pregnancy in Cameroon.

Methods: Between March and August 2015, 795 pregnant women attending 8 urban and 12 rural hospitals in Cameroon for antenatal (ANC) or other care were interviewed on first trimester medication use using structured questionnaires. Multivariate logistic regression was used to analyse the association of 18 sociodemographic factors with medication use.

Results: A total of 582 (73.2%) women took at least one orthodox (Western) medication during the first trimester, 543 (68.3%) women a non-pregnancy related orthodox medication, and 336 (42.3%)women a pregnancy related orthodox medication. 44% of the women took anti-infectives including antimalarials (33.6%) and antibiotics (20.8%). The other most common medications were analgesics (48.8%) and antianaemias (38.6%). Sulfadoxine/ pyrimethamine, contraindicated in the first trimester of pregnancy, was the most commonly used antimalarial(13% of women).0.2% of women reported antiretroviral use. Almost 80% of all orthodox medications consumed by women were purchased from the hospital. 12.8% of the women self-prescribed. Health unit and early gestational age at ANC booking were consistent determinants of prescribing of non-pregnancy related, pregnancy related and anti-infective medications. Illness and opinion on the safety of orthodox medications were determinants of the use of non-pregnancy related medications and anti-infectives. Age and parity were associated only with non-pregnancy related medications.

Conclusion: This study has confirmed the observations of studies across Africa indicating the increasing use of medications during pregnancy. This is an indication that access to medicine is improving and more emphasis now must be placed on medication safety systems targeting pregnant women, especially during the first trimester when the risk of teratogenicity is highest.

Keywords: Medication, pregnancy, drug safety, drug use, pharmacoepidemiology, determinants, pharmacovigilance, Cameroon

Background

Pregnant women are excluded from clinical trials for medication efficacy, since the fetus is particularly vulnerable to adverse effects. This means that at the time of marketing, there is no information on human safety in pregnancy. Since premarketing teratogenicity testing in animals is not enough to predict risks in humans, for the majority of medications the safety of their use during pregnancy is still not clearly defined [1]. Safety information needed by women and clinicians in order to be able to weigh the risks and benefits of different treatment options must therefore come from post-marketing pharmacoepidemiological studies. Within this context, epidemiological studies investigating medication use and safety in pregnancy are of paramount importance.

Minimal attention has been given to the subject of medication use and safety during pregnancy in developing countries which, ironically, have higher rates of adverse maternal/fetal outcomes, greater drug quality control

* Correspondence: zawuol@gmail.com; zawuo@biakahc.org
[1]Department of Nursing, School of Health Sciences, Biaka University Institute of Buea-Cameroon, PO BOX 77, Buea, Cameroon
[3]Office of the Deputy Vice Chancellor i/c Research/Cooperation/Quality, Biaka Universit Institute of Buea, PO Box 77-SWR, Buea, Cameroon
Full list of author information is available at the end of the article

problems compared to developed countries, and less resources to care for the babies born with problems relating
to their exposure in utero. In Cameroon for example,
WHO (2017) [2] statistics showed a maternal mortality
rate of 596/100.000 (ranking 14th in the world) and a neonatal mortality rate of 87.9/1000 (21 times higher than
that in the UK). Drug safety constraints in Sub-Saharan
Africa countries like Cameroon include: lack of strict control mechanisms as to which drugs are accepted or not accepted into the country, hence circulation of substandard,
counterfeit, and contaminated drugs [3]; lack of stringent
prescription regulations, e.g in Cameroon nurses are
allowed to prescribe highly specialized medications such
as psychotropics [4]; high rate of self-medication; availability of most medications over-the-counter; and common
use of traditional herbs [5] which are believed by many
users to be more potent than orthodox medicine and to
have no adverse effects [6]. In such a system, there are
high chances of pregnant women consuming potentially
teratogenic medications, including those categorized as
contraindicated in pregnancy.

While data on medication use are critical in understanding the depth of medication safety concerns, understanding the determinants of medication use can
provide valuable insights as to which subgroup of
women could be at higher risk of consuming potentially
teratogenic medications [7]. Such data could be valuable
to public health authorities in designing targeted interventions. The few studies conducted in Africa have
found setting type (urban/rural), history of negative
pregnancy outcome, illness during pregnancy, gravidity,
pregnancy planning and level of education of healthcare
provider to be significant predictors of medication use
[8, 9]. As determinants of medication use could vary
from context to context [10], it is difficult to extrapolate
data across different contexts.

This medication use survey provides data on the
prevalence, types and determinants of orthodox medication use by pregnant women in Cameroon, the first survey of this population. Results regarding herbal or
traditional medication use will be reported separately.

Methods
This cross sectional hospital based medication use survey was conducted during a six month period (March to
August 2015) in twenty hospitals across rural and urban
settings of the southwest region of Cameroon. Taking
into consideration the total number of live births in
South West Cameroon for 2013 (12,861 births of approximately 6,687 urban and 6,174 rural), a 6 months
data collection period, and a 50% response distribution
(worst case scenario), maximum sample size needed was
estimated at approximately 374 for both urban and rural
strata.

We used a two stage cluster sampling technique: in
the first step, eligible hospitals were randomly selected
and in the second step, all eligible women within the selected hospitals attending during the study period were
invited to participate.

Both private and government hospitals were eligible to
participate if they had an annual delivery rate of over
one hundred and two hundred for rural and urban settings respectively. Out of forty-one eligible hospitals
(twenty-two urban and nineteen rural), 20 were randomly selected.

All pregnant women attending the selected hospitals
on the days the researchers were in attendance (registered for antenatal clinics or not) were eligible to participate. To limit recall bias and to target the period within
first trimester, only women with a gestation of three to
seven months were eligible to participate in the survey.
The pregnant women were recruited as they came for
antenatal visits or in a small number of cases, for hospital consultation. Out of eight hundred and seventeen
eligible women approached, seven hundred and
ninety-five agreed to participate in the study (97.3% response rate).The observed distribution of the women
into urban (55.2%) and rural (44.8%) settings of residence matched the expected distribution in the general
population. Similarly, the proportion of women sampled
in each health district within the data collection period
was comparable to that of 2013 delivery data.

Existing literature on medication use and safety were
reviewed to facilitate the design of a questionnaire to be
used by interviewers (Additional file 1). The questionnaire
was designed to facilitate recall (e.g. the woman had to define the three months of her first trimester (exposure
period of interest) prior to completing the section on
medication exposure; the section on medication exposure
was followed by a section on first trimester illnesses so as
to validate data on exposure given (for example, if a
woman reported having malaria during the first trimester,
one would verify whether she reported taking an antimalarial in the previous section on medication exposure).

A picture guide of orthodox and traditional medications was developed to facilitate recall. In Cameroon, patients have individual hospital books which they bring
along during hospital visits. Antenatal care (ANC) files
kept in the hospitals contain data only on medications
prescribed during routine ANC visits. Hence medication
data for other hospital visits could only be obtained from
hospital books. When available, the data collectors used
antenatal files and the hospital books to complement
and validate data obtained from interviews. In a
sub-study involving 84 participants to evaluate the relevance of using the hospital books (Table 1), we observed
that 10.3% of the exposures would have been missed
without the use of hospital books.

Table 1 Comparison of source of medication exposure (N=84 Women)[a]

Medication mentioned in interview but not found in hospital book n (%)	Medications found in hospital book but not mentioned during interview n (%)	Medications mentioned during interviews and also found in hospital book n (%)	Total n (%)
51 (16.0)	33 (10.3)	236 (73.8)	320 (100)

[a] Excluding those without a hospital book and those that did not take medications according to the hospital book

In order to ensure standardized collection of data, eight nurses working in the areas of research and education were trained as data collectors and provided with a guidance note to assist them during data collection. A pilot study enabled the data collectors to feed back to adjust the questionnaire and various aspects of the data collection process.

Actual data collection took place from the months of March to August 2015. Using the predesigned questionnaire, the data collectors conducted one-on-one interviews for consented women in private rooms of the hospital to obtain data on first trimester medication exposure.

Following the approach of Baraka et al (2014) [10], orthodox medications were grouped as pregnancy related medications and non-pregnancy related medications. Pregnancy related medications were defined as routine medications taken not for ill-health, but to support the health of the mother and the developing fetus. These included anti-anemias, mineral supplements and vitamins.

The Anatomical Therapeutic Chemical Classification System of the WHO was used to classify drugs into therapeutic classes. Drugs were also classified according to the old version of United States Food and Drug Administration (FDA) pregnancy risk classification (A, B, C, D or X; see foot note in Fig 6). The FDA classification of each drug was verified from various sources including normal Google search, the Internet Drug Index (RxList) and Drugs .com. Drugs for which no FDA class could be obtained were classified as category "U".

Epi-info 3.1 was used for data entry and cleaning while all data analyses were conducted using SPSS version 22. Prevalence of medication use was determined by dividing the number of women who took at least one medication by the total number of participating women. Differences in the prevalence of medication use within categorical variables were tested using the Pearson Chi-squared test of independence with significance level set at 0.05. Multivariatelogistic regression was used to identify the determinants of medication use. Using backward conditional logistic regression, all the variables were initially included in the model. Then, variables were removed from the model based on significance level set at 0.10, if their removal did not significantly worsen the overall prediction of the model [11]. Variables (all categorical) entered into the model were: health unit (individual primary or secondary/tertiary healthcare facility), setting of hospital (urban/rural), maternal age (13-17 years, 18-25 years, 26-35 years and 36-45 years), marital status, highest level of education attained, living conditions, level of alcohol consumption, gravidity, parity, previous pregnancy termination, gestational age at interview, gestational age at first booking, pregnancy planning, gestational age at pregnancy awareness, opinion on the safety of orthodox medication, safety advice and illness during first trimester. We investigated determinants for general orthodox medication use, pregnancy related medication use, and anti-infectives use. Results were reported as adjusted odds ratios and 95%CI. Determinants of medication use were defined as those variables retained in the final logistic regression model.

Results

A total of twenty hospitals (eight urban and twelve rural) were involved in this study with a sample size of seven hundred and ninety-five participants (four hundred and thirty-nine urban and three hundred and fifty-six rural, Table 2). Table 2 presents data on the general characteristics of the women and their association with medication intake.

The age of the women ranged from thirteen to forty-five years, with the highest academic level for most being primary (25.8%) or secondary (41.4%) (Table 2).

Three quarters (75.1%) of the women lived in houses with pit/external toilets. About a third (36.9%) of the women were in their first pregnancy. Only 25% of the women registered for ANC within the first trimester. Some women (5.5%) although they had visited the hospital had not registered for ANC.

Based on the definition of pregnancy planning as used in this study, 37.7% of the women did not engage in sexual intercourse with the intention of getting pregnant. However, the majority (59.9%) of the women said they were aware of their pregnancy within the first month of gestation.

More than half (54.5%) reported they consume alcohol in pregnancy.

Table 2 Factors associated with maternal use of orthodox medication (N=795)

Factor	Total n (%) 795(100)	At least one orthodox medication n (%) 582(73.2)	Chi Sq.	df	P-value
Health unit			135.0	19	0.000
A[r,p]	43(5.4)	21 (48.8)			
B[r,g]	37(4.7)	30 (81.1)			
C[r,g]	29(3.6)	23 (79.3)			
D[r,g]	22(2.8)	20 (90.9)			
E[u,p]	29(3.6)	27 (93.1)			
F[u,g]	39(4.9)	23 (59.0)			
G[r,g]	36(4.5)	19 (52.8)			
H[r,g]	35(4.4)	28 (80.0)			
I[r,g]	26(3.3)	22 (84.6)			
J[u,g]	44(5.5)	32 (72.7)			
K[u,p]	50(6.3)	49 (98.0)			
L[u,g]	15(1.9)	14 (93.3)			
M[u,g]	67(8.4)	52 (77.6)			
N[u,p]	18(2.3)	17 (94.4)			
O[r,g]	108(13.6)	45 (41.7)			
P[r,g]	21(2.6)	18 (85.7)			
Q[r,g]	45(5.7)	42 (93.3)			
R[r,g]	56(7.0)	39 (69.6)			
S[r,g]	49(6.2)	36 (73.5)			
T[u,g]	26(3.3)	25 (96.2)			
Health Districts			43.9	6	0.000
Fontem[a]	43(5.4)	21 (48.8)			
Mbonge	66(8.3)	53 (80.3)			
Kumba	90(11.3)	70 (77.8)			
Muyuka	97(12.2)	69 (71.1)			
Buea[a]	194(24.4)	164 (84.5)			
Tiko[a]	174(21.9)	105 (60.3)			
Limbe	131(16.5)	100 (76.3)			
Setting type			1.4	1	0.235
Urban	439(55.2)	314 (71.5)			
Rural	356(44.8)	268 (75.3)			
Age (years)			1.9	3	0.594
13-17	41(5.2)	24 (58.5)			
18-25	380(47.8)	285 (75.0)			
26-35	335(42.1)	243 (72.5)			
36-45	39(4.9)	30 (76.9)			
Marital status		()	2.5	4	0.645
Married	486(61.1)	352 (72.4)			
Divorced	6(0.8)	4 (66.7)			
Engaged	64(8.1)	44 (68.8)			
Cohabitating (No formal engagement)	68(8.6)	54 (79.4)			
Single	171(21.5)	128 (74.9)			
Level of Education			33.9	4	0.000
Never went to school	19(2.4)	13 (68.4)			
Primary[a]	205(25.8)	123 (60.0)			

Table 2 Factors associated with maternal use of orthodox medication (N=795) *(Continued)*

Factor	Total n (%) 795(100)	At least one orthodox medication n (%) 582(73.2)	Chi Sq.	df	P-value
Secondary	329(41.4)	245 (74.5)			
High School	129(16.2)	101 (78.3)			
University/Professional[a]	113(14.2)	100 (88.5)			
Living condition			13.8	2	0.001
House with Pit /external toilet[a]	597(75.1)	417 (69.8)			
Renting self-contained studio	104(13.1)	86 (82.7)			
Renting or Own a self-contained House	94(11.8)	79 (84.0)			
Level of Alcohol consumption in pregnancy			0.4	3	0.937
Do not drink Alcohol	362(45.5)	264 (72.9)			
Drink Occasionally	324(40.8)	237 (73.1)			
1-2 bottles of beer/glass of wine a week	86(10.8)	65 (75.6)			
Greater than 1 bottles of beer/glass of wine a day	23(2.9)	16 (69.6)			
Gravidity			4.6	4	0.332
1	293(36.9)	221 (75.4)			
2	197(24.8)	145 (73.6)			
3	152(19.1)	114 (75.0)			
4	94(11.8)	64 (68.1)			
≥5	59(7.4)	38 (64.4)			
Parity			7.5	3	0.057
0	323(40.6)	236 (73.1)			
1	202(25.4)	155 (76.7)			
2	145(18.2)	111 (76.6)			
≥3	125(15.7)	80 (64.0)			
Terminations/miscarriages			1.9	2	0.385
0	424(53.3)	308 (72.6)			
1	56(7.0)	40 (71.4)			
2	22(2.8)	13 (59.1)			
GA at interview			7.6	3	0.056
4th month	212(26.7)	168 (79.2)			
5th month	230(28.9)	171 (74.3)			
6th month	294(37.0)	203 (69.0)			
7th month	59(7.4)	40 (67.8)			
GA at ANC booking			72.8	3	0.000
< 13 weeks[a]	199(25.0)	184 (92.5)			
13 - 24 weeks[a]	529(66.5)	369 (69.8)			
25 - 28 weeks	23(2.9)	12 (52.2)			
Not registered for ANC[a]	44(5.5)	17 (38.6)			
Pregnancy planning		()	2.0	2	0.372
Yes	474(59.6)	353 (74.5)			
No	300(37.7)	216 (72.0)			
Unknown	21(2.6)	13 (61.9)			
GA of pregnancy awareness			1.1	3	0.749
1st month	476(59.9)	346 (72.7)			
2nd month	131(16.5)	97 (74.0)			
≥3th month	32(4.0)	26 (81.3)			
Unknown	156(19.6)	113 (72.4)			

Table 2 Factors associated with maternal use of orthodox medication (N=795) *(Continued)*

Factor	Total n (%) 795(100)	At least one orthodox medication n (%) 582(73.2)	Chi Sq.	df	P-value
Number of diseases/ailments			162.6	6	0.000
0[a]	139(17.5)	52 (37.4)			
1[a]	152(19.1)	90 (59.2)			
2	142(17.9)	115 (81.0)			
3[a]	116(14.6)	104 (89.7)			
4[a]	108(13.6)	100 (92.6)			
5[a]	67(8.4)	61 (91.0)			
≥6	71(8.9)	60 (84.5)			
Number (types) of acute conditions			31.8	6	0.000
0	146(18.4)	56 (38.4)			
1[a]	154(19.4)	50 (32.5)			
2	145(18.2)	71 (49.0)			
3[a]	129(16.2)	74 (57.4)			
4[a]	106(13.3)	62 (58.5)			
5	61(7.7)	23 (37.7)			
≥6	54(6.8)	20 (37.0)			
Number (types) of chronic conditions			7.7	2	0.023
0	696(87.5)	300 (43.1)			
1[a]	89(11.2)	52 (58.4)			
≥2	10(1.3)	4 (40.0)			
Season			0.0	1	0.933
Dry	738 (92.8)	540 (73.2)			
Rainy	57(7.2)	42 (73.7)			
Opinion on safety of Orthodox medicationduring pregnancy			1.3	3	0.026
Yes, it is always safe	551(69.3)	395 (71.7)			
Yes, safe but depends[a]	157(19.7)	129 (82.2)			
No, never safe	21(2.6)	15 (71.4)			
I don't know	66(8.3)	43 (65.2)			
Participant received medication safety advice during current pregnancy			18.4	2	0.000
Yes[a]	468(58.9)	369 (78.8)			
No[a]	287(36.1)	187 (65.2)			
Can't remember	40(5.0)	26 (65.0)			

[a]Statistical significance as calculated from the adjusted standardised residuals
r Rural hospital, *u* Urban hospital, *p* Private hospital, *g* Government hospital
Chi Sq Chi-squared value based on test of independence, *df* degrees of freedom
P = 0.05 indicates a statistically significant association based on the Chi-squared test of independence

First trimester orthodox medication use

Almost three quarters (73.2%, n=582) women took at least one orthodox medicationduring the first trimester of pregnancy (Table 2). Out of the five hundred and eighty-two women who took an orthodox medication,30.9% took a non-pregnancy related orthodox medication only and 4.9% took a pregnancy related orthodox medication only (Fig. 1), most women taking both categories.

Fifteen different classes of medications were reported by the women (Fig. 2). Analgesics, antianaemias, antimalarials, antibacterials and mineral supplements were the top five classes of medications consumed. Ferrous sulphate (Fefol) was the most commonly used iron and folic acid prophylactic supplement containing 65mg of elemental iron and 0.4mg of folic acid.

With the high burden of infectious diseases in Cameroon, we paid particular attention to the anti-infectives data. 44.9% of women took one or more anti-infectives. Antimalarials (33.6%) followed by antibacterials (20.8%) were the most commonly consumed categories of anti-infectives (Fig. 3). Sulfadoxine/pyrimethamine and Quinine; and Amoxicillin and Metronidazole were the most commonly

Table 3 Logistic regression model for predicting consumption of non-pregnancy related orthodox medication (N=795)

Variables	Crude model					Adjusted model			
	Exposed (%)	OR	95% C.I		P-value	OR	95% C.I		P-value
			Lower	Upper			Lower	Upper	
Health unit(20)[b]					0.000[a]				0.000[a]
Maternal age (years)					0.095[a]				0.049[a]
18-25	71.3	1	-	-	-	1	-	-	ref
13-17	53.7	0.5	0.2	0.9		0.1	0.0	0.8	
26-35	66.3	0.8	0.6	1.1		0.6	0.4	1.1	
36-45	71.8	1.0	0.5	2.1		1.3	0.5	3.8	
Parity					0.107[a]				0.006[a]
0	68.7	1	-	-	-	1	-	-	ref
1	70.8	1.1	0.8	1.6		2.9	1.0	8.6	
2	71.7	1.2	0.8	1.8		4.0	1.3	12.7	
≥3	59.2	0.7	0.4	1.0		1.5	0.5	4.9	
Gestational age at ANC booking					0.000[a]				0.001[a]
13 - 24 weeks	65.8	1	-	-	-	1	-	-	ref
< 13 weeks	83.9	2.7	1.8	4.1		2.6	1.3	5.2	
25 - 28 weeks	52.2	0.6	0.2	1.3		1.6	0.4	6.4	
Not registered for ANC	36.4	0.3	0.2	0.6		0.3	0.1	0.8	
Illness during first trimester					0.000[a]				0.000[a]
No	32.8	1	-	-	-	1	-	-	ref
Yes	79.4	7.9	5.5	11.3		11.1	6.0	20.4	
Opinion on safety of orthodox medication					0.180[a]				0.078[a]
Yes, it is always safe	67.2	1	-	-	-	1	-	-	ref
Yes, safe but depends	75.2	1.5	1.0	2.2		0.7	0.4	1.3	
No, never safe	66.7	1.0	0.4	2.5		0.1	0.0	0.8	
I don't know	62.1	0.8	0.5	1.4		0.5	0.2	1.3	

[a] Overall statistical significance of variable within model
[b] See Additional file 2 for complete table showing statistics for all health units
OR Odds ratio, CI Confidence interval, r Rural hospital, u Urban hospital, p Private hospital, g Government hospital

consumed antimalarials and antibacterials respectively (Figs. 4 and 5).

FDA pregnancy risk classification of drugs

Most of the women took a category B (74.4%) or C (61.5%) medication (Fig. 6). A potentially teratogenic medication was defined as those belonging to FDA categories C, D or X. There was no intake of a category X medication. However, out of the five hundred and eighty-two women who took orthodox medications, a large proportion (65.5%) took a category C and/or D drug. Projected to the entire sample of 795, this corresponded to 48% of women. Drugs belonging to category D included: phenobarbital (one exposure), ibuprofen (nineteen exposures), diclofenac (eleven exposures), fluconazole (five exposures), and magnesium (three exposures). Antimalarials constituted the bulk of this proportion as they are mainly classified as FDA category C. When antimalarials were excluded, the overall consumption of potentially teratogenic medications reduced to 17% of the total study sample.

Sources and prescribers of orthodox medications

Almost 80% of all orthodox medications consumed by women were purchased from the hospital. Other sources were regular market (10.1%), commercial pharmacy (6.1%), medicine store (5.1%) and unknown (0.9%).

The majority (82%) of women took medications based on prescription from their healthcare provider in the hospital, but 12.8% of the women self-prescribed at least one medication, and 3.7% took at least one medication recommended by a friend or relative.

Determinants of orthodox medication use

Determinants of use were determined for three groups of orthodox medications: non-pregnancy related (Table 3), pregnancy related (Table 4) and anti-infectives (Table 5).

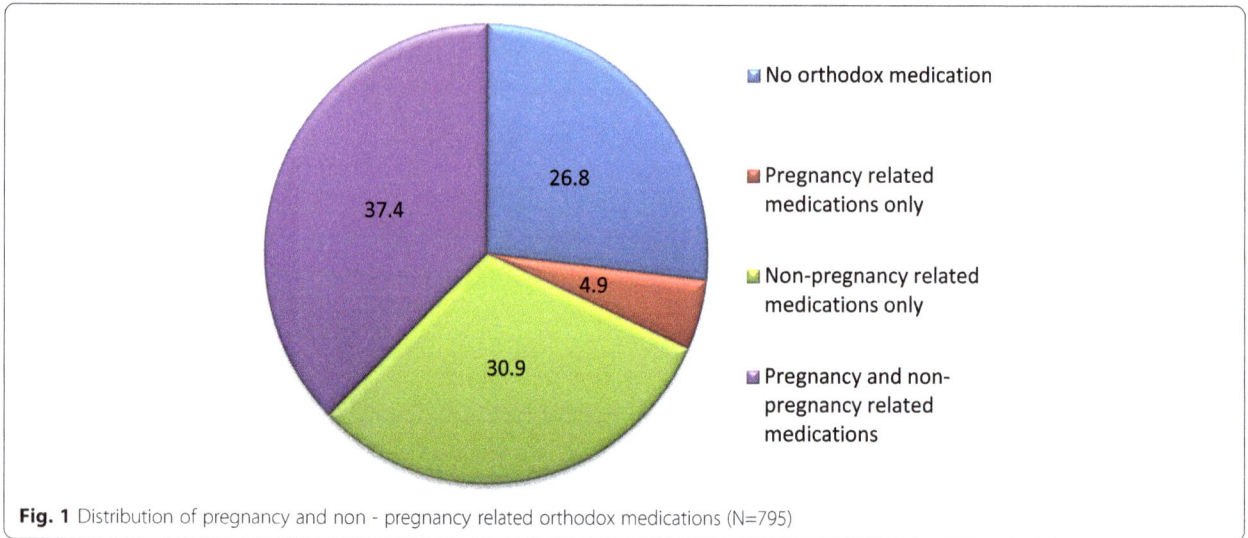

Fig. 1 Distribution of pregnancy and non - pregnancy related orthodox medications (N=795)

Health unit and gestational age at ANC booking were constant detrminants across the three categories. Women who booked for ANC early (within first trimester) were more likely to take any of the three groups of orthodox medications ((AOR: 2.6; CI=1.3-5.2); (AOR: 1.4; CI=0.9-2.4); (AOR: 2.7; CI=1.6-4.5); for non-pregnancy related medications, pregnancy related medications and anti-infectives respectively). The variation in medication use by Health Unit was wide (Table 2) and persisted after adjusting for other factors (Tables 3, 4, 5, see Additional file 2 for complete table showing all health units). Parity and age were associated with non-pregnancy related orthodox medications (Table 3). Younger women (<17years) were less likely (AOR: 0.1; CI=0.0-0.8), while multiparous women were more likely (e.g. those with a parity of 2 (AOR: 4.0; CI=1.3-12.7)) to take a non-pregnancy related orthodox

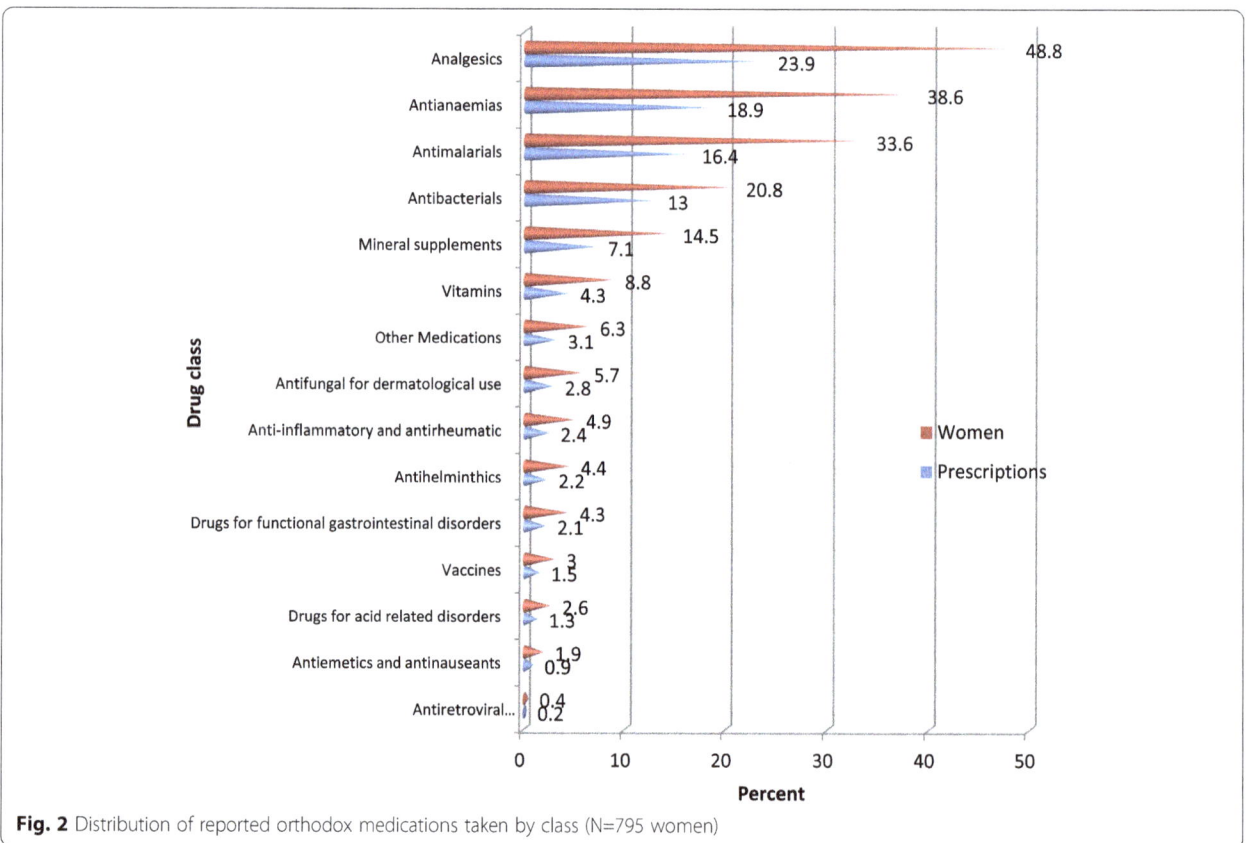

Fig. 2 Distribution of reported orthodox medications taken by class (N=795 women)

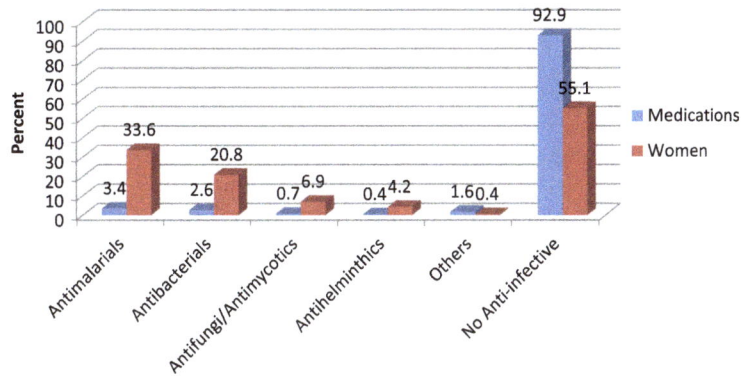

Fig. 3 Frequency of consumption of class of anti-infectives (N=795 women)

medication. High level of education, receipt of safety advice, and rural setting type were associated with more use of pregnancy related medication (Table 4). Illness and opinion on the safety of orthodox medications were associated with use of seen as predictors for non-pregnancy related medications and anti-infectives, but not pregnancy related medications.

Discussion

This study showed that the overall prevalence of first trimester orthodox medication consumption among pregnant women in SW Cameroon was 73.2%. When narrowed down to non-pregnancy related orthodox medications, the rate of consumption stood at 68.3%. It is apparent that these prevalences are high compared to those reported in Africa and other developing countries. Out of 1,268 women interviewed during ANC visits in 8 hospitals in Ethiopia, only 29.9% reported at least one drug exposure during the first trimester [12]. This low prevalence of drug exposure compared to the current study could be as a result of recall bias in the Ethiopian study as most women were in their third trimester. Two other studies in Brazil and Pakistan, based on sample sizes of approximately four thousand, reported an overall first trimester

exposure prevalence of 22.2% and 11.0% respectively [13, 14]. In the Brazilian study, women were interviewed within 24hrs of delivery. As this period is farther away from the first trimester, coupled with the stress of delivery, it may have been difficult for these women to recall first trimester exposures. The study in Pakistan reviewed only prescriptions given to women during ANC visits - hence over-the-counter medications and medications prescribed elsewhere (e.g. by GP) would have been missed. One study in China [15], based on prospectively collected data reported a similar prevalence (75%) to that seen in our study.

Unlike non-pregnancy related orthodox medications with a high prevalence, first trimester use of pregnancy related orthodox medications in this study was low (42.3%), suggesting underuse of these medications. This observation appears to be true also in other African countries. Based on the entire pregnancy, prevalencesof 42% and 34% have been reported in Nigeria [16] and Ethiopia [12] respectively. Two studies in Nigeria [17] and Tanzania [18] reported higher prevalences (76%, and 94% respectively) of folic acid intake. However, these results were based on exposures across the entire pregnancy and are likely to decrease when restricted to the

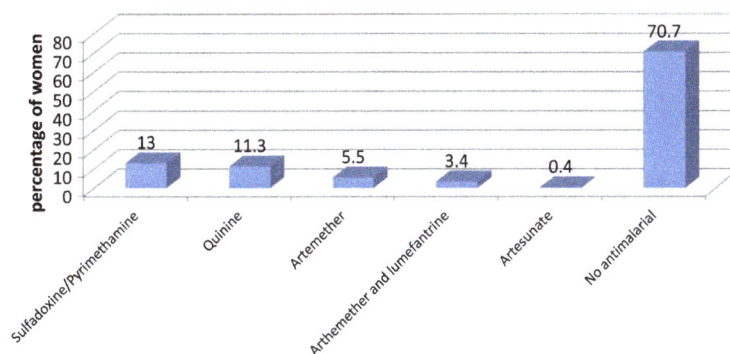

Fig. 4 Exposure of women to antimalarials (N=795). NB 30% of women who took a non sulfadoxine/pyrimethamineantimalaria did not report any malaria illness

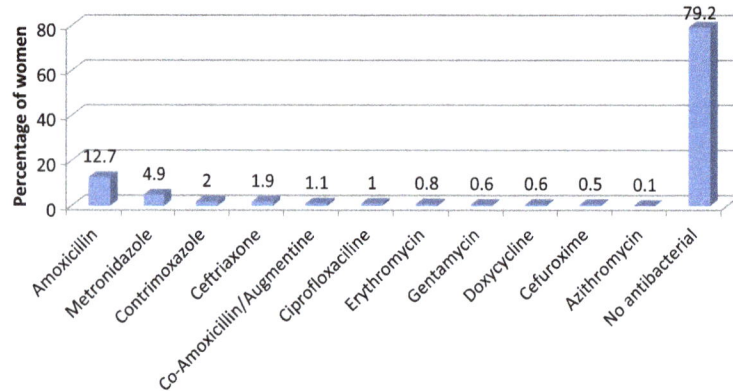

Fig. 5 Exposure of women to antibacterials

first trimester as studies in Africa have always reported a far greater proportion (about 40% greater) of medication exposure in the second and third trimesters compared to the first trimester [12, 19]. In our study, 75% of the women registered for ANC after the first trimester. Almost half (46%) of the women booked for ANC late (after 18 weeks), despite WHO recommendations to book by 17 weeks [20], and the women were dependent almost solely on medication given at the hospital. This could help explain the low first trimester intake of pregnancy-related medications which are mainly given during ANC visits.

The most commonly reported group of orthodox medications were analgesics. This seems to corroborate a similar study in Nigeria [16]. As observed in this study and as is the case in sub-Saharan Africa, the intake of analgesics was very high. This could be explained by the high prevalence of infectious diseases in sub- Saharan Africa often associated with fever for which analgesics are indicated. In fact, the intake of analgesics such as paracetamol when one suspects malaria is so common that when the women in our study were asked what paracetamol was indicated for, a few said "it is an accompaniment of antimalarial."

Anti-anaemias were the most common pregnancy related medications and second most consumed group of medications. Achidi and colleagues (2005) [21] reported that 70% of women registering at their first ANC clinic in SW Cameroon suffer from anaemia. Blood loss is one of the main causes of maternal mortality in sub-Saharan Africa. This is mainly due to infections (mainly malaria) that reduce blood haemoglobin levels and blood loss during delivery (post-partum haemorrhage (PPH)) [22]. Anti-anaemias are, therefore, more highly consumed in sub-Saharan

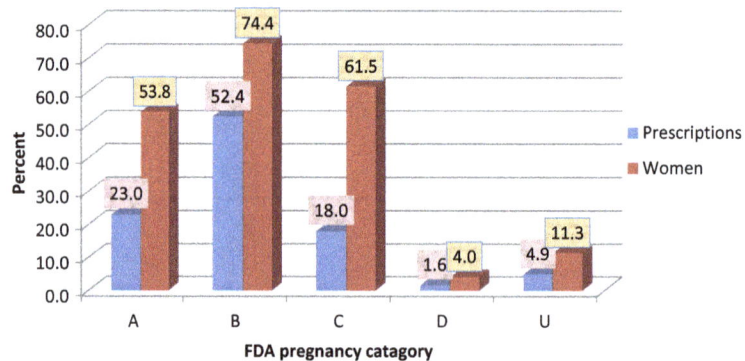

'FDA Pregnancy Category System (FDA)

Category	Description
A	Controlled studies show no risk. Adequate, well-controlled studies in pregnant women have failed to demonstrate risk to the fetus.
B	No evidence of risk in humans. Either animal study shows risk, but human findings do not; or, if no adequate human studies have been performed, animal findings are negative for risk.
C	Risk cannot be ruled out. Human studies are lacking, and animal studies are either positive for fetal risk or lacking as well. However, potential benefits may justify potential risk.
D	Positive evidence of risk. Investigational or postmarketing data show risk to the fetus. Nevertheless, potential benefits may outweigh the potential risk.
X	Contraindicated in pregnancy. Studies in animals or humans, or investigational or postmarketing reports, have shown fetal risk, which clearly outweighs any possible benefit to the patient.

Fig. 6 Othodox medication by FDA pregnancy categories (N=582) (based only on women who took orthodox medication, FDA category U=Undefined)

Table 4 Logistic regression model for predicting consumption of pregnancy related orthodox medication (N=795)

Variables	Crude model					Adjusted model			
	Exposed (%)	OR	95% C.I		P-value	OR	95% C.I		P-value
			Lower	Upper			Lower	Upper	
Health unit(20)[b]					0.000[a]				0.000[a]
Highest level of Education					0.000[a]				0.072[a]
Secondary	37.4	1	-	-	-	1	-	-	ref
Never went to school	38.0	1.0	0.7	1.5		0.9	0.5	1.4	
Primary	26.3	0.6	0.2	1.7		0.2	0.0	0.6	
High School	45.0	1.4	0.9	2.1		1.0	0.5	1.7	
University/Professional	63.7	2.9	1.9	4.6		1.4	0.7	3.0	
Gestational age at ANC booking					-				0.004[a]
13 - 24 weeks	39.5	1	-	-	0.000[a]	1	-	-	ref
< 13 weeks	59.8	2.3	1.6	3.2		1.4	0.9	2.4	
25 - 28 weeks	8.7	0.1	0.0	0.6		0.4	0.1	1.9	
Not registered for ANC	13.6	0.2	0.1	0.6		0.2	0.1	0.6	
Participant received safety advice					0.001[a]				0.057[a]
Yes	47.6	1	-	-	-	-	-	-	ref
No	34.5	0.6	0.4	0.8		0.6	0.4	0.9	
Can't remember	35.0	0.6	0.3	1.2		0.7	0.2	2.1	
Setting type					0.609[a]				0.042[a]
Urban	41.5	1	-	-	-	1	-	-	ref
Rural	43,3	1.1	0.8	1.4		3.3	1.0	10.2	

[a]Overall statistical significance of variable within model
[b] See Additional file 2 for complete table showing statistics for all health units
OR Odds ratio, CI Confidence interval, r Rural hospital, u Urban hospital, p Private hospital, g Government hopsital

Table 5 Logistic regression model for predicting consumption of anti-infectives (N=795)

Variables	Crude model					Adjusted model			
	Exposed (%)	OR	95% C.I		P-value	OR	95% C.I		P-value
			Lower	Upper			Lower	Upper	
Health unit(20)[b]					0.000[a]				0.001[a]
Gestational age at ANC booking					0.00[a]				0.000[a]
13 - 24 weeks	42.2	1	-	-	-	1	-	-	ref
< 13 weeks	62.8	2.3	1.7			2.7	1.6	4.5	
25 - 28 weeks	17.4	0.3	0.1			0.6	0.1	2.4	
Not registered for ANC	11.4	0.2	0.1			0.3	0.1	0.9	
Illness during first trimester									
No	20.6	-	-	-	-	-	-	-	ref
Yes	52.5	4.2	2.9	6.3	0.000[a]	3.7	2.1	6.4	0.000[a]
Opinion on safety of orthodox medication					0.098[a]				0.056[a]
Yes, it is always safe	46.6	1	-	-	-	1	-	-	ref
Yes, safe but depends	45.9	1.0	0.7	1.4		0.6	0.4	1.1	
No, never safe	33.3	0.6	0.2	1.4		0.2	0.0	1.2	
I don't know	31.8	0.5	0.3	0.9		0.4	0.2	1.0	

[a]Overall statistical significance of variable within model
[b] See Additional file 2 for complete table showing statistics for all health units
OR Odds ratio, CI Confidence interval, r Rural hospital, u Urban hospital, p Private hospital, g Government hospital

African countries than elsewhere in the world. The observed prevalence (38.6%) of anti-anaemias in this study was, therefore, very low compared to the expected70% prevalence of anaemia. Again, the low intake of anti-anaemias by women in our study could be related to late ANC registration as these drugs are usually prescribed during the ANC visit as prophylaxis.

Sub-Saharan Africa is known to have the largest burden of infectious diseases in the world. It was not surprising, therefore, that anti-infectives were widely used in this study population and that anti-malarials and anti-bacterials were the 3rd and 4th most commonly used orthodox medications by 33.6% and 20.8% of women respectively. However, when compared to the 11-17% prevalence of anti-malarialsinother studies [15, 16, 18] in Nigeria and Tanzania with a similar context to Cameroon, the rates reported here appear to be very high. These studies in Nigeria and Tanzania also reported a 5-15% prevalence of anti-bacterials use. While these studies had a limitation of focusing only in urban areas with possibly lower rates of disease compared to rural areas (although no urban-rural differences in anti-infective use were observed in the current study), the values reported seem surprisingly low compared to the current study.

Sulfadoxine/pyrimethamine (FDA category C), which is contraindicated during the first trimester and which is uniquely indicated as malaria prophylaxis from the second trimester [23], was the most commonly used anti-malarial (13% of women) during the first trimester. Analyses of the data from this study suggest that these drugs were actually used to treat malaria and not taken as preventive. This is in contrast to the observation in Tanzania where, based on the entire pregnancy period, artemether/lumefantrine was the most common anti-malarial (8.9% of women) used to treat malaria [18]. However, the Tanzanian study also found that 1.5% of women took Sulfadoxine/pyrimethamine for the treatment of malaria. When used to treat malarial infection, this anti-malarial has a huge potential to develop resistance – a major problem WHO has been struggling to deal with since the drug was first recommended as malaria prophylaxis in pregnancy in 1998 [24]. Given that most of these medications were obtained from the hospital, it is likely that the health personnel are the main contributors to this questionable decision with regard to risk/benefit analysis. There are, of course, many other reasons for this error to occur such as not knowing whether the woman was pregnant, or lack of well trained nurses on the use of these medications. However, one has to be careful about the accuracy of reporting by the women. It is possible that some women reported later use as first trimester; although this problem would not have been unique to Sulfadoxine/pyrimethamine.

Important also to highlight is the fact that almost one-third (30%) of women who did not report any malaria illness took a non-prophylactic antimalarial. Indeed, in countries like Cameroon where health care is paid from private pockets, it is common knowledge that patients could be loaded with unnecessary medications in a bid to fill the coffers of the hospital. Nevertheless, it remains a priority to ensure access to antimalarials for all pregnant women as this is essential for their health and survival, and that of their babies.

Most of the women got their orthodox medications mainly from the hospital, as also found in Nigeria [6]. This is an important finding which suggests that safety measures can be particularly targeted at hospitals rather than pharmacies or other sources. However, as indicated in this study, there was a missed opportunity during general consultation when healthcare providers insufficiently prescribed pregnancy related medications and seemingly failed to get the women to register for ANC.

More than two-thirds of women were of the opinion that orthodox medicines are always safe, indicating that women assume safety of medication and professionals need to introduce the element of balancing benefits and risks.

Based on FDA risk classification, it was reassuring to know that women in this study were not exposed to any known teratogenic medications (FDA category X). However, it was noted that up to 17% (excluding women exposed to antimalarials) of women were exposed to at least one FDA category C or D medication (potentially teratogenic).

Our study is the first in Africa to have critically examined a variety of sociodemographic determinants for medication use, and to have divided pregnancy-related and non-pregnancy related medications which were found to have different determinants. Only two studies in Ethiopia have attempted to examine predictors of medication use in pregnancy using a multivariate approach but have major limitations, and it is difficult to compare the results with our own. We found, perhaps not surprisingly, that medication intake is greater where there is illness, but we found that there were determinants of medication intake over and above illness, which suggest differences in behaviour, knowledge or attitudes. This was true of both pregnancy and non-pregnancy related medication. How early the woman booked for ANC was also a strong determinant, particularly of pregnancy related medications. Young maternal age was associated with much lower use of non-pregnancy related medications, but this did not apply specifically to anti-infectives. Women with one or two previous pregnancies were more likely to take non-pregnancy related medications than women in their first pregnancy, or those with three or more previous children, but again this did not apply specifically to anti-infectives.

Health unit was a constant determinant for intake of any of the three categories of orthodox medication suggesting that health units differ in their prescribing behaviour, irrespective of illness status and sociodemographic characteristics of individual women. In Cameroon, private and government hospitals differ in many aspects, including the cost of services (private hospitals being more expensive) and the quality of services (private hospitals giving more attention to patients). Nurses are the highest staff level in health centres, compared to tertiary hospitals which have doctors and specialists).

Those with a primary education were less likely to take pregnancy related medications; It is possible that the more educated a woman is, the more likely she is to understand why she has to take a medication when she is not sick. However, ability to pay may also play a part. Those who had received safety advice were also more likely to take pregnancy related medications. Perhaps as pregnancy related medications are to be taken for a longer period during pregnancy than most orthodox medications, women need safety advice to reassure them. Women in rural areas were more likely to take pregnancy related medications, perhaps because these medications are highly subsidised in government health centres (primary health units) which are the only hospitals in most rural areas, whereas tertiary health units with less subsidised drugs are in urban areas.

Strengths and limitations

This study had many strengths as well as limitations. The study is based on interviews with women and, therefore, all medications reported were consumed rather than only prescribed. The sample was designed to be representative of pregnant women in SW Cameroon, with respect both to urban/rural residence, and different types of health facility attended, while other studies in Africa have used less representative samples [12, 14, 15].

Recall bias was limited as the period of interview was mainly within the second trimester. A few women interviewed at the 7th month of gestation reported lower intake of medication, however, this was not significant in multivariate analysis. Additionally, participants' hospital books were used to complement data reported during interviews and medication picture guides were used to enhance recall. In a validation analysis, it was verified that the hospital books did provide some data which would not have been available based on interviews alone (about 10% of reported medications). Variable availability of hospital books across different health units may have exacerbated differences in medication rates. Although no formal validation was conducted for the use of medication picture guides, the data collectors reported that the picture guides did help the women to recall the medications they took. Even with these measures in

place, limitations of memory, particularly of short term drug use could not be ruled out. Some women faced the problem of recalling precisely when the first trimester was. And it is also possible that some women just said what they might have thought the interviewer wanted to hear. The use of many data collectors could have introduced interviewer bias. However, the interviewers all went through a standardized training which included pilot testing and validation of the interview process.

Difficulties in dealing with sensitive subjects such as HIV limited the amount of exposure information provided. According to the Cameroon 2011 Demographic Health Survey [25], 5.3% of women are infected with HIV. The rate of 0.2% observed in the current study shows a severe under reporting. Unfortunately, as anti-retrovirals are given as routine medications mainly in HIV treatment centres, information on anti-retroviral exposures are not found in the women's hospital records. In the Cameroon Prevention of Mother to Child Transmission programme, all HIV positive pregnant women attending ANC are placed on anti-retroviral therapy, but it is difficult to tell if there is any linkage between exposure data at the HIV treatment centres and ANC care units. Therefore, it may have been possible to obtain some data from the ANC files, but there were challenges in accessing these files such as hospital restriction. HIV infection in Cameroon, as is the case with many countries, still carries a stigma. Anti-retrovirals during pregnancy constitute an important topic in pharmacovigilance as the medications have several safety concerns, but are vital during pregnancy to prevent maternal to fetal transmission [26]. Future studies would have to devise means of overcoming the barrier of fear of stigmatisation, such as recruiting the pregnant women during their visit to HIV treatment centres or obtaining permission to access ANC notes.

Conclusion

Our study confirms the observations of studies across Africa indicating the increasing use of medications during pregnancy, including those that are potentially teratogenic. On the other hand, we also found evidence of under-prescription of medications beneficial for pregnancy. There is an urgent need for public health authorities in Cameroon to put in place medication safety systems targeting pregnant women, especially during the first trimester when the risk of teratogenicity is highest, avoiding unnecessary or contraindicated medication, ensuring that appropriate treatments needed for the health of the pregnant woman and her baby are received, and weighing risks and benefits carefully. Further research is needed about the knowledge and attitudes of health professionals, and pharmacovigilance should track pregnancy outcomes in relation to medication exposures in pregnancy.

Abbreviations
ANC: Antenatal Care; FDA: Food and Drug Administration; GP: General Practitioner; HIV: Human Immunodeficiency Virus; OTC: Over the Counter; PPH: Post Partum Haemorrhage; SW: South West; UK: United Kingdom; WHO: World Health Organisation

Acknowledgments
We are grateful to Ulster University whose Vice Chancellor PhD Research Scholarship to AZL made this project possible. We are also grateful to the Cameroon Public Health SW Regional Delegation for providing all the necessary administrative support. Finally we thank Health Research Foundation (HRF) Cameroon for providing us with office space and resources to host the project.

Synopsis
This study found high levels of medication use in pregnancy in Cameroon, highlights medication safety issues, and finds underuse of medications beneficial for pregnancy.

Funding
AZL received the Ulster University Vice Chancellor PhD Research Scholarship. The scholarship covered for tuition fees and a £13,500 annual stipend. During field work for this study in Cameroon, part of the scholarship was used to cover for accommodation and subsistence for AZL. No other funding was received for this study.

Authors' contributions
AZL, HD, MLand KC conceptualized the study. AZL conducted the literature review, coordinated data collection and data analysis with technical inputs from HD, MM and KC, NMM, SEM, LDN, PBN, OA, and DE did feasibility study and participated as data collectors. AZL, HD drafted the manuscript with full inputs from all other authors. All authors read and approved the final manuscript.

Competing interests
We declare no competing interests.

Author details
[1]Department of Nursing, School of Health Sciences, Biaka University Institute of Buea-Cameroon, PO BOX 77, Buea, Cameroon. [2]Centre for Maternal, Fetal and Infant Research, Institute for Nursing and Health Research, Ulster University, Shore Rd Newtownabbey, BT370QB Ulster, Ireland. [3]Office of the Deputy Vice Chancellor i/c Research/Cooperation/Quality, Biaka Universit Institute of Buea, PO Box 77-SWR, Buea, Cameroon.

References

1. Adam MP, Polifka JE, Friedman JM. Evolving knowledge of the teratogenicity of medications in human pregnancy. In American Journal of Medical Genetics Part C: Seminars in Medical Genetics 2011157(3):175–182). Wiley Subscription Services, Inc., A Wiley Company.
2. World Health Organization. World health statistics: monitoring health for the SDGs, sustainable development goals. In World health statistics 2017: monitoring health for the SDGs, sustainable development goals; 2017.http://www.who.int/gender-equity-rights/knowledge/world-health-statistics-2017/en/. Accessed 18 Sept 2017.
3. Onwujekwe O, Kaur H, Dike N, Shu E, Uzochukwu B, Hanson K, Okoye V, Okonkwo P. Quality of anti-malarial drugs provided by public and private healthcare providers in south-east Nigeria. Malar J. 2009;8(1):22.
4. World Health Organisation. Mental Health Atlas Available at. [WHO website]. 2011 http://www.who.int/mental_health/evidence/atlas/profiles/cmr_mh_profile.pdf. Accessed 18 Sept 2017.
5. Tripathi V, Stanton C, Anderson FW. Traditional preparations used as uterotonics in Sub-Saharan Africa and their pharmacologic effects. Int J Gynecol Obstet. 2013;120(1):16–22.
6. Fakeye TO, Adisa R, Musa IE. Attitude and use of herbal medicines among pregnant women in Nigeria. BMC Complement Altern Med. 2009;9(1):53.
7. Yang T, Walker MC, Krewski D, Yang Q, Nimrod C, Garner P, Fraser W, Olatunbosun O, Wen SW. Maternal characteristics associated with pregnancy exposure to FDA category C, D, and X drugs in a Canadian population. Pharmacoepidemiol Drug Saf. 2008;17(3):270–7.
8. Mohammed MA, Ahmed JH, Bushra AW, Aljadhey HS. Medications use among pregnant women in Ethiopia: A cross sectional study; 2013.
9. Admasie C, Wasie B, Abeje G. Determinants of prescribed drug use among pregnant women in Bahir Dar city administration, Northwest Ethiopia: a cross sectional study. BMC Pregnancy Childbirth. 2014;14(1):325.
10. Baraka M, Steurbaut S, Coomans D, Dupont AG. Determinants of medication use in a multi-ethnic population of pregnant women: a cross-sectional study. Eur J Contracept Reprod Health Care. 2014;19(2):108–20.
11. SPSS Regression 17.0. http://www.helsinki.fi/~komulain/Tilastokirjat/IBM-SPSS-Spec-Regression.pdf. Accessed 30 Sept 2018.
12. Kebede B, Gedif T, Getachew A. Assessment of drug use among pregnant women in Addis Ababa, Ethiopia. Pharmacoepidemiol Drug Saf. 2009;18(6):462–8.
13. Rohra DK, Das N, Azam SI, Solangi NA, Memon Z, Shaikh AM, Khan NH. Drug-prescribing patterns during pregnancy in the tertiary care hospitals of Pakistan: a cross sectional study. BMC Pregnancy Childbirth. 2008;8(1):24.
14. Bertoldi AD, Dal Pizzol TD, Camargo AL, Barros AJ, Matijasevich A, Santos IS. Use of medicines with unknown fetal risk among parturient women from the 2004 Pelotas Birth Cohort (Brazil). J Pregnancy. 2012;2012:257597.
15. Zhu X, Qi X, Hao J, Huang Z, Zhang Z, Xing X, Cheng D, Xiao L, Xu Y, Zhu P, Tao F. Pattern of drug use during the first trimester among Chinese women: data from a population-based cohort study. Eur J Clin Pharmacol. 2010;66(5):511–8.
16. Eze UI, Eferakeya AE, Oparah AC, Enato EF. Assessment of prescription profile of pregnant women visiting antenatal clinics. Pharm Pract (Granada). 2007;5(3):135–9.
17. Gharoro EP, Igbafe AA. Pattern of drug use amongst antenatal patients in Benin City, Nigeria. Med Sci Monit. 2000;6(1):CR84–7.
18. Mosha D, Mazuguni F, Mrema S, Abdulla S, Genton B. Medication exposure during pregnancy: a pilot pharmacovigilance system using health and demographic surveillance platform. BMC Pregnancy Childbirth. 2014;14(1):322.
19. Potchoo Y, Redah D, Gneni MA, Guissou IP. Prescription drugs among pregnant women in Lome, Togo, West Africa. Eur J Clin Pharmacol. 2009; 65(8):831–8.
20. World Health Organization. Antenatal care report of a technical working group. Geneva: World Health Organization; 1994. p. 31.
21. Achidi EA, Kuoh AJ, Minang JT, Ngum B, Achimbom BM, Motaze SC, Ahmadou MJ, Troye-Blomberg M. Malaria infection in pregnancy and its effects on haemoglobin levels in women from a malaria endemic area of Fako Division, South West Province, Cameroon. J Obstet Gynaecol. 2005; 25(3):235–40.

22. Say L, Chou D, Gemmill A, Tunçalp Ö, Moller AB, Daniels J, Gülmezoglu AM, Temmerman M, Alkema L. Global causes of maternal death: a WHO systematic analysis. Lancet Global Health. 2014;2(6):e323–33.
23. World Health Organisation. Intermittent preventive treatment in pregnancy. (2017). http://www.who.int/malaria/areas/preventive_therapies/pregnancy/en/. Accessed 10 Oct 2017.
24. World Health Organization. WHO Evidence Review Group: Intermittent Preventive Treatment of malaria in pregnancy (IPTp) with Sulfadoxine-Pyrimethamine (SP). Geneva: WHO Headquarters; 2012. http://www.who.int/malaria/mpac/sep2012/iptp_sp_erg_meeting_report_july2012.pdf?ua=1. Accessed 18 Sept 2017
25. Cameroon, D. (2011) Preliminary report [PR13](in French). 2011.https://dhsprogram.com/publications/publication-fr260-dhs-final-reports.cfm. Accessed 10 Oct 2017.
26. Kourtis AP, Lee FK, Abrams EJ, Jamieson DJ, Bulterys M. Mother-to-child transmission of HIV-1: timing and implications for prevention. Lancet Infect Dis. 2006;6(11):726–32.

19

Inequities in utilization of prenatal care: a population-based study in the Canadian province of Manitoba

Maureen I. Heaman[1]* (iD), Patricia J. Martens[2,3]^, Marni D. Brownell[2,3], Mariette J. Chartier[2,3], Kellie R. Thiessen[1], Shelley A. Derksen[3] and Michael E. Helewa[4]

Abstract

Background: Ensuring high quality and equitable maternity services is important to promote positive pregnancy outcomes. Despite a universal health care system, previous research shows neighborhood-level inequities in utilization of prenatal care in Manitoba, Canada. The purpose of this population-based retrospective cohort study was to describe prenatal care utilization among women giving birth in Manitoba, and to determine individual-level factors associated with inadequate prenatal care.

Methods: We studied women giving birth in Manitoba from 2004/05–2008/09 using data from a repository of de-identified administrative databases at the Manitoba Centre for Health Policy. The proportion of women receiving inadequate prenatal care was calculated using a utilization index. Multivariable logistic regressions were used to identify factors associated with inadequate prenatal care for the population, and for a subset with more detailed risk information.

Results: Overall, 11.5% of women in Manitoba received inadequate, 51.0% intermediate, 33.3% adequate, and 4.1% intensive prenatal care ($N = 68,132$). Factors associated with inadequate prenatal care in the population-based model ($N = 64,166$) included northern or rural residence, young maternal age (at current and first birth), lone parent, parity 4 or more, short inter-pregnancy interval, receiving income assistance, and living in a low-income neighborhood. Medical conditions such as multiple birth, hypertensive disorders, antepartum hemorrhage, diabetes, and prenatal psychological distress were associated with lower odds of inadequate prenatal care. In the subset model ($N = 55,048$), the previous factors remained significant, with additional factors being maternal education less than high school, social isolation, and prenatal smoking, alcohol, and/or illicit drug use.

Conclusion: The rate of inadequate prenatal care in Manitoba ranged from 10.5–12.5%, and increased significantly over the study period. Factors associated with inadequate prenatal care included geographic, demographic, socioeconomic, and pregnancy-related factors. Rates of inadequate prenatal care varied across geographic regions, indicating persistent inequities in use of prenatal care. Inadequate prenatal care was associated with several individual indicators of social disadvantage, such as low income, education less than high school, and social isolation. These findings can inform policy makers and program planners about regions and populations most at-risk for inadequate prenatal care and assist with development of initiatives to reduce inequities in utilization of prenatal care.

Keywords: Prenatal care, Pregnancy, Delivery of health care, Socioeconomic factors, Cohort studies

* Correspondence: Maureen.Heaman@umanitoba.ca
^Deceased
[1]College of Nursing, Rady Faculty of Health Sciences, University of Manitoba, 89 Curry Place, Winnipeg, MB R3T 2N2, Canada
Full list of author information is available at the end of the article

Background

Prenatal care is important to achieving a healthy pregnancy and birth and positively influencing the health of the fetus and child [1]. The Marmot Review [2], "Fair Society, Healthy Lives," emphasized the importance of ensuring high quality maternity services across the social gradient. Despite the emphasis placed on the value of prenatal care, a portion of the childbearing population continues to receive inadequate prenatal care, defined as receiving no prenatal care, initiating care later than the first trimester, or, given a first trimester start of care, receiving less than the recommended number of visits [3]. In the United States (U.S), 11.2% of women received inadequate prenatal care in 2004 [4], while in 2016, 77.1% of women began prenatal care in the first trimester of pregnancy, 4.6% began care late (in the third trimester), and 1.6% had no prenatal care, with significant disparities by race/ethnicity [5]. In Canada, national population-level data are not collected on utilization of prenatal care and therefore the rate of inadequate prenatal care is not included as an indicator in the Perinatal Health Reports published by the Public Health Agency of Canada [6, 7]. One older study reported an 8.9% rate of inadequate prenatal care in the Canadian province of Manitoba in 1987/88 [8], while another reported a rate of 6.9% from 1991 to 2000 [9], using different measures of prenatal care utilization. Given that Canada has a universal health care system, and women are not required to pay for prenatal care, these findings suggest inequities in utilization of prenatal care and the existence of barriers other than cost of care. Marmot defines inequity as an inequality or difference that is not fair or just, and is preventable and avoidable [10].

Inadequate prenatal care is a well-recognized risk factor for adverse pregnancy outcomes [11, 12]. In a study of over 28 million births in the U.S., inadequate prenatal care was associated with an increased risk of preterm birth, stillbirth, and early and late neonatal death [11]. In addition, there is growing evidence of an association between prenatal care utilization and subsequent use of postpartum care [13] and well child visits [14, 15]. Thus, efforts to reduce inequities in utilization of prenatal care may contribute to improved maternal and child outcomes. Although several studies on factors associated with inadequate prenatal care have been conducted in the U.S. and other high-income countries [16], the results are not necessarily generalizable to the Canadian population, with its different health care system and racial/ethnic composition. Only a few studies have explored use of prenatal care in the Canadian context [8, 17–22].

In previous work, members of our research team conducted a population-based ecologic study of women having singleton live births in Manitoba from 1991 to 2000 to identify neighborhood-level determinants of prenatal care utilization [9]. We found wide regional variations in the proportion of women receiving inadequate prenatal care, with rates ranging from 1.1 to 21.5% across 498 geographic areas. There was a geographic concentration of high rates of inadequate prenatal care in the inner-city of Winnipeg and in northern Manitoba, areas known to be more socio-economically deprived. After adjusting for individual characteristics of age and parity, women living in areas with the highest proportion of the population who were unemployed, Aboriginal, recent immigrants, single parent families, or having less than 9 years of education, or who lived in areas with the lowest average household income, had the highest rates of inadequate prenatal care [9]. This earlier study provided initial evidence of inequities in use of prenatal care. The purpose of the current population-based study was to expand our understanding of individual-level factors associated with inadequate prenatal care in Manitoba.

Since 2000, new initiatives with the potential to improve use of prenatal care have been implemented in Manitoba, such as the Healthy Baby program [23–25] and regulation of the profession of midwifery [26], creating a need for an updated study of prenatal care utilization. There have also been a number of improvements and additions to the databases housed in the Population Research Data Repository at the Manitoba Centre for Health Policy (MCHP) that allow researchers to significantly improve upon the approach used in the earlier population-based studies of prenatal care [8, 9]. Because physicians used to bill for provision of prenatal care using a global tariff instead of claiming reimbursement for each visit, earlier studies had to rely on hospital abstracts to identify prenatal care visits, which were abstracted from the prenatal record; these data had a high percent of missing information (12–15%), and coding of visits was restricted to one digit, therefore limiting the recorded number of prenatal care visits to a maximum of 8 (with a code of 9 indicating missing data). As of 2001, the medical claims system was revised to have physicians submit claims for reimbursement for the initial prenatal visit and each subsequent visit. Around the same time, space for coding of prenatal care visits in the discharge abstracts was increased to two digits. These changes made determination of the timing and number of prenatal care visits more accurate. In addition, earlier research in Manitoba was limited to only a few individual level variables available in the data files, such as age and parity, necessitating greater reliance on area-level variables derived from the Canadian Census. With the incorporation of data files from Healthy Child Manitoba and Manitoba Families at MCHP, individual level variables such as achievement of high school education, social risk factors (social isolation, single parent status) and health behaviors (smoking, alcohol and drug use) from the Families First screen [27] and receipt of income assistance could be studied.

The current population-based study therefore updates and extends our previous work. The objectives of this study were:

1. To describe rates of inadequate, intermediate, adequate, and intensive prenatal care utilization among women giving birth in the province of Manitoba from 2004/05 to 2008/09 and to examine trends over time;
2. To describe variation in rates of inadequate prenatal care by geographical region; and
3. To determine factors associated with inadequate prenatal care.

Methods
Study design, setting, and inclusion criteria
This was a population-based retrospective cohort study of all women giving birth in hospital in Manitoba over a five-year time period, from 2004/05 to 2008/09. We included women with live births, stillbirths, and singleton or multiple births, in order to provide a population-level examination of prenatal care utilization across the spectrum of types of births. In 2006, Manitoba had a population of 1,148,401 people, and the metro area population for the capital city of Winnipeg was 694,668 people [28]. There were approximately 14,000 to 15,000 births per year in Manitoba during the time frame of this study, and women received prenatal care from obstetricians (41%), family physicians (35%), midwives (4.7%) or a mix of providers (19.1%) in 2008/09 [29]. The provincial Ministry of Health provides comprehensive universal health care coverage for essentially all residents of Manitoba.

Data sources
We analyzed data from existing administrative databases available in the Manitoba Population Research Data Repository (hereafter referred to as the Repository) housed at the MCHP in the University of Manitoba. This Repository is an extensive, person-level, linkable but de-identified collection of administrative databases for all permanent residents of Manitoba, covering both health and social services records. The validity and utility of information in the repository has been well documented [30–32]. The specific data files analyzed for this project were as follows:

- Hospital Abstracts file includes information on all hospitalizations of Manitoba residents, including birth hospitalization information and date of

initiation of prenatal care and number of visits abstracted from the prenatal care record.
- Medical Claims/Medical Services file includes information on claims for physician visits, including the service provided, the date of service and a diagnosis code on all ambulatory care contacts for residents of Manitoba, as well as information about physicians' specialties.
- Drug Program Information Network file includes information on all prescription medications dispensed in the community to Manitoba residents, including prenatal use of prescription medications.
- Manitoba Health Insurance Registry includes information on all Manitobans registered for health care in the province (including demographics such as age of mother and place of residence) and can be used to derive marital status, number of children, and residential postal code, and to determine when residents have moved into or out of the province.
- Canada Census public access file includes area-level sociodemographic information such as average household income, attributed to the population at an aggregate level via the residential six-digit postal code.
- Families First Screen file from Healthy Child Manitoba includes information on 39 social, biological, and demographic risk factors collected by public health nurses within a week of the newborn's discharge from hospital.
- Employment and Income Assistance data file from Manitoba Families includes information on Manitoba residents who receive support from the Income Assistance Program, a provincial program of last resort for people who need help to meet basic personal and family needs.

A detailed description of the databases can be found online [33].

Variables
Outcome variable: Utilization of prenatal care
The Society of Obstetricians and Gynecologists of Canada (SOGC) recommends that women receive prenatal care visits every 4 to 6 weeks in early pregnancy, every 2 to 3 weeks after 30 weeks' gestation, and every 1 to 2 weeks after 36 weeks' gestation [34], while the American Academy of Pediatrics (AAP) and American College of Obstetricians and Gynecologists (ACOG) recommend that women with an uncomplicated first pregnancy be examined every 4 weeks for the first 28 weeks of pregnancy, every 2 to 3 weeks until 36 weeks gestation, and weekly thereafter, while parous women may be seen less frequently [35]. Several indices have been developed to measure the adequacy of prenatal care use, taking into account

the month prenatal care began, the number of prenatal visits, and the gestational age at delivery [36, 37]. We selected the Revised Graduated Index of Prenatal Care Utilization (R-GINDEX) [36] for use in this study as it improves on earlier indices and performed well in one of our previous studies [38]. The R-GINDEX is based on the ACOG recommendation for prenatal care visits, and assigns women to one of six categories of care: "no care," "inadequate," "intermediate," "adequate," "intensive," and "missing." For example, at 40 weeks gestation, a woman who began prenatal care in the first 3 months and received between 13 to 16 visits would be categorized as having adequate care, whereas a woman who began care between 1 to 6 months of pregnancy and had less than 8 visits would be categorized as having inadequate care. The intensive care category includes women who have an unexpectedly large number of prenatal care visits, which may indicate potential morbidity or complications.

Information on three birth–related outcomes was used to calculate the R–GINDEX: the gestational age of the infant (obtained from hospital abstracts), the trimester during which prenatal care began, and the total number of prenatal visits during pregnancy. We recorded weeks gestation at the first prenatal care visit and total number of visits from both the hospital abstracts and medical claims files, and used the lower number of weeks gestation and the higher number of visits to reduce the possibility of misclassification of R-GINDEX categories.

Independent variables

We selected several independent variables that might be associated with utilization of prenatal care based on a review of the literature and availability of variables in the Repository. Maternal age group, young maternal age (< 20 years) at first birth, and parity were obtained from the Hospital Abstracts, while information on maternal education less than grade 12 and a composite variable of smoking, alcohol and/or illicit drug use during pregnancy were obtained from the Families First Screen. Table 1 provides a description of the additional independent variables and how they were defined and calculated. We included selected maternal pre-existing medical conditions and complications of pregnancy because a previous study found that women with medical risks during pregnancy made more prenatal visits [39].

Data analysis

Rates of prenatal care utilization were calculated for each of the five fiscal years, in order to describe and compare the proportion of women in the no care, inadequate, intermediate, adequate, and intensive categories of prenatal care over time. Thereafter, we combined no care with inadequate prenatal care into one variable for the remaining analyses. Geographical comparisons of

rates of inadequate prenatal care between regions of the province were conducted, and the Manitoba provincial average was used as the reference point to determine statistically high, similar, or low rates. A linear trend analysis determined if there was a statistically significant trend in rates of inadequate prenatal care over time, using the Cochran-Armitage Trend Test. Statistical significance for all analyses was defined as $p < 0.05$.

Univariable logistic regression analyses were conducted to determine geographic, socio-demographic and pregnancy-related factors associated with inadequate prenatal care (compared to the reference category of intermediate/adequate prenatal care). Unadjusted odds ratios (uORs) and 95% confidence intervals (CI) of the association between each independent variable and the outcome were calculated. Women with intensive prenatal care were excluded from these analyses. We assessed multicollinearity among the independent variables based on variation inflation factors (VIFs) and tolerance levels (TLs), with multicollinearity defined as VIFs > 2.5 and TLs < 0.40 [40]. Variables with significant uORs were entered into multivariable regression models in order to determine adjusted ORs (aORs) and 95% CI. Two multivariable models were generated: one model for all women in the population giving birth from 2004/05 to 2008/09 (after exclusions), and a second model based on a subset of women having the Families First screen, which captures approximately 80% of the population [27]. Because data missing from the Families First screen may not be random, we reported proportions of missing data for these variables and included the missing category in the regression analyses. The c statistic, or area under the receiver operating characteristic (ROC) curve, was calculated to measure the ability of the models to correctly classify those with and without inadequate prenatal care [41]. The statistical analyses were conducted using SAS Software Version 9.2.

Lastly, because some women had more than one delivery during the period of study, we conducted a sensitivity analysis to remove the effect of multiple deliveries (or observations that were not independent). For women with more than one delivery, we randomly selected one delivery per woman and excluded the other deliveries, and then re-ran the multivariable logistic regression analysis.

Results
Participants
There were a total of 70,612 deliveries in Manitoba from 2004/05 to 2008/09. We excluded maternal delivery records that could not be linked to a newborn birth record (0.74%), with a recorded gestation out of range, defined as < 18 or > 45 weeks (0.83%), with a recorded birth

Table 1 Description of additional independent variables

Variable	Description
Income Assistance	A woman was considered to have received income assistance if she was coded as having received income assistance anytime during the period of seven months prior to the month of the baby's delivery to one month after the baby's delivery (excludes: women living in First Nations communities, stillbirths, out of province births)
Marital Status	
Single Parent	A woman was considered a single (or lone) parent if she was identified as the sole primary care giver for the child on the Families First Screen.
Married or Partnered	A woman giving birth was considered married/partnered if either a marriage was reported to Manitoba Health OR if according to the Families First Screen, she was not a single parent.
Unknown marital status	A woman giving birth was considered to have an unknown marital status if the single parent question on the Families First Screen was left blank or no Families First Screen was done and there was no marriage reported to Manitoba Health.
Income quintile	Income quintiles were developed by assigning average household income from the 2006 Statistics Canada Census to dissemination areas and then ranking these from highest to lowest. Dissemination areas were then grouped into five groups or quintiles (1 being poorest and 5 being wealthiest). Each quintile contained approximately 20% of the population.
Diabetes	A woman was considered to have diabetes if in the three years prior to giving birth she had: 1) one or more hospitalizations with diagnosis code 250 (ICD–9–CM) or E10–E14 (ICD–10–CA) in any diagnosis field over three years of data OR 2) two or more physician claims with diagnosis code 250 over three years of data OR 3) one or more prescriptions for diabetic drugs – Insulins and Analogues (A10A); Blood Glucose Lowering Drugs excluding Insulin (A10BA02, A10BB01, A10BB02, A10BB03, A10BB09, A10BB12, A10BB31, A10BD03, A10BF01, A10BG02, A10BG03, A10BX02, A10BX03) over three years of data OR 4) one or more hospitalizations with gestational diabetes code in the gestation period (ICD–9–CM: 648.8, ICD–10–CA: O24)
Hypertension	A woman was considered to have hypertension if in the one year prior to giving birth she had: 1) at least one physician visit or one hospitalization (ICD–9–CM codes 401–405 or ICD–10–CA codes I10–I13, I15) OR 2) two or more prescriptions for hypertension drugs – Antihypertensives (C02AB01, C02AB02, C02AC01, C02CA04, C02CA05, C02DB02, C02DC01, C02KX01, C02LA01, C02LB01, G04CA03); Diuretics (C03AA03, C03BA04, C03BA11, C03CA01, C03CA02, C03CC01, C03DA01, C03DB01, C03DB02, C03EA01); Beta Blocking Agents (C07AA02, C07AA03, C07AA05, C07AA06, C07AA12, C07AB02, C07AB03, C07AB04, C07AB07, C07AG01, C07BA05, C07BA06, C07CA03, C07CB03); Calcium Channel Blockers (C08CA01, C08CA02, C08CA04, C08CA05, C08CA06, C08DA01, C08DB01); Agents Acting on the Renin–Angiotensin System (C09AA01, C09AA02, C09AA03, C09AA04, C09AA05, C09AA06, C09AA07, C09AA08, C09AA09, C09AA10, C09BA02, C09BA03, C09BA04, C09BA06, C09BA08, C09CA01, C09CA02, C09CA03, C09CA04, C09CA06, C09CA07, C09DA01, C09DA02, C09DA03, C09DA04, C09DA06, C09DA07) OR 3) At least one physician visit or one hospitalization in the gestation period (ICD–9–CM code 642 or ICD–10–CA codes O10–O16)
Antepartum hemorrhage	A woman was considered to have had an antepartum hemorrhage by the presence of: 1) One or more hospitalizations (ICD–9–CM 641, 641.0, 641.1, 641.2, 641.3, 641.8, 641.9; ICD 10– CA O44,O45, O46) in the gestation period indicating antepartum hemorrhage OR 2) One or more physician visits (ICD–9–CM 641, 641.0, 641.1, 641.2, 641.3, 641.8, 641.9) in the gestation period indicating antepartum hemorrhage.
Maternal Psychological distress	A woman was considered to have psychological distress if, in the two years prior to giving birth (or hospital discharge in case of a stillbirth), she had: 1) one or more hospitalizations with a diagnosis for depressive disorder, affective psychoses, neurotic depression, or adjustment reaction (ICD–9–CM codes 296.2–296.8, 300.4, 309, 311; ICD–10–CA codes F31, F32, F33, F341, F38.0, F38.1, F41.2, F43.1, F43.2, F43.8, F53.0, F93.0) OR 2) one or more physician visits with a diagnosis for depressive disorder, affective psychoses, or adjustment reaction (ICD–9–CM codes 296, 309, or 311) OR 3) one or more hospitalizations with a diagnosis for anxiety disorders (ICD–9–CM code 300; ICD–10–CA codes F32.0, F34.1, F40, F41, F42, F44, F45.0, F451, F452, F48, F68.0, F99) OR 4) one or more prescriptions for an antidepressant or mood stabilizer (ATC codes N03AB02, N03AB52, N03AF01, N05AN01, N06A) OR 5) one or more physician visits with a diagnosis for anxiety disorders (ICD–9–CM code 300) and one or more prescriptions for an antidepressant or mood stabilizer (ATC codes N03AB02, N03AB52, N03AF01, N05AN01, N06A) OR 6) one or more hospitalizations with a diagnosis for anxiety states, phobic disorders, or obsessive–compulsive disorders (ICD–9–CM codes 300.0, 300.2, 300.3; ICD–10–CA codes F40, F41.0, F41.1, F41.3, F41.8, F41.9, F42) OR 7) three or more physician visits with a diagnosis for anxiety disorders (ICD–9–CM code 300)
Short inter-pregnancy interval	A short inter-pregnancy interval was defined if the time between the last delivery and conception of the most recent pregnancy was less than 12 months, further divided into two categories: (i) of less than 180 days and (ii) 180–365 days. The date of the last delivery was determined from the Manitoba Health Insurance Registry while conception of the most recent pregnancy was determined from the Hospital Abstract Database.
Social isolation	A woman was considered to have social isolation (defined as lack of social support and/or isolation related to culture, language or geography) if this was identified on the Families First Screen.

Note: Manitoba implemented ICD-10-CA/CCC coding classification system in April 2004

weight < 400 g and gestation > 22 weeks (0.06%), and with a maternal Personal Health Identification Number (PHIN) not found on Manitoba Health Registry (0.01%) or not covered by Manitoba Health Registry during pregnancy (2.66%). We excluded midwifery cases having a home birth (0.8%) since prenatal care was not well recorded for those cases. We also excluded midwifery cases of mothers delivered in hospital who were missing a prenatal care record (0.06%), because medical claims data could not be used to determine prenatal care visits as midwives are reimbursed via salary. Lastly, we excluded 211 deliveries that were missing data on the variables required to calculate the R-GINDEX category. These exclusions resulted in a final sample size of 68,132 deliveries, of which 927 of the deliveries were multiple births.

Utilization of prenatal care

From 2004/05 to 2008/09, the rate of no prenatal care ranged from 0.4 to 0.5%, inadequate care from 9.9 to 12.0%, intermediate care from 50.1 to 51.6%, adequate care from 32.2 to 34.1% and intensive care from 3.6 to 4.3% (Table 2).

Overall, 11.5% of women had either no care or inadequate prenatal care (hereafter referred to as a combined variable of inadequate prenatal care), and there was a significant increase in the rate of inadequate prenatal care from 10.5 to 12.5% over time (Table 3). Three-quarters (74.5%) of women initiated prenatal care in the first trimester, 22.7% in the second trimester, and 2.6% in the 3rd trimester, while overall 0.5% of women did not receive any prenatal care.

Regional variation in prevalence of inadequate prenatal care

There was significant variation in rates of inadequate prenatal care by geographic district across the province and the city of Winnipeg (Fig. 1). The primarily northern regions of Interlake, North Eastman, Parkland, Nor-Man, and Burntwood all had rates of inadequate prenatal care that were significantly higher than the Manitoba average (Figs. 2 & 3). As well, rates of inadequate prenatal care also varied across the Winnipeg community areas, with the inner-city areas of Inkster, Point Douglas, and

Downtown having rates that were significantly higher than the Winnipeg average (Figs. 4 & 5).

Factors associated with Inadequate prenatal care

The proportions of maternal characteristics among deliveries with inadequate prenatal care, adequate/intermediate prenatal care, and intensive prenatal care are presented in Table 4. We excluded deliveries with intensive prenatal care ($n = 2799$) from the regression analyses because a high proportion of women with preexisting conditions or pregnancy complications received intensive care, and these deliveries were therefore judged to be inappropriate to include as part of the reference group. None of the variance inflation factors were > 2.5 (most were < 1.5) and none of the tolerance values were < 0.4 for the variables, indicating that multicollinearity was not a problem in the models.

In the first model of all deliveries in the population ($N = 64,166$), shown in Table 5, women were significantly more likely to receive inadequate prenatal care if they lived in the northern (aOR 2.72) or south rural (aOR 1.15) regions of the province compared to the urban areas (the major cities of Winnipeg and Brandon). Women in younger age groups had higher odds of inadequate prenatal care (12–17 years, aOR 1.96; 18–19 years, aOR 1.60; 20–24 years, aOR 1.32) compared to the reference category of 25–29 years, while those 30–34 years had lower odds of inadequate prenatal care (aOR 0.90). Women who were less than or equal to 19 years at their first birth were also at higher odds of inadequate prenatal care (aOR 1.38) compared to women whose first birth was at age 20 or higher. Women who lived in census dissemination areas with an average household income in the 3 lowest income quintiles had higher odds of inadequate prenatal care, compared to those who lived in an area with the highest income quintile. At an individual level, women receiving income assistance had over twice the odds (aOR 2.15) of receiving inadequate prenatal care than women who were not on income assistance. Women were also more likely to have inadequate prenatal care if they were a single parent (aOR 1.85), had a parity of 4 or higher (aOR 2.29), or a short inter-pregnancy interval of either less than 180 days (aOR 3.11) or 180–365 days

Table 2 Utilization of prenatal care in Manitoba, 2005/06 to 2008/09 (N = 68,132 deliveries)

Category of prenatal care utilization	2004/05 N = 12,808 n (%)	2005/06 N = 13,216 n (%)	2006/07 N = 13,640 n (%)	2007/08 N = 14,134 n (%)	2008/09 N = 14,334 n (%)	Total N = 68,132 n (%)
No prenatal care	68 (0.5)	67 (0.5)	55 (0.4)	62 (0.4)	59 (0.4)	311 (0.5)
Inadequate prenatal care	1273 (9.9)	1363 (10.3)	1513 (11.1)	1646 (11.7)	1726 (12.0)	7521 (11.0)
Intermediate prenatal care	6578 (51.4)	6752 (51.1)	6835 (50.1)	7298 (51.6)	7316 (51.0)	34,779 (51.0)
Adequate prenatal care	4339 (33.9)	4502 (34.1)	4613 (33.8)	4555 (32.2)	4713 (32.9)	22,722 (33.3)
Intensive prenatal care	550 (4.3)	532 (4.0)	624 (4.6)	573 (4.1)	520 (3.6)	2799 (4.1)

Table 3 Rate of combined no care and inadequate prenatal care in Manitoba, 2005/06 to 2008/09 (N = 68,132 deliveries)

Category of prenatal care utilization	2004/05 N = 12,808 n (%)	2005/06 N = 13,216 n (%)	2006/07 N = 13,640 n (%)	2007/08 N = 14,134 n (%)	2008/09 N = 14,334 n (%)	Total N = 68,132 n (%)
Inadequate and no prenatal care*	1341 (10.5)	1430 (10.8)	1568 (11.5)	1708 (12.1)	1785 (12.5)	7832 (11.5)

*The rate significantly increased over time ($p < .0001$) based on Cochran-Armitage Trend Test

(aOR 2.26). A variety of medical conditions contributing to an at-risk pregnancy were associated with lower odds of inadequate prenatal care: multiple birth (aOR 0.40), diabetes (aOR 0.47), hypertension (aOR 0.76), antepartum hemorrhage (aOR 0.71), and maternal depression or anxiety (AOR 0.80). The c statistic for the first model was 0.83, indicating that the model explained 83% of the area under the ROC curve. Therefore the model had good ability to correctly classify those with and without inadequate prenatal care.

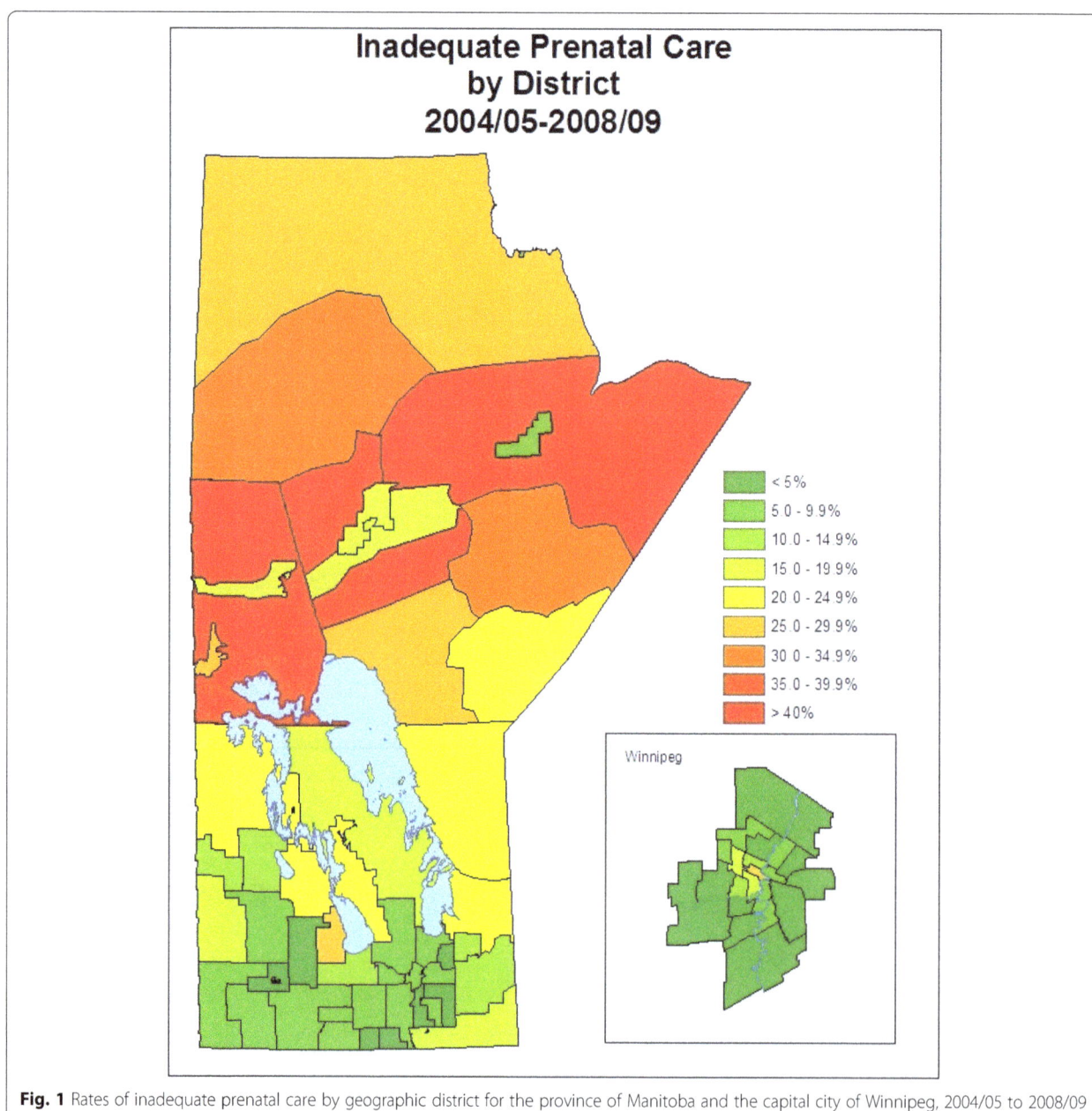

Fig. 1 Rates of inadequate prenatal care by geographic district for the province of Manitoba and the capital city of Winnipeg, 2004/05 to 2008/09

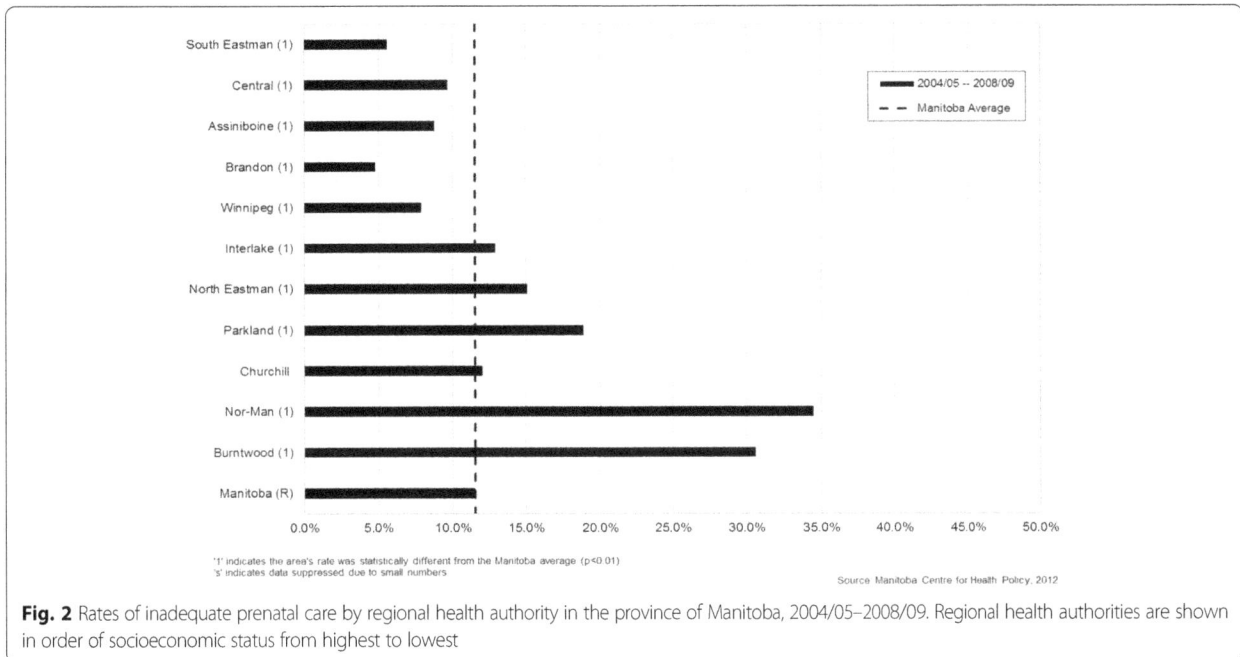

Fig. 2 Rates of inadequate prenatal care by regional health authority in the province of Manitoba, 2004/05–2008/09. Regional health authorities are shown in order of socioeconomic status from highest to lowest

In a second model incorporating deliveries which had Families First screening data ($N = 55,048$), the previous factors associated with inadequate prenatal care remained significant, with additional significant factors consisting of maternal education of less than high school (aOR 1.93), social isolation (aOR 1.21), and the composite variable of smoking, alcohol, and/or illicit drug use during pregnancy (aOR 1.43) (Table 5). The c statistic for this model was 0.81.

Sensitivity analysis

There were 52,144 women and 68,132 deliveries in our original analysis, with 27% of the women having more than one delivery in the five year time frame. After randomly selecting one delivery per woman and re-running the first model ($N = 48,925$), the results remained similar, with aORs of similar magnitude and significance (results available upon request). The only exception was that the aOR for age group 30–34 years became non-significant in the sensitivity analysis (aOR 0.906, 95% CI 0.818–1.004).

Discussion

The results of this study describe patterns of utilization of prenatal care in the Canadian province of Manitoba, confirm that inequities in use of prenatal care persist, and identify factors associated with inadequate prenatal care that will help inform policy makers and program planners about which populations and regions are most at-risk for inadequate prenatal care. These findings fill an important gap in knowledge related to utilization of prenatal care in Canada, given the lack of

surveillance data on prenatal care at a national level in this country.

In terms of utilization, our findings showed that a high proportion of women in Manitoba (11.5%) had inadequate prenatal care, and the rate significantly increased over time from 10.5 to 12.5% during 2004/05 to 2008/09. This rate of 11.5% is higher than that of 6.9% reported in our earlier study [9], which may be a result of using different prenatal care utilization indices – GINDEX [42] versus R-GINDEX [36] - and of improvements in capturing prenatal care utilization in the administrative databases. The higher rates may also reflect changes in provision of health care (e.g., fewer family physicians providing prenatal care) [29] and population trends (e.g., higher proportion of immigrants) [43], although the exact reasons require further exploration. Our population-based rate of 11.5% is much higher than the 4.1% rate of inadequate prenatal care reported by Debessai et al. [17] using data from the Canadian Maternity Experiences Survey [44]. The lower rate reported by Debessai et al. was based on self-report data from a survey of 6421 women in Canada, which may be prone to recall bias, as women may have overestimated their use of prenatal care, and selection bias, as women most at risk of inadequate prenatal care may not have participated in the survey. Findings from the Canadian Maternity Experiences Survey do, however, provide some explanation for the high rates of inadequate prenatal care in Manitoba, as Manitoba had the highest proportion of women who reported not getting prenatal care as early as they wanted (18.6%) compared to the other provinces [44].

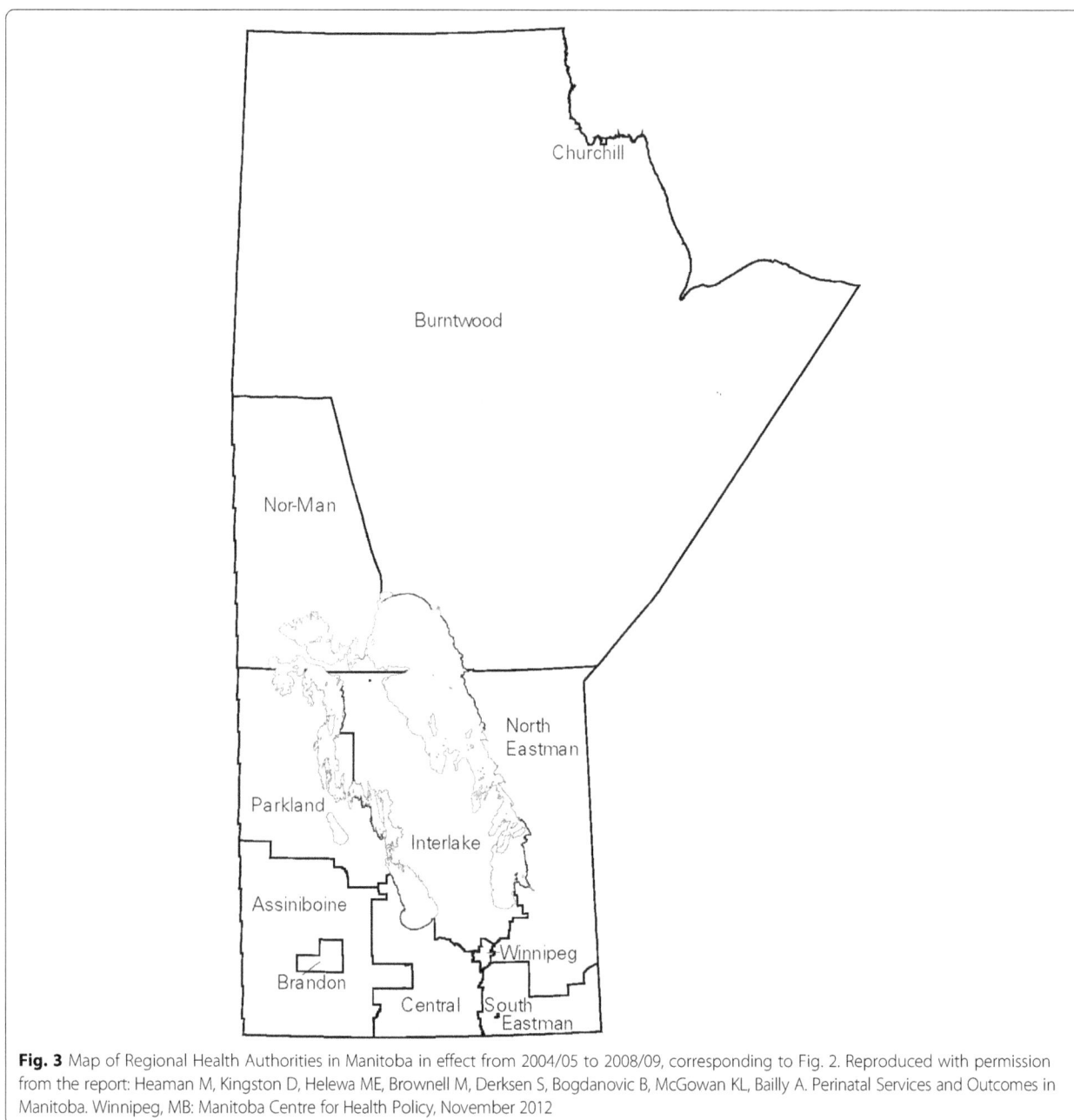

Fig. 3 Map of Regional Health Authorities in Manitoba in effect from 2004/05 to 2008/09, corresponding to Fig. 2. Reproduced with permission from the report: Heaman M, Kingston D, Helewa ME, Brownell M, Derksen S, Bogdanovic B, McGowan KL, Bailly A. Perinatal Services and Outcomes in Manitoba. Winnipeg, MB: Manitoba Centre for Health Policy, November 2012

Studies from the U.S. and Europe found that a lack of health insurance was an important risk factor for inadequate prenatal care [45, 46]. Somewhat surprisingly, given our universal health care system, the Manitoba rate of inadequate prenatal care of 11.5% was similar to the rate of 11.2% reported in the U.S. using data from 2004 [4]. However, caution needs to be used in comparing these rates because we used the R-GINDEX, whereas the U.S. rate was calculated from birth certificate data using the Adequacy of Prenatal care Utilization Index (APNCU) [47], and rates vary depending on which index is used [47]. Although women in a universal health care system

do not have to pay for prenatal care visits, other economic, psychosocial, attitudinal and structural barriers have been shown to negatively influence access to care among women in Manitoba, such as stress and family problems, having an unplanned pregnancy, the costs of transportation and child care, not knowing where to get care or having a long wait for care, and fear of apprehension of the infant by the child welfare agency [18]. Similar barriers have been reported in other studies [48–50], suggesting that health insurance is only one of many factors influencing use of prenatal care. However, only 0.5% of women in Manitoba had no prenatal care, providing

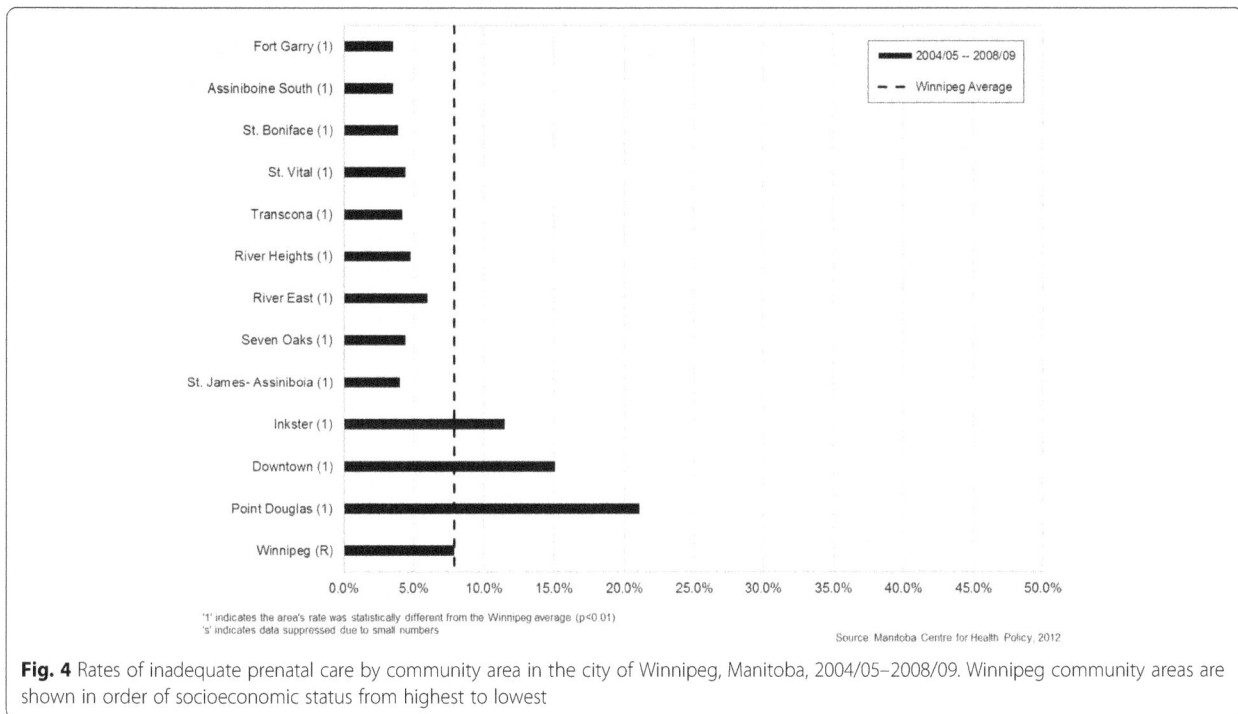

Fig. 4 Rates of inadequate prenatal care by community area in the city of Winnipeg, Manitoba, 2004/05–2008/09. Winnipeg community areas are shown in order of socioeconomic status from highest to lowest

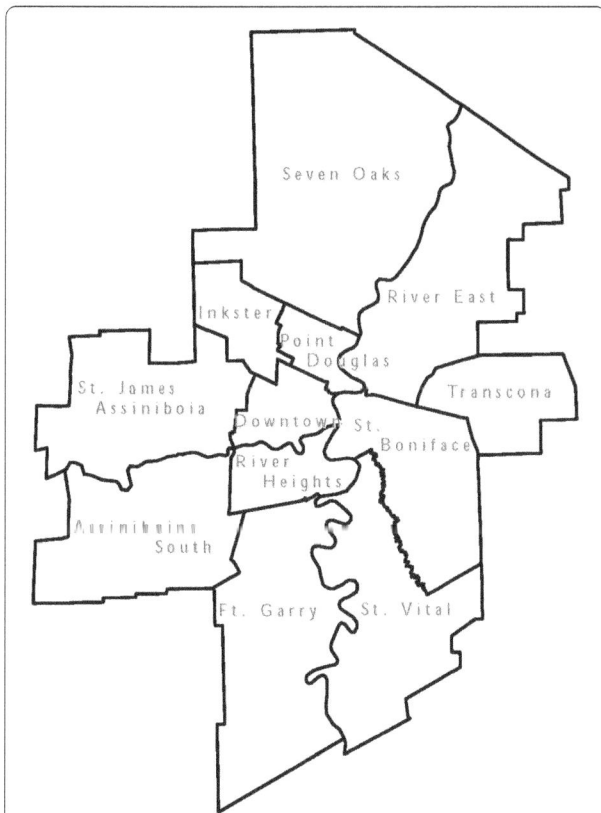

Fig. 5 Map of Community Areas in the city of Winnipeg, corresponding to Fig. 4. Reproduced with permission from the report: Heaman M, Kingston D, Helewa ME, Brownell M, Derksen S, Bogdanovic B, McGowan KL, Bailly A. Perinatal Services and Outcomes in Manitoba. Winnipeg, MB: Manitoba Centre for Health Policy, November 2012

evidence that the majority of women (95.5%) accessed at least some prenatal care. Our rate of 0.5% is lower than the rate of 1.0% of women who had no prenatal care in a hospital register based study in Finland, another country which offers free prenatal care [51]. Our Manitoba rate of no prenatal care was also lower than the U.S. rates of 1.9% in 2008 [52] and 1.6% in 2016 [5].

Our findings showed wide variation in rates of inadequate prenatal care across geographic regions in Manitoba, indicating the persistence of inequities in use of prenatal care similar to the findings of our previous study [9]. The northern regions of the province and inner-city areas in Winnipeg continued to have the highest rates of inadequate prenatal care, and are known to be more socioeconomically deprived. In addition, northern or rural residence was a significant independent factor associated with inadequate prenatal care in the regression models. Possible reasons for this finding might include less access to health care services and prenatal care providers in northern and rural areas of the province, compounded by problems of distance to travel for care. Utilization of prenatal care also followed a clear social gradient, with rates of inadequate prenatal care steadily increasing from a low of 4.8% in the most affluent neighborhoods (income quintile 5) to a high of 21.3% in the poorest neighborhoods (income quintile 1). Living in a neighborhood with the lowest average household income was associated with almost twice the odds (aOR=1.92) of inadequate prenatal care compared to living in a neighborhood with the highest average household income.

Table 4 Proportions (%) of maternal characteristics among deliveries with inadequate prenatal care, adequate/intermediate prenatal care, and intensive prenatal care for women giving birth in Manitoba from 2004/05 to 2008/09

Characteristic	Entire population of women giving birth (after exclusions) N = 68,132			Subset of population of women giving birth who had a Families First screen N = 57,603		
	Inadequate/ No prenatal care N = 7832	Intermediate/Adequate prenatal care N = 57,501	Intensive prenatal care N = 2799	Inadequate/No prenatal care N = 4482	Intermediate/Adequate prenatal care N = 50,566	Intensive prenatal care N = 2555
Marital status						
Single parent	18.8	77.0	4.2	18.0	77.8	4.3
Married/partnered	5.4	90.1	4.6	4.7	90.7	4.6
Unknown	30.9	66.7	2.4	23.0	73.8	3.3
On Income Assistance						
Yes	26.2	70.3	3.4	24.2	72.1	3.7
No	8.9	86.9	4.2	4.7	90.7	4.6
Income Quintile -neighborhood						
Q1 (lowest)	21.3	75.2	3.6	14.9	80.7	4.4
Q2	13.2	82.7	4.0	8.0	87.5	4.5
Q3	7.0	87.8	5.2	6.0	88.8	5.3
Q4	5.3	90.6	4.1	5.0	91.0	4.0
Q5 (highest)	4.8	91.3	3.9	4.7	91.3	3.9
Maternal Age Group						
12–17 years	27.0	68.9	4.1	22.0	71.4	6.5
18–19 years	24.4	72.7	2.8	18.0	78.5	3.5
20–24 years	16.6	79.8	3.6	11.8	84.0	4.2
25–29 years	9.4	86.7	3.9	6.4	89.4	4.1
30–34 years	6.9	89.0	4.1	4.8	91.0	4.2
35+	7.1	87.0	5.8	5.4	88.6	6.0
Region of Residence						
North	31.4	66.6	2.0	19.3	78.2	2.5
South Rural	10.8	85.3	3.9	6.7	89.2	4.1
Urban (Winnipeg/ Brandon)	7.7	87.7	4.7	7.6	87.7	4.7
Maternal Age at First Birth						
< = 19 years	25.4	71.5	3.1	19.4	76.8	3.8
20+ years	6.1	89.4	4.5	4.6	90.8	4.6
Number of births						
Multiple birth	5.2	83.1	11.7	4.1	83.5	12.4
Singleton birth	11.6	84.4	4.0	7.8	87.8	4.3
Parity						
0–3	9.9	85.9	4.2	6.8	88.7	4.5
4+	31.7	65.9	2.4	26.4	70.9	2.7
Inter-Pregnancy Interval						
< 180 days	35.6	62.8	1.6	28.3	70.0	1.8
180–365 days	20.3	77.5	2.3	14.5	83.1	2.5
366+ days	10.9	85.3	3.8	7.7	88.4	3.9
First child	7.5	87.2	5.3	5.1	89.3	5.6

Table 4 Proportions (%) of maternal characteristics among deliveries with inadequate prenatal care, adequate/intermediate prenatal care, and intensive prenatal care for women giving birth in Manitoba from 2004/05 to 2008/09 *(Continued)*

Characteristic	Entire population of women giving birth (after exclusions) N = 68,132			Subset of population of women giving birth who had a Families First screen N = 57,603		
	Inadequate/ No prenatal care N = 7832	Intermediate/Adequate prenatal care N = 57,501	Intensive prenatal care N = 2799	Inadequate/No prenatal care N = 4482	Intermediate/Adequate prenatal care N = 50,566	Intensive prenatal care N = 2555
Diabetes						
Yes	8.6	81.7	9.7	4.4	84.5	11.1
No	11.7	84.6	3.7	8.0	88.0	4.1
Hypertension						
Yes	7.1	82.3	10.7	4.3	84.4	11.4
No	11.9	84.6	3.5	8.1	88.1	3.7
Antepartum hemorrhage						
Yes	9.9	82.0	8.0	6.8	84.3	8.9
No	11.6	84.5	3.9	7.8	88.0	4.2
Maternal psychological distress						
Yes	10.6	82.9	6.5	8.2	85.0	6.9
No	11.6	84.6	3.7	7.7	88.3	4.0
Education						
Less than Grade 12	–	–	–	17.2	78.9	3.9
High school or better	–	–	–	3.5	91.8	4.7
Unknown	–	–	–	15.0	81.2	3.8
Social isolation						
Yes	–	–	–	10.9	83.7	5.4
No	–	–	–	5.8	89.6	4.6
Unknown	–			16.5	79.9	3.6
Smoking, alcohol and/or illicit drug use during pregnancy						
Yes	–	–	–	12.6	83.0	4.4
No	–	–	–	4.2	91.3	4.6
Unknown	–	–	–	17.3	78.9	3.7

Inadequate prenatal care was associated with several individual-level indicators of social disadvantage, such as low income (receiving income assistance), education less than high school, being a single parent, and being assessed as socially isolated. This association between inadequate prenatal care and social disadvantage is similar to findings from other developed countries such as New Zealand [53], England [54, 55] and Belgium [39] and with findings of a systematic review of determinants of prenatal care in high income countries [16]. We also found that young maternal age, high parity, and smoking, alcohol or drug use were factors associated with inadequate prenatal care, congruent with the findings of other studies [11, 16, 39].

To our knowledge, two of our variables have not been studied in previous work and add new knowledge on factors associated with inadequate prenatal care:

short inter-pregnancy interval and young maternal age (< 20 years) at first birth. Birth spacing can be measured using inter-pregnancy interval, defined as the time between the last delivery and conception of the current pregnancy [56, 57]. Our results showed that a short inter-pregnancy interval of either less than 180 days, or between 180 and 365 days were both associated with an increased odds of inadequate prenatal care (aOR of 3.11 and 2.26 respectively). Women with closely spaced pregnancies may lack the time or energy to seek prenatal care due to child care responsibilities, or may view prenatal care as unnecessary given the short time since the previous pregnancy. Young maternal age (< 20 years) at first birth was associated with increased odds of inadequate prenatal care (aOR = 1.38). Although young maternal age at first birth is likely at least partly a proxy for lower socioeconomic status,

Table 5 Factors associated with inadequate prenatal care among women giving birth in Manitoba from 2004/05 to 2008/09, compared to women having intermediate or adequate prenatal care, using multivariable logistic regression (adjusted odds ratios [aOR] and 95% confidence intervals [CI])

Variable	Model 1* (N = 64,166) aOR (95% CI)	Model 2** (N = 55,048) aOR (95% CI)
Marital status		
Single parent	1.85 (1.69–2.02)	1.47 (1.33–1.63)
Married/partnered	Reference	Reference
Unknown	3.08 (2.89–3.03)	2.24 (1.93–2.59)
On Income Assistance		
Yes	2.15 (2.00–2.30)	1.81 (1.65–1.98)
No	Reference	Reference
Income Quintile -neighborhood		
Q1 (lowest)	1.92 (1.72–2.13)	1.60 (1.14–1.82)
Q2	1.65 (1.47–1.84)	1.34 (1.18–1.52)
Q3	1.27 (1.13–1.44)	1.12 (0.99–1.28)
Q4	1.03 (0.91–1.17)	0.98 (0.86–1.12)
Q5 (highest)	Reference	Reference
Age Group		
12–17 years	1.96 (1.70–2.27)	2.04 (1.68–2.48)
18–19 years	1.60 (1.41–1.80)	1.50 (1.28–1.76)
20–24 years	1.32 (1.22–1.43)	1.31 (1.19–1.44)
25–29 years	Reference	Reference
30–34 years	0.90 (0.83–0.98)	0.89 (0.80–0.98)
35+	0.98 (0.88 1.10)	0.99 (0.87–1.12)
Region of Residence		
North	2.72 (2.52–2.98)	2.53 (2.21–2.98)
South Rural	1.15 (1.41–1.62)	1.30 (1.19–1.41)
Urban (Winnipeg/Brandon)	Reference	Reference
Maternal Age at First Birth		
< 20 years	1.38 (1.28–1.49)	1.32 (1.20–1.45)
20+ years	Reference	Reference
Number of births		
Multiple birth	0.40 (0.29–0.56)	0.52 (0.35–0.75)
Singleton birth	Reference	Reference
Parity		
0–3	Reference	Reference
4+	2.29 (2.09–2.50)	2.59 (2.31–2.91)
Inter-Pregnancy Interval		
< 180 days	3.11 (2.79–3.48)	3.47 (3.01–4.01)
180–365 days	2.26 (2.06–2.50)	2.45 (2.17–2.77)
366+ days	1.48 (1.37–1.61)	1.53 (1.39–1.69)
First child	Reference	Reference
Diabetes		
Yes	0.47 (0.41–0.53)	0.50 (0.41–0.61)
No	Reference	Reference

Table 5 Factors associated with inadequate prenatal care among women giving birth in Manitoba from 2004/05 to 2008/09, compared to women having intermediate or adequate prenatal care, using multivariable logistic regression (adjusted odds ratios [aOR] and 95% confidence intervals [CI]) *(Continued)*

Variable	Model 1* (N = 64,166)	Model 2** (N = 55,048)
	aOR (95% CI)	aOR (95% CI)
Hypertension		
Yes	0.76 (0.66–0.85)	0.72 (0.62–0.83)
No	Reference	Reference
Antepartum hemorrhage		
Yes	0.71 (0.63–0.81)	0.71 (0.60–0.83)
No	Reference	Reference
Maternal psychological distress		
Yes	0.80 (0.79–0.85)	0.76 (0.69–0.83)
No	Reference	Reference
Education		
Less than Grade 12	–	1.93 (1.76–2.12)
High school or better	–	Reference
Unknown	–	1.53 (1.33–1.76)
Social isolation		
Yes	–	1.21 (1.03–1.42)
No	–	Reference
Smoking, alcohol and/or illicit drug use during pregnancy		
Yes	–	1.43 (1.31–1.56)
No	–	Reference
Unknown	–	1.03 (0.87–1.23)

*Model 1: Entire population of women giving birth in Manitoba (after exclusions). Value of c statistic for Model 1 = 0.83
**Model 2: Subset of population of women giving birth in Manitoba who had a Families First screen. Value of c statistic for Model 2 = 0.81

and is associated with number of children in the family, its independent association with inadequate prenatal care in the multivariable regression analyses in this study demonstrates having her first child at a young age may continue to influence a woman's prenatal care utilization in subsequent pregnancies. In other research, young maternal age at first birth was associated with increased risks of poor health, social and education outcomes among children of prior teen mothers, similar to risks found for children of teen mothers [58].

Our findings also showed that medical conditions such as multiple birth, hypertensive disorders, antepartum hemorrhage, diabetes, and prenatal psychological distress were associated with lower odds of inadequate prenatal care, which suggests that pregnant women with medical risks may seek out more prenatal care, or may have more prenatal care due to increased follow-up and/or referrals to specialists, or more prenatal care may have led to more diagnoses. A higher proportion of women with these conditions received intensive prenatal care compared to those without the condition, as shown in Table 4. Similarly, Beeckman et al. [39] found that

women with medical risks during pregnancy made 12% more prenatal visits compared to those without medical risk, while Petrou [59] reported that pregnant women in England and Wales with high risk status at booking had slightly more visits. A study conducted by Krans et al. [60] in Michigan showed that women with high medical risk pregnancies and dual high medical and high psychosocial risk pregnancies were more likely to receive "adequate plus" prenatal care. However, high psychosocial risk pregnancies were more likely to receive inadequate prenatal care.

Strengths and limitations of the study

This study has several strengths. This study used administrative data to describe utilization of prenatal care and factors associated with inadequate care for the population of women giving birth in Manitoba. Linked administrative databases are a powerful resource for studying important public health issues [30]. However, one important limitation of administrative data is the frequent lack of individual-level socioeconomic information [30]. We were able to overcome that limitation through using highly reliable individual-level information on receipt of income assistance, in addition to ecologic measures such as area-based household income. We were also able to assess social and health behavior factors recorded in the Families First screen.

However, our study also has limitations. This was an observational study, so cause and effect cannot be inferred. In the multivariable regression analyses, multiple individual comparisons could lead to Type 1 error, creating a potential limitation regarding any single factor being studied. In addition, administrative data may be subject to a certain degree of coding errors and incomplete data, which may be random or contain systematic biases. For example, the Families First screening data were available for approximately 80% of the population, and excluded women living in First Nations communities and women having a stillbirth. The completeness of data on number of prenatal visits may be lower for women in some isolated northern communities or other locations where they may be served by salaried physicians, resulting in an over-estimation of rates of inadequate prenatal care.

We selected the R-GINDEX to categorize prenatal care utilization, which is one of several available indices. As previously described, the R-GINDEX is based on the ACOG recommendations for number of visits for low risk pregnant women. Alexander and Kotelchuck note that the effectiveness of this standard has not been assessed through rigorous scientific testing, nor has adequacy of care for women with high risk pregnancies been operationalized [61]. The R-GINDEX is strictly a measure of utilization and only reflects the quantity of prenatal care; it does not measure the content, clinical adequacy, or quality of prenatal care. As well, inaccurate ascertainment of gestational age may affect assignment to a prenatal care utilization category. Our measure of prenatal care also did not take into account use of other maternal health services which may supplement prenatal care, such as participation in the Healthy Baby community support program or prenatal classes.

We were unable to examine maternal characteristics such as unplanned pregnancy, stress and homelessness, which were not captured in the administrative databases. In addition, this study was limited to women having a hospital birth, and excluded the small proportion of women having a home birth with a midwife (0.8%) due to lack of reliable information on number of prenatal visits from the midwifery data. We used firstborn child as the reference category for interpregnancy interval in order to include the full spectrum of birth orders and retain primiparous women in the analysis, based on work by Auger and colleagues [56]. We recognize that some investigators consider the appropriate unexposed category to be women with longer interpregnancy intervals,

particularly for studies examining the association between interpregnancy interval and birth outcomes [57]. Lastly, although other studies have found that immigrant women [17, 62] and First Nations women [19, 63] are at higher risk of inadequate prenatal care, the Repository does not include individual-level information on race/ethnicity or immigrant status, so we were unable to study the association of these factors with use of prenatal care. Caution needs to be used in generalizing the results of this study to other Canadian provinces which may have different proportions of First Nations and immigrant women in the population than Manitoba, and different proportions of types of prenatal care providers.

Implications for practice

Marmot contends that universal health coverage is an important step toward improving access to primary health care, but will not by itself reduce health inequities without also taking action on the social determinants of health [64]. The results of this study confirm that several social determinants of health are associated with inadequate use of prenatal care, such as low income, low education, and rural or northern region of residence. Work to improve social determinants of health needs to be done both within the health sector, and through complementary activities outside health care related to housing, income, education and employment [64]. The Chief Public Health Officer of Canada [1] emphasized the need to address the broader social issues affecting pregnant women, such as low income, homelessness, and substance use, and stated, "Programs that work to break down barriers to prenatal care through community outreach have shown some success through targeting distressed communities and individuals" (p. 52).

Public health interventions to improve prenatal care utilization are important because of the potential to reduce unfavorable births outcomes [12]. Studies in the provinces of Manitoba and Newfoundland have shown that participation in prenatal support programs may improve birth outcomes [24, 25, 65]. Handler and Johnson [66] refer to prenatal care as "a critical anchor of the reproductive/perinatal health continuum for women who do become pregnant, often providing a woman's first encounter with the health care delivery system" (p. 2221) The factors associated with inadequate prenatal care in this study offer some direction for improving use of prenatal care through strategies such as reduction of teenage pregnancy, optimal birth spacing, cessation of smoking and drug abuse, provision of social support, and providing an income supplement during pregnancy such as the Manitoba Prenatal Benefit [25]. Other authors have recommended paying special attention to socially vulnerable women to reduce variations in use of prenatal care [39, 67] or more systematic attention to the roles of social disadvantage [68], and using a multidisciplinary approach [69]. In Manitoba, we have built on the results of our previous work [9, 18, 70, 71] by implementing health system improvements to reduce inequities in access to and use of prenatal care in inner-city Winnipeg [72, 73].

Conclusion

Inequities exist in utilization of prenatal care in the province of Manitoba, with wide variations in rates of inadequate prenatal care across geographic regions. Inadequate prenatal care was associated with several individual indicators of social disadvantage, such as low income, education less than high school, and social isolation. Knowledge of these inequities in utilization of prenatal care will help inform policy makers and program planners about which regions and populations are most at-risk for inadequate prenatal care and assist with development of initiatives to reduce inequities in utilization of prenatal care.

Abbreviations

AAP: American Academy of Pediatrics; ACOG: American College of Obstetricians and Gynecologists; aOR: Adjusted Odd Ratio; APNCU: Adequacy of Prenatal Care Utilization Index; CI: Confidence Interval; GINDEX: Graduated Index of Prenatal Care Utilization; HIPC: Health Information Privacy Committee; MCHP: Manitoba Centre for Health Policy; PHIN: Personal Health Identification Number; R-GINDEX: Revised Graduated Index of Prenatal Care Utilization; ROC: Receiver operating characteristic; SOGC: Society of Obstetricians and Gynecologists of Canada; TL: Tolerance Levels; U.S.: United States; uOR: Unadjusted Odd Ratio; VIF: Variation Inflation Factors

Acknowledgements

We would like to acknowledge the valuable contributions of Dr. Patricia Martens, Co-Principal Investigator (deceased), to the planning, implementation and interpretation of the results of this project. We would also like to extend our sincere thanks to our collaborators for their input: Ms. Deborah Maladrewicz, Information Management & Analytics, Manitoba Health, Seniors & Active Living; Dr. Rob Santos, Healthy Child Manitoba Office; Ms. Dawn Ridd, Manitoba Health, Seniors and Active Living; Ms. Kristine Robinson, former Clinical Midwifery Specialist, Winnipeg Regional Health Authority; and Ms. Elisabeth Dolin, former Maternal and Newborn Health Services Consultant, Manitoba Health. Thanks to Ms. Leah Crockett for developing the maps.

The authors acknowledge the Manitoba Centre for Health Policy for use of data contained in the Population Research Data Repository under project HIPC# 2009/2010 - 28. The results and conclusions are those of the authors and no official endorsement by the Manitoba Centre for Health Policy, Manitoba Health, Seniors and Active Living, or other data providers is intended or should be inferred. Data used in this study are from the Population Research Data Repository housed at the Manitoba Centre for Health Policy, University of Manitoba and were derived from data provided by Manitoba Health, Seniors and Active Living, Healthy Child Manitoba, and Manitoba Families.

Funding

This study was funded by a Canadian Institutes of Health Research (CIHR) Operating Grant: Maternal and Child Health, in partnership with Public Health Agency of Canada – Health Surveillance and Epidemiology Division (Funding reference number MCH - 97591), $100,000, 07/2009–06/2011, for the project, "Predictors and Outcomes of Prenatal Care: Vital Information for Future Service Planning." The funding body did not have a role in design of the study or collection, analysis and interpretation of data or in writing the manuscript. The following authors were recipients of career support funding during the project:
Dr. Heaman: CIHR Chair in Gender & Health.
Dr. Martens: CIHR/Public Health Agency of Canada (PHAC) Applied Public Health Chair.
Dr. Brownell: MCHP Population-based Child Health Research Award funded by the Government of Manitoba.

Authors' contributions

MIH wrote the grant application, directed the implementation of the study protocol, and had overall responsibility for the research. PJM, MDB, MJC, and MEH contributed to conception and design of the study. SAD was the programmer analyst for the study. KRT assisted MIH with preparation of the submission to Health Research Ethics Board and the Health Information Privacy Committee. MIH, PJM, MDB, MJC, MEH, KRT and SAD contributed to interpretation of the results. MIH drafted the manuscript. All authors provided feedback on the draft manuscript, and read and approved the final manuscript.

Competing interests

The authors declare that they have no competing interests.

Author details

[1]College of Nursing, Rady Faculty of Health Sciences, University of Manitoba, 89 Curry Place, Winnipeg, MB R3T 2N2, Canada. [2]Department of Community Health Sciences, Max Rady College of Medicine, Rady Faculty of Health Sciences, University of Manitoba, S113 - 750 Bannatyne Avenue, Winnipeg, MB R3E 0W3, Canada. [3]Manitoba Centre for Health Policy, University of Manitoba, 408-727 McDermot Avenue, Winnipeg, MB R3E 3P5, Canada. [4]Department of Obstetrics, Gynecology and Reproductive Sciences, Max Rady College of Medicine, Rady Faculty of Health Sciences, University of Manitoba, WR120-735 Notre Dame Avenue, Winnipeg, MB R3E 0L8, Canada.

References

1. The Chief Public Health Officer of Canada: The Chief Public Health Officer's Report on the State of Public Health in Canada 2009: Growing Up Well - Priorities for a Healthy Future. http://publichealth.gc.ca/CPHOreport. Accessed 10 Oct 2017.
2. The Marmot Review. Fair Society, Healthy Lives. February 2010. http://www.instituteofhealthequity.org/resources-reports/fair-society-healthy-lives-the-marmot-review/fair-society-healthy-lives-full-report-pdf.pdf . Accessed 10 Oct 2017.
3. D'Ascoli PT, Alexander GR, Petersen J, Kogan MD. Parental factors influencing patterns of prenatal care utilization. J Perinatol. 1997;17:283–7.

4.   Martin JA, Hamilton BE, Sutton PD, Ventura SJ, Menacker F, Kirmeyer S. Births: final data for 2004. NatlVital StatRep. 2006;55:1–101.

5.   Martin JA, Hamilton BE, Osterman MJK, Driscoll AK, Drake P. Births: final data for 2016. Natl Vital Stat Rep. 2018;67:1–55.

6.   Public Health Agency of Canada. Canadian Perinatal Health Report, 2008 Edition. Ottawa: Author. p. 2008.

7.   Public Health Agency of Canada. Perinatal Health Indicators for Canada 2013: A report of the Canadian perinatal surveillance system. Ottawa, 2013.

8.   Mustard CA, Roos NP. The relationship of prenatal care and pregnancy complications to birthweight in Winnipeg, Canada. Am J Public Health. 1994;84:1450–7.

9.   Heaman MI, Green CG, Newburn-Cook CV, Elliott LJ, Helewa ME. Social inequalities in use of prenatal care in Manitoba. J Obstet Gynaecol Can. 2007;29:806–16.

10. Marmot M, Friel S, et al. Closing the gap in a generation: health equity though action on the social determinants of health. Lancet. 2008;372:1661–9.

11. Partridge S, Balayla J, Holcroft CA, Abenhaim HA. Inadequate prenatal care utilization and risks of infant mortality and poor birth outcome: a retrospective analysis of 28,729,765 U.S. deliveries over 8 years. Amer J Perinatol. 2012;29:787–93.

12. Cox RG, Zhang L, Zotti ME, Graham J. Prenatal care utilization in Mississippi: racial disparities and implications for unfavorable birth outcomes. Matern Child Health J. 2011;15:931–42. https://doi.org/10.1007/s10995-009-0542-6.

13. Chu SY, Callaghan WM, Shapiro-Mendoza CK. Postpartum care visits – 11 states and new York City, 2004. CDC MMWR Morb Mortal Wkly Rep. 2007;56:1312–6.

14. Chi DL, Momany ET, Jones MP, Kuthy RA, Askelson NM, Wehby GL, Damiano PC. An explanatory model of factors related to well baby visits by age three years for medicaid-enrolled infants: a retrospective cohort study. BMC Pediatr. 2013;13(1).

15. Cogan LW, Josberger RE, Gesten FC, Roohan PJ. Can prenatal care impact future well-child visits? The experience of a low income population in New York state Medicaid managed care. Matern Child Health J. 2012;16:92–9. https://doi.org/10.1007/s10995-010-0710-8.

16. Feijen-De Jong EI, Jansen DE, Baarveld F, Van Der Schans CP, Schellevis FG, Reijneveld SA. Determinants of late and/or inadequate use of prenatal healthcare in high-income countries: a systematic review. EurJ Public Health. 2012;22:904–13.

17. Debessai Y, Costanian C, Roy M, El-Sayed M, Tamim H. Inadequate prenatal care use among Canadian mothers: findings from the maternity experiences survey. J Perinatol. 2016;36:420–6. https://doi.org/10.1038/jp.2015.218 Epub 2016 Jan 21.

18. Heaman M, Moffatt M, Elliott L, Sword W, Helewa M, Morris H, Gregory P, Tjaden L, Cook C. Barriers, motivators and facilitators related to prenatal care utilization among inner-city women in Winnipeg, Canada: a case-control study. BMC Pregnancy and Childbirth. 2014;14:227.

19. Heaman MI, Gupton AL, Moffatt ME. Prevalence and predictors of inadequate prenatal care: a comparison of aboriginal and non-aboriginal women in Manitoba. J Obstet Gynaecol Can. 2005;27:237–46.

20. Hiebert S. The utilization of antenatal services in remote Manitoba first nations communities. Int J Circumpolar Health. 2001;60:64–71.

21. Sword W. Prenatal care use among women of low income: a matter of "taking care of self". QualHealth Res. 2003;13:319–32.

22. Tough SC, Newburn-Cook CV, Faber AJ, White DE, Fraser-Lee NJ, Frick C. The relationship between self-reported emotional health, demographics, and perceived satisfaction with prenatal care. Int J Health Care Qual Assur Inc Leadersh Health Serv. 2004;17:26–38.

23. Healthy Child Manitoba. Healthy baby. http://www.gov.mb.ca/healthychild/healthybaby/ Accessed 10 Oct 2017.

24. Brownell MD, Chartier M, Au W, Schultz J. Program for expectant and new mothers: a population-based study of participation. BMC Public Health. 2011;11:691. https://doi.org/10.1186/1471-2458-11-691.

25. Brownell MD, Chartier M, Nickel NC, Chateau D, Martens PJ, Sarkar J, et al. Unconditional prenatal income supplement and birth outcomes. Pediatrics 2016;137(6). pii: e20152992. doi: https://doi.org/10.1542/peds.2015-2992.

26. Thiessen K, Heaman M, Mignone J, Martens P, Robinson K. Trends in midwifery use in Manitoba. J Obstet Gynaecol Can. 2015;37:707–14.

27. Brownell M, Chartier M, Santos R, Au W, Roos N, Girard D. Evaluation of a newborn screen for predicting out-of-home placement. Child Maltreatment. 2011;16:239–49.

28. Statistics Canada. 2006 Census of Population 2006. http://www12.statcan.ca/census-recensement/2006/index-eng.cfm. Accessed 10 Oct 2017.

29. Heaman M, Kingston D, Helewa ME, Brownell M, Derksen S, Bogdanovic B, McGowan KL, Bailly A. Perinatal services and outcomes in Manitoba. Winnipeg, MB: Manitoba Centre for Health Policy. 2012. http://mchp-appserv.cpe.umanitoba.ca/reference/perinatal_report_WEB.pdf. Accessed 10 Oct 2017.

30. Jutte DP, Roos LL, Brownell MD. Administrative record linkage as a tool for public health research. Annu Rev Public Health. 2011;32:91–108. https://doi.org/10.1146/annurev-publhealth-031210-100700.

31. Roos LL, Nicol PJ. A research registry: uses, development, and accuracy. J Clin Epidemiol. 1999;52:39–47. https://doi.org/10.1016/S0895-4356(98)00126-7.

32. Roos LL, Brownell M, Lix L, Roos NP, Walld R, MacWilliam L. From health research to social research: privacy, methods, approaches. Soc Sci Med. 2008;66:117–29.

33. Manitoba Centre for Health Policy. Manitoba Population Research Data Repository Data List. http://umanitoba.ca/faculties/health_sciences/medicine/units/chs/departmental_units/mchp/resources/repository/datalist.html. Accessed 10 Oct 2017.

34. Society of Obstetricians and Gynaecologists of Canada (SOGC). SOGC Clinical Practice Guidelines: Healthy beginnings: guidelines for care during pregnancy and childbirth. Ottawa: SOGC; 1998.

35. American Academy of Pediatrics and American College of Obstetricians and Gynecologists. Guidelines for perinatal care. 7th ed. Elk Grove Village, IL: author; 2012.

36. Alexander GR, Kotelchuck M. Quantifying the adequacy of prenatal care: a comparison of indices. Public Health Rep. 1996;111:408–18.

37. Kogan MD, Alexander GR, Jack BW, Allen MC. The association between adequacy of prenatal care utilization and subsequent pediatric care utilization in the United States. Pediatrics. 1998;102:25–30.

38. Heaman M, Newburn-Cook C, Green C, Elliott L, Helewa M. Inadequate prenatal care and its association with adverse pregnancy outcomes: a comparison of indices. BMC Pregnancy and Childbirth. 2008;8:15.

39. Beeckman K, Louckx F, Putman K. Determinants of the number of antenatal visits in a metropolitan regions. BMC Public Health. 2010;10:527.

40. Hosmer DW, Lemeshow S. Applied logistic regression. New York: Wiley; 2000.

41. The area under an ROC curve. http://gim.unmc.edu/dxtests/roc3.htm. Accessed 10 Oct 2017.

42. Alexander GR, Cornely DA. Prenatal care utilization: its measurement and relationship to pregnancy outcome. Am J Prev Med. 1987;3:243–53.

43. Manitoba Labour and Immigration. Manitoba immigration facts - 2014 statistical report. 2015. https://www.immigratemanitoba.com/wp-content/uploads/2015/09/MIF-2014_E_Web_Programmed.pdf. Accessed 23 Oct 2018.

44. Public Health Agency of Canada. What Mothers Say. Ottawa: The Canadian maternity experiences survey; 2009.

45. Ayoola AB, et al. Time of pregnancy recognition and prenatal care use: a population-based study in the United States. Birth. 2010;37:37–43.

46. Delvaux T, Buekens P, Godin I, Boutsen M. Barriers to prenatal care in Europe. Am J Prev Med. 2001;21:52–9.

47. Kotelchuck M. An evaluation of the Kessner adequacy of prenatal care index and a proposed adequacy of prenatal care utilization index. Am J Public Health. 1994;84:1414–20.

48. Downe S, Finlayson K, Walsh D, Lavender T. 'Weighing up and balancing out': a meta-synthesis of barriers to antenatal care for marginalised women in high-income countries. BJOG. 2009;116:518–29. https://doi.org/10.1111/j.1471-0528.2008.02067.x.

49. Phillippi JC. Women's perceptions of access to prenatal care in the United States: a literature review. J Midwifery Womens Health. 2009;54:219–25. https://doi.org/10.1016/j.jmwh.2009.01.002.

50. Sword W. A socio-ecological approach to understanding barriers to prenatal care for women of low income. J Adv Nurs. 1999;29:1170–7.

51. Raatikainen K, Heiskanen N, Heinonen S. Under-attending free antenatal care is associated with adverse pregnancy outcomes. Public Health. 2007;7:268. https://doi.org/10.1186/1471-2458-7-268 PMCID: PMC2048953.

52. United States (U.S.) Department of Health and Human Services. Expanded Data From the New Birth Certificate, 2008. National vital statistics reports. 2011; 59(7).

53. Corbett S, Chelimo C, Okesene-Gafa K. Barriers to early initiation of antenatal care in a multi-ethnic sample in South Auckland. New Zealand NZ Med J. 2014;127:53–61.

54. Raleigh VS, Hussey D, Seccombe I, Hallt K. Ethnic and social inequalities in women's experience of maternity care in England: results of a national survey. J R Soc Med. 2010;103:188–98. https://doi.org/10.1258/jrsm.2010.090460.

55. Rowe RE, Magee H, Quigley MA, Heron P, Brocklehurst P. Social and ethnic differences in attendance for antenatal care in England. Public Health. 2008; 122:1363–72.

56. Auger N, Daniel M, Platt RW, Luo ZC, Wu Y, Choinière R. The joint influence of marital status, interpregnancy interval, and neighborhood on small for gestational age birth: a retrospective cohort study. BMC Pregnancy Childbirth. 2008;8:7. https://doi.org/10.1186/1471-2393-8-7.

57. Wendt A, Gibbs CM, Peters S, Hogue C. Impact of increasing inter-pregnancy interval on maternal and infant health. Paed Per Epid. 2012;26(1): 239–58.

58. Jutte DP, Roos NP, Brownell MD, Briggs G, MacWilliam L, Roos LL. The ripples of adolescent motherhood: social, educational and medical outcomes for children of teen and prior teen mothers. Acad Pediatr. 2010; 10:293–301. https://doi.org/10.1016/j.acap.2010.06.008.

59. Petrou S, Kupek E, Vause S, Maresh M. Clinical, provider and sociodemographic determinants of the number of antenatal visits in England and Wales. Soc Sci Med. 2001;52:1123–34.

60. Krans EE, Davis MM, Schwarz EB. Psychosocial risk, prenatal counseling and maternal behavior: findings from PRAMS, 2004-2008. Am J Obstet Gynecol. 2013;208:141 e141–7.

61. Alexander GR, Kotelchuck M. Assessing the role and effectiveness of prenatal care: history, challenges, and directions for future research. Public Health Rep. 2001;116:306–16.

62. Heaman M, Bayrampour H, Kingston D, Blondel B, Gissler M, Roth C, Alexander S, Gagnon A. Migrant women's utilization of prenatal care: a systematic review. Matern Child Health J. 2013;17:816–36.

63. Di Lallo S. Prenatal care through the eyes of Canadian aboriginal women. Nurs Womens Health. 2014;18:38–46.

64. Marmot M. Universal health coverage and social determinants of health. Lancet. 2013;382:1227–8.

65. Canning PM, Frizzell LM, Courage ML. Birth outcomes associated with prenatal participation in a government support programme for mothers with low incomes. Child Care Health Dev. 2010;36:225–31. https://doi.org/10.1111/j.1365-2214.2009.01045.x.

66. Handler A, Johnson K. A call to revisit the prenatal period as a focus for action within the reproductive and perinatal care continuum. Matern Child Health J. 2016;20:2217–27.

67. Sutherland G, Yelland J, Brown S. Social inequalities in the organization of pregnancy care in a universally funded public health care system. Matern Child Health J. 2012;16:288–96.

68. Gavin AR, Nurius P, Logan-Greene P. Mediators of adverse birth outcomes among socially disadvantaged women. J Women's Health. 2012;21:634–42.

69. Bryant AS, Worjoloh A, Caughey AB, Washington AE. Racial/ethnic disparities in obstetrical outcomes and care: prevalence and determinants. Am J Obstet Gynecol. 2010;202:335–43. https://doi.org/10.1016/j.ajog.2009.10.864.

70. Heaman MI, Sword W, Elliott L, Moffatt M, Helewa ME, Morris H, Gregory P, Tjaden L, Cook C. Barriers and facilitators related to use of prenatal care by inner-city women: perceptions of health care providers. BMC Pregnancy Childbirth. 2015;15:2.

71. Heaman M, Sword W, Elliott L, Moffatt M, Helewa M, Morris H, Tjaden L, Gregory P, Cook C. Perceptions of barriers, Facilitators and Motivators related to use of Prenatal Care: A Qualitative Descriptive Study of Inner-City Women in Winnipeg. SAGE Open Med. 2015;3:2050312115621314.

72. Heaman M, Tjaden L, Chang ZM, Morris M, Helewa M, Elliott L, Moffatt M, Sword W, Kingston D. Quantitative evaluation of the Partners in Inner-City Integrated Prenatal Care Project [abstract]. J Obstet Gynaecol Can. 2016;38:488.

73. Heaman M, Tjaden L, Chang ZM, Morris M, Helewa M, Elliott L, Moffatt M, Sword W, Kingston D. Evaluation of the Partners in Inner-City Integrated Prenatal Care Project: perspectives of women and health care providers [abstract]. J Obstet Gynaecol Can. 2016;38:487–8.

74. Manitoba Centre for Health Policy, University of Manitoba. Policies on Use and Disclosure. http://umanitoba.ca/faculties/health_sciences/medicine/units/chs/departmental_units/mchp/resources/access_policies.html. Accessed 10 Oct 2017.

20

The effect of exercise during pregnancy on gestational diabetes mellitus in normal-weight women: a systematic review and meta-analysis

Wai-Kit Ming [1,2,3†], Wenjing Ding[1†], Casper J. P. Zhang[4], Lieqiang Zhong[1], Yuhang Long[1], Zhuyu Li[1], Cong Sun[1], Yanxin Wu[1], Hanqing Chen[1], Haitian Chen[1] and Zilian Wang[1*] (iD)

Abstract

Background: Gestational diabetes mellitus (GDM) is one of the most common complications during pregnancy, and it has both short- and long-term adverse effects on the health of mothers and fetuses. To investigate the effect of exercise during pregnancy on the occurrence of GDM among normal-weight pregnant women.

Methods: We searched for studies published between January 1994 and June 2017 that appeared in the Web of Science, Scopus, ClinicalTrials.gov or Cochrane library databases. Randomized controlled trials that investigated the preventive effect of exercise on GDM in normal-weight women were included. Interventions including any confounding factors (e.g., dietary) were excluded. We extracted maternal characteristics, the diagnostic criteria of GDM, and basic information for intervention and obstetric outcomes. The primary outcome was the occurrence of GDM, and the secondary outcomes included gestational weight gain, gestational age at birth, birth weight, and the odds of cesarean section. A meta-analysis was conducted based on calculations of pooled estimates using the random-effects model.

Results: Eight studies were included in this systematic review and meta-analysis. Exercise during pregnancy was shown to decrease the occurrence of GDM [RR = 0.58, 95% CI (0.37, 0.90), $P = 0.01$ and RR = 0.60, 95% CI (0.36, 0.98), $P = 0.04$ based on different diagnosis criteria, respectively] in normal-weight women. Regarding secondary outcomes, exercise during pregnancy can decrease gestational weight gain [MD = − 1.61, 95% CI (− 1.99, − 1.22), $P<0.01$], and had no significant effects on gestational age at birth [MD = − 0.55, 95% CI (− 1.57, 0.47), $P = 0.29$], birth weight [MD = − 18.70, 95% CI (− 52.49, 15.08), $P = 0.28$], and the odds of caesarean section [RR = 0.88, 95% CI (0.72, 1.08), $P = 0.21$], respectively.

Conclusions: Exercise during pregnancy can ostensibly decrease the occurrence of GDM without reducing gestational age at delivery and increasing the odds of cesarean section in normal-weight women.

Keywords: Exercise, Gestational diabetes mellitus, Systematic review, Meta-analysis

* Correspondence: wangzil@mail.sysu.edu.cn
†Wai-Kit Ming and Wenjing Ding contributed equally to this work.
[1]Department of Obstetrics and Gynaecology, The First Affiliated Hospital of
Sun Yat-sen University, Guangzhou, China
Full list of author information is available at the end of the article

Background

Gestational diabetes mellitus (GDM) is a common complication of pregnancy; based on the diagnosis criteria published by the International Association of Diabetes and Pregnancy Study Groups (IADPSG), the estimated prevalence of GDM worldwide is 17.8% [1]. In 2013, the World Health Organization (WHO) adopted the IADPSG evidence-based criteria as their standard for GDM diagnosis [2, 3]; these criteria use lower thresholds for several indices (i.e., a fasting glucose ≥5.1 mmol/l, or a one-hour result ≥10.0 mmol/l, or a two-hour result ≥8.5 mmol/l, using a 75 g oral glucose tolerance test) than previously accepted, therefore yielding more cases of GDM [4]. Gestational diabetes mellitus is more common among women who are overweight or of advanced maternal age, have a history of GDM and macrosomia, and who have a family history of diabetes [5–8].

Gestational diabetes mellitus can affect the health of mothers and their offspring due to transient abnormalities in carbohydrate metabolism [1, 5, 9, 10]. Women with GDM are at higher risk of experiencing fetal demise, fetal malformation, preterm birth, macrosomia, polyhydramnios, infection, and cesarean section than the general population [11–15]. Furthermore, both women with GDM and their infants are more likely to become overweight or obese [16, 17] and develop type 2 diabetes mellitus (T2DM) [10], cardiovascular diseases (CVD) and neuropsychological deficits later in life than the normal group [1, 17, 18].

Recent studies have demonstrated that GDM could be modified by lifestyle interventions such as exercise and diet control [19]. Exercise is characterized as planned, structured, repetitive movement that has a specific goal (e.g., health improvement). It is a subcategory of physical activity, which refers to any movement that involves energy expenditures and the use of skeletal muscles [20]. Exercise is deemed to be an important component of lifestyle intervention for GDM [21]. Regular exercise reduces the risk of T2DM, CVD, and metabolic syndrome in non-pregnant patients [22, 23]. The Royal College of Obstetricians and Gynecologists (RCOG) recommends that to accrue health benefits, healthy pregnant women should engage at least 30 min of moderate-intensity exercise at least four times per week [24]. However, only a small proportion of pregnant women achieve this goal.

Several meta-analyses support the evidence that exercise protects against GDM. Da Silva et al. concluded that leisure-time physical activity during pregnancy played a protective role against the development of GDM [25]; another meta-analysis of randomized controlled trials (RCTs) found that exercise prevents GDM in normal-weight and overweight women [26]; yet another meta-analysis of the association between exercise and preterm birth also showed that exercise lowers the occurrence of GDM in overweight or obese women [27].

Objectives

The majority of the GDM population comprises women of normal weights (based on pre-pregnant body mass index [BMI]). However, the existing systematic reviews and meta-analyses focused on the over-weight or obese population [28]. Exclusively on the normal-weight population, there are few reviews of pregnancy outcomes and one recent paper focused on the exercise during pregnancy in the normal-weight population and the risk of preterm birth [29]. To our knowledge, no published reviews have examined GDM in such population. Evidence of how exercise influencing GDM in normal-weight women could inform first-line treatments of GDM in clinical practice. Earlier meta-analyses of all-weight populations did not rule out the impact of maternal weight on GDM given that overweight and obese populations are at high risk of GDM and their status may be attributed to a variety of factors. Here, we synthesized available evidence of RCTs of exercise during pregnancy in preventing GDM in normal-weight women.

Methods

We conducted a systematic review and meta-analysis and reported our findings according to the Preferred Reporting Items for Systematic Reviews and Meta-Analyses (PRISMA) statement.

Search strategy

We searched Web of Science, Scopus (including Pubmed, MEDLINE and Embase), ClinicalTrials.gov and the Cochrane Library for articles published between January 1994 and June 2017, using the following combinations of keywords: ('activit*' OR 'fitness' OR 'exercise' OR 'sport*' OR 'physical activit*' OR 'physical exercise') AND ('pregnancy' OR 'wom*') AND ('trial*') AND ('diabetes' OR 'gestational diabetes' OR 'gestational diabetes mellitus' OR 'GDM' OR 'glucose'). The integrated search strategy is shown in Additional file 1: Textbox 1. These search terms were reviewed by a trained librarian and a physician. Reference citations for relevant articles were additionally screened to identify possible missing publications.

Study selection

Studies were included if they satisfied the following conditions: 1) they consisted of randomized controlled trials; 2) interventions used in the study included at least one type of exercise; 3) the occurrence of GDM was reported for both the intervention and control groups; 4) subjects were pregnant women with a pre-pregnancy BMI or a mean pre-pregnancy BMI ranging from 18.5–24.9 kg/m^2. Publications were excluded if they met any of the following conditions: 1) they integrated interventions of other factors (e.g., dietary) confounding the independent effects of exercise on the occurrence of GDM; 2) the pre-pregnancy BMI or the mean pre-pregnancy BMI of each group was less than 18.5 kg/m^2 or equal to or greater than 25 kg/m^2; 3) papers were literature reviews, case reports or protocols; 4) only the abstract or conference contents were published, or the studies lacked specific data.

Data extraction and outcome measures

Two reviewers (W.D., W.M.) independently searched the literature and extracted data from all eligible studies. Any discrepancy in crosschecks was resolved by a third reviewer and by discussion between all participating authors. The following data were extracted if available: 1) study characteristics (authors, publication year, country, affiliation of the authors, number of subjects, and gestational period); 2) exercise intervention (type, frequency, duration, and intensity); 3) pregnancy outcomes (GDM, gestational weight gain [GWG], caesarean section, gestational age, and birth weight). The primary outcome was the occurrence of GDM, and the secondary outcomes included gestational age at birth, cesarean section, birth weight, and GWG.

Assessment of risk of Bias

Quality assessment was based on the criteria outlined in the Cochrane Handbook for Systematic Reviews of Interventions and consisted of 1) randomization; 2) concealment of allocation; 3) blinding of the outcome assessment (blinding of participants and healthcare providers was impossible owing to the nature of exercise); 4) incomplete outcome data; 5) selective reporting and 6) other potential bias.

Data synthesis

Data analysis was conducted using Review Manager 5.3 (RevMan 5.3). Relative risks (RRs) or mean differences (MDs) with 95% confidence intervals (CIs) were used to calculate pooled effects. Relative risks were reported for dichotomous outcomes (i.e., the occurrence of GDM and cesarean section), and MDs were reported for continuous outcomes (i.e., gestational age at birth, gestational weight gain, and birth weight). Heterogeneity was assessed using the Cochran Q statistic ($P < 0.1$), qualified with Higgins I^2 statistics. A p-value less than 0.05 in the two-tailed tests was considered to be statistically significant.

Results

Study selection and characteristics

We identified 5077 publications in four databases. Upon screening the titles and abstracts, the full texts of 21 studies were reviewed. Of these studies, 13 were excluded due to the following reasons: the pre-pregnancy BMI of the patients did not meet the inclusion criteria (7 studies) [30–36], the patients underwent lifestyle interventions including dietary changes (3 studies) [37–39], there were no control groups (2 studies) [40, 41], or the studies were only observational (2 studies) [42, 43]. Eight RCTs [44–51], including a total of 3256 pregnant women, were eligible for this meta-analysis. The detailed selection procedure is shown in Fig. 1. The publication bias in the primary outcome was assessed by a funnel plot, and the results revealed that such bias existed (Fig. 2).

The general characteristics of the included RCTs are listed in Table 1. All trials were conducted in European countries. The sample sizes ranged from 83 to 962. With the exception of Stafne et al. [50], all of the interventions adopted comprehensive exercise programs of light-to-moderate intensity that were performed three times per week. The duration of each exercise period ranged from 35 to 60 min. Seven trials started in the first trimester and continued to the end of the third trimester [44–49, 51], and only one trial spanned the 20th through 36th weeks of gestation [50]. Pregnant women in the control group received regular antenatal care in all trials.

All studies reported the occurrence of GDM, gestational age at birth and birth weight; in addition, gestational weight gain was reported in five studies [45–47, 49, 51]; and the likelihood of caesarean section was reported in seven studies [44, 45, 47–51].

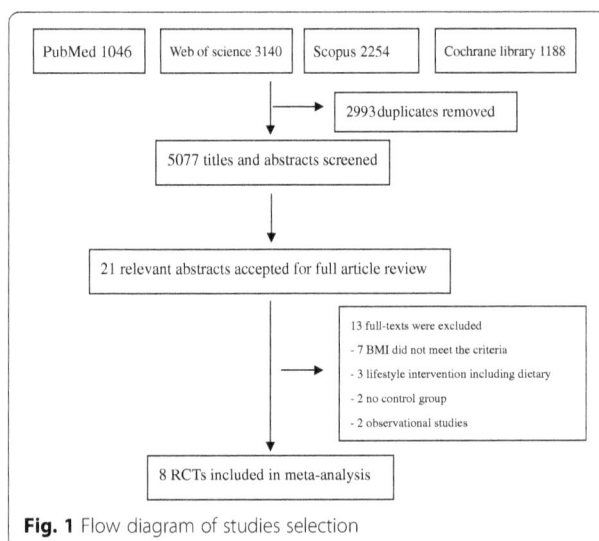

Fig. 1 Flow diagram of studies selection

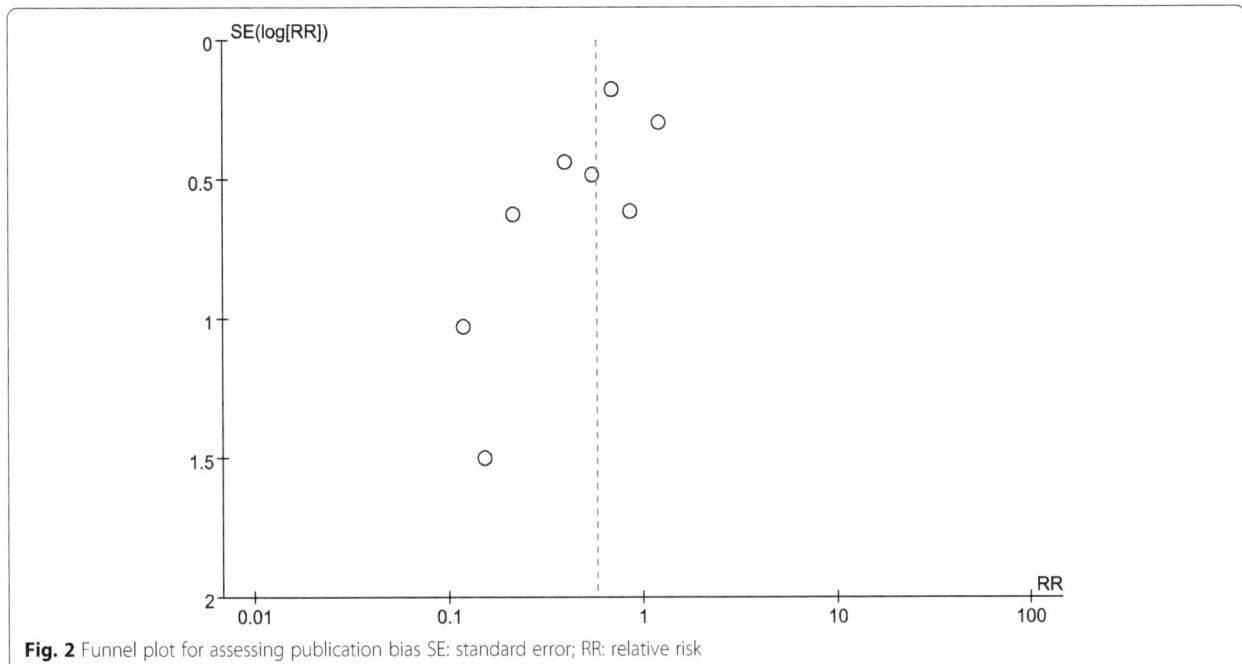

Fig. 2 Funnel plot for assessing publication bias SE: standard error; RR: relative risk

Risk of Bias in the included studies

Due to the nature of the exercise, blinding of personnel and participants was impractical. We accordingly excluded the blinding component from the bias assessment. Overall, the included trials displayed specific methodological bias (Fig. 3). Five trials showed a low risk of randomization based on the use of a computer random number generator [45–47, 50, 51], and one trial showed a high risk of bias (i.e., randomization is based on the sequence of entering study) [48], and two trials did not report this aspect. Three trials reported that the group allocation was concealed from the staff who conducted the assessment [45, 50, 51]. In terms of incomplete outcome data, three trials reported a full description of participants and follow-up status during the trial [45, 50, 51]. Only one trial was associated with a low risk of selective reporting bias of its outcomes [44].

Synthesis of results

Primary outcome: The occurrence of GDM

The diagnostic criteria for GDM varied among the eight RCTs (among these eight studies, one of the RCT with two criteria, as a result, we decided to did additional analysis as two RCTs): two were based on WHO criteria [50, 51], one was based on IADPSG criteria [51], one was based on National Diabetes Data Group (NDDG) criteria [44], one was based on criteria defined by the authors (self-reported criteria) [49]; and four studies did not report their diagnostic criteria [45–48]. Notably, one trial determined the occurrence of GDM based on the WHO criteria (before 2013) as well as the IADPSG

criteria [denoted as "Barakat(a) 2013" and "Barakat(b) 2013," respectively] (Table 1).

The analysis included 1472 women in the intervention group and 1509 women in the control group. Barakat et al. [51] was analyzed as two separate trials due to different diagnosis criteria used. Exercise during pregnancy significantly decreased the occurrence of GDM [RR = 0.58, 95% CI (0.37,0.90), $P = 0.01$ and RR = 0.60, 95% CI (0.36, 0.98), $P = 0.04$ based on different diagnosis criteria, respectively] in normal-weight women. The absolute risk reduction was 3.66% and 2.53%, respectively. The heterogeneity across included studies was high ($I^2 = 46\%$ and 52%, $P = 0.07$ and 0.04) (Figs. 4 and 5).

Secondary outcomes

Exercise had no significant impact on gestational weight gain [MD = – 1.61, 95% CI (– 1.99, – 1.22), $P<0.01$; Additional file 2: Figure S1], gestational age at birth [MD – = 0.55, 95% CI (– 1.57, 0.47), $P = 0.29$; Additional file 3: Figure S2], birth weight [MD = – 18.70, 95% CI (– 52.49, 15.08), $P = 0.28$; Additional file 4: Figure S3], and the odds of caesarean section [RR = 0.88, 95% CI (0.72, 1.08), $P = 0.21$; Additional file 5: Figure S4].

Discussion

Main findings

This meta-analysis of eight studies that included 2981 pregnant women suggests that exercise during pregnancy has a significant protective impact on the occurrence of GDM, and decrease gestational weight gain. Exercise during pregnancy does not reduce the gestational age of

Table 1 Characteristics of randomized controlled trials included in the systematic review and meta-analysis ($n = 9$)

Authors	Year	Country	Subjects(N) IG	CG	Intervention description Type of exercise	Gestational period (weeks)	Duration (minutes)	Frequency (times/week)	Intensity	Parameters Maternal	Neonatal	Diagnosis criteria
Barakat et al. [45]	2013	Spain	107	93	mobilization exercises, aerobic dance, and muscle training.	from 9 to 13 weeks to the end of the third trimester	50–60	3	Light-moderate	√	√	Not mentioned.
Barakat et al. (a) [51]	2013	Spain	210	218	aerobic exercises, muscle strength and flexibility	weeks 10 to 12 of pregnancy to the end of the third trimester	50–55	3	moderate	√	√	WHO
Barakat et al. (b) [51]	2013	Spain	210	218	aerobic exercises, muscle strength and flexibility	weeks 10 to 12 of pregnancy to the end of the third trimester	50–55	3	moderate	√	√	IADPSG
Barakat et al. [49]	2011	Spain	40	43	two land aerobic sessions and one aquatic activities session.	from week 6–9 to the end of the third trimester	35–45	3	Light-moderate	√	√	Self-reported
Cordero et al. [44]	2014	Spain	101	156	two on land and one as an aquatic activity	weeks 10 and 14 to the end of the third trimester	50–60	3	Light-moderate	√	√	NDDG
Stafne et al. [50]	2012	Norway	375	327	aerobics, resistance, stretching	between 20 and 36 gestation weeks	60	1	Moderate	√	√	WHO
Tomić et al. [48]	2013	Croatia	166	168	aerobic exercise	From 6 to 8 gestation week till the week of delivery	50	3	Moderate	√	√	WHO
Ruiz et al. [47]	2013	Spain	481	481	aerobics exercise and resistance exercises	From week 9 to week 38–39	50–55	3	Light-moderate	√	√	Not mentioned
Barakat et al. [46]	2014	Spain	152	138	toning and joint mobilization exercises and resistance exercises	From week 8–10 to week 38–39	55–60	3	Moderate	√	√	Not mentioned

IG intervention group, *CG* control group

Barakat et al. (a) = analysis with World Health Organization criteria; Barakat et al. (b) = analysis with International Association for Diabetes in Pregnancy Study Group criteria

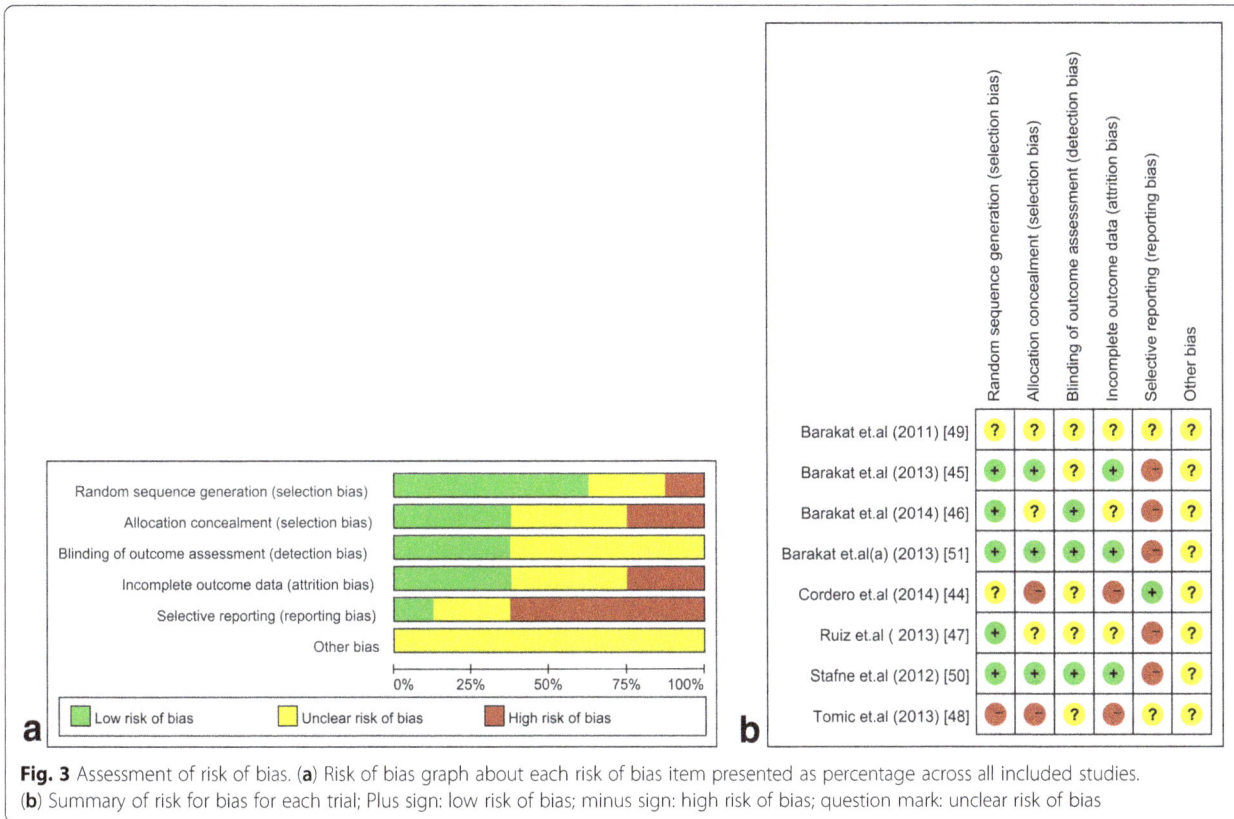

Fig. 3 Assessment of risk of bias. (**a**) Risk of bias graph about each risk of bias item presented as percentage across all included studies. (**b**) Summary of risk for bias for each trial; Plus sign: low risk of bias; minus sign: high risk of bias; question mark: unclear risk of bias

delivery or increase the odds of cesarean section in mostly normal-weight pregnant women. The mean gestational age at delivery, birth weight, and the odds of cesarean section are similar in women who exercise regularly and women who receive routine prenatal care. Summary of findings was shown in Additional file 6: Table S1.

Comparisons with the existing literature

Recently, Shepherd et al. described the effect of combined exercise and diet intervention on preventing GDM in detail, and suggested that combined diet and exercise interventions can reduce risks of GDM [52]. The meta-analysis conducted by Sanabria-Martinez et al., which included all BMI categories, showed that structured exercise during pregnancy could prevent GDM and prevent excessive weight gain [28]. Another meta-analysis performed by Magro-Malosso et al. demonstrated that aerobic exercise during pregnancy, with or without dietary intervention, could reduce the incidence of GDM in overweight and obese women [27].

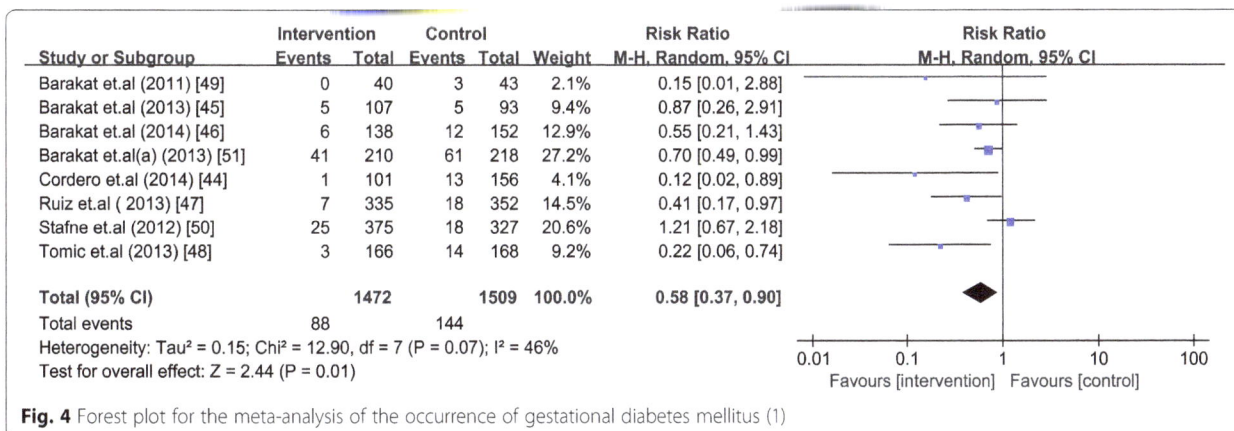

Fig. 4 Forest plot for the meta-analysis of the occurrence of gestational diabetes mellitus (1)

Study or Subgroup	Intervention Events	Total	Control Events	Total	Weight	Risk Ratio M-H, Random, 95% CI	Risk Ratio M-H, Random, 95% CI
Barakat et.al (2011) [49]	0	40	3	43	2.6%	0.15 [0.01, 2.88]	
Barakat et.al (2013) [45]	5	107	5	93	10.5%	0.87 [0.26, 2.91]	
Barakat et.al (2014) [46]	6	138	12	152	13.8%	0.55 [0.21, 1.43]	
Barakat et.al(b) (2013) [51]	29	210	32	218	22.6%	0.94 [0.59, 1.50]	
Cordero et.al (2014) [44]	1	101	13	156	4.9%	0.12 [0.02, 0.89]	
Ruiz et.al (2013) [47]	7	335	18	352	15.2%	0.41 [0.17, 0.97]	
Stafne et.al (2012) [50]	25	375	18	327	20.2%	1.21 [0.67, 2.18]	
Tomic et.al (2013) [48]	3	166	14	168	10.3%	0.22 [0.06, 0.74]	
Total (95% CI)		**1472**		**1509**	**100.0%**	**0.60 [0.36, 0.98]**	
Total events	76		115				

Heterogeneity: Tau^2 = 0.22; Chi^2 = 14.55, df = 7 (P = 0.04); I^2 = 52%
Test for overall effect: Z = 2.06 (P = 0.04)

0.01   0.1   1   10   100
Favours [intervention]   Favours [control]

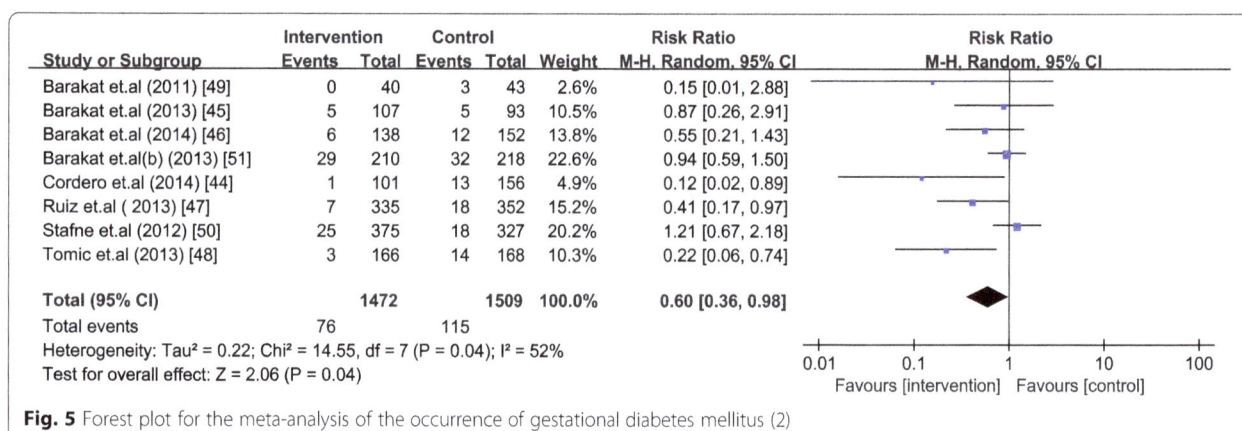

Fig. 5 Forest plot for the meta-analysis of the occurrence of gestational diabetes mellitus (2)

Recently, Di Mascio et al., in a meta-analysis of nine trials—including 2059 normal-weight women—showed that exercise during pregnancy was not associated with an increased risk of preterm birth. However, these authors found that exercise was correlated with a significantly lower incidence of GDM, cesarean delivery, and hypertensive disorders [29]. All of these studies support our findings. On the other hand, a meta-analysis conducted in 2014 suggested that physical exercise had no significant effect on lowering the occurrence of GDM. However, this study included only 947 pregnant women. In addition, exercise during pregnancy can also decrease the risk of gestational hypertension, preterm birth, cesarean delivery and macrosomia, which can significantly decrease the perinatal morbidity and mortality [53, 54].

Strengths and limitations
To the best of our knowledge, this study is the first meta-analysis focused on normal-weight women to examine the relationship between exercise/physical activity and the occurrence of GDM. This meta-analysis included all eight RCTs on the topic that have been published so far, with a larger sample size (2981 women) than earlier meta-analyses. Individual studies did not affect the overall results because of the similar sample size of each included study. These key factors are essential for assessing the validity of a meta-analysis.

However, our analysis has some limitations. The baseline characteristics (e.g., maternal age, occupation, educational level, household income, etc.) of the participants across the included studies were not balanced. Furthermore, compliance with the intervention and the effect of exercise might have varied due to differences in maternal education levels, parity, residence, and lifestyle habits before pregnancy; no included study reported adherence and compliance with the exercise regimens. Only one trial was stratified by pre-pregnancy BMI when assessing

outcomes [47]; therefore, the mean BMI of the women included in all of the RCTs was in the normal range, but some of the studies might have included a small proportion of underweight, overweight, or obese women. The result of funnel plot suggested possible publication bias, which indicated the effect of exercise during pregnancy on decreasing the risks of GDM was likely reported in published studies, yielding over-estimation of the true effect. Moreover, the method for objectively monitoring physical activity is needed. Cordero et al. [44] used a heart rate monitor to modulate the intensity of exercise, but such set-up has not yet proofed as the best site for pregnant women.

Conclusions and interpretation
Over a decade, healthcare professionals have mainly focused on overweight/obese women's exercise during pregnancy related to GDM. However, there is a considerable proportion of GDM women having a normal pre-pregnancy BMI. Also, the majority group in the whole pregnancy population is those with normal pre-pregnancy BMI. From a cost-effectiveness perspective, we need to be more concerned about those women with a normal pre-pregnancy BMI. Our study shows light-to-moderate exercise for 30–60 min, three times a week, during pregnancy is safe and worthy of promotion in normal-weight women with uncomplicated, single pregnancies. This type of exercise could significantly decrease the occurrence of GDM and gestational weight gain, which is associated with adverse outcomes like gestational hypertension, preeclampsia. Besides, exercise during pregnancy is not associated with a reduction of mean gestational age at delivery or an increase in the odds of cesarean delivery. Therefore, our findings support the RCOG recommendations that women with uncomplicated pregnancies should engage in 30 min of moderate physical activity at least four times per week in all trimesters. Our finding indicates that the physical

activity intervention in normal pre-BMI women could be a cost-effective or cost-saving management among the pregnancy population with normal pre-pregnancy BMI. Future studies should include larger cohorts to examine the association between exercise pattern (frequency and intensity) and glucose level, and to identify exercise amount and intensity that are suitable for the pregnancy population.

Abbreviations
BMI: Body mass index; CI: Confidence interval; CVD: Cardiovascular diseases; GDM: Gestational diabetes mellitus; GWG: Gestational weight gain; IADPSG: The International Association of Diabetes and Pregnancy Study Groups; NDDG: National Diabetes Data Group; OR: Odds risk; PRISMA: Preferred reporting items for systematic reviews and meta-analyses; RCOG: Royal College of Obstetricians and Gynecologists; RCT: Randomized controlled trials; SMD: Standard mean differences; T2DM: Type 2 diabetes mellitus; WHO: World Health Organization

Authors' contributions
ZW contributed to discussion and reviewed and edited the manuscript. WM and WD designed the study, searched the published work, extracted articles, analysed data, and drafted the manuscript. CJPZ interpreted the data, and reviewed and edited the manuscript. LZ selected articles, extracted data, and commented on drafts. YL, ZL, CS, YW, HC1 and HC2 commented and edited the manuscript. HC2 would correspond to the author furthest up on the author list.

Competing interest
The authors declare that they have no competing interests.

Author details
[1]Department of Obstetrics and Gynaecology, The First Affiliated Hospital of Sun Yat-sen University, Guangzhou, China. [2]Harvard Medical School, Harvard University, Boston, MA, USA. [3]Division of Pharmacoepidemiology and Pharmacoeconomics, Brigham and Women's Hospital, Boston, MA, USA. [4]School of Public Health, The University of Hong Kong, Hong Kong, China.

References
1. Metzger BE, Lowe LP, Dyer AR, Trimble ER, Chaovarindr U, Coustan DR, et al. Hyperglycemia and adverse pregnancy outcomes. N Engl J Med. 2008; 358(19):1991–2002.
2. Organization, W.H., Diagnostic criteria and classification of Hyperglycaemia first detected in pregnancy. 2013.
3. Metzger BE, Gabbe SG, Persson B, Buchanan TA, Catalano PA, Damm P, et al. International association of diabetes and pregnancy study groups recommendations on the diagnosis and classification of hyperglycemia in pregnancy. Diabetes Care. 2010;33(3):676–82.
4. Sacks DA, Hadden DR, Maresh M, Deerochanawong C, Dyer AR, Metzger BE, et al. Frequency of gestational diabetes mellitus at collaborating centers based on IADPSG consensus panel-recommended criteria: the hyperglycemia and adverse pregnancy outcome (HAPO) study. Diabetes Care. 2012;35(3):526–8.
5. Chodick G, Elchalal U, Sella T, Heymann AD, Porath A, Kokia E, et al. The risk of overt diabetes mellitus among women with gestational diabetes: a population-based study. Diabet Med. 2010;27(7):779–85.
6. Getahun, D., M.J. Fassett and S.J. Jacobsen, Gestational diabetes: risk of recurrence in subsequent pregnancies. Am J Obstet Gynecol, 2010. 203(5): p. 467.e1–6.
7. Petry CJ. Gestational diabetes: risk factors and recent advances in its genetics and treatment. Br J Nutr. 2010;104(6):775–87.
8. Cypryk K, Szymczak W, Czupryniak L, Sobczak M, Lewinski A. Gestational diabetes mellitus - an analysis of risk factors. Endokrynol Pol. 2008;59(5):393–7.
9. O'Sullivan JB. Body weight and subsequent diabetes mellitus. JAMA. 1982; 248(8):949–52.
10. Bellamy L, Casas JP, Hingorani AD, Williams D. Type 2 diabetes mellitus after gestational diabetes: a systematic review and meta-analysis. Lancet. 2009;373(9677):1773–9.
11. Landon MB, Spong CY, Thom E, Carpenter MW, Ramin SM, Casey B, et al. A multicenter, randomized trial of treatment for mild gestational diabetes. N Engl J Med. 2009;361(14):1339–48.
12. Crowther CA, Hiller JE, Moss JR, McPhee AJ, Jeffries WS, Robinson JS. Effect of treatment of gestational diabetes mellitus on pregnancy outcomes. N Engl J Med. 2005;352(24):2477–86.
13. Wendland EM, Torloni MR, Falavigna M, Trujillo J, Dode MA, Campos MA, et al. Gestational diabetes and pregnancy outcomes--a systematic review of the World Health Organization (WHO) and the International Association of Diabetes in pregnancy study groups (IADPSG) diagnostic criteria. BMC Pregnancy Childbirth. 2012;12:23.
14. Ferrara A, Kahn HS, Quesenberry CP, Riley C, Hedderson MM. An increase in the incidence of gestational diabetes mellitus: northern California, 1991-2000. Obstet Gynecol. 2004;103(3):526–33.
15. Langer O, Mazze R. The relationship between large-for-gestational-age infants and glycemic control in women with gestational diabetes. Am J Obstet Gynecol. 1988;159(6):1478–83.
16. Clausen TD, Mathiesen ER, Hansen T, Pedersen O, Jensen DM, Lauenborg J, et al. Overweight and the metabolic syndrome in adult offspring of women with diet-treated gestational diabetes mellitus or type 1 diabetes. J Clin Endocrinol Metab. 2009;94(7):2464–70.
17. Yogev Y, Visser GH. Obesity, gestational diabetes and pregnancy outcome. Semin Fetal Neonatal Med. 2009;14(2):77–84.
18. Ben-Haroush A, Yogev Y, Hod M. Epidemiology of gestational diabetes mellitus and its association with type 2 diabetes. Diabet Med. 2004; 21(2):103–13.
19. Clapp IF. Effects of diet and exercise on insulin resistance during pregnancy. Metab Syndr Relat Disord. 2006;4:84–90.
20. Organization, W.H., Global recommendations on physical activity for health. 2017.
21. Sanabria-Martinez G, Garcia-Hermoso A, Poyatos-Leon R, Gonzalez-Garcia A, Sanchez-Lopez M, Martinez-Vizcaino V. Effects of exercise-based interventions on neonatal outcomes: a meta-analysis of randomized controlled trials. Am J Health Promot. 2016;30(4):214–23.
22. Colberg SR, Sigal RJ, Fernhall B, Regensteiner JG, Blissmer BJ, Rubin RR, et al. Exercise and type 2 diabetes: the American College of Sports Medicine and the American Diabetes Association: joint position statement executive summary. Diabetes Care. 2010;33(12):2692–6.
23. Hawley JA, Lessard SJ. Exercise training-induced improvements in insulin action. Acta Physiol (Oxf). 2008;192(1):127–35.
24. Royal College of Obstetricians and Gynaecologists. Exercise in Pregnancy. London: Statement No. 2006:4.
25. da Silva SG, Ricardo LI, Evenson KR, Hallal PC. Leisure-time physical activity in pregnancy and maternal-child health: a systematic review and meta-analysis of randomized controlled trials and cohort studies. Sports Med. 2017;47(2):295–317.

26. Yu Y, Xie R, Shen C, Shu L. Effect of exercise during pregnancy to prevent gestational diabetes mellitus: a systematic review and meta-analysis. J Matern Fetal Neonatal Med. 2017:1–6.

27. Magro-Malosso ER, Saccone G, Di Mascio D, Di Tommaso M, Berghella V. Exercise during pregnancy and risk of preterm birth in overweight and obese women: a systematic review and meta-analysis of randomized controlled trials. Acta Obstet Gynecol Scand. 2017;96(3):263–73.

28. Sanabria-Martinez G, Garcia-Hermoso A, Poyatos-Leon R, Alvarez-Bueno C, Sanchez-Lopez M, Martinez-Vizcaino V. Effectiveness of physical activity interventions on preventing gestational diabetes mellitus and excessive maternal weight gain: a meta-analysis. Bjog-An Int J Obstet Gynaecol. 2015;122(9):1167–74.

29. Di Mascio D, Magro-Malosso ER, Saccone G, Marhefka GD, Berghella V. Exercise during pregnancy in normal-weight women and risk of preterm birth: a systematic review and meta-analysis of randomized controlled trials. Am J Obstet Gynecol. 2016;215(5):561–71.

30. Korpi-Hyovalti EA, Laaksonen DE, Schwab US, Vanhapiha TH, Vihla KR, Heinonen ST, et al. Feasibility of a lifestyle intervention in early pregnancy to prevent deterioration of glucose tolerance. BMC Public Health. 2011;11:179.

31. Gray-Donald K, Robinson E, Collier A, David K, Renaud L, Rodrigues S. Intervening to reduce weight gain in pregnancy and gestational diabetes mellitus in Cree communities: an evaluation. CMAJ. 2000;163(10):1247–51.

32. Rakhshani A, Rakhshani A, Nagarathna R, Mhaskar R, Mhaskar A, Thomas A, Gunasheela S. The effects of yoga in prevention of pregnancy complications in high-risk pregnancies: a randomized controlled trial. Prev Med. 2012;55(4):333–40.

33. Hopkins SA, Baldi JC, Cutfield WS, McCowan L, Hofman PL. Exercise training in pregnancy reduces offspring size without changes in maternal insulin sensitivity. J Clin Endocrinol Metab. 2010;95(5):2080–8.

34. Korpi-Hyovalti E, Heinonen S, Schwab U, Laaksonen DE, Niskanen L. Effect of intensive counselling on physical activity in pregnant women at high risk for gestational diabetes mellitus. A clinical study in primary care. Prim Care Diabetes. 2012;6(4):261–8.

35. Nobles C, Marcus BH, EJRd S, Braun B, Whitcomb BW, Solomon CG, et al. Effect of an exercise intervention on gestational diabetes mellitus: a randomized controlled trial. Obstet Gynecol. 2015;125(5):1195–204.

36. Price BB, Amini SB, Kappeler K. Exercise in pregnancy: effect on fitness and obstetric outcomes-a randomized trial. Med Sci Sports Exerc. 2012;44(12):2263–9.

37. Shuang Wang JMHY. Lifestyle intervention for gestational diabetes mellitus prevention: A cluster-randomized controlled study. Chronic Diseases and Translational Medicine. 2015;1:169–74.

38. Sagedal LR, Overby NC, Bere E, Torstveit MK, Lohne-Seiler H, Smastuen M, et al. Lifestyle intervention to limit gestational weight gain: the Norwegian fit for delivery randomised controlled trial. BJOG. 2017;124(1):97–109.

39. Sagedal LR, Vistad I, Overby NC, Bere E, Torstveit MK, Lohne-Seiler H, et al. The effect of a prenatal lifestyle intervention on glucose metabolism: results of the Norwegian fit for delivery randomized controlled trial. BMC Pregnancy Childbirth. 2017;17(1):167.

40. Yeo S. A randomized comparative trial of the efficacy and safety of exercise during pregnancy: design and methods. Contemp Clin Trials. 2006;27(6):531–40.

41. White E, Pivarnik J, Pfeiffer K. Resistance training during pregnancy and perinatal outcomes. J Phys Act Health. 2014;11(6):1141–8.

42. Leng J, Liu G, Zhang C, Xin S, Chen F, Li B, et al. Physical activity, sedentary behaviors and risk of gestational diabetes mellitus: a population-based cross-sectional study in Tianjin, China. Eur J Endocrinol. 2016;174(6):763–73.

43. Morkrid K, Jenum AK, Berntsen S, Sletner L, Richardsen KR, Vangen S, et al. Objectively recorded physical activity and the association with gestational diabetes. Scand J Med Sci Sports. 2014;24(5):e389–97.

44. Cordero Y, Mottola MF, Vargas J, Blamco M, Barakat R. Exercise is associated with a reduction in gestational diabetes mellitus. Med Sci Sports Exerc. 2015;47(7):1328–33.

45. Barakat R, Perales M, Bacchi M, Coteron J, Refoyo I. A program of exercise throughout pregnancy. Is it safe to mother and newborn? Am J Health Promot. 2014;29(1):2–8.

46. Barakat R, Palaez M, Montejo R, Refoyo I, Coteron J. Exercise throughout pregnancy does not cause preterm delivery: a randomized, controlled trial. J Phys Act Health. 2014;11(5):1012.

47. Ruiz JR, Perales M, Pelaez M, Lopez C, Lucia A, Barakat R. Supervised exercise-based intervention to prevent excessive gestational weight gain: a randomized controlled trial. Mayo Clin Proc. 2013;88(12):1388–97.

48. Tomic V, Sporis G, Tomic J, Milanovic Z, Zigmundovac-Klaic D, Pantelic C. The effect of maternal exercise during pregnancy on abnormal fetal growth. Croat Med J. 2013;54(4):362–8.

49. Barakat R, Cordero Y, Coteron J, Luaces M, Montejo R. Exercise during pregnancy improves maternal glucose screen at 24–28 weeks: a randomised controlled trial. Br J Sports Med. 2012;46(9):656–61.

50. Stafne SN, Salvesen KA, Romundstad PR, Eggebo TM, Caelsen SM, Morkved S. Regular exercise during pregnancy to prevent gestational diabetes: a randomized controlled trial. Obstet Gynecol. 2012;119(1):29–36.

51. Barakat R, Pelaez M, Lopez C, Lucia A, Ruiz JR. Exercise during pregnancy and gestational diabetes-related adverse effects: a randomised controlled trial. Br J Sports Med. 2013;47(10):630–6.

52. Shepherd R, Gomersall J.C., Tieu J., Han S., Crowther C.A., Middleton P. Combined diet and exercise interventions for preventing gestational diabetes mellitus (Review). Cochrane Database of Systematic Reviews 2017, Issue 11. Art. No.: CD010443.

53. Magro-Malosso ER, Saccone G, Di Tommaso M, Roman A, Berghella V. Exercise during pregnancy and risk of gestational hypertensive disorders: a systematic review and meta-analysis. Acta Obstet Gynecol Scand. 2017;96(8):921–31.

54. Berghella V, Saccone G. Exercise in pregnancy. Am J Obstet Gynecol. 2017s; 216(4):335–7.

21

Attitude, knowledge and informed choice towards prenatal screening for Down Syndrome: a cross-sectional study

Melania Elena Pop-Tudose[1*], Dana Popescu-Spineni[2,3], Petru Armean[2] and Ioan Victor Pop[1]

Abstract

Background: Down Syndrome screening test is a bridge between knowledge and uncertainty, safety and risk, unpredictability and desire to know in order to gain control. It may be accepted either not to have a baby with Down syndrome, or to prepare to have a baby with this condition. Every woman should understand that it is an option and should be encouraged to make their own decisions based on information and personal values. The implications and possible subsequent scenarios differentiate this type of test from the common biochemical tests performed during pregnancy, of paramount importance being the right to make informed choices. The aim of this study was to investigate the knowledge and attitude towards prenatal Down syndrome screening in order to asses to what extent the Romanian women make informed choices in this area.

Methods: A cross-sectional study was carried out that included 530 postpartum women, clients of Romania' south-east region maternities, during April–September 2016. The level of knowledge and the attitude concerning the Down syndrome screening were evaluated using a questionnaire. Data were analyzed using SPSS version 20.0.

Results: 48.1% of the women have never heard about any tests for Down Syndrome and from those 51.9% who have heard, only 14.2% made an informed choice, 78.9% had a positive attitude for screening, 88% were classified as having insufficient knowledge and 68.3% made a value-consistent decision to accept or decline prenatal screening. A higher knowledge level was associated with a higher education level and the urban residence. The information satisfaction and confidence in the overall value of screening were predictive factors of positive attitude. More informed choices were made by women monitored by an obstetrician in a private practice.

Conclusions: The prenatal screening tests for Down Syndrome were mostly unknown and the women who accepted or not to perform a test were insufficiently knowledgeable that means that the ethical concept of the informed choice wasn't followed. In our opinion the Romanian Health System needs to improve the antenatal policy by developing an adequate information strategy at the reproductive population level based on a network of trained specialists.

Keywords: Attitude, Down syndrome, Informed consent, Knowledge, Prenatal screening

Background

The incidence of Down Syndrome (DS) or trisomy 21 [1] is 1 in 650 to 1000 live births, representing the most common genetic cause of mental retardation (moderate to severe), the most common chromosomal disease of the newborn, but also the most compatible with survival of all autosomal trisomies. It is characterized by a particular facial aspect and may associate organic malformations, often cardiac. Persons with DS who benefit from special care may be socially integrated and live more than 60 years [2, 3]. Taking into account that it is caused mainly by a meiotic accident, all pregnant women have the risk of delivering a DS baby, a risk that increases steeply with maternal age [2]. Starting with 2007 the American College of Obstetrics and Gynecology (ACOG) recommends that screening for DS (DSS) to be available for all pregnant women regardless of age [4].

* Correspondence: melaniaelena_tudose@yahoo.ro
[1]Department of Medical Genetics, "Iuliu Hațieganu" University of Medicine and Pharmacy, Pasteur Louis Street No.6, 400349 Cluj-Napoca, Romania
Full list of author information is available at the end of the article

There is a wide range of DSS tests, with rates of prediction obtained either with a single test or combinations of several, thus offering multiple options. The latest technological advancement is Non-invasive Prenatal Test (NIPT), an investigation based on the analysis of free circulating fetal DNA in the maternal blood. It has a high predictability potential, that recommends it as a next in line screening in case of a positive traditional DSS, in order to avoid invasive methods [5, 6].

In Romania prenatal care is free of charge and it is part of primary care performed by family physicians. The Romanian health system refuses to include the midwife in the prenatal care team and the obstetricians can monitor healthy pregnant women only in private units. Traditional screening tests applied in Romania in the 1st trimester are the double test and/or the combined test (weeks 11–14 of amenorrhea), in the 2nd trimester the triple (between weeks 15–20) test and pregnancy morphology. These tests are not covered financially by the state and they are not part of the basic prenatal care package.

DSS identifies a condition that has no treatment yet, therefore deprived of the concept of prevention, which leads to a different meaning and multiple implications that require an altogether different approach [7]. In many countries the traditional DSS has become a routine practice [8, 9], attracting criticism because of its use by obstetricians as a "simple blood test", performed without an informed consent [10]. Studies have shown a manipulation tendency by specialists in the sense of test acceptance, by infusing a feeling of responsibility for the normal development of the fetus [11, 12]. Sometimes the manipulation is pushed to the extreme by presenting DSS as mandatory without any information, mostly under the pressure of time [13]. The very presentation of the test as routine is manipulative, as it determines its perception and acceptance as a standard [14]. Even worse, the pregnant women often let to their obstetrician the choice of tests to be performed [12], based on the assumption that all of them are for their own good and interest, with scientifically documented benefits [15].

The main argument in favor of DSS is that is offers the possibility of an informed choice by the future parents [11]. The concept of informed choice in DSS context is based on both relevant knowledge and personal beliefs and values, all reflected in the behavior toward this type of test [16, 17]. The level and the amount of information provide the basis of autonomy, it marks and orients the choice [13]. Providing biased, inaccurate, incomplete or insufficient information, either deliberately, because of haste, ignorance, or to protect the mother, is against all ethical principles, with devastating consequences over time [7, 15, 18, 19]. This prompts for the necessity to present DSS in full and without bias, and also DS in all its aspects, negative and positive, with the

implications and progress up to date [20–22], in a manner adapted to the level of education and the social-spiritual profile of the audience [11]. Obviously, such a presentation cannot be a stereotype but individualized, which requires time and specialists trained to deliver such information [19, 23]. Most studies show that in fact the pregnant women are not sufficiently informed and have limited knowledge about the aspects of the DSS process (the majority does not have the basic knowledge) and very rarely their beliefs, personal values, preferences and their need to deliberate are taken into account [9, 24–26].

The decision to take DSS is important and hard, given the possible scenarios, the probabilistic uncertainty and the impossibility to anticipate or guarantee results [23]. Both the decision and the choice of the type of testing should belong to woman or to both parents and not to local policies or to the doctor [24]. The range of options should also include the option of no testing [23, 27]. The ethics of DSS will obviously depend on the social policy and context [11].

Unfortunately the policies and screening programs influence DSS absorption [8, 12], many countries aiming at maximizing absorption, not informed absorption though, which justifies the questions raised: does DSS serve its purpose, does it observe informed choice, or not? [27]. This study started from the hypothesis that those women who have heard about at least one DSS test have a positive attitude but most probably have insufficient knowledge in order to make informed choices.

Methods

This was a cross-sectional study, carried out in 7 maternities of the South East region of Romania, during April–September 2016. Questionnaires were administered to the postpartum women on days 3–4 after delivery and included 4 sections: attitude and information satisfaction (18 items), knowledge (24 items), demographic data (7 items), as well as data related to pregnancy follow-up (7 items) (Additional file 1). The items used were adapted from two previous studies Rostant et al. [13] and Pruksanusak et al. [28] that have been validated in Australia and Thailand. Reliability of the knowledge and attitude measures were assessed on a group of 20 volunteers by Cronbach's alpha coefficient and we obtained 0.82 for knowledge scale and 0.87 for the attitude scale. We excluded women with cognitive deficits or other conditions that would prevent them from understanding the nature and purpose of the study and/or from providing requested information, as well as mothers whose babies were premature, had died, or had impaired health. Every questionnaire was accompanied by an information sheet and filling the questionnaire was considered a consent to participate. For participants under age of 16, verbal informed consent was obtained from one of their parents and the parental consent was witness by the institution's staff. The questionnaires were handed out personally by the main researcher to 610 postpartum women of which: 80 returned an unfilled questionnaire, meaning a refusal to participate, 530 (76.4%) accepted to fill in but 255 (48.1%) of them had never heard about any DSS tests and answered partially (demographic and follow up questions) and only 275 (51.9%) heard about them and completed the whole questionnaire. Data were processed with the IBM SPSS 20.0 (IBM Corp., Armonk, NY, USA). We checked for normal distribution using Chi-Square Test, Kolmogorov-Smirnov and Shapiro-Wilk tests, we applied Spearman's Rank-Order Correlation, Cross Tabulation, Mann-Whitney U and Kruskal Wallis H tests and we performed PCA (Principal Component Analyses) for the attitude and informational satisfaction scale. Statistical significance was set at $p < 0.05$. Knowledge was measured by a scale consisting of 24 items. The scale was based on answers of "yes", "no" and "do not know" about these tests. An answer showing accurate knowledge (which can be yes or no, depending on the question) received 1 point and an answer showing the lack of knowledge or "do not know" was scored with 0 points. The women with a total score of equal or less than 8 were classified as having a low level of knowledge, the women with a score between 9 and 16 were classified as having an average level and the women with a score between 17 and 24 were classified as having a high level of knowledge. We have taken into account the fact that in order to make an informed choice, it is necessary to have a level of knowledge above average. Data obtained through surveys of attitude, based on likert scale, were divided into 3 categories according to the scores obtained: negative attitude (disagreement), neutral, and positive attitude (agreement). We also analyzed the concordance between attitude and survey behavior (consistency value), and the existence of informed choice. For consistency the van den Berg et al. [26] model was used, assessing the concordance of behavior (taking, not taking the survey) with attitude (positive, negative). For the assessment of informed choice we made the correlation between the value consistency and the level of knowledge after the same model.

Results

Initially, data were collected from 530 post-partum women but after we had analyzed the questionnaires we divided the participants into two groups: Group I included 255 (48.1%) women who had never heard about any DSS and from whom we received only demographic and follow up data and the Group II with 275 (51.9%) women who had heard of at least one DSS. The mean age of the Group I was 25.91 years (SD = 6.51, range 14 to 43), three-quarters of them were from rural areas and had a low level of education and about a quarter of them were Roma (Table 1).

Table 1 Demographic characteristics (N = 530)

Category	Group I N = 255 Number %		Group II N = 275 Number %	
Age				
14–24	114	44.7	78	28.4
25–34	113	44.3	167	60.17
35–44	28	11	30	10.9
Ethnicity				
Romanian	189	74.1	268	97.5
Roma	61	23.9	5	1.8
Other	5	2	2	0.7
Religion				
Christian	241	94.5	268	97.5
Other	14	5.5	7	2.5
Education level				
Low	187	73.3	61	22.2
Medium	63	24.7	147	53.5
High	5	2	67	24.3
Residence				
Urban	74	29	149	54.2
Rural	181	71	126	45.8
No. of children				
1	87	34.1	153	55.6
2	75	29.4	98	35.6
≥3	93	36.5	24	8.7
Abortion/miscarriage				
Yes	105	41.2	104	37.2
No	150	58.8	171	62.2

Only half of them had been followed-up by an obstetrician (nearly a quarter alternatively with a familly doctor), but less than a quarter of them did not follow-up their pregnancy with anyone and only less than a quarter had a private care (Table 2).

Because the study's aim was to investigate the knowledge, attitude and informed choice towards prenatal DSS, we concentrated our research on Group II, who had heard of at least one screening test.

The mean age of the Group II was 27.88 years (SD = 5.45, range 15 to 44). More than three quarters of the women (N = 221, 80.4%) had undergone one or more tests, and less than one quarter (N = 54, 19.6%) were not tested. Overall, almost all the respondents (N = 252, 97.6%) had been followed up by an obstetrician, half of them only by the obstetrician and the other half by obstetrician and family physician (alternatively). About three quarters of the women (N = 193, 70.2%) resorted to private medical services, more precisely half of them used only private services and about a quarter both

Table 2 Data related to follow-up and information (N = 530)

Category	Group I N = 255 Number %		Group II N = 275 Number %	
Follow-up				
Family doctor	78	30.6	23	8.4
Obstetrician	75	29.4	134	48.9
Both	49	19.2	118	48.7
None	53	20.8	0	0
Where				
Private Services	33	12.9	116	42.2
State Services	146	57.3	82	29.8
Both	23	9	77	28
None	53	20.8	0	0
Time allocated by the specialist for DSS presentation				
0 min	N/A	N/A	27	9.8
≤10 min	N/A	N/A	169	61.5
15-20 min	N/A	N/A	37	13.5
≥30 min	N/A	N/A	43	15.3
Using teaching aids				
Yes	N/A	N/A	49	17.8
No	N/A	N/A	226	82.2
Took at least one test				
Yes	N/A	N/A	149	17.8
No	N/A	N/A	126	82.2

private and state insurance services (alternatively). A small percentage appealed only to the family physician and more than a quarter used strictly state ensured services. For more than a half of the participants, the time allocated on presenting DSS was equal or less than 10 min. The average time of DSS presentation by specialists was 12.23 min (Median = 10, SD = 15.26, range 0 to 120 min).

Women's knowledge

The mean knowledge score was 10.9 (range 0 to 22, SD = 4.77). None of the respondents obtained the maximum score, whilst 2.9% (N = 8) had no knowledge of these tests. The classification by 3 levels of knowledge showed that more than half of the participants (N = 157, 57.1%) had an average level of knowledge about DSS, more than a quarter (N = 85, 30.9%) a low level, and only a small proportion (N = 33, 12%) a high level considered sufficient for an informed choice. Thus, starting from the concept that informed choice implies adequate information, above the average, we considered that 88% (N = 244) of the participants had insufficient knowledge to abide by this concept.

We found that knowledge increased significantly ($\chi2 = 49.51$, df = 2, $p < 0.001$) by undergoing the DSS process, due to the higher level of general education

($\chi2 = 30,63$, df = 4, $p < 0.001$), due to a follow-up with an obsterician ($\chi2 = 20.46$, df = 2, $p < 0.001$), accessing private services ($\chi2 = 21.65$, df = 2, $p < 0.001$) and increasing the time allocated to DSS presentation by specialists ($\chi2 = 10.31$, df = 2, $p = 0.006$). We also found significant differences related to the living background, the urban participants had better knowledge than the rural ones (U = 8142, $p < 0.05$) and among the group given teaching aids (video, brochures, leaflets) (U = 4134, $p = 0.002$), that scored higher compared with those who had no visual or information materials. There was a positive correlation, though weak, between knowledge and women's age ($r = 0.12$, < 0.05). We found no correlations with the number of live children or abortions/miscarriages. For a better comprehension of the differences related to the demographic and follow up variables, a comparison of the medians is given in Table 3.

Women's attitude

The mean attitude score was 20.36 (range 0 to 22, SD = 3.39). More than three quarters (N = 217, 78.95%) had a positive attitude to DSS, almost a quarter (N = 56, 20.4%) were neutral, and only 0.7% (N = 2) had a negative attitude. Attitude was not influenced significantly by any demographic variable, though mild correlations were found in relation to follow-up. Those women followed up in a private practice, by an obstetrician who allocated more time to presentations and explanations about DSS, were more positive ($r = 0.18$, $r = 0.16$, $r = 0.12$, $p < 0.05$). We found significant differences between those who underwent at least one DSS and those who did not (U = 4335, $p < 0.001$); the former had a more positive attitude. We investigated the relation between the knowledge level and the attitude of those who took at least one test. As Table 4 shows, the two variables were correlated (phi = 0.27), better knowledge slightly increasing the positive attitude tendency.

Further on we performed the PCA for attitude and informational satisfaction scale of the questionnaire completed by the women who had at least one DSS (N = 221). Three factors were initially extracted with an Eigen value ≥1. After oblim extraction and scatter plot analysis we chose only two factors that explained 55% of the variance. The first factor was the attitude towards the adequate information (39.8%) and the second the attitude towards the overall benefits of the test (15.2%).

The value consistency and the informed choice

Starting from the fact that an informed choice is based on the level of knowledge of the subject and the personal values and beliefs reflected in the attitude and the behavior towards DSS, we searched for a concordance between the attitude toward DSS and the women's behavior (taking or not the test), as well as the degree of informed choice.

Table 3 Median scores of knowledge survey related to demographic and follow-up variables (N^c=275)

Variables	N	Median (IQR)	Test statistics	p-value
Took at least one test				
Yes	221	12(6)	2868.0[a]	0.000
No	54	6.5(5)		
Age				
14–24	78	10(7)		
25–34	167	12(7)	5.872[b]	0.050
35–44	30	12(6)		
Residence				
Urban	149	14(5)	8142.0[a]	0.032
Rural	126	9(5)		
Education level				
Low	61	8(6)	30.503[b]	0.000
Medium	120	11(7)		
High	55	14(4)		
Follow-up				
Family doctor	23	6(7)	22.489[b]	0.000
Obstetrician	134	12(6)		
Both	118	11(7)		
Where				
State services	82	8.5(7)	22.325[b]	0.000
Private services	116	13(6)		
Both	77	11(6)		
Teaching aids				
Yes	49	13(5)	4134.0[a]	0.002
No	226	11(7)		
Time allocated by the specialist for DSS presentation				
0 min	27	7(6)	24.820[a]	0.000
≤ 10 min	169	11(7)		
15–20 min	37	13(7)		
≥30 min	42	13(5)		

[a]Mann Whitney Test
[b]Kruskal Wallis Test ($p \leq 0.05$)
[c]Women who heard about at least one DSS

Table 4 The relationship between knowledge and attitude of those who took at least one DSS (N^a=221)

Attitude			
Knowledge	Neutral N (%)	Positive N (%)	Test
Low	16 (7.2)	31 (14.2)	$\chi2 = 15.49$, df = 2, $p < 0.001$
Medium	17 (7.7)	125 (56.5)	
High	2 (0.9)	30 (13.6)	
Total	35 (15.8)	186 (84.2)	

[a]No negative attitude was found in women who were submitted to at least one DSS

Summing up the number (N^a) of participants whose behavior was according with their attitude (Table 5), we found that in almost three quarters (N^a = 188, 68.3%) the attitude rhymed with behavior. A neutral attitude cannot be taken into account when referring to informed consent, therefore neutral cases were excluded (N = 275–56 = 219). We found that only 14.2% (N^a = 31) of participants (Table 6), who were pro-active, made an informed choice, according with behavior and based on a sufficient level of knowledge, while more than three quarters (N^b = 188, 85.8%) made a choice without being informed.

We analyzed the two groups (informed and uninformed choice) in relation to their independent variables (demographic, follow-up, information). Significant differences were found between the two groups regarding the education level (H = 10.90, p = 0.004), the specialist (U = 5240.5, $p < 0.05$) and the health unit (U = 5331.5, $p < 0.05$) where they followed- up their pregnancy. However, no significant difference ($p \geq 0.05$) was seen in terms of age, background, number of children or lost pregnancies, nor to the training length of time or teaching aids.

Discussion

We didn't expect to find so many women who had never heard about at least one DSS. Analyzing their demographic profile we can see that most of them came from rural places, had a low education and an inadequate follow-up in pregnancy. It's a fact that suggests to us that there is a possible discrimination in terms of health care services accessing.

However, as we expected, over three quarters of women who had heard about at least one DSS, had a high positive attitude towards DSS, a result in line with other studies: Pruksanusak et al. [28], Gourounti and Sandall [16], Rostant et al. [13], and van den Berg et al. [26]. Moreover, our hypothesis was reinforced by the poor level of knowledge found, as few of the women succeeded in completing the knowledge test with high scores that would sustain an informed choice. In fact the analysis of informed choice, based on the knowledge level and value-consistent decisions, evidenced that only 14.2% of the pro-active study women could qualify as informed for making a choice.

Table 5 Attitude towards having DSS of the women who accepted/declined the test offer

Attitude	Acceptors N (%)	Decliners N (%)	Total N (%)
Positive	186[a] (67.6)	31[b] (11.3)	217 (78.9)
Neutral	35 (12.7)	21 (7.6)	56 (20.4)
Negative	0[b] (0)	2[a] (0.7)	2 (0.7)
Total	221 (79.5)	54 (20.5)	275 (100%)

[a]These categories represent value-consistent decisions
[b]These categories represent value-inconsistent decisions

Table 6 Value (in-) consistency and knowledge about DSS (N^c=219)

Knowledge			
	Insufficient N (%)	Sufficient N (%)	Total N (%)
Value consistency	157[b] (71.7)	31[a] (14.2)	188 (85.8)
Value inconsistency	30[b] (13.7)	1[b] (0.5)	31 (14.2)
Total	187 (85.4)	32 (14.6)	219 (100%)

[a]These categories represent informed choice
[b]These categories represent uninformed choice
[c]without the neutral participants

Our study along with the Australian [13], Thai [28] and Greek [16] studies found a poor knowledge level, only the Dutch study [26], found that the majority of the participants had sufficient knowledge about DSS but this may be due to the fact that study participants received "an information booklet about DSS" before the administration of the questionnaire. There are a number of similarities between our results and those of the above-mentioned studies, but also differences regarding the possible influences. Our study as well as those by Rostant et al. and van den Berg et al. found a higher tendency to be positive in the women who had undergone at least one DSS. We could state, like Rostant et al., that this may be because those women benefited from additional information from specialists. More than that, like in the Australian study, the strongest predictive factor of positive attitude was the good information process. On the other hand, Rostant et al. and we identified a positive correlation between attitude, older age and higher education level, in contrast with Pruksanu-sak et al., who reported younger age and lower education as correlated with positive attitude. In our study, knowledge was positively correlated mainly with average to high level of general education, pregnancy monitored by a specialist, preferably in a private practice, a longer time allocated to DSS presentation, and also with age and teaching aids, handouts, especially the emphasis on explaining fully the DSS process. In the studies mentioned (except Gourounti and Sandall), higher levels of education and older age were also found positive for the knowledge process. Unlike in our study, Rostant et al. found that undergoing the whole DSS process was negatively associated with knowledge levels, but like us they found a positive association between knowledge level and private follow-up, use of teaching aids and urban background. For the women qualified as making an informed choice – 14.6% in our study, 44% in Gourounti and Sandall, and 68% in van den Berg et al. – the common predictors were the high level of education and a good financial status, the latter expressed in our study by access to private care, which is considered expensive in our country.

This study, the first in Romania on this topic, had the main objective to investigate the level of knowledge, the attitude and the degree of informed choice about DSS. Because nearly half of the participants had never heard about any DSS, the remained group for the investigation was smaller than we anticipated so that it cannot be considered representative for the region explored. However, our findings can represent a big warning for the authorities to rethink the prenatal care policies. We also consider that we've already opened a door for a future extensive study based on our methods that could investigate a large group of pregnant women to find out how well they are informed about all possible investigations in pregnancy.

Conclusions

For those women who have never heard of DSS, we can talk about violating the human right to be informed and implicitly about obstructing the right to have a choice which can be a good subject for another research.

Furthermore, a mediocre level of knowledge, as we identified in those who heard about at least one DSS, is insufficient regarding to the concept of informed choice, and most probably the almost dominant positive attitude was related to maternal responsibility and the wish to fulfill it by accepting the investigations proposed.

On the other hand, the high rate of "don't know" responses (41.1%) showed that the respondents did not want to give answers arbitrarily, nor they didn't want to appear ignorant. In support of this statement is the fact that after questionnaire completion an impressive number of women asked for the correct answers and other additional information, which our researcher provided by handing out leaflets and informative materials. This suggests that women want to be informed and the usual practice to offer specific information in a routine obstetric consulting is not a proper one.

In conclusion, this study suggests that DSS is mostly unknown and women who accepted or not to perform a test were insufficiently knowledgeable which means that the ethical concept of the informed choice wasn't followed. It also underlines the necessity of introducing DSS as an option on the list of the maternity insurance services. In our opinion, the Romanian healthcare system is subpar in this field and it is required to develop an information strategy for the reproductive population based on a network of trained specialists (midwives, genetic counselors) to provide women with adequate information to enable them to make an informed choice and facilitate their decision-making process.

Abbreviations
ACOG: American College of Obstetrics and Gynecology;
DNA: Deoxyribonucleic acid; DS: Down syndrome; DSS: Down' syndrome

Attitude, knowledge and informed choice towards prenatal screening for Down Syndrome...

219

screening; NIPT: Non-invasive Prenatal Test; PCA: Principal Component Analyses; SPSS: Statistical package for the social sciences

Acknowledgements
The authors are grateful to all the women who by their participation made this study possible.

Authors' contributions
Concept, literature search and writing the manuscript: MEP-T, IVP; Design: MEP-T, PA; Supervision: IVP, PA; Resources and materials, Data collection and/ or processing, Analysis and/or interpretation: MEP-T, DP-S; Critical review: All authors read and approved the final manuscript.

Competing interests
The authors declare that they have no competing interests.

Author details
[1]Department of Medical Genetics, "Iuliu Hațieganu" University of Medicine and Pharmacy, Pasteur Louis Street No.6, 400349 Cluj-Napoca, Romania. [2]Department of Specific Disciplines, Faculty of Midwifery and Nursing, "Carol Davila" University of Medicine and Pharmacy, Bucharest, Romania. [3]"Francisc I. Rainer" Anthropology Research Centre, Bucharest, Romania.

References
1. Online Mendelian Inheritance in Man, OMIM (TM). Down syndrome. Baltimore: Johns Hopkins University. Number:#190685: Updated 23 November 2016. Available from http://omim.org/entry/190685. Last accessed 15 Nov 2017
2. Palomaki GE, Lee JE, Canick JA, McDowell GA, Donnenfeld AE. Technical standards and guidelines: prenatal screening for Down syndrome that includes first-trimester biochemistry and/or ultrasound measurements. Genet Med. 2009;11(9):669–81. https://doi.org/10.1097/GIM. 0b013e3181ad5246.
3. Foley KR, Taffe J, Bourke J, Einfeld SL, Tonge BJ, Trollor J, Leonard H. Young people with intellectual disability transitioning to adulthood: do behaviour trajectories differ in those with and without Down syndrome? PLoS One. 2016;11(7):e0157667. https://doi.org/10.1371/journal.pone.0157667.
4. Wilson KL, Czerwinski JL, Hoskovec JM, Noblin SJ, Sullivan CM, Harbison A, et al. NSGC practice guideline: prenatal screening and diagnostic testing options for chromosome aneuploidy. J Genet Couns. 2013;22:4–15. https:// doi.org/10.1007/s10897-012-9545-3.
5. Spencer K. Screening for Down syndrome. Scand J Clin Lab Invest. 2014; 74(Suppl 244):41–7. https://doi.org/10.3109/00365513.2014.936680.
6. ACOG Committee on Practice Bulletins. Practice bulletin no. 163: screening for fetal aneuploidy. Obstet Gynecol. 2016;127(5):e123–37. https://doi.org/10. 1097/AOG.0000000000001406.
7. De Jong A, de Wert GM. Prenatal screening: an ethical agenda for the near future. Bioethics 2015;29(1):46–55. https://doi.org/10.1111/bioe.12122.

8. Crombag NM, Vellinga YE, Kluijfhout SA, Bryant LD, Ward PA, Iedema-Kuiper R, et al. Explaining variation in Down's syndrome screening uptake: comparing the Netherlands with England and Denmark using documentary analysis and expert stakeholder interviews. BMC Health Serv Res. 2014;14:437. https://doi.org/10.1186/1472-6963-14-437.
9. West H, Bramwell R. Do maternal screening tests provide psychologically meaningful results? Cognitive psychology in an applied setting. J Reprod Infant Psychol. 2006;24(1):61–9. https://doi.org/10.1080/02646830500475278.
10. Bryant LD, Green JM, Hewison J. The role of attitudes towards the targets of behaviour in predicting and informing prenatal testing choices. Psychol Health. 2010;25:1175–94. https://doi.org/10.1080/ 08870440903055893.
11. Gottfreðsdóttir H, Arnason V. Bioethical concepts in theory and practice: an exploratory study of prenatal screening in Iceland. Med Health Care Philos. 2011;14(1):53–61. https://doi.org/10.1007/s11019-010-9291-y.
12. Vassy C, Rosman S, Rousseau B. From policy making to service use. Down's syndrome antenatal screening in England, France and the Netherlands. Soc Sci Med. 2014;106:67–74. https://doi.org/10.1016/j.socscimed.2014.01.046.
13. Rostant K, Steed L, O'Leary P. Survey of the knowledge, attitudes and experiences of Western Australian women in relation to prenatal screening and diagnostic procedures. Aust N Z J Obstet Gynaecol. 2003;43(2):134–8. https://doi.org/10.1046/j.0004-8666.2003.00041.x.
14. Constantine ML, Allyse M, Wall M, De Vries R, Rockwood TH. Imperfect informed 45 consent for prenatal screening: lessons from the quad screen. Clin Ethics. 2014;9(1):17–27. https://doi.org/10.1177/1477750913511339.
15. Rowe H, Fissher J, Quinlivan J. Women who are well informed about prenatal genetic 52 screening delay emotional attachment to their fetus. J Psychosom Obstet Gynecol. 2008;30(1):34–41. https://doi.org/10.1080/ 01674820802292130.
16. Gourounti K, Sandall J. Do pregnant women in Greece make informed choices about antenatal screening for Down's syndrome? A questionnaire survey. Midwifery. 2008;24(2):153–62. https://doi.org/10.1016/j.midw.2006.09.001.
17. Erenbourg A, Stephenson J, Pandya P, Jones P, Dowie J. Decision support in Down's syndrome screening using multi-criteria decision analysis: a pilot study. Epidemiol Biostat Public Health. 2013;10(3):1–13. https://doi.org/10.2427/8941.
18. Sahin NH, Ilkay G. Congenital anomalies: parents' anxiety and women's concern before prenatal testing and women's opinion towards the risk factors. J Clin Nurs. 2008;17(6):827–36. https://doi.org/10.1111/j.1365-2702.2007.02023.x.
19. Raffle AE. Information about screening - is it to achievehigh uptake or to ensure informed choice? Health Expect. 2001;4(2):92–8. https://doi.org/10. 1046/j.1369-6513.2001.00138.x.
20. Skirton H, Barr O. Antenatal screening: informed choice and parental consent report. 2008. https://www.mentalhealth.org.uk/learning-disabilities/publications/antenatal-screening-informed-choice-and-parental-consent-report. Accessed 6 Sept 2017.
21. Seavilleklein V. Challenging the rhetoric of choice in prenatal screening. Bioethics. 2009;23(1):68–77. https://doi.org/10.1111/j.1467-8519.2008.00674.x.
22. Garcia E, Timmermans DR, van Leeuwen E. The impact of ethical beliefs on decisions about prenatal screening tests: searching for justification. Soc Sci Med. 2008;66(3):753–64. https://doi.org/10.1016/j.socscimed.2007.10.010.
23. Muller C, Cameron LD. Trait anxiety, information modality, and responses to communications about prenatal genetic testing. J Behav Med. 2014;37:988–99. https://doi.org/10.1007/s10865-014-9555-8.
24. Knutzen DM, Stoll KA, McClellan MW, Deering SH, Foglia LM. Improving knowledge about prenatal screening options: can group education make a difference? J Matern Fetal Neonatal Med. 2013;26(18):1799–803. https://doi.org/10.3109/14767058.2013.804504.
25. Jaques AM, Halliday JL, Bell RJ. Do women know that prenatal testing detects fetuses with Down syndrome? J Obstet Gynaecol. 2004;24(6):647–51. https://doi.org/10.1080/01443610400007885.
26. van den Berg M, Timmermans DRM, ten Kate LP, van Vugt JMG, van der Wal G. Are pregnant women making informed choices about prenatal screening? Genet Med. 2005;7(5):332–8. https://doi.org/10.1097/01.GIM. 0000162876.65555.AB.

27. Garcia E, Timmermans DRM, van Leeuwen E. Reconsidering prenatal screening: an empirical–ethical approach to understand moral dilemmas as a question of personal preferences. J Med Ethics. 2009;35(7):410–4. https://doi.org/10.1136/jme.2008.026880.

28. Pruksanusak N, Suwanrath C, Kor-Anantakul O, Prasartwanakit V, Leetanaporn R, Suntharasaj T, et al. A survey of the knowledge and attitudes of pregnant Thai women towards Down syndrome screening. J Obstet Gynaecol Res. 2009;35(5):876–81. https://doi.org/10.1111/j.1447-0756.2009.01035.x.

22

Barriers and facilitators to the provision of optimal obstetric and neonatal emergency care and to the implementation of simulation-enhanced mentorship in primary care facilities in Bihar, India: a qualitative study

Melissa C. Morgan[1,2,3*] (iD), Jessica Dyer[4], Aranzazu Abril[5], Amelia Christmas[6], Tanmay Mahapatra[7], Aritra Das[7] and Dilys M. Walker[2,4,8]

Abstract

Background: Globally, an estimated 275,000 maternal deaths, 2.7 million neonatal deaths, and 2.6 million third trimester stillbirths occurred in 2015. Major improvements could be achieved by providing effective care in low- and middle-income countries, where the majority of these deaths occur. Mentoring programs have become a popular modality to improve knowledge and skills among providers in low-resource settings. Thus, a detailed understanding of interrelated factors affecting care provision and mentorship is necessary both to improve the quality of care and to maximize the impact of mentoring programs.

Methods: In partnership with the Government of Bihar, CARE India and PRONTO International implemented simulation-enhanced mentoring in 320 primary health clinics (PHC) across the state of Bihar, India from 2015 to 2017, within the context of the AMANAT mobile nurse mentoring program. Between June and August 2016, we conducted semi-structured interviews with 20 AMANAT nurse mentors to explore barriers and facilitators to optimal care provision and to implementation of simulation-enhanced mentorship in PHCs in Bihar. Data were analyzed using the thematic content approach.

Results: Mentors identified numerous factors affecting care provision and mentorship, many of which were interdependent. Such barriers included human resource shortages, nurse-nurse hierarchy, distance between labor and training rooms, cultural norms, and low skill level and resistance to change among mentees. In contrast, physical resource shortages, doctor-nurse hierarchy, corruption, and violence against providers posed barriers to care provision alone. Facilitators included improved skills and confidence among providers, inclusion of doctors in training, increased training frequency, establishment of strong mentor-mentee relationships, administrative support, and nursing supervision and feedback.

(Continued on next page)

* Correspondence: Melissa.Morgan@ucsf.edu; Melissa.Morgan@lshtm.ac.uk
[1]Department of Pediatrics, University of California San Francisco, 550 16th Street, Box 1224, San Francisco, CA 94158, USA
[2]Institute for Global Health Sciences, University of California San Francisco, 550 16th Street, Box 1224, San Francisco, CA 94158, USA
Full list of author information is available at the end of the article

(Continued from previous page)

Conclusions: This study has identified many interrelated factors affecting care provision and mentorship in Bihar. The mentoring program was not designed to address several barriers, including resource shortages, facility infrastructure, corruption, and cultural norms. These require government support, community awareness, and other systemic changes. Programs may be adapted to address some barriers beyond knowledge and skill deficiencies, notably hierarchy, violence against providers, and certain cultural taboos. An in-depth understanding of barriers and facilitators is essential to enable the design of targeted interventions to improve maternal and neonatal survival in Bihar and related contexts.

Keywords: Nurse mentoring, Nurse mentorship, Obstetric care, Neonatal care, Rural health, Bihar, India

Background

Globally, an estimated 275,000 maternal deaths, 2.7 million neonatal deaths, and 2.6 million third trimester stillbirths, defined as fetal death at ≥28 weeks of gestation, occurred in 2015 [1–3]. Direct obstetric causes accounted for 86% of maternal deaths, among which postpartum hemorrhage (PPH) was the principal cause [1]. Preterm birth complications (35%), intrapartum-related events (24%), and infection (15%) were the leading causes of neonatal death [2]. Risk of mortality is highest in labor and on the day of birth, during which time 46% of maternal deaths and stillbirths and 36% of neonatal deaths occur [4]. To help reduce preventable deaths during this critical period, the World Health Organization advocates for all births to be attended by a a skilled health provider [5]. Further, estimates suggest that trained midwives, who are regulated under international standards, have the competencies to provide 87% of essential maternal and newborn healthcare services [6].

In 2015, India alone accounted for 23% and 26% of global maternal and neonatal deaths, respectively [1, 2]. In an effort to improve survival among mothers and newborns, the Indian Government launched two initiatives to promote institutional deliveries across the country. Established in 2005, Janani Suraksha Yojana (JSY) provided cash incentives to pregnant women, facilitated by Accredited Social Health Activists (ASHA), to deliver in health facilities [7, 8]. In 2011, the Government of India started Janani Sishu Suraksha Karyakram (JSSK), which provides free delivery and neonatal care as well as transport to and from health facilities [9]. To maximize impact, these initiatives focused on states with relatively high rates of fertility and neonatal mortality, such as Bihar in northeastern India, which has also been found to be the poorest region in all of South Asia [10]. Between 2002 and 2016, the institutional delivery rate across India increased from 19% to 79% [11], and in Bihar, from 20% to 64% [12]. However, while the rate of institutional delivery has risen, the quality of care in facilities is often suboptimal and coverage inadequate, especially in rural areas [13–16].

In partnership with the Government of Bihar, CARE India implemented a mobile nurse mentoring program called AMANAT (Hindi for 'emergency obstetric and neonatal readiness') in 2012 [17]. Through this program, trained nurse mentors visited primary health clinics (PHC) in pairs, conducting week-long visits to four PHCs every month over a period of 7 to 8 months to train nurse midwives. In 2014, CARE India partnered with PRONTO International to incorporate simulation and team training into the AMANAT program [18]. PRONTO is a highly realistic, simulation-based obstetric and neonatal emergency training program designed for low-resource settings [19, 20]. Simulation-enhanced mentoring was implemented in 320 PHCs across Bihar between 2015 and 2017, as described in detail elsewhere [21].

Mentoring programs have become a popular training model to address deficiencies in knowledge and skills among skilled birth attendants, typically employing a combination of bedside teaching, didactic lectures, skills stations, and simulations. However, little is known about the obstacles and enablers of this training model. Further, essential maternal and neonatal health interventions are not successfully implemented in many low- and middle-income countries due to underlying constraints, particularly regarding workforce, financing, and service delivery [22]. An in-depth understanding of interrelated factors affecting care delivery and mentoring in such contexts is necessary both to improve the quality of care and to maximize the impact of mentoring programs. This study aimed to qualitatively explore barriers and facilitators to the provision of optimal obstetric and neonatal emergency care and to the implementation of simulation-enhanced mentorship in primary care facilities in Bihar.

Methods
Setting

Bihar has a population of over 100 million, of which 87% is rural [12]. According to the most recently available estimates, the maternal mortality ratio was 274 (2013) and the neonatal mortality rate was 37 (2016) [7, 12], compared to 248 and 25, respectively, for India as a whole [1, 23]. In Bihar, each PHC serves an average population of 45,000 [24]. Obstetric and newborn care at PHCs are provided by nurses with either an Auxiliary Nurse Midwifery (ANM) or a General Nursing and Midwifery (GNM) qualification, which entail two years and three and a half years of training, respectively, following completion of secondary school [25].

Data Collection

We conducted semi-structured interviews with 20 nurse mentors, purposively selected from the total pool of 120 AMANAT nurse mentors who had provided simulation-enhanced mentoring. Participants were selected based on the following criteria: 1) nurse mentor employed by AMANAT at the time of interview, and 2) completed ≥1 phase of AMANAT (equivalent to 8 months). Participants were selected from intervention sites across 11 districts to gain maximum diversity and generate richer information (Additional file 1). Participants were recruited until thematic saturation was achieved [26]. Interviews were conducted between June and August 2016. Duration ranged from 40 to 60 minutes. The interview guide (Additional file 2) was developed in English, translated to Hindi, and translated back to English in a blinded manner to ensure accuracy and equivalence [27]. Interviews were conducted in the language of the participant's preference, either English or Hindi. Interviews were conducted by a co-author (AA) and an Indian research assistant. Both were females who had received training in qualitative research skills. Two pilot interviews were conducted to identify unclear interview questions, allowing refinement of the interview guide. These were not included in the final analysis. Questions were open-ended to allow participants to expand upon topics they felt were important, allowing the interviewer to ask new questions on emerging themes. Interviews were held in private rooms at PHCs to ensure anonymity and confidentiality.

Data Analysis

Interviews were transcribed and, where necessary, translated to English by three Indian research assistants. Transcriptions were done following the True Verbatim method to accurately capture meanings, perceptions, and context [28]. To ensure data quality, two independent staff double-checked all transcriptions and translations. Data were analyzed using the thematic content approach [26], consisting of four steps: 1) familiarization; 2) identifying codes and themes; 3) coding the data; 4) organizing codes and themes. The thematic content approach is broadly used in qualitative research and aims to present the main elements of the participants'

descriptions [26]. The first author (MM) and one interviewer (AA) read all transcripts and developed the preliminary coding scheme together. Two interviews were double-coded by the first author and a co-author (JD). Any inconsistencies were discussed and resolved to develop the final coding framework. The first author coded all remaining interviews. New themes, which could not be placed within the established coding framework, were also included [29, 30]. The consolidated criteria for reporting qualitative research [31] guided reporting for this study (Additional file 3).

Results

We interviewed 20 nurse mentors. Table 1 shows the participant characteristics.

We use the main themes emerging from the data to structure the presentation of material from the interviews,

Table 1 Participant characteristics (N=20)

Characteristic	n (%)
Female	20 (100)
Age, years (median, range)	24 (22-33)
Time working as mentor, months (median, range)	12 (9-18)
State of birth	
Delhi	7 (35)
West Bengal	4 (20)
Kerala	3 (15)
Maharashtra	2 (10)
Bihar	2 (10)
Other (Odisha, Uttar Pradesh)	2 (10)
Previous clinical experience	
Nursing school only	10 (50)
Worked as staff nurse	10 (50)
Previous teaching experience	
None	16 (80)
Nursing school tutor	2 (10)
Other (lecturer, nurse educator)	2 (10)
Primary reason for becoming a nurse mentor	
Gain teaching experience	9 (45)
Gain clinical experience	5 (25)
Wanted to work in Bihar	4 (20)
Salary	2 (10)
Career plans after this mentoring phase	
Continue mentoring in AMANAT program	14 (70)
Pursue master's degree	3 (15)
Apply for different mentoring program	1 (5)
Apply for clinical nursing position	1 (5)

broadly classified as barriers (Table 2) and facilitators (Table 3).

Barriers

Physical resources (care provision)

Over three-quarters of participants cited lack of physical resources, including supplies and equipment, as a barrier to care provision. Resources that were often unavailable or non-functional included autoclaves (for sterilization), gloves, labor tables, intravenous catheters, and suction bulbs.

"Here [beginning of the program], they are not using any instruments and they are conducting deliveries even without gloves." (Age 24, 12 months mentoring)

Several participants described persistent shortages of uterotonics, antibiotics, intravenous fluids, and antihypertensive agents. When medications were out of stock, patients or their family members were asked to purchase medications from outside pharmacies or, in emergency cases, nurses sometimes purchased medications for patients.

"Once there was a patient with severe pre-eclampsia... We used to ask them to make something available, but they used to not make it available at all... Her BP was very high, so what could we do? We had to give her nifedipine. We had magnesium sulfate in that place, but what to do about nifedipine? We did not have nifedipine there. We can't leave the patient, as her BP is so high... and how can we refer her with this high BP? We had to reduce her BP, so we went to get nifedipine from the outside." (Age 22, 9 months mentoring)

"Drugs were not at all available, so we ourselves have to go to store, tell the MOIC [Medical Officer In-Charge] about the drugs which are missing, medicines which are missing... We have to go and speak

Table 2 Barriers to care provision and mentorship

Theme	Area(s) affected
Physical resources	Care provision
Facility layout	Care provision, mentorship
Human resources	Care provision, mentorship
Doctor-nurse hierarchy	Care provision
Nurse-nurse hierarchy	Care provision, mentorship
Corruption and fear	Care provision
Cultural issues	Care provision, mentorship
Low baseline skill level	Care provision, mentorship
Resistance to change	Mentorship

Table 3 Facilitators of care provision and mentorship

Theme	Area(s) affected
Improved skills and confidence through training	Care provision, mentorship
Refresher training, increased training frequency	Care provision, mentorship
Establishment of strong mentor-mentee relationships	Care provision, mentorship
Administrative support	Care provision
Nursing supervision and feedback	Care provision

because the nurses would say, 'Sister, we are fed up of telling them again and again, nothing is happening.'" (Age 23, 9 months mentoring)

Facility layout (care provision and mentorship)

Mentors stated that distance between labor rooms and training rooms, where simulations were often conducted, was a common barrier to timely provision of emergency care and to mentorship.

"Our training room... it was far from the labor room... we had to see the patient and also the training too... we did not get to know when a patient came in full dilatation and her delivery was done in the ward... ASHA came and shouted at us so much, saying, 'Did you come here to see patients or to kill them? Patient's delivery is happening in the ward and you all are not seeing it." (Age 22, 9 months mentoring)

Human resources (care provision and mentorship)

One-quarter of participants described staffing shortages as a significant barrier to both care provision and mentorship. They explained it was common in PHCs for a single nurse to cover the outpatient department, immunization duties, emergency room, and labor room. Further, participants stated that heavy delivery loads made it difficult to find time to conduct simulations. In addition, several explained that mentees were frequently assigned to night duty before or after training, leading to fatigue with a negative effect on work performance.

Doctor-nurse hierarchy (care provision)

Nearly three-quarters of participants stated that many doctors in PHCs failed to follow evidence-based care guidelines, citing this a major barrier to care provision. Further, doctors frequently argued with nurses who attempted to follow such guidelines.

"I think they [mentees] are not... trusting in our mean doctors... In complication management, what we are

Barriers and facilitators to the provision of optimal obstetric and neonatal emergency care...

225

telling them [mentees], doctors are telling some other things... so they are in conflict to listen to us or the doctor." (Age 24, 10 months mentoring)

"'Sir [speaking to doctor], this is... PPH is happening, so we have to give'... He [doctor] will tell, 'No, no, give dexamethasone'... We told him, 'Actually sir, let's not give dexamethasone... What if we start RL [Ringer's lactate] today... as it has been given in the guidelines that we should do all these steps.' Then he [doctor] told, 'You don't have to teach us... we know how we should manage.'" (Age 22, 9 months mentoring)

Almost half of participants stated that doctors were unwilling to treat complications, instead instructing nurses to immediately refer such patients. Several participants felt this was due to doctors lacking of a sense of responsibility for patient care.

"If there is a complication, they [male doctors] will not see the patient. They will ask the sister and then just order... 'Ok, you want this medication to be written, I'll write this'... attitude is there. And if there is a female [doctor]... she will be getting so much irritated... 'Why are you calling every time? This is not normal process, natural process. You have 35 years' experience, do nicely.'... They are fighting with sisters like that." (Age 22, 18 months mentoring)

"Some MOICs and some doctors have even told us in a way like, if the mentees face any problem, then refer the patient as fast as possible. If the patient dies, then it will be out of our boundary that the patient will die." (Age 23, 10 months mentoring)

"If something happens here, the public will tell me only that, 'You did not take care well'... Doctors also, even before we do anything, keep telling, 'Refer the patient, refer the patient'... like this it happens here, so I feel that doctors should be more involved in patients' care." (Age 26, 18 months mentoring)

Over one-third of participants described doctors refusing to conduct rounds or see patients. Others stated that doctors were very slow to come even in emergency situations; for example, taking 10 to 15 minutes to attend to an asphyxiated newborn requiring resuscitation.

"They don't even touch the patient... because they get paid even without touching... nobody is there to tell them... Already they are given a big position and considered in a high position... So why would they go out of the way and do hard work without any government

pressure." (Age 23, 10 months mentoring)

"[Doctors] don't have any tension... [my] first time in Bihar, I saw two gynecologists posted in one hospital. But in that hospital also, if we are calling other after PPH... the doctor is coming after one and a half hours, where the person is going to be just collapsed." (Age 22, 18 months mentoring)

Several participants felt that some doctors were rude and disrespectful toward nurses.

"Some doctors we have fought so much... They are making fun of us in public. They are not respecting us sometimes... we have a fight with many doctors." (Age 22, 18 months mentoring)

"'You can't refer instead of me, you are not doctor... You can't refer because you are only [a] mentor in this facility.' Like that he was directly blaming me." (Age 23, 18 months mentoring)

Nurse-nurse hierarchy (care provision and mentorship)
Participants described the age gap between mentors and staff in PHCs as a significant barrier to mentorship. Over half felt that older mentees commonly perceived younger mentors as lacking experience and, as a result, were resistant to learning from them. Notably, 80% of participants had no prior teaching experience and 50% had recently graduated from nursing school (Table 1).

"She [mentee] told me that, 'I have 23 years' experience, you were not born [at] that time I started working, so don't teach me!'" (Age 23, 11 months mentoring)

"Like this age gap... they [mentees] used to not accept us, they used to cross question us... In starting in one of our PHCs... [mentee said] 'These are like kids only, what they will teach us?' But later on, when we started interacting with them... they were telling, 'You really are teaching us new things we didn't know.'" (Age 24, 12 months mentoring)

Several participants also discussed barriers to care provision related to seniority level and nursing qualifications. In particular, nurses with GNM degrees tended to have less respect for those with ANM degrees. As a result, some mentees were not able to practice the skills they had learned.

"We had a mentee who was really intelligent and she was of young age and she had a will to learn, and she learned all but she was not able to do her work... If she starts doing it [communication techniques], obviously,

everyone will start praising her, so her senior will not allow to do her work." (Age 24, 9 months mentoring)

Corruption (care provision)

Half of participants described various forms of corruption affecting patient care. Several stated that nurses collected money directly from patients for conducting deliveries. As a result, senior nurses often did not allow junior nurses to conduct deliveries. Participants explained that administrators commonly condoned this practice because they received a portion of these incentives.

"It's the same ego problem, even if we tell them... in 3 weeks, you have to do this much deliveries, then they would take us to the side sometimes and say that the one who has duty, they only do, they do not let us do it... there is some issue with money, like that who does the delivery gets some money." (Age 22, 12 months mentoring)

"If I say that, 'We should talk to the manager that your mentee is doing like this.' I would like to tell you that the manager is also taking money from someone, incentive from someone, so why will he stop the money... some percentage is divided, so why will they [laughs], you know, spoil their incentives."(Age 22, 18 months mentoring)

In addition, participants described that it was common for nurses to run private clinics in their own homes to make extra money. Nurses with private clinics often prioritized these activities over their duties in the respective PHC, and many would refer patients with complications to their clinics instead of to the nearest district hospital. A monetary incentive was typically provided to doctors and MOICs to allow these practices to take place.

"It's very common... everybody knows this.... they themselves would tell their rate, for normal delivery we take 5000, for complicated delivery we take 8000. In fact, some mentees were so... I don't know... should I call them greedy?... There is a complication... she would say, 'Go to my clinic, I will come.' After the training, she would go to her clinic, and we would come to know the complication, which we had referred [to the district hospital], happened in her clinic."(Age 23, 10 months mentoring)

Further, participants described that ASHAs received financial incentives to discourage patients from going to district hospitals and to instead bring patients to nurses' private clinics. They stated that some ASHAs conducted vaginal exams to earn extra money, despite lack of training and being warned against this practice by supervisors in PHCs.

"ASHA used to say sometimes that, 'No, these people are doing like this. We go to DH [district hospital], so much problems occur, it is very far and it is expensive also. So, it is better it happens here. We'll conduct your delivery'... they will tell like that... they will go to private practice like the nurses are doing now... they will tell like this... 'You will go to there, you will spend so much money- 5000 directly... We'll get 4000, 3000, and we'll do everything.'"(Age 22, 9 months mentoring)

"If the ASHA does PV [per vaginal] from home and comes, they would get money for it... They were not doing it properly and that was the problem... sometimes... after doing PV only, the ASHA used to bring... so that they did not have to wait for long time, they will bring after full dilatation, will get the delivery done... they will get the money and also the patient."(Age 22, 9 months mentoring)

One participant explained that some administrators instructed providers not to record complications occurring in PHCs. Another described how some staff working in PHCs sold government-issued equipment and commodities for personal monetary gain.

"We'll ask them to write all the complications... but when we go after three weeks, not many complications would have occurred... Then we came to know through the nurses that MOIC and BHM [Block Health Manager] had forced them, saying, 'Don't write any complication. We don't want any complication.'" (Age 22, 9 months mentoring)

"Some persons from the PHCs are getting many things from the government, they are getting many equipments, many things, but they are selling in the private areas. They are selling and getting more money from that." (Age 22, 18 months mentoring)

Fear (care provision)

Several participants stated that nurses in PHCs feared being blamed by doctors or authorities or being punished by patients' families if something goes wrong. As a result, nurses often refused to manage complicated patients, instead referring them to another facility.

"[Before simulation training] mentees would not even enter the delivery room... because of fear that they won't be able to do it alone or what would happen... 'If anything goes wrong then the public and the doctor would beat us.'" (Age 26, 18 months mentoring)

Barriers and facilitators to the provision of optimal obstetric and neonatal emergency care...

227

"They are afraid in some at the higher authorities... and in some local peoples... they are fearing... because if anything happens to the patient, they kill that nurse... In Bihar, many PHCs [are] like that... If complicated cases come, they are not managed." (Age 33, 18 months mentoring)

Cultural issues (care provision and mentorship)

Participants described an overall lack of awareness about the value of medical care during childbirth in Bihar. In addition, misconceptions surrounding the use of intra-uterine contraceptive devices (IUCD) were prevalent in local communities.

"People from Bihar itself, not from anywhere... they are saying like, 'Everyone, dogs, cows are giving birth so, yes, human beings are also giving birth, there is not much to think so much to have a tension so much... We don't need all these things." (Age 22, 18 months mentoring)

"Even if one [woman with IUCD] has bleeding, now then, the whole village would come to know and it would become taboo... that IUCD would lead to bleeding, then cancer, this and that, even now people say the same thing, 'No, no, no, we don't want to put anything inside... cancer would happen'... We would give counseling you know, we would concentrate much on pre-counseling, post-counseling, then we made it as a routine after patient delivered, but still that taboo... exactly because this thing was spread in their village, that it would lead to cancer, there would be more bleeding, they can't have child, can't have boy child, womb would turn." (Age 23, 10 months mentoring)

In addition, participants stated that preference for male children was common in Bihar. This led to neglect of female newborns, with some families threatening or even abusing nurses who attempted to resuscitate them.

"We have got abused while resuscitating a female baby... 'Why do you want to give life to her?... Before we have three baby, four baby, all the four are females, and now which delivery took place, even that is female... These people who have come from outside- because of them, this happened... That sister, if she would have conducted the delivery, we would have got a male'... So, we faced all this." (Age 23, 10 months mentoring)

Participants also discussed several cultural barriers to simulation-enhanced mentorship. They explained that, among local communities, belief that male doctors are not allowed in the labor room was widespread. As a result, some mentees felt ashamed or uncomfortable acting as patients in simulations when male staff were present. For religious reasons, some mentees refused to lie on the labor table during simulations and others were reluctant to enter the labor room. One participant described a situation where a mentee had psychosomatic symptoms after acting as the patient in a PPH simulation, which was perceived as a bad omen by fellow mentees.

"Sometimes they have rituals... Once, one mentee... it was a PPH scenario and there was bleeding, it was the artificial blood. After going home, she started having some problems like headache and knee pain... she became very scared that, 'No, today in the PPH [simulation], I bled so much. Because of that, I had so much problem at home.' So, all the mentees started having this thought... that this is a bad omen. With lots of difficulty we explained to them... after that, for two days, we only acted as patients then we told them, 'Sister, it is nothing, you see, do and see. Nothing happened to us.'" (Age 24, 9 months mentoring)

Low baseline skill level (care provision and mentorship)

Participants explained that low baseline skill level among mentees, coupled with longstanding use of non-evidence-based practices, posed barriers to both care provision and mentorship.

"Yes, actually really it's very bad things. The practices they are using... to initiate cry in baby... They are applying oil and tapping." (Age 24, 18 months mentoring)

"The problem is with the malpractices they follow from the last 20 years... they have learned some wrong practices, and society has given them a good name." (Age 24, 9 months mentoring)

Resistance to change (mentorship)

Finally, participants described how resistance to change made mentorship challenging, especially at the beginning. In some cases, mentees refused to participate in training sessions due to arrogance and disinterest.

"One of our facilities... it was one of our worst facilities actually... because the mentees, the administration, all were very rigid... rigid as in their behavior, in the system they didn't want to change. In everything, there was an excuse." (Age 23, 10 months mentoring)

"[Mentees] would be sitting around saying, 'It is not our duty hours, so why should we work?' At the beginning, they used to think like that only... Some of them did not change at all... like, 'I know everything, I don't need to learn.'" (Age 22, 9 months mentoring)

Facilitators

Improved skills and confidence through training (care provision and mentorship)

All participants agreed that training and mentorship improved providers' skills and confidence, particularly with regard to managing common obstetric and neonatal complications, and that this was a key facilitator of evidence-based care provision and successful mentorship.

"The first time they [mentees] were going [into the] labor room... they will say, 'I can't do delivery... never I would I have been doing,' and now they are calling us, they are managing PPH, they are managing pre-eclampsia, they are managing eclampsia, they are managing birth asphyxia." (Age 22, 18 months mentoring)

"A lot of changes have occurred in their knowledge and their practices. Earlier, in the beginning, mentees used to be a lot behind, they used to feel scared that, 'We can't do this, we can't do this'... I mean they were scared to talk to MOIC... 'Sir, how will we refer this patient?' or 'How will we do?'... they started doing everything by themselves very well... everything!" (Age 22, 9 months mentoring)

"[Previously] they are not bothering about the patient is bleeding or baby is not crying, anything they are not taking it serious[ly] because they are telling, 'It's luck, it's her luck or the baby's luck, he is going, he is not alive, so what to do with them'... But after that, we have seen that they have managed... complications about birth asphyxia, meconium or PPH." (Age 24, 10 months mentoring)

All participants agreed that simulation was a valuable aspect of training, particularly for teaching mentees how to manage complications seen less frequently in PHCs, such as shoulder dystocia and pre-eclampsia. The majority of participants felt that simulation was more effective than other training methods; however, they stressed the importance of providing lectures and skills stations to improve understanding of new content areas prior to conducting simulations in those areas.

"Simulations... I think this is a very great idea... teaching somebody who has experience of 25 to 30 years and now we have to change his practice... After doing simulation, they'll [mentees] learn how we are doing and what else we can do... Because if we are teaching them like, 'You have to do this, this, and this,' they'll not understand, they'll not even do that thing. But after doing simulation, they'll remember all we have done... so we have to do these things in real life also." (Age 23, 11 months mentoring)

"I'll frankly say, after the lunch, my mentees will sleep for classroom training... But when we do the simulation, they [say], 'Oh my god! What scenario will she give? What scenario?'... their mind starts working." (Age 22, 18 months mentoring)

"In college, we used to read from books and, by reading, we would learn something and forget something. But here practically when we did things... we understood it deep, as in what it is. I didn't have to open [a] book and read... to learn why is it like this, practically we did and the concept got cleared... I think simulation is better than anything because theory, anything would not go in their mind." (Age 23, 9 months mentoring)

Nearly all participants felt that doctors should also participate in training in order to ensure they are aware of current, evidence-based guidelines for obstetric and neonatal care. One explained that doctors in some PHCs participated in a clinical guidelines workshop that was very helpful because, after the workshop, doctors started listening to the nurses and asking questions.

"When we ask[ed] them something or had to refer, then they [doctors] used to tell by themselves that, 'No, no, we should not do this.' For example, like when there is an asphyxiated baby, they say, 'There is no role for dexamethasone here'... And that oxytocin should not be given before. In the beginning... they used to order to give misoprostol and methergin after every delivery. After that, they came to know and they used to say, 'No, no, there is no role of that and we should give only oxytocin.'" (Age 22, 9 months mentoring)

In addition, several participants felt that nurses who are not participating in the mentoring program should be included in training when possible. Related suggestions included pairing mentees with non-mentee nurses during work shifts and incorporating a short training session for both at the beginning of the mentoring period to cover basic skills, such as measuring vital signs and using a partograph.

Refresher training and increased training frequency (care provision and mentorship)

One-quarter of participants recommended refresher training and increased training frequency to improve both care provision and mentorship, explaining that mentees commonly forgot what they had previously learned following the three-week gaps between monthly mentoring visits.

"They [mentees] say, 'Sister, if this... training is done again or revision is done, then we will completely re-member it.' So, I asked that [mentee], 'What happened now?' Then she said... 'Sister, you have taught us pulse or anything, but if we do not know the basic then what do we do?' One mentee even said that, 'It was 30 years already and I still did not know how to measure BP [blood pressure].... I used to feel very ashamed, but due to this training, I learned many basic things that I used to feel shy about to do.'" (Age 24, 9 months mentoring)

"When we leave one facility and go to the other and go back to that facility after three weeks, then some changes happen again. If the gap is reduced, then it will be so much better... because some changes start oc-curring during the week, but after that the training gets completed, and then they forget those things in the three-week gap. Then again, after three weeks, we have to start from bringing about new changes." (Age 26, 18 months mentoring)

One mentor discussed use of unplanned follow-up visits during non-mentoring weeks to motivate mentees who were not practicing, additionally noting the value of employing a combination of strictness and kindness to promote behavior change.

"We used to go see what is happening... We thought that no follow up was happening at night of the third week, so they used to go at any time be it night, morning, or evening and they got used to it that people will come for visit at any time and if something is not done, they would be scolded... We had to be strict with them because, with love, we could only change the behaviors... We decided that I would be strict one and sister the loving one... so that they could share their problem with her... and I am strict, so they would be a little scared... At least they should be scared of one and other one should be good." (Age 22, 9 months mentoring)

Establishment of strong mentor-mentee relationships (care provision and mentorship)

Almost half of participants discussed the value of estab-lishing strong relationships, based upon mutual respect and trust, with mentees. Role modeling and companion-ship were also seen as key components in building such relationships.

"When we were given the ToT [training of trainers], then we were told that we have to maintain good relationship no matter how because, if it is maintained, then only

they would listen to you... In the first week, any of the days, we used to do cleaning, organizing, and seeing this, that the mentors are doing it even though they come and go in big cars, means in spite of being in a better position they are doing it, then we should also be doing it... We all used to eat together, feed each other, we never thought anything otherwise." (Age 22, 9 months mentoring)

Participants also described the importance of being approachable and promoting open communication with mentees.

"They [mentees] used to call us ma'am, actually, in starting but later we told them no use of this ma'am and all because we are really a facilitator, not a teacher... so that whatever doubts and whatever they have, they can come to us." (Age 24, 12 months men-toring)

"In the beginning, it took a lot of time to develop a relationship... then after that, so much more... They [mentees] started sharing everything with us like, 'All these things are happening here'... and if there was any complication in the night, also, they used to call us freely that, 'Sister, there is a case like this, what should we do?'" (Age 22, 9 months mentoring)

Administrative support (care provision)

Nearly three-quarters of participants discussed the im-portance of administrative support for improved care provision, particularly with regard to repair of broken equipment and replenishment of out-of-stock supplies and medications. One mentor recommended assigning experienced administrators to cover PHCs whose staff had not yet received mentoring.

"We used to tell our district manager to come in this QI [quality improvement] meeting, as the gaps were more... the district manager was also not taking things seriously... When the feedback started going, then everyone started taking things seriously... When the QI meeting was there, then the MOIC felt guilty that in his PHC things were not available." (Age 22, 9 months mentoring)

Nursing supervision and feedback (care provision)

Several participants discussed the importance of nurs-ing supervision and provision of performance feed-back by local governmental employees, particularly during non-mentoring weeks (when mentors were not present), to encourage mentees to practice newly learned skills.

"They [mentees] will practice during the mentoring week, but during the non-mentoring week, they will not

practice until their own superiors create pressure... One thing is there should be some pressure from the administrative level. That does not happen. So, I mean, only during the mentoring week, they learn well, they understand well at that time itself. But later when we come again, we had to revise the same chapter again." (Age 24, 9 months mentoring)

One participant suggested appointing the most skilled and knowledgeable mentee at each PHC to serve as leaders, supervising other mentees and providing feedback to program staff.

"The best mentee should be made the leader, so that they can supervise and should report what is not going on... this can help in sustaining [the effects of training]." (Age 26, 18 months mentoring)

Discussion

This study has demonstrated that there are a wide variety of barriers and facilitators to the provision of high quality obstetric and neonatal emergency care and to the implementation of simulation-enhanced mentorship in PHCs in Bihar, many of which are interdependent. Many of the barriers were related to the broader systemic context, and thus not directly addressed by the mentoring program. Others were related to the working culture in PHCs and providers' knowledge, skills, and practices, which may be affected by simulation-enhanced mentorship.

Barriers

Shortages of physical and human resources, coupled with high patient volume in PHCs, posed significant barriers to both care provision and mentorship. Similar resource constraints have been reported globally [32, 33] and in Bihar [24, 34]. Despite establishment of 1,045 new institutions offering GNM courses and 1,362 new institutions offering ANM courses across India between 2009 and 2015 [35, 36], estimates suggested shortages of approximately 1.3 million GNMs (178%) and 670,000 ANMs (185%) in 2015 [37]. Improved utilization of ASHAs and Ayurvedic, Yoga and Naturopathy, Unani, Siddha and Homoeopathy doctors may help relieve this burden by providing basic healthcare services, particularly at the community level [38]. Barriers related to doctor-nurse and nurse-nurse hierarchy were also prevalent in PHCs. Problems with doctors stemmed from disrespect, disagreement regarding clinical guidelines, and poor sense of responsibility for patient care; whereas among nurses, differences in age, seniority, or nursing qualifications were commonly implicated. Other studies have similarly noted hierarchical issues affecting the quality of healthcare in India [39, 40]. In this program, the fact that the mentors were young, with limited

clinical and teaching experience, was an important limitation to their ability to effectively mentor.

Various forms of corruption affecting care provision were identified, including side payments for doctors and nurses and financial incentives for ASHAs. Corruption in healthcare has been recognized as a common problem in India [41–43]. Several reports have acknowledged corruption, primarily in the form of providers demanding side payments from patients, as a barrier to the success of the JSY and JSSK programs [44–46]. Such practices not only have negative financial consequences for patients; they may also hinder appropriate management and referral of patients with complications. Fear of blame and physical assault in response to poor outcomes was another significant barrier to care provision, leading providers to frequently refer complicated cases. Violence against providers has been increasing globally, due to mistrust of the medical profession, corruption and lack of faith in the judicial system, rising cost of healthcare, and insufficient security in many facilities [47–51]. In India, additional causes include low health literacy, poor quality of service, and widespread belief that patients' families may perpetrate violence with impunity [49–51]. These factors create an environment where providers are disinclined to communicate details about medical emergencies to patients and their families, leading to a sense of perceived neglect that may trigger violence. A training or mentorship program that focuses on empathy and effective communication with patients may help to address this systemic issue [49, 50]. The next iteration of the PRONTO simulation curriculum in Bihar has been adapted accordingly.

Lack of awareness about the value of medical care during childbirth was found to be common in Bihar. A related study similarly identified that prevalent perception of childbirth as a 'natural event,' which does not require healthcare, was a key factor impeding the uptake of JSY services in other high-focus states [46]. Preference for male infants was another cultural barrier, which frequently led to neglectful care of female newborns. Recent demographic data supports this finding, additionally determining that sex-selective abortion is common in Bihar [12]. Finally, this study identified widespread misconceptions regarding use of IUCDs, including beliefs that they cause irregular bleeding, cancer, and infertility. Similar findings have been reported elsewhere in India [52]. In 2016, the contraceptive prevalence rate in Bihar was 24%, compared to 54% nationally, and the rate of IUCD use was 0.5%, compared to 1.5% nationally [11, 12]. A study in Bihar found that lack of trained providers, community awareness, and accessibility to quality services were the main causes for low acceptance of IUCDs, and suggested that mobile family planning units with trained and skilled providers may promote use in remote areas [53].

Facilitators

Improved skills and confidence, inclusion of doctors in training, and increased training frequency were seen as key facilitators of evidence-based care provision and successful mentorship. A study in India found that a 16-week training program for medical officers increased the proportion of trainees performing basic emergency obstetric care [54]. Comparable findings have also been seen in other programs focusing on obstetric and neonatal provider training in low-resource settings, including Making it Happen [55], Helping Babies Breathe (HBB) [56, 57], and the Dakshata Initiative [58]. Unlike AMANAT, these programs were much shorter in duration (1-2 days), utilized mannequins (as opposed to patient actors), and were generally conducted outside trainees' usual workplaces. A study of HBB training in Tanzania found that the pass percentage for knowledge tests decreased from 89% to 69% eight weeks after initial training, improving to 90% following refresher training [56]. A more recent study of HBB in India and Kenya found that the successful completion rate for skills evaluations decreased from 99% to 81% seven months after initial training [57]. Similarly, participants in this study felt that knowledge and skills declined between monthly visits, and increased training frequency and refresher training were recommended. A nurse mentoring study in Uganda also noted the value of refresher training [59]. A study in Indonesia found that peer review and follow-up training led to enhanced consolidation of provider knowledge and skills [60].

Establishment of strong mentor-mentee relationships was identified as a key facilitator of mentorship, encouraging mutual respect, trust, and self-reflection among mentees. Role modeling, approachability, and open communication were seen as vital aspects of this relationship. A study in the U.S. similarly identified open communication and accessibility; mutual respect and trust; goals and challenges; passion and inspiration; caring personal relationship; knowledge exchange; independence and collaboration; and role modeling as central components of an effective mentoring relationship [61]. The aforementioned Ugandan study also noted the importance of role modeling, approachability, and establishing rapport [59]. As shown in this study, this can be challenging if there are significant gaps in age and experience between mentors and mentees.

Administrative support was an additional facilitator of care provision, particularly with regard to achieving sustainable improvements. Panda and Thakur similarly suggested that management practices, including decision making norms, knowledge, and experience of administrators, are critical to ensure the successful delivery of public health services in India [62]. Finally, nursing supervision and feedback were identified as additional facilitators of mentoring. In Tanzania, a study suggested identifying champion mentees at each site to receive additional and continued distance mentorship, who could provide refresher trainings and assist with follow-up [63]. Similarly, one participant in this study recommended appointing lead mentees at each site to supervise other nurses and provide programmatic feedback. Routine maternal and perinatal mortality audits, including consistent cause of death classification and use of best practice guidelines to monitor performance, have also been shown to promote improved care at the facility level in low-resource settings [64].

Limitations

This study has several limitations. Participants had experience mentoring in PHCs during the AMANAT program, but had not served as primary providers in PHCs; thus, any preconceptions they had about Bihar could have introduced information bias. However, all participants had at least 9 months of mentoring experience in four or more PHCs. Further, two participants were from Bihar and their responses were not notably different compared to those from other states. Feedback regarding the mentoring program was not obtained from government officials or doctors working in PHCs; however, interviews were conducted with nurse mentees. These findings will be presented in a future manuscript. As the interviewers were members of the PRONTO team who were involved in training mentors, respondents may have provided answers to please the interviewers. To increase content validity, a local Hindi interviewer was present at all interviews and participants were ensured their responses were completely confidential in nature.

Overall recommendations

Many of the identified obstacles were interdependent, affecting both care provision and mentorship, including those related to human resources, hierarchy, cultural beliefs, and provider practices and behaviors. These factors are particularly important to recognize and to address when possible, as they negatively affect both the quality of facility-based care and the impact of mentorship. Simulation-enhanced mentoring programs may be contextually tailored to address key barriers beyond deficiencies in providers' knowledge and skills, notably hierarchical issues in facilities, violence against providers, and cultural taboos regarding provision of delivery care by male doctors. This suggests that simulation-enhanced mentoring is an appropriate training model to improve obstetric and neonatal care at primary care facilities in Bihar.

Conclusions

This study has identified numerous barriers and enablers to the provision of obstetric and neonatal emergency care and to the implementation of simulation-enhanced mentorship in Bihar. The mentoring program was not designed to address some obstacles, including resource shortages, facility infrastructure, corruption, and cultural norms, as these require government support, community awareness, and other systemic changes. Mentoring programs may be adapted to address some aspects of care provision beyond provider knowledge and skills, notably hierarchy in facilities, violence against providers, and certain cultural taboos, while simultaneously building confidence in simulation training. An in-depth understanding of key barriers and facilitators is essential to enable the design of contextually-targeted interventions to improve survival among mothers and newborns in Bihar and elsewhere in India.

Abbreviations

AMANAT: Aapathekalin Matritva Aevum Naavjat Sishu Tatparta (Hindi for 'emergency obstetric and neonatal readiness'); ANM: Auxiliary Nurse Midwifery (degree); ASHA: Accredited Social Health Activist; BHM: Block Health Manager; BP: Blood pressure; GNM: General Nursing and Midwifery (degree); HBB: Helping Babies Breathe; IUCD: Intrauterine contraceptive device; JSSK: Janani Sishu Suraksha Karyakram; JSY: Janani Suraksha Yojana; MOIC: Medical Officer In-Charge; PHC: Primary health clinic; PPH: Postpartum hemorrhage; QI: Quality improvement; ToT: Training of trainers

Acknowledgements
Special thanks to the nurse mentors who participated in this study. We thank Praicey Thomas, Shravan Kumar, Swarna Yadav, Rebecka Thananki, and Rohit Srivastava for their work on this study.

Funding
This study was funded by the Bill and Melinda Gates Foundation. The sponsor was not involved in study design, data collection, analysis, data interpretation, or manuscript writing.

Authors' contributions

MM conceptualized and designed the study, created the study tools, analyzed and interpreted the data, and wrote and revised the manuscript. JD assisted with study tool design, managed the study, assisted with data analysis and interpretation, and reviewed and edited the manuscript. AA assisted with study tool design, conducted interviews, assisted with data analysis and interpretation, and reviewed and edited the manuscript. AC supervised PRONTO training, implemented the study, provided expert local opinion for study tool design and data analysis, and reviewed and edited the manuscript. TM managed the AMANAT program, supervised data collection, and reviewed and edited the manuscript. AD managed the AMANAT program, supervised data collection, and reviewed and edited the manuscript. DW is the principal investigator for the overarching evaluation of PRONTO training in Bihar and made significant contributions to all aspects of study design and manuscript preparation. All authors read and approved the final manuscript.

Competing interests

DW is a founding member of PRONTO International and part of the Board of Directors. All other authors declare that they have no competing interests.

Author details

[1]Department of Pediatrics, University of California San Francisco, 550 16th Street, Box 1224, San Francisco, CA 94158, USA. [2]Institute for Global Health Sciences, University of California San Francisco, 550 16th Street, Box 1224, San Francisco, CA 94158, USA. [3]Maternal, Adolescent, Reproductive, and Child Health Centre, London School of Hygiene & Tropical Medicine, Keppel Street, London WC1E 7HT, UK. [4]Pronto International, 5419 Greenwood Avenue North, Seattle, WA 98103, USA. [5]Médecins Sans Frontières, Nou de la Rambla 26, 08001 Barcelona, Spain. [6]Pronto International; State RMNCH+A Unit, C-16 Krishi Nagar, A.G. Colony, Patna, Bihar 80002, India. [7]CARE India, 14 Patliputra Colony, Patna, Bihar 800013, India. [8]Department of Obstetrics, Gynecology, and Reproductive Sciences, University of California San Francisco, 1001 Potrero Ave, San Francisco, CA 94110, USA.

References

1. Kassebaum NJ, Barber RM, Bhutta ZA, Dandona L, Gething PW, Hay SI, et al. Global, regional, and national levels of maternal mortality, 1990–2015: a systematic analysis for the Global Burden of Disease Study 2015. Lancet. 2016;388:1775–812.
2. Liu L, Oza S, Hogan D, Chu Y, Perin J, Zhu J, et al. Global, regional, and national causes of under-5 mortality in 2000–15: an updated systematic analysis with implications for the Sustainable Development Goals. Lancet. 2016;388:3027–35.
3. Lawn JE, Blencowe H, Waiswa P, Amouzou A, Mathers C, Hogan D, et al. Ending preventable stillbirths: rates, risk factors, and acceleration towards 2030. Lancet. 2016;387:587–603.
4. Lawn JE, Blencowe H, Oza S, You D, Lee ACC, Waiswa P, et al. Progress, priorities, and potential beyond survival. Lancet. 2014;384:189–205.
5. World Health Organization. Maternal mortality: fact sheet. 2016. http://www.who.int/mediacentre/factsheets/fs348/en/. Accessed 2018 Apr 28.
6. United Nations Population Fund, International Confederation of Midwives, World Health Organization. The State of the World's Midwifery: A Universal Pathway. A Woman's Right to Health. 2014. https://www.unfpa.org/sites/default/files/pub-pdf/EN_SoWMy2014_complete.pdf. Accessed 2017 Nov 11.
7. Office of the Registrar General & Census Commissioner. Fact Sheet: Bihar. Annual Health Survey 2012-13. New Delhi; 2013. http://www.censusindia.gov.in/vital_statistics/AHSBulletins/AHS_Factsheets_2012-13/FACTSHEET-Bihar.pdf. Accessed 2017 Nov 11

8. Ministry of Health & Family Welfare. Janani Suraksha Yojana: Guidelines for Implementation. 2015. http://www.ilo.org/dyn/travail/docs/683/JananiSurakshaYojanaGuidelines/MinistryofHealthandFamilyWelfare.pdf. Accessed 2018 Apr 28.

9. Ministry of Health and Family Welfare. Guidelines for Janani Sishu Suraksha Karyakram (JSSK). https://www.nhp.gov.in/janani-shishu-suraksha-karyakaram-jssk_pg. Accessed 2018 Apr 28.

10. Oxford Poverty & Human Development Initiative. Multidimensional Poverty Index 2016 Highlights ~ South Asia. Oxford, UK; 2016. https://www.ophi.org.uk/wp-content/uploads/MPI2015-SOUTH-ASIA-HIGHLIGHTS_June.pdf. Accessed 2017 Nov 8

11. Ministry of Health and Family Welfare, International Institute for Population Sciences. National Family Health Survey (NFHS-4), 2015-16: India Fact Sheet. Mumbai; 2017. http://rchiips.org/NFHS/pdf/NFHS4/India.pdf. Accessed 2018 Mar 23

12. Ministry of Health and Family Welfare, International Institute for Population Sciences. National Family Health Survey (NFHS-4), India, 2015-16: Bihar. Mumbai; 2017. https://dhsprogram.com/pubs/pdf/FR338/FR338.BR.pdf. Accessed 2018 Mar 23

13. Powell-Jackson T, Mazumdar S, Mills A. Financial incentives in health: New evidence from India's Janani Suraksha Yojana. J Health Econ. 2015;43:154–69.

14. Ng M, Misra A, Diwan V, Agnani M, Levin-Rector A, De Costa A. An assessment of the impact of the JSY cash transfer program on maternal mortality reduction in Madhya Pradesh. India. Glob Health Action. 2014;7:24939.

15. Randive B, Diwan V, De Costa A. India's Conditional Cash Transfer Programme (the JSY) to Promote Institutional Birth: Is There an Association between Institutional Birth Proportion and Maternal Mortality? PLoS One. 2013;8:e67452.

16. Das A, Rao D, Hagopian A. India's Janani Suraksha Yojana: Further review needed. Lancet. 2011;377:295–6.

17. Das A, Nawal D, Singh MK, Karthick M, Pahwa P, Shah MB, et al. Impact of a Nursing Skill-Improvement Intervention on Newborn-Specific Delivery Practices: An Experience from Bihar, India Birth. 2016;43:328–35.

18. Das A, Nawal D, Singh MK, Karthick M, Pahwa P, Shah MB, et al. Evaluation of the mobile nurse training (MNT) intervention - a step towards improvement in intrapartum practices in Bihar. India BMC Preg Childbirth. 2017;17:266.

19. Walker DM, Cohen SR, Estrada F, Monterroso ME, Jenny A, Fritz J, et al. PRONTO training for obstetric and neonatal emergencies in Mexico. Int J Gynaecol Obs. 2012;116:128–33.

20. Walker D, Fritz J, Olvera M, Lamadrid H, Cohen S, Fahey J. PRONTO Low-Tech Obstetric Simulation and Team Training in Mexico Improves Patient Outcomes, and Evidence-Based Care at Birth. Obs Gynecol. 2014;123(Suppl 1):S176–7.

21. Vail B, Spindler H, Morgan MC, Cohen SR, Christmas A, Sah P, et al. Care of the mother-infant dyad: a novel approach to neonatal resuscitation simulation training in Bihar. India BMC Preg Childbirth. 2017;17:252.

22. Dickson KE, Simen-Kapeu A, Kinney MV, Hulcho L, Vesel L, Lackritz E, et al. Every Newborn: Health-systems bottlenecks and strategies to accelerate scale-up in countries. Lancet. 2014;384:438–54.

23. United Nations Inter-agency Group for Child Mortality Estimation. Levels and Trends in Child Mortality: Report 2017. New York; 2017. http://www.childmortality.org/files_v21/download/IGME report 2017 child mortality final.pdf. Accessed 2018 Mar 24

24. Ministry of Health and Family Welfare. Rural health statistics in India 2016. 2016. https://data.gov.in/catalog/rural-health-statistics-2016. Accessed 2018 Mar 13.

25. Indian Nursing Council. Types of nursing programs. http://www.indiannursingcouncil.org/nursing-programs.asp?show=prog-type. Accessed 2018 Mar 20.

26. Green J, Thorogood N. Qualitative Methods for Health Research. 3rd ed. London: SAGE; 2014.

27. Regmi K. Understanding the Processes of Translation and Transliteration in Qualitative Research. Int J Qual Methods. 2010;9:16–26.

28. Poland BD. Transcription Quality as an Aspect of Rigor in Qualitative Research. Qual Inq. 1995;1:290–310.

29. Keenan KF, Van Teijlingen E, Pitchforth E. The analysis of qualitative research data in family planning and reproductive health care. J Fam Plann Reprod Health Care. 2005;31:40–3.

30. Graneheim UH, Lundman B. Qualitative content analysis in nursing research: Concepts, procedures and measures to achieve trustworthiness. Nurse Educ Today. 2004;24:105–12.

31. Tong A, Sainsbury P, Craig J. Consolidated criteria for reporting qualitative research (COREQ): a 32-item checklist for interviews and focus groups. Int J Qual Health Care. 2007;19:349–57.

32. Raykar NP, Yorlets RR, Liu C, Goldman R, Greenberg SLM, Kotagal M, et al. The How Project: understanding contextual challenges to global surgical care provision in low-resource settings. BMJ Glob Health. 2016;1:e000075.

33. Raykar NP, Yorlets RR, Liu C, Greenberg SLM, Kotagal M, Goldman R, et al. A qualitative study exploring contextual challenges to surgical care provision in 21 LMICs. Lancet. 2015;385:S15.

34. Chauhan M, Sharma J, Negandhi P, Reddy S, Sethy G, Neogi S. Assessment of newborn care corners in selected public health facilities in Bihar. Indian J Public Health. 2016;60:341–2.

35. Central Bureau of Health Intelligence. National health profile 2015. New Delhi; 2015. https://www.thehinducentre.com/multimedia/archive/02557/National_Health_Pr_2557764a.pdf. Accessed 19 Oct 2018.

36. Central Bureau of Health Intelligence. Chapter 6. In: Health infrastructure, National Health Profile 2009. New Delhi; 2009. http://www.cbhidghs.nic.in/WriteReadData/l892/11%20Health%20Infrastructure8356493923.pdf. Accessed 19 Oct 2018.

37. Patel V, Parikh R, Nandraj S, Balasubramaniam P, Narayan K, Paul VK, et al. Assuring health coverage for all in India. Lancet. 2015;386:2422–35.

38. Hazarika I. Health workforce in India: assessment of availability, production and distribution. WHO South-East Asia J Public Heal. 2013;2:106–12.

39. Kalyan G, Vatsa M. Neonatal Nursing: An Unmet Challenge in India. Indian J Pediatr. 2014;81:1205–11.

40. Campbell-Yeo M, Deorari A, Mcmillan D, Singhal N, Vatsa M, Aylward D, et al. Identification of barriers and facilitators for education of nurses in care of sick and at- risk newborn babies in India. 2013. https://www.newbornwhocc.org/pdf/APW-WHO-SEARO-Shastri-Report.pdf. Accessed 2018 Mar 15.

41. Chattopadhyay S. Corruption in healthcare and medicine: Why should physicians and bioethicists care and what should they do? Indian J Med Ethics. 2013;10:153–9.

42. Berger D. Corruption ruins the doctor-patient relationship in India. BMJ. 2014;348:g3169.

43. Kumar S. Health care is among the most corrupt services in India. BMJ. 2003;326:10.

44. Shukla S. India probes corruption in flagship health programme. Lancet. 2012;379:698.

45. Rai SK, Dasgupta R, Das M, Singh S, Devi R, Arora N. Determinants of utilization of services under MMJSSA scheme in Jharkhand 'Client Perspective': A qualitative study in a low performing state of India. Indian J Public Health. 2011;55:252–9.

46. Vellakkal S, Reddy H, Gupta A, Chandran A, Fledderjohann J, Stuckler D. A qualitative study of factors impacting accessing of institutional delivery care in the context of India's cash incentive program. Soc Sci Med. 2017;178:55–65.

47. Jawaid S. Patient satisfaction, patient safety and increasing violence against healthcare professionals. Pakistan J Med Sci. 2015;31:1–3.

48. Bawaskar H. Violence against doctors in India. Lancet. 2014;384:955–6.

49. Ambesh P. Violence against doctors in the Indian subcontinent: A rising bane. Indian Heart J. 2016;68:749–50.

50. Nagpal N. Incidents of violence against doctors in India: Can these be prevented? Natl Med J India. 2017;30:97–100.

51. Kar SP. Addressing underlying causes of violence against doctors in India. Lancet. 2017;389:1979–80.

52. Mishra N, Panda M, Pyne S, Srinivas N, Pati S, Pati S. Barriers and enablers to adoption of intrauterine device as a contraceptive method: A multi-stakeholder perspective. J Fam Med Prim Care. 2017;6:616.

53. Moharana P, Kumari N, Trehan S, Sahani N. Mobile family planning unit: An innovation for expanding accessibility to family planning services in Bihar. Indian J Public Health. 2014;58:289.

54. Evans C, Maine D, McCloskey L, Feeley F, Sanghvi H. Where there is no obstetrician - increasing capacity for emergency obstetric care in rural India: An evaluation of a pilot program to train general doctors. Int J Gynecol Obstet. 2009;107:277–82.

55. Raven J, Utz B, Roberts D, Van Den Broek N. The "Making it Happen" programme in India and Bangladesh. BJOG. 2011;118(Suppl 2):100–3.

56. Goudar SS, Somannavar MS, Clark R, Jocelyn M, Revankar AP, Fidler HM, et al. Stillbirth and Newborn Mortality in India After Helping Babies Breathe. Pediatr. 2013;131:e344–52.

57. Bang A, Patel A, Bellad R, Gisore P, Goudar SS, Esamai F, et al. Helping Babies Breathe (HBB) training: What happens to knowledge and skills over time? BMC Preg Childbirth. 2016;16:364.

58. Jhpiego. Improving Quality of Maternal and Newborn Health in India: Fact Sheet July 2016. 2016. https://www.jhpiego.org/wp-content/uploads/2016/10/MNH-factsheet_-July-2016_final.pdf. Accessed 2018 Mar 13.

59. Mubeezi MP, Gidman J. Mentoring student nurses in Uganda: A phenomenological study of mentors' perceptions of their own knowledge and skills. Nurse Educ Pract. 2017;26:96–101.

60. McDermott J, Beck D, Buffington ST, Annas J, Supratikto G, Prenggono D, et al. Two models of in-service training to improve midwifery skills: How well do they work? J Midwifery Women's Health. 2001;46:217–25.

61. Eller L, Lev E, Feurer A. Key components of an effective mentoring relationship: a qualitative study. Nurse Educ Today. 2014;34:815–20.

62. Panda B, Thakur HP. Decentralization and health system performance - a focused review of dimensions, difficulties, and derivatives in India. BMC Health Serv Res. 2016;16(Suppl 6):561.

63. Ojemeni MT, Niles P, Mfaume S, Kapologwe NA, Deng L, Stafford R, et al. A case study on building capacity to improve clinical mentoring and maternal child health in rural Tanzania: The path to implementation. BMC Nurs. 2017;16:57.

64. Kerber KJ, Mathai M, Lewis G, Flenady V, Erwich JJHM, Segun T, et al. Counting every stillbirth and neonatal death through mortality audit to improve quality of care for every pregnant woman and her baby. BMC Preg Childbirth. 2015;15(Suppl 2):S9.

23

Incidence and factors associated with outcomes of uterine rupture among women delivered at Felegehiwot referral hospital, Bahir Dar, Ethiopia: cross sectional study

Dawud Muhammed Ahmed[1*], Tesfaye Setegn Mengistu[2] and Aemiro Getu Endalamaw[3]

Abstract

Background: Maternal mortality is a major public health challenge in Ethiopia. Uterine rupture is an obstetrical emergency with serious undesired complications for laboring mothers resulting in fatal maternal and neonatal outcomes. Uterine rupture has been contributing to high maternal morbidity and mortality. However, there is limited research on the factors and management outcomes of women with uterine rupture. Understanding the factors and management outcomes might delineate strategies to support survivors. Therefore the aim of this study is to assess the incidence and factors associated with outcomes of uterine rupture among laboring mothers at Felegehiwot Referral Hospital in Bahir Dar City, Northwest Ethiopia.

Methods: This is a cross sectional study with retrospective facility based data collection technique. All pregnant women who were managed for ruptured uterus at Felegehiwot referral hospital from September 11 2012 to August 30 2017 were included. The chart numbers of the women collected from operation theatre registers. Their case folders retrieved from the medical records room for analysis. Using structured check list, information on their sociodemography, booking status, clinical features at presentation and the place of attempted vaginal delivery was extracted. Data on the intraoperative findings, treatment, and associated complications and outcomes also collected. The collected data cleaned, coded and entered into EPI- Info version (7.1.2.0) and then exported in to SPSS Version 20.0 for analysis. Statistical comparison was done using chi square (x^2). Strength of association between the explanatory variables and outcome variables described using odds ratio at 95% CI and P value less than 0.05. The results presented in tables.

(Continued on next page)

* Correspondence: muftidawud67@gmail.com
[1]Obstetrics and Gynecology, Bahir Dar University, College of Medicine and Health Sciences, P. O box: 79, Bahir Dar, Ethiopia
Full list of author information is available at the end of the article

(Continued from previous page)

Results: We studied 239 cases of uterine rupture in the 5 years period. Mothers without previous cesarean delivery including eight primigravidas took 87% of the cases. From all study participants, 54 of mothers (22.6%) developed undesired outcomes whereas 185(77.4%) discharged without major sequel. More than half (56.9%) arrived in hypovolemic shock. Total abdominal hysterectomy was the commonest procedure accounting for 61.5%. Duration of surgery was less than 2 h in 67.8% of the procedures. Anemia is the commonest complication (80.3%) followed by wound infection and VVF (11.7% each). There were 5 maternal deaths (2.1%). Mothers who had prolonged operation time (> 2 h) (AOR: 2.2, 95% CI: 1.10, 4.63) were significantly associated with undesired maternal outcomes after management of uterine rupture.

Conclusion: Incidence of ruptured uterus and its complications were high in the study area. It reflects the need for improvement in obstetric care and strong collaboration with referring health facilities to ensure prompt referral and management.

Keywords: Ruptured uterus, Felegehiwot referral hospital, Undesired outcomes

Background

Uterine rupture is tearing of the uterine wall either partially or completely during pregnancy or delivery. This leads to extrusion of the fetus and /or placenta in to the maternal abdomen and massive hemorrhage especially when the rupture is of unscarred uterus [1–4], Uterine rupture contributes significantly to both fetal and maternal mortality, serous morbidities and loss of fertility from hysterectomy. The severity of fetal and maternal morbidity depends on the extent of uterine rupture [1, 5–7]. There is wide variation in incidence between developed and developing countries. In developing countries [8] the incidence is high due to socio economic factors, cultural practices and lack of access to antenatal and intra-partum care. This can be evidenced by the greater number of un-booked obstetric emergencies, often originating from rural areas with poor antenatal care [9], poor obstetric care [10, 11], few comprehensive emergency care facilities [2, 12], and poor socioeconomic status of the community [6, 13].

In Ethiopia for every 1000 births there are about 4 maternal deaths [14]. Uterine rupture with or without obstructed labor is the leading cause of maternal mortality accounting for 36% of the total maternal mortality [15]. This may be a reflection of high prevalence of home delivery [5, 15], especially in the rural areas. Majority of pregnant women in Ethiopia stay at home laboring for 2–3 days and come to health facility when they are seriously ill [15].

Previous caesarean section had been one of the leading cause of uterine rupture in developed countries, while uterine rupture from unscarred uterus is more prevalent in less and least developed countries [1, 7]. Studies conducted in the developing world give strong evidence that uterine rupture is a major health problem in these countries with the rate being high in rural areas [13]. A major factor in uterine rupture in developing countries is obstructed labour due to inadequate access to medical care [2, 3, 16, 17]. Also the high incidence of contracted

pelvis among black African women is found to be a high risk factor for obstetric complications. Other risk factors for uterine rupture include grand multiparity, instrumental delivery, and use of uterotonic drugs to induce or augment labour [5, 13]. Rarely placenta percreta and intrauterine manipulations such as internal podalic version and breech extraction can result in uterine rupture [1].

The type of surgical intervention on the uterus is dependent on the type and extent of rupture, hemodynamic status of the mother, desire for future fertility, presence of gross infection and experience of the surgeon. This could be total or subtotal abdominal hysterectomy, uterine repair with or without tubal ligation [3, 17–20]. Uterine repair should be reserved for women who have low transverse rupture, no extension of the tear to broad ligaments, cervix or vagina, easily controllable hemorrhage, good general condition, desire for future child bearing and no evidence of gross infection. Hysterectomy is appropriate for those with one of the above intra operative findings [17].

Uterine rupture is associated with a number of acute and long term complications. These include anemia, need for transfusion, bladder injury, wound infection, sepsis and death [19]. Complications like obstetric fistula, foot drop, psychological trauma, permanent loss of fertility are some of the long term outcomes [17, 18].Acute renal failure from pre renal azotemia is also possible following massive hemorrhage [9, 21].Among these, the most commonly encountered complication is hemorrhage leading to anemia [3, 5, 18, 19].

Not only this, Loss of fertility in communities where reproduction is considered the very essence of womanhood has grave socio cultural implications like divorce, and loss of economic support [3, 18].

Patients with fistula are living leaking urine or feces through the vagina. They have to continue living thereafter unclean, outcast, smelling of urine and faces. This is a cause for separate from their families, worsening poverty, malnutrition and almost unendurable suffering [22].

Maternal death as a consequence of uterine rupture occurs at a rate of 0–1% in modern developed nations, but the mortality rates in developing countries are 5–10% [17].

The determinant factors for maternal outcome of uterine rupture differ across geographical boundaries due to the difference in socio-demographic status, and the availability and accessibility of skilled birth attendant and health system effectiveness [5].

Once diagnosis of uterine rupture is entertained, the time spent for successful surgical intervention should be very short and all available resources should be quickly mobilized for favorable outcome of both mother and new born [17, 18].Late arrival and treatment increase the maternal and fetal morbidity and mortality [18]. Difficulty performing an exact diagnosis at the arrival of the patient with a severe diagnosis like uterine rupture may worsen the condition [13]. Immediate surgery and blood replacement plays major role in maternal survival [13, 18]. The main causes of maternal mortality in rupture uterus are failure to diagnose the condition at the first referral center and arrival at the tertiary center in a moribund condition [23]. The immediate cause of death in such condition includes puerperal sepsis [18] and hypovolemic shock [19].

Prognosis for the fetus is even worse than the mother [18]. Studies in different parts of developing countries indicated high fetal case fatality rate [2, 5, 18, 24];complete uterine rupture being associated with the highest fetal death rate [18].

Initiation of labor at health institutions, early referral [2], and treatment of hypovolumia and prevention of postoperative anemia is recommended to decrease maternal death secondary to uterine rupture [5, 24]. In addition proper monitoring of labour and improvement of comprehensive emergence obstetric care at all levels of health care are recommended to avoid unnecessary delays in care [3].Early diagnosis and active surgical management will go a long way in reducing maternal and fetal mortality [9].

Uterine rupture remains an important clinical problem in northern Ethiopia. Changes in the cultural preference for home delivery, better transport and referral systems, and improved obstetric training and hospital management of laboring women are needed [20].

Currently the federal ministry of health of Ethiopia is improving obstetric care by scaling up of skilled personnel attended delivery; universal primary education, infrastructure and human resource development [15, 20, 25]. Despite these strategies births assisted by skilled provider in our country is 28% [14]. This

indicates the need for further research and implementation of programs to improve health status of the country.

Statement of the problem

The incidence of uterine rupture has regional and sub-regional variability posing a major public health problem in under developed countries [1, 7]. The rate of pregnancy-related uterine rupture in women with unscarred uterus is 0.012% (1 in 8434) for women living in industrialized countries and 0.11% (1 in 920) for women living in developing countries [17].

In low resource settings multiple factors including educational status of women, ignorance, poverty, regular antenatal care checkup, home delivery, prolonged (dysfunctional) and obstructed labor had been identified risk factors of uterine rupture [21, 26]. Similarly evidences showed that previous cesarean delivery, mal-presentations [7, 27], induction and augmentation of labor [27], grand multiparty [7, 28], neglected labor, breech extraction, uterine instrumentation are predisposing factors for uterine rupture [7].

Evidences showed that abdominal pain, vaginal bleeding, loss of fetal station, non-reassuring fetal heart rate, shock and fetal bradycardia are most common indicators of uterine rupture [29]which needs prompt diagnosis and treatment before progressing serious maternal and perinatal outcomes [7, 30, 31]. Hemorrhage [7, 31], hypovolemic shock, need for blood transfusion [31], bladder injury, need for hysterectomy, and a maternal death are some of maternal consequences/outcomes while, admission to neonatal intensive care unit, fetal hypoxia or anoxia, and neonatal death are some of neonatal outcomes [7]. However, maternal/neonatal morbidity and mortality following uterine rupture depend on the level of medical care [7].

Although uterine rupture is preventable condition, it has also been one of the leading cause of maternal mortality in Ethiopia [15, 26]. The federal ministry of health is providing curative health services to the community as one of the priorities, and, as a consequence, the number of government hospitals in the country has increased from 126 to 31. It is also trying to change the cultural preference of home delivery through better transport, access to prenatal care, obstetric training and exempted service charges for laboring mothers (2014 FMOH Bulletin). As part of this improvement Bahir dar university launched residency programs in Obstetric in 2014 using Felege hiwot referral hospital as affiliated site. There is a 24 h blood transfusion service and intensive care unit in the hospital. Despite all these, evidences are lacking as to the magnitude and factors for the outcome of uterine rupture in this area. In addition there was no effort to measure changes in management outcome as a result of improvement of obstetric services. Therefore the aim of this study is to identify factors associated with outcomes of uterine rupture among laboring mothers at Felegehi-wot Referral Hospital in Bahir Dar City, Northwest Ethiopia.

Literature review

Uterine rupture has continued to be a catastrophic feature of obstetric practice especially in the low-resource settings [28].

There are some studies conducted in Ethiopia. Among these a prospective study over a period of 2 years at Debre Markos hospital found the incidence of ruptured uterus to be 3.8%. Susceptible groups were age 25 to 29 years and grand multiparas (> 5). Complete type uterine rupture accounted for 88.6%. In more than half (54.3%) of the cases the site of rupture was anterior. The commonest procedure performed was hysterectomy (81.4%). The postoperative complication rate was 24.3%. Sepsis was the leading cause of death [16].

But more recently a review of uterine rupture cases at Ayder Referral hospital in Mekelle, northern Ethiopia between 2009 and 2013 found a rate of uterine rupture of 1 in 110 deliveries. Predisposing factors in order of their frequency were cephalopelvic disproportion (74%), previous cesarean delivery (11%), and fetal malpresentation (9%). The presenting symptoms were pain, sudden cessation of contractions during labor and vaginal bleeding. The vast majority of ruptured uterus occurred from unscarred uterus; only five patients had undergone a previous cesarean delivery. The mean gravidity was 3.6. Less than two-thirds had received any prenatal care. Almost all patients came to Ayder from referring health facilities. One patient who had unrecognized ureteric injury and persistent anemia died. Perinatal mortality was 94% [20].

Analysis of the causes, complications and management outcomes of ruptured uterus in Dar-es-Salaam, Tanzania shows the incidence to be 2.25 per 1000 deliveries. The leading causes identified were obstructed labor, previous cesarean delivery and use of uterotonic drugs for induction and augmentation of labor. Most of these patients were referrals from municipal hospitals and all attended antenatal follow up at least once. There were 21 maternal deaths and 157 perinatal deaths giving case fatality rate of 12.9 and 96.3% respectively. The commonest maternal complication was hemorrhage (34.4%) followed by sepsis, VVF and blood transfusions. Subtotal hysterectomy is the most common performed procedure (73.6%), repair with BTL (12.3%), repair only (12.3%) and total hysterectomy (1.8%). Most operations were made by obstetricians [3].

Rupture of the gravid uterus is still a significant cause of maternal mortality and morbidity in Nnamdi Azikiwe University Teaching Hospital, Nnewi, Anambra State Southeast Nigeria. The incidence was 1 in 161 deliveries. The commonest age range of occurrence was 30–34 years. Contrary to widespread belief that uterine rupture is a disease of multiparous women, in this study women of low parity predominate. Most of the ruptures were as a result a combination of risk factors like previous caesarean section with concurrent use of oxytocic. The commonest procedure performed was uterine repair only [32].

A 10 year retrospective study in the same hospital showed an incidence of 0.84%. All the patients were multiparous and 63.8% were unbooked. Majority were Traumatic (iatrogenic) ruptures (72.1%). Uterine repair with (55.8%) or without (34.9%) bilateral tubal ligation was the commonest surgery performed. The case fatality rate and perinatal mortality rate were 16.3 and 88.4% respectively. Average duration of hospitalization following surgery was 10.3 days [28].

There is also a retrospective study describing the factors influencing the management and the prognosis of ruptured uterus in a level III maternity care center of a third world country (Cocody University Hospital Center, Abidjan-Cote d'Ivoire). There were 513 cases of ruptured uterus between January 2002 and December 2014 giving an incidence of 0.95%. Most cases occurred in women with unscarred uterus (76.8%). Radical hysterectomy was done in 35.3% of all women. Uterine repair was done more commonly for women from the communes of Abidjan and its suburbs (71%). Maternal mortality rate was 5.8% and factors like the type of surgery ($p = 0.000$), the time of uterine rupture ($p = 0.000$) and the transportation distance ($p = 0.000$) were significantly associated. Fetal mortality was 94.1% [8].

Study done in Sweden showed increased risk of uterine rupture (during their second delivery) in women who underwent a cesarean delivery compared with women who delivered vaginally in their first birth. Additional factors associated with increased risk of uterine rupture were induction of labor, high (> or = 4000 g) birth weight, post term (> or = 42 weeks) births, high (> or = 35 years) maternal age, and short (< or = 164 cm) maternal stature [33].

Researchers found the incidence of ruptured uterus to be 0.116% in one of the tertiary care hospital in Turkey. Trial of labor after cesarean was the most common cause of uterine rupture accounting for 31.1% of the cases. Vaginal Bleeding was the main symptom at presentation (44.3%). Lower uterine segment (isthmus) was the most vulnerable part of uterus (39.3%) for rupture. Women with delayed surgical intervention and older patients with increased parity were likely to have longer hospitalization periods [34].

One research in Zurich with special interest on effect of uterine fundal pressure on uterine rupture revealed previous uterine surgery as the main risk factor for uterine rupture in the whole study population. Risk factors in women with unscarred uterus were uterine fundal pressure (UFP), abnormal placentation, and age at delivery > 40 years. The only factor which can be modified is Uterine Fundal Pressure [35].

Population based study in Sweden reported the overall rate of uterine rupture among women with an attempted vaginal birth in their second delivery to be 0.91/1000. The rate of uterine rupture among women who attempted vaginal birth after a caesarean section was 9.00/1000 compared with a uterine rupture rate of 0.18/1000 among women without a history of caesarean delivery. Compared with women who experienced a spontaneous onset of delivery, women whose second delivery was induced faced a doubled increase in risk of uterine rupture. Induction of labor was associated with a doubled risk of uterine rupture both among women with a previous caesarean and among women who did not have previous caesarean. High maternal age, induction of labour, and high birth weight increased the risk of uterine rupture. The neonatal death rate was 51.09/1000. This was more than 60 fold increase compared with neonatal death rate among women without uterine rupture (1.4/1000) [36].

A population based study aimed at determining trends, risk factors and pregnancy outcome in women with uterine rupture compared all singleton deliveries with and without uterine rupture between 1988 and 2009. Uterine rupture occurred in 0.06% of all deliveries; 59% in women with a previous cesarean delivery. There was a gradual increase in the rate of uterine rupture from 1988 (0.01%) to 2009 (0.05%). Independent risk factors for uterine rupture were: previous CD, preterm delivery (< 37 weeks), malpresentation, parity, and dystocia during the first and second stages of labor. In addition, Uterine rupture was noted as an independent risk factor for perinatal mortality [37].

Rupture of gravid uterus brings about potentially hazardous risks. Regular antenatal care, hospital deliveries and vigilance during labor with quick referral to a well-equipped center may reduce the incidence of this condition [34]. There is therefore a dire need for education of women on health-related issues, utilization of available health facilities, adequate supervision of labour and provision of facilities for emergency obstetric care [28].

Uterine rupture is a complication that can be eliminated under conditions of best obstetric practice. To attain this objective, use of misoprostol in primary health facilities should be stopped or proper management of the medication instituted. The survival of patients after uterine rupture depends on the time interval between rupture and intervention, and the availability of blood products for transfusion [38].

Justification of the study

Maternal and fetal morbidity and mortality is high in Ethiopia. Ruptured uterus contributes significantly to maternal mortality. In spite of this, there has been paucity of evidences on factors associated with management outcome of mothers who had uterine rupture. This study documents common complications and factors related with management outcomes of uterine rupture in FHRH. Therefore, the result of this study helps policy makers, program, planners, governmental and non-governmental organization implementers and maternal health service providers/practitioners to provide evidence based interventions which will contribute in maternal morbidity and mortality reduction in the hospital and the region as well. Most importantly, since there are limited research evidences on uterine rupture in the study area, this study serves as a baseline work for other researchers interested to work on the risk factors and outcomes of women who had uterine rupture.

General objectives

The objective of the study is to assess the incidence of uterine rupture and factors associated with outcomes of uterine rupture among women delivered in Felegehiwot referral hospital in Bahir Dar City, Northwest Ethiopia.

Specific objectives

- To determine the incidence of uterine rupture among women delivered at Felege hiwot referral hospital in the study period
- To identify complications after management of uterine rupture
- To identify factors associated with outcome of clients managed for uterine rupture in FHRH

Methods
Study area and period

Institutional based cross-sectional study was conducted from May 1 to 30, 2017 in Bahir Dar City, Felege Hiwot Referral Hospital. Bahir Dar is the capital city of Amhara National Regional State (ANRS), located 565 km Northwest of Addis Ababa. FHRH is one of the 42 governmental Hospitals in Amhara Regional state. The hospital serves for more than 5,000,000 populations in its catchment area (ANRHB 2015). The hospital has one big maternity ward which possesses around 74 beds. There are about 6000 deliveries per year, 30% of which is cesarean deliveries (prenatal report, 2016). There are 7 obstetricians, 27 residents and 25 midwives currently working in the department of obstetrics. As it is a referral hospital most of the clients are referral cases from health centers and district hospitals.

Study design
Cross sectional study with retrospective facility based data collection was used.

Source population
Women who had uterine rupture (reached through their charts documented during the procedure).

Study population
Women who had uterine rupture in the time from September 11 2012 to August 30 2017 were included.

Inclusion and exclusion criteria
Inclusion criteria
All women who had diagnosed with uterine rupture and managed at FHRH from 2012 to 2017 were included.

Exclusion criteria
Women who had uterine rupture and managed at other health facilities and referred to FHRH for complications like transfusion, ICU admission and Women who had ruptured uterus from medical termination of pregnancy in the second trimester, and those cases with missed data on outcome variable and major factors (parity, age, duration of labor, place of labor, operation factors...) were not included in the study.

Sample size determination
A single population proportion formula using the assumptions of 95% confidence level and 5% margin of error was used to estimate the sample size. Estimated proportion of laboring at home among ruptured cases i.e. 57% ($P = 0.57$) was used (Astatikie et al. [5]). Substituting the above assumption in the formula, the required sample size is calculated to be 376.

$n = \overline{(Z\alpha/_2)^2 xp(1\text{-}p)}/d^2$; Where

n = Sample size

Z a/$_2$ = Confidence level at 95% = **1.96**

P = Proportion of population which is 57%

Factor	Proportion	Sample size	Reference
Labor at home	57%	**376**	Astatikie G et al. 2017 [5]
Hypovolemic shock	34.3%	346	"
Post op anemia	21.9%	262	"

Sampling procedure
First the main registration book of the Operation room where all emergencies registered according to their order was used to list all uterine rupture cases. Each of the cases included. The names of the mother's selected

were checked from the charts and data was collected daily.

Study variables
Dependent Variable:
Outcome of uterine rupture
Independent variables

– **Socio-demographic variables:** age, address
– **Obstetric factors:** Parity, ANC status, previous cesarean delivery, obstructed labor, referral from health facility, induction and augmentation, place of trial of labor, blood pressure at arrival, anemia, duration of labor, type of rupture, type of surgical procedure and duration of surgery.

Measurement
The outcome variable was measured as desired outcome and undesired outcomes. The desired outcome was also measured as cured without major sequel (Yes, No). Women were classified as having undesired management outcome when she had developed one of the following condition: death, permanent organ injury, obstetric fistula, wound dehiscence, Sepsis, ICU admission.

Maternal death secondary to uterine rupture is defined as death of the mother from uterine rupture, its complications or management.

Sepsis: a woman will be declared she has sepsis if she is diagnosed and treated as recorded in the patient chart.

Operation time is defined prolonged if it took more than 2 h.

Senior resident is a physician who is on fourth year of training in gynecology and obstetrics.

Source of admission is recorded as it is written from admission note.

Table 1 Socio demographic characteristics of uterine rupture in Felegehiwot Referral hospital from September 2012 to August 2017(n = 239)

Variables	Frequency	Percent
Age of study participants		
< =16	0	0.0
17–39	229	95.8
≥ 40	10	4.2
Total	239	100.0
Address of study participants		
Awi	69	28.9
Bahir dar Zuria	28	11.7
Metekel zone	2	0.8
West Gojjam	53	22.2
South Gondar	87	36.4
Total	239	100.0

Table 2 Obstetric variables of uterine rupture in Felegehiwot Referral hospital from September 2012 to August 2017($n = 239$)

Variables	Frequency	Percent
Gravidity		
Primi gravida	8	3.3
Multi gravida	157	65.7
Grand multi gravida	74	31.0
Total	239	100.0
Gestational age		
Preterm	16	6.7
Term	164	68.6
Post term	30	12.6
Unknown	29	12.1
Total	239	100.0
Antenatal care		
No	53	22.2
< 4	68	28.5
≥ 4	118	49.4
Total	239	100
Previous cesarean delivery		
Yes	31	13
No	208	87
Total	239	100
Source of admission to FHRH		
Home	14	5.9
health center	188	78.7
district hospital	27	11.3
FHRH	10	4.2
Total	239	100.0
Duration of labor		
< 24 h	191	79.9
24–48	41	17.2
> 48	7	2.9
Total	239	100.0
Diagnosis on referral		
uterine rupture	42	17.6
CPD/OL	94	37.6
Second stage	31	13.0
IUFD	28	11.7
other	23	9.6
No referral	21	8.8
Total	239	100.0
Time of arrival		
Day	164	68.6
Night	75	31.4
Total	239	100.0

Table 2 Obstetric variables of uterine rupture in Felegehiwot Referral hospital from September 2012 to August 2017($n = 239$) (Continued)

Variables	Frequency	Percent
Blood pressure on arrival		
Non recordable	53	22.2
< 90/60mmhg	83	34.7
$\geq$ 90/60mmhg	103	43.1
Total	239	100.0
Diagnosis on admission to FHRH		
uterine rupture	202	84.5
other diagnosis	37	15.5
Total	239	100

Time of arrival from 7:00 AM to 6:59 PM is labeled as "Day time", and 7:00 PM to 6:59 AM as "Night time".

Data collection

The folder numbers of the women who were managed for ruptured uterus over a 5 year period (September 11 2012–August 30 2017) was collected from operation theatre registers. Their case folders were retrieved from the medical records department. Using structured check list, information on their sociodemography, booking status, clinical features at presentation and the place of attempted vaginal delivery was extracted by the data collectors. Data on the intraoperative findings, treatment, associated complications and maternal outcomes were also collected. Check list checked by data collectors & supervisors on daily base for completeness.

Data processing and analysis

Data was entered in to Epi Info version 7.1.2.0 and then transported to SPSS version 20 software packages for analysis. Descriptive statistics such as mean, percentage and standard deviation, was determined. Bi variable logistic regression was used to determine the association between each independent variable and the outcome variable. The degree of association between dependent and independent variables was determined using the OR with CI of 95% and p-value of < 0.05.

Data quality control

Prior to data collection, the check list was tested to check the consistency of the checklist format and the ability of the data collector's performance. The checklist was modified based on the pretest results. One day training/ orientation how to carry out their duty was given for the data collectors.

Results

There were a total of 262 cases of uterine rupture at FHRH in 5 years period from 2012 to 2017. The total number of deliveries in the same period was 28,835. This gives an incidence of 0.9% (1 in 110). Among the uterine rupture cases, 10 charts were lost from card record room and additional 13 were rejected because of missing information. The final study population becomes 239. Response rate becomes 91%.

Socio demographic characteristics of study participants

Most of the study population (95.8%) was in the age group of 17–39. The mean age is 29.38 years. Most came from areas outside Bahir dar, Debub Gondar being the highest (36.4). There were 2 cases from Benshangul Gumuz region (Table 1).

Obstetric variables

Most are multigravidas with only eight uterine rupture cases among Primigravidas (3.3%). Most of the ruptures occurred on unscarred uterus (87%). Half of respondents have four and above Antenatal visits. 78% have attempted delivery at health centers. Ten uterine ruptures occurred at Felege Hiwot hospital. Uterine rupture was diagnosed correctly in 17.6% of cases up on referral. Most arrived with hypovolemic shock (Table 2).

Presenting symptoms

The three symptoms identified were abdominal pain (65.7), cessation of labor (56.5) and vaginal bleeding (45.65). The commonest presenting sign of uterine rupture is uterine tenderness (81.2%). Fetal heart sounds were positive in 12.6% of cases (Table 3).

Intra operative findings

Anterior lower segment is the commonest site of uterine rupture accounting for 56%. Total abdominal hysterectomy (61.5%) leads from procedures performed. There

Table 3 Clinical presentations among cases of uterine rupture in Felegehiwot Referral hospital from September 2012 to August 2017(n = 239)

Symptoms	Frequency	Percent
1. Abdominal pain	157	65.7
2. cessation of labor	135	56.5
3. vaginal bleeding	109	45.6
4. tenderness	194	81.2
5. easily palpable fetal parts	132	55.2
6. uterine contraction present	34	14.2
7. FHB positive	30	12.6
8. Palpable defect on uterus	56	23.4

Table 4 Operative findings among cases of uterine rupture in Felegehiwot Referral hospital from September 2012 to August 2017(n = 239)

Intra operative findings	Frequency	Percent
Type of rupture		
Complete	203	84.9
Incomplete	36	15.1
Total	239	100.0
Site of rupture		
Anterior lower segment	134	56.1
Posterior	19	7.9
Lateral	78	32.6
Fundal	8	3.3
Total	239	100.0
Bladder injury	8	3.3
Necrotic edges	55	23.0
Vaginal extension	64	26.8
Duration of surgery		
< =2 h	162	67.8
> 2 h	77	32.2
Total	239	100.0
Type of Procedure		
TAH	147	61.5
STAH	24	10.0
repair only	54	22.6
repair with BTL	14	5.9
Total	239	100.0
Surgeon		
consultant	174	72.8
resident	65	27.2
Total	239	100.0

were 8 bladder ruptures diagnosed intraoperative (Table 4).

Complications

Anemia is the commonest complication (80.3%) followed by wound infection and VVF. There were 5 maternal deaths (2.1%). Totally there were 54(22.6%) mothers who developed undesired outcomes (Table 5).

Perinatal outcome: 84.1% of mothers end up in still birth. In 16 charts nothing is documented about the status of the neonate.

Factors associated with outcomes of uterine rupture

In multi variable logistic regression analysis it is found that mothers with operation times more than 2 h (AOR: 2.260, 95% CI: 1.102, 4.638) were more likely to have undesired maternal outcomes than operation times less

Table 5 Complications among cases of uterine rupture in Felegehiwot Referral hospital from September 2012 to August 2017($n = 239$)

Complications	Frequency	Percent
Post op hemoglobin		
$\geq$ 12 g/dl	47	19.7
7-12 g/dl	169	70.7
$\leq$ 7 g/dl	23	9.6
Total	239	100.0
Transfusion		
No	59	24.6
1 units	38	16.0
2 units	97	40.6
3 units	24	10.0
4 units	15	6.3
> =5 units	6	2.5
Total	239	100
Wound infection	28	11.7
Hospital stay		
< 8 days	160	66.9
> =8 days	79	33.1
Total	239	100.0
Undesired outcomes		
ICU admission	5	2.1
VVF	28	11.7
Sepsis	12	5.0
Wound dehiscence	15	6.3
Death	5	2.1

than 2 h. Nearly one third (31.2%) of those cases whose operation time was more than 2 h, resulted in undesired outcomes. Gravidity, gestational age, place of attempted delivery, and time of arrival to Felegehiwot were not significantly associated with maternal outcomes (Table 6).

Discussion

The incidence of uterine rupture is 0.9% (1 in 110). This is lower than the 2012 incidence in this same hospital (2.9% or 1 in 35) and the prevalence found at Debre Markos hospital 2.24%(5) [39]. This may be as a result of establishment of functional district hospitals capable of managing these cases. But still it is higher when compared to incidence in other developing countries like 0.22% in Dar-es- Salaam, Tanzania and 0.057% in Imphal, India [3, 40]. This might be a reflection of delay in timely diagnosis of uterine rupture and referral once women reach health centers.

Most of the mothers in this study were referrals from health institutions (90%). This is similar with the study

in Dar selam, Tanzania where most patients were referrals from municipal hospitals. Despite the national report of high prevalence of home delivery in Ethiopia [5, 15] especially in the rural areas, in this study it shows only 5.9%. The low figure of home delivery in this study may be a reflection of inappropriate assignment of those with referral papers as if they tried labor at health institution. But the common scenario is visiting health centers when they are seriously ill after laboring for 2–3 days at home. This affects the true figure of the problem. The other possibility may be inadequate supervision of labour and emergency obstetric care. Uterine rupture was diagnosed correctly in only 17.6% of the cases by referring health institution. This may be because of either difficulty in diagnosing uterine rupture or ruptures occur on the way to Felegehiwot.

There were 10 cases of uterine rupture at Felege Hiwot, none of whom developed undesired outcome. This may be due to prompt diagnosis, blood transfusion whenever necessary and immediate laparotomy indirectly reflecting the improved obstetric practice at this referral hospital.

Most underwent Total abdominal hysterectomy (62% TAH), & 10% had STAH. Around 75% of mothers from areas outside Bahir dar underwent hysterectomy whereas half from Bahir dar and its surroundings. This findings are consistent with the finding from Cocody University Hospital Center, Abidjan-Cote d'Ivoire which shows more conservative surgeries by uterine suture in women from the communes of Abidjan and its suburbs (71%) versus 25% of women who came from inland towns [8]. However, in other studies the commonest procedure carried out was uterine repair only [9, 11, 13, 32]. Unstable hemodynamic status, more number of obstructed labors, presence of gross infection, and higher parities in our study may lead to hysterectomy.

Vesico Vaginal fistula (VVF) affected large proportion of mothers (11.7) who sustained uterine rupture similar with other studies [18]. However one study in India reveals a 2% risk [9]. The possible reason for this difference is high rate of obstructed labor in our study area, where as in India majority are following uterine scar.

Blood availability for transfusion as part of management of uterine rupture is lifesaving. In this regard 75.3% of study participants had blood transfusion and 40.6% got at least two units of cross matched blood. This is not usually possible in some countries. Even if all are anemic, only 57.1% of mothers got 500-1000 ml blood transfusion at Al-thawra hospital, the main hospital in Sana'a City, the capital of the Republic of Yemen. This better blood availability in our study may indicate strong commitment of Federal ministry of health and continuous work of student clubs in mobilizing the community to donate blood.

Table 6 Binary and multivariable logistic regression table for factors associated with outcome of uterine rupture in Felegehiwot hospital from September 2011 to August 2017($n = 239$)

Variables	UR management outcomes		COR (95% CI)	AOR (95% CI)
	Undesired n (%)	Desired n (%)		
Gravidity				
Primigravida	4 (7.4%)	4 (2.2%)	1.0	1.0
Multigravida	26 (48.1%)	131 (70.8%)	0.2 (0.04–0.84)	0.2 (0.03, 1.30)
Grandmultigravida	23 (42.6%)	45 (24.3%)	0.5 (0.11–2.23)	0.7 (0.11, 4.64)
Gestational age				
Preterm	5 (9.3%)	11 (5.9%)	1.0	1.0
Term	25 (46.3%)	139 (75.1%)	0.3 (0.12–1.23)	0.3 (0.08, 1.17)
Post term	8 (14.8%)	22 (11.9%)	0.8 (0.21–3.02)	0.5 (0.11, 2.46)
Unknown	16 (29.6%)	13 (7.0%)	2.7 (0.74–9.79)	2.6 (0.63,11.52)
Place of attempted delivery				
Home	6 (11.1%)	8 (4.3%)	1.0	1.0
Health Center	40 (74.1%)	148 (80.0%)	0.3 (0.11, 1.09)	0.6 (0.16, 2.47)
District hospital	8 (14.8%)	19 (10.3%)	0.5 (0.14,2.15)	0.8 (0.17, 4.24)
Time of arrival to FHRH				
Day	43 (79.6%)	121 (65.4%)	1.0	1.0
Night	11 (20.4%)	64 (34.6%)	0.4 (0.23,1.00)	0.4 (0.22,1.08)
Duration of surgery				
< =2 h	30 (55.6)	132 (71.4)	1.0	1.0
> 2 h	24 (44.4)	53 (28.6)	1.9 (1.06, 3.72) [*]	2.2 (1.10,4.63)

[*]statistically significant at P – value < 0.05

There were 5 maternal deaths (2.1%) as a result of uterine rupture in the study period. This is lower as compared with deaths at Debre Markos hospital (6.6%) and Cot devours (5.8%) [5, 8]. Early diagnosis and management of uterine rupture, widely available blood transfusion services as well as close follow up post operatively may have contributed for this reduction. In this regard the hospital being teaching institution for the residency program, interns and residents could have a significant role.

According to research done at Abidjan, Cote d'Ivoire, maternal mortality was significantly influenced by the type of surgery (p = 0.000), time of uterine rupture (p = 0.000) transportation distance (p = 0.000) [8]. In our study as well, four out of the five maternal deaths were from those treated with hysterectomies. This may be mainly due to the combination of more severe lesions in hysterectomies than repairs.

This study reveals that undesired outcomes were more likely to occur(two times) if time of operation took more than 2 h (AOR: 2.260, 95% CI: 1.102, 4.638). Nearly one third (31.2%) of those cases whose operation time was more than 2 h, resulted in undesired outcome. This may be attributed to the complexity of the lesion in ruptured uterus and poor patient condition.

The age, source of admission, duration of labor before arriving FHRH, site and type of rupture, gestational age, and previous operations were not significantly associated with outcomes of uterine rupture.

The fetal outcome was poor with around 84% of still births. This is similar with other studies in developing countries [11]. There is Poor documentation about the baby that make difficult to analyze other factors.

Conclusion

This study shows high incidence of uterine rupture with significant undesired outcomes in Northwest Ethiopia. It reflects the need for improvement in obstetric care and strong collaboration with referring health facilities to ensure prompt referral and management.

Limitations of the study

Since the study is retrospective, 23 charts could not be included in this study because of missed variables and lost charts. Prospective multicenter study in the future will alleviate the limitations of this study.

Abbreviations

ANC: Antenatal care; ANRHB: Amhara National regional Health Bureau; ANRS: Amhara National Regional State; AOR: Adjusted odds ratio; BTL: Bilateral tubal ligation; CD: Cesarean delivery; CPD: Cephalo pelvic disproportion; FHRH: Felegehiwot referral hospital; FMOH: Federal Ministry of Health; ICU: Intensive care unit; IUFD: Intra uterine fetal death; MD: Medical doctor; MPH: Master of Public health; NICU: Neonatal Intensive Care Unit; OL: Obstructed labor; RH: Reproductive health; SPSS: Statistical package for

Incidence and factors associated with outcomes of uterine rupture among women delivered...

245

social sciences; STAH: Sub total abdominal hysterectomy; TAH: Total abdominal hysterectomy; UFP: Uterine fundal pressure; VVF: Vesico vaginal fistula; WHO: World Health Organization

Acknowledgements
We would like to express our gratitude to department of Gynecology and Obstetrics, School of Medicine, College of Medicine and Health Sciences, Bahir-Dar University for giving us this opportunity.
We are also indented to Felegehiwot Referral Hospital and its staffs for their valuable time and genuine collaboration during this research process.

Funding
The fund for this research was obtained from Bahir Dar University. It was used for collecting data and writing the manuscript.

Authors' contributions
DMA wrote the proposal; over sought the data collection, analyzed the data and drafted the paper. TSM participated in the proposal development, reviewed and interpreted the analysis. AGE revised the paper upon reviewers' comments and wrote the final manuscript. All authors read and approved the final version of the manuscript.

Competing interests
The authors declare that they have no competing interests.

Author details
[1]Obstetrics and Gynecology, Bahir Dar University, College of Medicine and Health Sciences, P. O box: 79, Bahir Dar, Ethiopia. [2]Bahir Dar University College of Medicine and Health Sciences, Bahir Dar, Amhara Regional State, Ethiopia. [3]Marie Stops International Ethiopia, Bahir Dar, Ethiopia.

References
1. Hofmey GJ, Say L, Gulmezoglu AM. WHO systematic review of maternal mortality and morbidity: the prevalence of uterine rupture. BJOG. 2005;112: 1221–8.
2. Aliyu SA, Yizengaw TK, Lemma TB. Prevalence and associated factors of uterine rupture during labor among women who delivered in Debre Markos hospital north West Ethiopia. Intern Med. 2016;6(4).
3. Kidanto HL, Mwampagatwa I, Van Roosmalen J. Uterine rupture: a retrospective analysis of causes, complications and management outcomes at Muhimbili National Hospital in Dar Es Salaam, Tanzania. Tanzan J Health Res. 2012;14(3):220–5.
4. Gabbe G, Niebyl JR, JLSimpson MBL, Galan HL, Jauniaux ERM, et al. Obstetrics: normal and problem pregnancies. 7th ed; 2017.
5. Astatikie G, Limenih MA, Kebede M. Maternal and fetal outcomes of uterine rupture and factors associated with maternal death secondary to uterine rupture. BMC Pregnancy Childbirth. 2017;17:117.
6. Mukasa PK, Kabakyenga J, Senkungu JK, Ngonzi J, Kyalimpa M, van Roosmalen J. Uterine rupture in a teaching hospital in Mbarara, western Uganda, unmatched case- control study. Reprod Health. 2013;10:29.
7. Vladimir Revicky AM, Mukhopadhyay S, Mahmood T. A case series of uterine rupture: lessons to be learned for future clinical practice. J Obstet Gynaecol India. 2012;62(6):665–73.
8. Loue VA, Dia JM, Effoh DN, Adjoby RC, Konan JK, Gbary EA, Abauleth RY, Kouakou F, Boni SE. Management and prognosis of uterine rupture during labor in an under-medicalized country: about 513 cases collected at the Cocody University hospital center (Abidjan-cote d'Ivoire). Int J Reprod Contracept Obstet Gynecol. 2015;4(5):1277–82.
9. Sunitha K, Indira I, Suguna P. Clinical Study of Rupture Uterus - Assessment of Maternal and Fetal Outcome. J Dental Med Scie. 2015;14(3):39–45.
10. Dan K, Kaye OK, Nakimuli A, Osinde MO, Mbalinda SN, Kakande N. Lived experiences of women who developed uterine rupture following severe obstructed labor in Mulago hospital, Uganda. Reprod Health. 2014;11:31.
11. Nousheen Aziz SY. Analysis of uterine rupture at university teaching hospital Pakistan. Pak J Med Sci. 2015;31(4):920–4.
12. Igwegbe AO, Eleje GU, Udegbunam OI. Risk factors and perinatal outcome of uterine rupture in a low-resource setting. Niger Med J. 2013;54(6):415–9.
13. Ishraq Dhaifalah JS, Fingerova H. Uterine rupture during pregnancy and delivery among women attending the Al-Tthawra hospital in Sana'a city Yemen Republic. Biomed Pap Med Fac Univ Palacky Olomouc Czech Repub. 2006;150(2):279–83.
14. Survey EDaH. Key indicators report. In: CSACEa, editor. ICF. Addis Ababa; Rockville: CSA and ICF; 2016.
15. Yifru Berhan AB. Causes of maternal mortality in Ethiopia: a significant decline in abortion related death. Ethiop J Health Sci. 2014;24(0 suppl):15–28.
16. Admassu A. Analysis of ruptured uterus in Debre Markos hospital, Ethiopia. East Afr Med J. 2004;81(1):52–5 PubMed PMID: 15080517. Epub 2004/04/15. eng.
17. Gerard G, Nahum M, FACS. Uterine Rupture in Pregnancy: FACOG, FACS; 2016.
18. Yasmeen Khooharo JZY, Malik SH, Amber A, Majeed N, Malik NH, Pervez H, Majeed I, Majeed N. Incidence and management of rupture uterus in obstructed labour. J Ayub Med Coll Abbottabad. 2013;25:1–2.
19. Ahmed MA, Elkhatim GES, Ounsa MAA/GE, Mohamed EY. Rupture uterus in sudanese women: management and maternal complications. World J Pharm Pharmaceut Sci. 2015;4(04):1669–75.
20. Berhe Y, Gidey H, Wall LL. Uterine rupture in Mekelle, northern Ethiopia, between 2009 and 2013. Int J Gynaecol Obstet. 2015;130(2):153–6 PubMed PMID: 25935473. Epub 2015/05/04. eng.
21. Mahbuba IA. Uterine rupture -- experience of 30 cases at Faridpur medical college hospital. Faridpur Med Coll J. 2012;7(2):79–81.
22. AbouZahr CDC. Global burden of obstructed labour in the year 2000 evidence and information for policy (EIP). Geneva: World Health Organization; 2003.
23. Ofir K, Sheiner E, Levy A, Katz M, Mazor M. Uterine rupture: differences between a scarred and an unscarred uterus. Am J Obstet Gynecol. 2004; 19(1):425–9.
24. Amanael Gessesew MMM. Ruptured uterus-eight year retrospective analysis of the cause and management outcomes in Adigrat hospital Tigray region, Ethiopia. Ethiop J Health. 2002;16(3):241–5.
25. Noah Elias SA, Admasu K. Quarterly health bulletin policy and practice information for action. In: FDRoEMo, editor. Health. Addis Ababa; 2014.
26. Sinha M, Gupta R, Gupta P, Rani R, Kaur R, Singh R. Uterine rupture: a seven year review at a tertiary care hospital in New Delhi, India. Indian J Community Med. 2016;41(1):45–9.
27. Al-Jufairi ZA, Sandhu AK, Al-Durazi KA. Risk factors of uterine rupture. Saudi Med J. 2001;22(8):702–4 PubMed PMID: 11573117.
28. Igwegbe AO, Eleje GU, Udegbunam OI. Risk factors and perinatal outcome of uterine rupture in a low-resource setting. Niger Med J. 2013;54(6):415–9 PubMed PMID: 24665158. Pubmed Central PMCID: 3948966.
29. Nahum GG. Uterine rupture in pregnancy. Medscape. 2016.
30. Latika S. A 10 year analysis of uterine rupture at a teaching institution. J Obstet Gynecol India. 2006;56(6):502–6.
31. Guyot A, Carbonnel M, Frey C, Pharisien I, Uzan M, Carbillon L. [Uterine rupture: risk factors, maternal and perinatal complications]. J Gynecol Obstet

Biol Reprod 2010;39(3):238–245. PubMed PMID: 20392573. Rupture uterine : facteurs de risque, complications maternelles et foetales.

32. Mbamara SU, Obiechina N, Eleje GU. An analysis of uterine rupture at the Nnamdi Azikiwe University teaching hospital Nnewi, Southeast Nigeria. Niger J Clin Pract. 2012;15(4):448–52.

33. Kaczmarczyk M, Sparen P, Terry P, Cnattingius S. Risk factors for uterine rupture and neonatal consequences of uterine rupture: a population-based study of successive pregnancies in Sweden. BJOG. 2007;114(10):1208–14 PubMed PMID: 17877673.

34. Turgut A, Ozler A, Siddik Evsen M, Ender Soydinc H, Yaman Goruk N, Karacor T, et al. Uterine rupture revisited: predisposing factors, clinical features, management and outcomes from a tertiary care center in Turkey. Pak J Med Sci. 2013;29(3):753–7 PubMed PMID: 24353622. Pubmed Central PMCID: 3809304.

35. Sturzenegger K, Schaffer L, Zimmermann R, Haslinger C. Risk factors of uterine rupture with a special interest to uterine fundal pressure. J Perinat Med. 2016; PubMed PMID: 27235667.

36. Spencer C, Robarts P. Risk factors for uterine rupture and neonatal consequences of uterine rupture: a population-based study of successive pregnancies in Sweden. BJOG. 2008;115(3):415 author reply –6. PubMed PMID: 18190390.

37. Ronel D, Wiznitzer A, Sergienko R, Zlotnik A, Sheiner E. Trends, risk factors and pregnancy outcome in women with uterine rupture. Arch Gynecol Obstet. 2012;285(2):317–21 PubMed PMID: 21735183.

38. Egbe TO, Halle-Ekane GE, Tchente CN, Nyemb JE, Belley-Priso E. Management of uterine rupture: a case report and review of the literature. BMC Res Notes. 2016;9(492):2295–9.

39. Darlow K, Wolf H, Lawley R. Ruptured Uterus in Ethiopia: A series of 67 cases; GLOW book of abstracts liverpool. p. 29.

40. Aggrawal P, Terhase N. Unscarred uterine rupture: a retrospective study. Int J Reprod Contracept Obstet Gynecol. 2015;4(6):1997–9.

24

Multilevel analysis of factors associated with assistance during delivery in rural Nigeria: implications for reducing rural-urban inequity in skilled care at delivery

Bola Lukman Solanke[*] and Semiu Adebayo Rahman

Abstract

Background: Studies have observed rural-urban inequity in the use of skilled delivery in Nigeria. A number of studies have explicitly examined associated factors of assistance during delivery in rural areas. However, the studies so far conducted in rural Nigeria have investigated mainly individual-level characteristics with near exclusion of community-level characteristics. Also, most of the studies that have investigated community-level influence on use of maternal healthcare services in Nigeria did not isolate rural areas for specific research attention. The objective of this study was to investigate the individual-level and community-level characteristics associated with assistance during delivery in rural Nigeria.

Methods: The study analysed women data of 2013 Nigeria Demographic and Health Survey. A weighted sample size of 12,665 rural women was analysed. The outcome variable was assistance during delivery, dichotomised into 'skilled assistance' and 'unskilled assistance'. The explanatory variables are selected individual-level characteristics (maternal education, parity, age at first birth, religion, healthcare decision, employment status, access to mass media, and means of transportation); and selected community-level characteristics (community literacy level, community childcare burden, proportion of women employed outside agriculture, proportion of women who perceived distance to facility as a big problem, community poverty level, and geographical region). The mixed-effects logistic regression was applied.

Results: During the most recent deliveries, 23.0% of rural women utilised skilled assistance compared with 77.0% who utilised unskilled assistance. Maternal education, parity, religion, healthcare decision, access to mass media, and means of transportation were the individual-level characteristics that revealed significant effects on the likelihood of utilising skilled assistance during delivery, while community literacy level, community poverty level, community perception of distance to health facility, and geographic region were the community-level characteristics that revealed significant effects on the odds of using skilled assistance during delivery. Results of Intra-Class Correlation (ICC) supported significant community-level effects on the likelihood of using skilled assistance during delivery.

Conclusions: Assistance during delivery is influenced by individual-level and community-level characteristics. Health policies and programmes seeking to reduce rural-urban inequity in skilled delivery should endeavour to identify and address important factors at both the individual and community levels of the social environment.

Keywords: Skilled assistance, Individual-level, Community-level, Delivery, Rural women, Nigeria

* Correspondence: modebolasolanke@gmail.com; bsolanke@oauife.edu.ng
Department of Demography and Social Statistics, Faculty of Social Sciences,
Obafemi Awolowo University, Ile-Ife, Nigeria

Background

Rural areas in Nigeria have 51% population compared with 49% urban population [1], the rural areas also have higher incidences of pregnancies, child deliveries, and preventable maternal and child morbidities and mortality compared with the urban areas [2]. This makes the provision of maternal healthcare services across the continuum of maternal health care more compelling in the rural areas. However, evidence abounds that infrastructure for healthcare delivery particularly infrastructure for skilled care at delivery is markedly different between rural and urban areas, with the rural areas suffering infrastructural neglect in the country [3]. The existing rural health facilities in Nigeria are often bereft of adequate equipment, competent health personnel, and are largely inaccessible due to distance and poor road networks [2]. This situation which also exists in several sub-Saharan Africa countries often culminates not only in disparity in where rural and urban women deliver their babies [4], but also in disparity in the competency of persons providing assistance during delivery [5–7].

Assistance during delivery refers to the person attending child delivery. The person may be a 'skilled attendant' such as a doctor, nurse and midwife or an 'unskilled attendant' such as a traditional birth attendant, community extension worker, and friend/relative. The skills and competency of the person attending child delivery determine to a large extent whether complications during delivery are promptly identified and well-managed, as well as ensuring that hygienic practices are upheld during delivery [2]. While percentage of birth delivered by a skilled attendant in the urban areas of Nigeria increased from 65.4% in 2008 to 67.0% in 2013, the proportion in the rural areas of Nigeria, declined from 27.7% in 2008 to 22.7% in 2013 [8, 9]. This not only depict inequity in skilled care at delivery within Nigeria, it may continue to adversely affect birth outcome [10], exert negative impact on use of skilled delivery services by rural women [11], and may be a contributory factor to current poor maternal and newborn health in the country [2]. In addition, the situation of skilled delivery in Nigeria is a far cry from global expectation that all pregnant women irrespective of location be assisted by skilled attendants during delivery [12].

Health interventions in Nigeria such as the Midwives Service Scheme (MSS), which was established to improve human resources for health often, fail to reduce rural-urban disparity in skilled care at delivery due to challenges such as difficulty in retaining health personnel for rural health practice [13, 14]. The situation is aggravated by the unwillingness of many students undergoing medical training to take up future appointments in the rural and remote areas of the country [15]. Though, the World Health Organization (WHO) has made useful suggestions for recruiting and retaining rural health workforce [16], but achieving current and future human resource needs for sexual and reproductive health including maternal and child health in sub-Saharan Africa countries remains a huge challenge [17]. Thus, amid rural neglect and poor health delivery system, understanding the wide spectrum of factors affecting assistance during delivery remains relevant in reproductive health research in Nigeria.

Numerous studies across the world have confirmed that use of maternal healthcare services including assistance during delivery is mainly affected by a mixture of individual characteristics such as gender inequality [18, 19], maternal education [20], socio-economic inequality [21], spousal violence [22, 23], birth order and pregnancy wantedness [24], and community characteristics such as type of residence [25, 26], prevalence of larger family size [27], community education, community perception of distance to health facility, and community media saturation [28, 29]. Though, a number of studies have explicitly examined associated factors of assistance during delivery in rural areas [30–36], the studies so far conducted in rural Nigeria have investigated mainly individual-level characteristics with near exclusion of the community-level characteristics associated with assistance during delivery in rural areas [37–41]. Also, most of the studies that have investigated community-level influence on use of maternal healthcare services in Nigeria [28, 42–44] did not isolate rural areas for specific research attention.

This may undermine understanding the role of community-level characteristics (the characteristics of the social groups' individual belong) in influencing utilisation of skilled care at delivery, and how community-level characteristics may contribute to developing effective community-based responses that could address existing inequity in utilisation of skilled care at delivery in the country. Community-level characteristics represent a unique social context that not only affect how individuals perceived and respond to health or other issues in the social environment, but also exert independent effects on the health outcomes of individuals in the community. Such independent effects made it possible for two women with identical socio-demographic and health characteristics to have different likelihood of using or not using skilled care at delivery. Thus, community-level characteristics may affect assistance during delivery by moderating how individuals in the community perceive the relevance and quality of assistance during child delivery. Increasing numbers of studies have provided research evidence that such social context is crucial for improving health behaviour [45–49].

The objective of the study was therefore, to examine the individual-level and community-level characteristics associated with assistance during delivery in rural Nigeria. This was with the view to providing additional policy-relevant information for addressing current rural-urban inequity in skilled care at delivery, and promoting equity in utilisation of skilled care at delivery in the country. The study was guided by the research question: to what extent are individual-level and community-level characteristics associated with assistance during delivery in rural Nigeria? The socio-ecological theory of health behaviour provides the theoretical underpinning of the study. The theory asserts that human health behaviour such as the use of maternal healthcare service is influenced at multiple levels within the social and physical environment such as the individual, household, community, societal and policy environment levels [50].

Methods

Study context

The study location is Nigeria, the most populous country in Africa [1]. Nigeria has a weak health delivery system that contributes to adverse maternal and child health outcomes [10, 51]. Also, the health delivery system in the country is inadequately funded [52]. Average national indices of maternal and child health, particularly utilisation of crucial maternal healthcare services such as skilled care delivery in the country is among the poorest in sub-Saharan Africa [2]. In the 5 years preceding the 2013 Nigeria Demographic and Health Survey (NDHS), among women who had a live birth, 61% received antenatal care from a skilled health provider; a lower proportion (51%) reported the recommended four or more antenatal care visits; 36% had facility-delivery, and 38% of deliveries were attended by a skilled health provider [9]. These show that utilisation of maternal healthcare services in the country need improvement. The Integrated Maternal, Newborn and Child Health (IMNCH) Strategy currently being implemented in the country seeks to boost utilisation of essential maternal care services across the continuum of maternal health-care [2]. For instance, some of the IMNCH priority actions include increasing the coverage and quality of the Focused Antenatal Care; increasing demand for facility-based deliveries with skilled birth attendance; and ensuring that all mothers and newborns receive prompt postnatal check within 2 days. Nevertheless, the coverage of the IMNCH interventions is still very low particularly in rural and remote areas of the country [53]. The Federal Government has also made efforts to boost the funding of maternal and child health delivery in the country through The Subsidy Reinvestment and Empowerment Programme [51]. The programme has however recorded only marginal improvement in the situation of maternal, newborn and child health in the country, as drop out from the continuum of maternity care remain high in the country [54] with substantial rural-urban differentials in the use of maternal health-care services [55].

Some health practitioners have commenced advocacy for free maternal and child health in the country to further boost utilisation of maternal healthcare services [56]. Some other health professionals have also advocated for the implementation of Conditional Cash Transfer (CCT) Scheme in the country, as another means of encouraging maternal healthcare use, particularly among socially disadvantaged women [57]. In spite of this efforts, negative perception of public health facilities may have continue to hinder improved utilisation among women in the country [58]. The Community-based health insurance programme, another initiative designed to enhance access to healthcare in the country is yet to successfully commence in many communities in the country [59]. These have provided compelling need for further investigation of associated factors of maternal healthcare use in the country.

Data source and sample

This study was based on data collected from women of reproductive age in the 2013 NDHS. The 2013 NDHS is part of the series of cross-sectional Demographic and Health Survey (DHS) conducted across developing countries to provide reliable and internationally comparable information on the current state of fertility, childhood and adult mortality, family planning, and other sexual and reproductive health issues in developing countries. Relevant information about the design and implementation of the survey has been published [9]. In this study, only rural women were analysed. The study however, excluded women who were not currently married, and women who had no live birth in the 5 years preceding the survey. A weighted sample of 12,665 women were analysed in the study. A formal request to analyse the dataset was made to MEASURE DHS (the custodian of the DHS data) through online platform. Authorisation was granted.

Outcome variable

The outcome variable in the study was assistance during delivery. This was a dichotomous variable with 'skilled assistance' and 'unskilled assistance' as categories. Skilled assistance in the study refers to delivery assistance provided by a doctor, nurse, midwife, or auxiliary nurse/midwife. This was based on the classification of skilled and unskilled health provider adopted in the 2013 NDHS [9]. But in some other countries, auxiliary nurse/midwife may not be classified as a skilled health provider [60]. Unskilled assistance in the study refers to delivery assistance provided by community extension worker, traditional birth attendants, friends/relatives, and no one. The category of interest in the study was the skilled assistance category.

Explanatory and control variables

The explanatory variables in the study are individual-level and community-level characteristics. The individual-level characteristics analysed are maternal education, healthcare decision, parity, age at first birth, religion, employment status, access to mass media, and means of transportation. These characteristics were selected for analysis because previous studies have established their associations with utilisation of maternal healthcare services particularly in developing countries [20, 21, 23–26, 61–65]. Some of the variables were re-coded to suit the analytic framework of the study. Healthcare decision was based on whether women were involved in making decision about their own healthcare. Women who solely or jointly with male partner had final say on their healthcare decision were grouped as 'participation', while other women who had no say in the decision were grouped as 'no participation'. Women's access to the mass media was based on the frequency of listening to radio, watching television, or reading newspaper weekly. Women who did not listen to radio, watch television, or read newspaper during the week were grouped as 'no access', while those who listened to radio, watched television, or read newspaper at least once weekly were grouped as 'moderate' access. Women who listened to radio, watched television, or read newspaper more than once weekly were grouped as 'high' access. Women's parity was divided into primiparity (one child ever born), multiparity (two to four children ever born), and grand multiparity (five or more children ever born).

Six community-level characteristics were analysed in the study. These are community childcare burden (proportion of women who had five or more children), community literacy level (proportion of women who cannot read and write at all), community poverty level (proportion of women in the poorest household quintile), proportion of women employed outside agricultural sector, community perception of distance to health facility (proportion of women who perceived distance to health facility as a big problem), and geographic region. The community-level characteristics were derived by aggregating the selected characteristic at the cluster level and then dividing into suitable categories. This was done because the variables are not directly available in the DHS data. Most studies that have analysed community-level variables using DHS data adopted the method [28, 29, 48]. In addition, to the selected individual-level and community-level variables, three variables were selected for statistical control. These are household wealth quintile, number of antenatal

care visits, and timing of first antenatal care visits. The selection of these variables was guided by literature [24–27, 66].

Data analysis

Three levels of statistical analyses were employed. The univariate analysis describes assistance during delivery using the pie chart, while respondents' characteristics were presented using frequency distributions and percentages. At the bivariate level of analysis, cross tabulation of the research variables were carried out to show percentage of skilled assistance as changes in the categories of the explanatory variable occurs. This analytic level also describes the relationship between the variables using unadjusted binary logistic regression coefficient to reveal whether the relationships are positive or negative. Before the multivariate analysis was carried out, a Variance Inflation Factor (VIF) was calculated to detect extent of multi-collinearity of the independent variables using the mean VIF score. This was needed to determine the suitability of the selected variables for multivariate analysis. As a rule of thumb in regression analysis, a mean VIF score of less than 5 is tolerated, while a mean VIF score of 5–10 suggests that the regression coefficients might be inadequately estimated [67, 68]. At the multivariate level, the mixed-effects logistic regression was used to determine extent of variation in the use of skilled assistance attributable to individual-level and community-level characteristics. The mixed-effects logistic regression model consists of two parts, namely, the fixed effect and the random effect [43]. The model was specified as:

$$\log\left(\frac{\pi_{ij}}{1-\pi_{ij}}\right) = \beta_0 + \beta_1 x_{ij} + \beta_2 x_{2ij} + \dots + \beta_8 x_{8ij}$$
$$+ \beta_9 z_{1j} + \beta_{10} z_{2j} + \dots \beta_{14} z_{6j} + \mu_{0j}$$

Where:
π_{ij} is the log of odds of skilled assistance.
$(1 - \pi_{ij})$ is the log of unskilled assistance.
x and z are the explanatory variables for the likelihood of skilled assistance.
x_1 to x_8 are the individual-level characteristics.
z_1 to z_6 are the community-level characteristics.
β_0 is the overall intercept.
$\beta_1 \dots \beta_{14}$ are the regression coefficients for the explanatory variables x_1 to x_8, and z_1 to z_6.
u_{0j} is the community-level random effect (assumed to be normally distributed with mean equal to 0 and variance equal to $\sigma_{\mu 0^2}$).

The fixed effects were estimated using odds ratio of adjusted binary logistic regression, while the random effects were estimated using the Intra-Class Correlation (ICC) calculated as: $\frac{\tau}{\tau + \left[\frac{\mu^2}{3}\right]}$ where τ is the estimated community-level variance [43]. The ICC ranges from 0 to 1, with ICC of 1 indicating that women in the community have identical use of skilled assistance during delivery, and with ICC of 0 indicating that women in the community do not have identical use of skilled assistance in the community. Four models were fitted in the study. Model 1 included only individual-level characteristics, while Model 2 was based solely on community-level characteristics. Model 3 included both individual-level and community-level characteristics. Model 4 was the full model that included the explanatory and control variables. The models were fitted using the *xtmelogit* command of Stata version 12 [69]. Model adequacy was examined using the Wald chi-square which assesses the statistical significance of the model. The 5% alpha level was considered statistically significant. Analyses were performed using Stata version 12.

Results
Univariate results
Figure 1 presents distribution of respondents by assistance during delivery. As shown in the figure, during their most recent deliveries, slightly less than a quarter of respondents (23.0%) utilised 'skilled assistance' while the majority of respondents (77.0%) utilised 'unskilled assistance'. Table 1 presents respondents' socio-demographic profile. Nearly two-thirds of the respondents' had no formal education. However, among respondents with educational attainments, primary education was dominant. The majority of respondents were either multiparous (42.7%) or grand multiparous (41.7%) women. Reproductive age interval of 15–19 years was the dominant age interval at first birth among the respondents. The proportion of the respondents who had first birth at age twenty-five or older ages was less than one-tenth of the respondents. The majority of the respondents were employed during the

survey. However, slightly more than one-third of the respondents were unemployed during the survey. Muslim women compared with women practicing Christianity or other religions were dominant among respondents.

More than two-thirds of the respondents did not participate in their healthcare decision. Slightly more than two-fifths of respondents had no access to the mass media. However, nearly one-third of the women had 'high' access to the mass media. More than two-fifths of respondents either had no modern means of transportation or had animal-drawn cart as means of transportation. Motorcycle/scooter was the dominant modern means of transportation available to the respondents who reported a modern means of transportation. Higher proportions of the respondents were in the poorest (34.7%) and poorer (31.1%) wealth quintiles compared with the respondents in other wealth categories. Nearly half of the respondents (49.5%) had no antenatal care visits prior to their most recent deliveries, while nearly half of respondents reported some numbers of antenatal care visits. However, more than one-third of the respondents (37.6%) reported the recommended four or more antenatal care visits prior to their most recent deliveries. Distribution of respondents by timing of first antenatal care visits however revealed that nearly half of the respondents had their first antenatal care visit in the third trimester of pregnancy, while slightly more than one-third of respondents (35.6%) had their first antenatal care visit in the second trimester of pregnancy.

More than one-third of the respondents live either in communities with low (36.3%) or moderate (39.0%) childcare burden that is communities with low or medium proportion of high parous women but nearly one-quarter of the respondents live in communities with high childcare burden. In contrast, more than one-third of the respondents live in communities with either medium or high proportions of women who cannot read or write at all. Likewise, the distribution of respondents by community poverty level showed that the proportions of women who live in communities with either medium or high poverty level were more than one-third of respondents. The proportions of respondents employed outside agriculture were similar in the communities, though with slightly higher proportion of respondents living in communities with high proportion of women employed outside agriculture. More respondents live in communities where more than half of the women perceived distance to health facility as a big problem. Women from the northern region of the country were dominant among the respondents.

Bivariate results
Table 2 presents proportions of skilled assistance and the bivariate relationships between the research

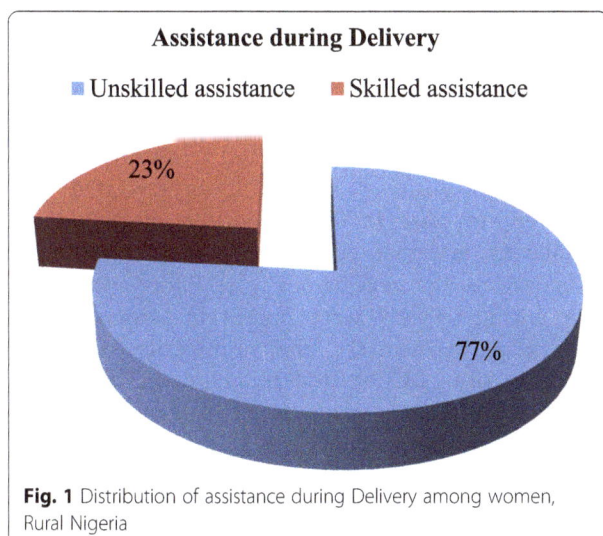
Fig. 1 Distribution of assistance during Delivery among women, Rural Nigeria

Table 1 Respondents socio-demographic characteristics, rural Nigeria, 2013

Characteristic	Number of women (n = 12,665)	Percentage
Maternal Education		
None	8100	64.0
Primary	2294	18.1
Secondary	1992	15.7
Higher	278	2.2
Parity		
Primiparity	1.979	15.6
Multiparity	5411	42.7
Grandmultiparity	5275	41.7
Age at first birth (years)		
14 or less	1248	9.8
15–19	7405	58.5
20–24	2999	23.7
25 or older	1013	8.0
Employment status		
Unemployed	4361	34.4
Employed	8304	65.6
Religion		
Christianity	3608	28.5
Islam	8816	69.6
Others	241	1.9
Healthcare decision		
No Participation	9139	72.2
Participate	3526	27.8
Access to mass media		
No access	5654	44.6
Moderate access	2860	22.6
High access	4151	32.8
Means of Transportation		
None/animal cart	5108	40.3
Boat/canoe	210	1.7
Bicycle	1710	13.5
Motorcycle/scooter	5064	40.0
Car/truck	573	4.5
Household wealth quintile		
Poorest	4400	34.7
Poorer	3937	31.1
Middle	2560	20.2
Richer	1306	10.3
Richest	462	3.7

Table 1 Respondents socio-demographic characteristics, rural Nigeria, 2013 *(Continued)*

Characteristic	Number of women (n = 12,665)	Percentage
Number of antenatal care visit		
No Visit	6279	49.5
1–3 Visits	1629	12.9
4 or more visits	4756	37.6
Timing of first antenatal visit		
1st Trimester	1831	14.5
2nd Trimester	4508	35.6
3rd Trimester	6326	49.9
Community childcare burden		
Low	4602	36.3
Medium	4934	39.0
High	3129	24.7
Community literacy level		
Low	3552	28.0
Medium	4522	35.7
High	4591	36.3
Community poverty level		
Low	3761	29.7
Medium	4237	33.4
High	4667	36.9
Proportion employed outside agriculture		
Low	4120	32.5
Medium	4156	32.8
High	4389	34.7
Proportion who perceived distance as a big problem		
Low	6556	51.8
High	6109	48.2
Geographic Region		
Northern region	10,303	81.4
Southern region	2362	18.6

Source: Author's analysis based on 2013 Nigeria Demographic and Health Survey

variables. Maternal education and assistance during delivery were positively and significantly related with consistent increase in the proportion of skilled assistance as maternal education improves from one lower level to the next higher level. Parity and assistance during delivery were negatively associated. As maternal parity increased from primiparity (one-CEB) to multiparity (4-CEB), and to grand multiparity (5 or more CEB), proportion of skilled assistance respectively decreased from 29.9 to 25.3%, and 18.9%. Age at first birth and assistance during delivery are positively and significantly related with the highest proportion of skilled assistance among women who

Table 2 Proportion of skilled assistance and unadjusted binary logistic regression coefficients showing bivariate relationships, Rural Nigeria, 2013

Characteristic	% of Skilled assistance	Coeff.	95% CI
Maternal education			
None[RC]	9.1	–	–
Primary	35.0	1.684*	1.476–1.891
Secondary	58.8	2.658*	2.450–2.866
Higher	87.0	4.205*	3.728–4.683
Parity			
Primiparity[RC]	29.9	–	–
Multiparity	25.3	−0.230**	−0.370, −0.091
Grandmultiparity	18.9	−0.604*	−0.746, −0.462
Age at first birth (years)			
14 or less[RC]	14.6	–	–
15–19	17.7	0.232**	0.036–0.428
20–24	33.5	1.080*	0.865–1.294
25 +	45.0	1.566*	1.278–1.855
Employment status			
Unemployed[RC]	16.8	–	–
Employed	26.7	0.591*	0.411–0.770
Religion			
Christianity[RC]	51.3	–	–
Islam	11.9	−2.053*	−2.280, −1.825
Others	20.8	−1.388*	−2.002, −0.774
Healthcare decision			
No participation[RC]	16.3	–	–
Participation	41.4	1.287*	1.124–1.451
Access to mass media			
No access[RC]	12.9	–	–
Moderate access	20.5	0.556*	0.341–0.770
High access	39.5	1.487*	1.298–1.676
Means of transportation			
None/animal cart[RC]	21.6	–	–
Boat/canoe	15.2	−0.430	−0.955, 0.094
Bicycle	15.3	−0.423**	−0.682, −0.164
Motorcycle/scooter	25.4	0.211**	0.030–0.391
Car/truck	47.0	1.167*	0.887–1.447
Household wealth quintile			
Poorest	4.8	–	–
Poorer	16.1	1.333*	1.081–1.586
Middle	38.4	2.509*	2.235–2.782
Richer	58.3	3.317*	3.011–3.622
Richest	78.2	4.258*	3.834–4.682
Number of antenatal care visits			
No visit	5.6	–	–

Table 2 Proportion of skilled assistance and unadjusted binary logistic regression coefficients showing bivariate relationships, Rural Nigeria, 2013 *(Continued)*

Characteristic	% of Skilled assistance	Coeff.	95% CI
1–3 visits	22.4	1.583*	1.352–1.814
4 or more visits	47.1	2.711*	2.496–2.925
Timing of first antenatal care visit			
1st trimester	51.9	–	–
2nd trimester	37.7	−0.576*	−0.745, −0.408
3rd trimester	4.8	−3.066*	−3.297, −2.835
Community childcare burden			
Low	36.1	–	–
Medium	16.5	−1.051*	−1.398, −0.704
High	15.2	−1.150*	−1.524, −0.776
Community Literacy Level			
Low	56.5	–	–
Medium	17.0	−1.850*	−2.128, −1.573
High	3.9	−3.462*	−3.772, −3.153
Community Poverty Level			
Low	52.9	–	–
Medium	18.4	−1.606*	−1.903, −1.309
High	3.9	−3.315*	−3.627, −3.004
Proportion employed outside agriculture			
Low	22.0	–	–
Medium	23.3	0.074	−0.286, 0.434
High	24.7	0.152	−0.216, 0.520
Proportion who perceived distance as a big problem			
Low	13.1	–	–
High	34.3	1.244*	0.936–1.552
Geographic region			
Northern region	14.8	–	–
Southern region	60.6	2.180*	1.891–2.470

Notes: Coeff. (Coefficient), RC (Reference Category), *$p < 0.01$, **$p < 0.05$

had their first birth at age 25 years or older ages (45.0%). Likewise, employment status was positively and significantly associated with assistance during delivery ($\beta = 0.591$; CI: 0.411–0.770). Employed women had higher skilled assistance compared with unemployed women (26.7% vs. 16.8%).

Religion was negatively associated with assistance during delivery. Christian women compared with Muslim and other women had higher prevalence of skilled assistance. The relationship between healthcare decision and assistance during delivery was significantly positive ($\beta = 1.287$; CI: 1.124–1.451) with higher prevalence of skilled assistance among women who participated in the decision compared with women who did not participate in the decision (41.4% vs. 16.3%). Access to mass media and assistance during delivery were significantly positively related. As access to mass media improve from 'none' to 'moderate' and 'high', the proportion of skilled delivery increased from 12.9 to 20.5%, and 39.5% respectively. Means of transportation had mixed relationship with assistance during delivery. The relationship was negative among women whose means of transportation were boat/canoe or bicycle but positive among women whose means of transportation were motorcycle/scooter or car/truck. However, the proportion of skilled assistance was highest among women whose means of transportation were car or truck (47.0%).

Household wealth quintile had significant positive relationship with assistance during delivery. As wealth quintile improved from one lower wealth group to another higher wealth group, the proportion of skilled assistance progressively improved. For instance, proportion of skilled assistance improved from 38.4% among women in 'middle' wealth group to 58.3% among women in 'richer' wealth group. Antenatal care visits relates positively with assistance during delivery. The proportion of skilled assistance was 5.6% among women who had no antenatal care visit but increased to 22.4% among women who had 1–3 antenatal care visits. It further increased to 47.1% among women who had the recommended four or more antenatal care visits. Timing of first antenatal care visit was negatively associated with assistance during delivery with lowest proportion of skilled assistance (4.8%) among women whose first antenatal care visits took place in the third trimester of pregnancy compared with 51.9% of skilled assistance among women whose first antenatal care visit took place within the first trimester of pregnancy.

Community childcare burden was negatively associated with assistance during delivery with reduction in the proportions of skilled assistance as childcare burden increases in the communities. The relationship between community literacy level and assistance during delivery was also negative with lowest proportion of skilled assistance (3.9%) among women in communities with high proportion of women who cannot read or write at all. Community poverty level was negatively associated with assistance during delivery. The proportion of skilled assistance was highest among women who live in communities with low proportion of women in the poorest wealth group. Proportion of women employed outside agricultural sector relates positively with assistance during delivery. The proportion of skilled assistance increased as the proportion of women employed outside agriculture improved. For instance, the proportion of skilled assistance was higher among women who live in communities with high proportion of women employed outside agricultural sector compared with women in communities with low proportion of women employed outside agriculture (24.7% vs. 22.0%). Community perception of distance to health facility was positively associated with assistance during delivery with lower proportion of skilled assistance (13.1%) among women who live in communities with low perception of distance to health facility as a big problem to accessing healthcare. Likewise, geographic region and assistance during delivery were significantly positively related ($\beta = 2.180$; CI: 1.891–2.470). Southern women compared with their northern counterpart had higher use of skilled assistance (60.6% vs. 14.8%).

Multivariate results

Prior to fitting the multivariate models, the VIF computed revealed a mean VIF score of 3.36. This not only confirms that the explanatory variables were not significantly multi-collinear, it also suggest that the variables were sufficient for adequate estimation of the regression coefficients. The variables were then included in the mixed-effects analyses. Table 3 presents the fixed-effects on the likelihood of skilled assistance during delivery. The Wald chi-square confirm that all the fitted models were statistically significant ($p < 0.01$). In Model 1 (Wald $\chi^2 = 288.3$; $p < 0.01$), six individual-level characteristics, namely, maternal education, parity, religion, healthcare decision, access to mass media, and means of transportation had significant effects on the likelihood of skilled assistance. For instance, grand multiparous women were 48.2% less likely to utilise skilled assistance compared with primiparous women (OR = 0.518: CI: 0.420–0.640). In contrast, women who participated in healthcare decision were 43.5% more likely to utilise skilled assistance compared with women who did not participate in healthcare decision (OR = 1.435; CI: 1.215–1.693).

In Model 2 (Wald $\chi^2 = 333.4$; $p < 0.01$), four community-level characteristics, namely, community literacy level, community poverty level, community perception of distance to health facility, and geographic region revealed significant independent effects on the likelihood of skilled assistance. For instance, women in communities with high proportion of women who cannot read or write at all were less likely to utilise skilled assistance compared with women in communities with low proportion of women who cannot read or write at all (OR = 0.072; CI: 0.040–0.128). Likewise, women in communities with high proportion of women in poorest wealth group were less likely to utilise skilled assistance compared with women in communities with low proportion of women in poorest wealth group (OR = 0.159; CI: 0.090–0.282). The inclusion of both individual-level and community-level characteristics in Model 3 (Wald $\chi^2 = 367.9$; $p < 0.01$) reinforced the

Table 3 Odds ratio of adjusted binary logistic regression showing fixed effects on the likelihood of skilled assistance

Characteristic predicting skilled assistance	Model 1 (Wald $\chi^2 = 288.3$; $p < 0.001$)		Model 2 (Wald $\chi^2 = 333.4$; $p < 0.001$)		Model 3 (Wald $\chi^2 = 367.9$; $p < 0.001$)		Model 4 (Wald $\chi^2 = 474.9$; $p < 0.001$)	
	Odds Ratio	95% CI	Odds Ratio	95% CI	Odds Ratio	95% CI	Odds Ratio	95% CI
Maternal education								
None[RC]	–	–			–	–	–	–
Primary	1.994*	1.623–2.450			1.481*	1.215–1.806	1.205	0.996–1.458
Secondary	3839*	2.583–5.706			2.703*	2.120–3.447	1.840*	1.464–2.313
Higher	4.131*	3.184–5.358			13.114*	7.533–22.831	5.793*	3.474–9.660
Parity								
Primiparity[RC]	–	–			–	–	–	–
Multiparity	0.538*	0.440–0.657			0.532*	0.437–0.648	0.575*	0.476–0.695
Grand multiparity	0.518*	0.420–0.640			0.506*	0.411–0.624	0.564*	0.462–0.689
Age at first marriage (years)								
14 years or less[RC]	–	–			–	–	–	–
15–19 years	0.843	0.654–1.086			0.839	0.654–1.077	0.811	0.635–1.035
20–24 years	1.104	0.840–1.453			1.044	0.798–1.366	0.981	0.755–1.275
25 years or older	1.121	0.800–1.571			1.033	0.743–1.437	0.945	0.685–1.304
Employment Status								
Unemployed[RC]	–	–			–	–	–	–
Unemployment	1.169	0.991–1.378			1.094	0.931–1.286	1.033	0.883–1.208
Religion								
Christianity[RC]	–	–			–	–	–	–
Islam	0.317*	0.237–0.423			0.741**	0.560–0.982	0.750**	0.577–0.974
Traditional/others	0.354**	0.188–0.664			0.558	0.299–1.040	0.712	0.390–1.300
Healthcare Decision								
No Participation[RC]	–	–			–	–	–	–
Participation	1.435*	1.215–1.693			1.290**	1.100–1.513	1.213**	1.041–1.413
Access to mass media								
None[RC]	–	–			–	–	–	–
Moderate	1.138	0.932–1.388			1.039	0.856–1.260	0.934	0.774–1.127
High	1.817*	1.506–2.193			1.562*	1.304–1.871	1.255**	1.055–1.494
Means of Transportation								
None/animal cart[RC]	–	–			–	–	–	–
Boat/canoe	0.513**	0.293–0.900			0.386*	0.226–0.659	0.392*	0.234–0.659
Bicycle	0.966	0.748–1.249			1.028	0.800–1.321	1.052	0.824–1.341
Motorcycle/scooter	1.425*	1.207–1.683			1.383*	1.177–1.626	1.222**	1.046–1.429
Car/truck	2.169*	1.566–3.003			1.984*	1.447–2.719	1.438**	1.055–1.960
Community childcare burden								
Low[RC]			–	–	–		–	–
Medium			0.886	0.623–1.260	1.071	0.759–1.511	1.079	0.796–1.462
High			0.752	0.505–1.116	0.936	0.635–1.380	0.978	0.694–1.378
Community literacy level								
Low[RC]			–	–	–	–	–	–
Medium			0.208*	0.136–0.319	0.389*	0.256–0.591	0.489*	0.339–0.706
High			0.072*	0.040–0.128	0.170*	0.095–0.302	0.346*	0.208–0.575

Table 3 Odds ratio of adjusted binary logistic regression showing fixed effects on the likelihood of skilled assistance *(Continued)*

Characteristic predicting skilled assistance	Model 1 (Wald χ^2 = 288.3; p < 0.001)		Model 2 (Wald χ^2 = 333.4; p < 0.001)		Model 3 (Wald χ^2 = 367.9; p < 0.001)		Model 4 (Wald χ^2 = 474.9; p < 0.001)	
	Odds Ratio	95% CI	Odds Ratio	95% CI	Odds Ratio	95% CI	Odds Ratio	95% CI
Community poverty level								
Low[RC]	–	–	–	–	–	–	–	–
Medium			0.382*	0.252–0.579	0.447*	0.299–0.670	0.602**	0.421–0.860
High			0.159*	0.090–0.282	0.213*	0.122–0.370	0.402*	0.241–0.670
Proportion employed outside agriculture								
Low[RC]	–	–	–	–	–	–	–	–
Medium			1.065	0.747–1.518	1.064	0.749–1.511	0.932	0.683–1.274
High			1.416	0.982–2.043	1.331	0.923–1.919	1.084	0.783–1.502
Proportion who perceived distance as big problem								
Low[RC]	–	–	–	–	–	–	–	–
High			2.774*	1.999–3.850	2.433*	1.770–3.345	1.815*	1.374–2.397
Geographic region								
Northern[RC]	–	–	–	–	–	–	–	–
Southern			2.103*	1.399–3.162	1.750**	1.163–2.634	1.818**	1.265–2.611
Household wealth quintile								
Poorest[RC]							–	–
Poorer							1.261	0.990–1.606
Middle							1.630**	1.227–2.166
Richer							1.819**	1.296–2.552
Richest							2.834*	1.761–4.560
Number of antenatal care visits								
None[RC]							–	–
1–3							1.430	0.991–2.064
4+							2.602*	1.803–3.756
Timing of first antenatal visit								
1st trimester[RC]							–	–
2nd trimester							0.802**	0.680–0.946
3rd trimester							0.252*	0.173–0.369

Notes: *p < 0.001, **p < 0.05

statistical significance of the individual-level and community-level characteristics which showed significant effects in the earlier models.

In the full model (Wald χ^2 = 474.9; p < 0.01), the inclusion of the three control variables did not result in any substantial change in the pattern of the fixed effects on assistance during delivery. In the model, the likelihood of utilising skilled assistance increased significantly as maternal education improved. For instance, women who attained higher education were nearly six times more likely to use skilled assistance compared with uneducated women (OR = 5.793: CI: 3.474–9.660). Likewise, multiparous women (OR = 0.575; CI: 0.476–0.695) and grand multiparous women (OR = 0.564; CI: 0.462–0.689) were less likely to utilise skilled assistance compared

with primiparous women. Also, Muslim women were 25% less likely to utilise skilled assistance compared with Christian women (OR = 0.750; CI: 0.577–0.974). Women who participated in healthcare decision were 21.3% more likely to utilise skilled assistance compared with women who did not participate in healthcare decision (OR = 1.213; CI: 1.041–1.413). Access to mass media revealed significant effect on the odds of skilled assistance. Women who had high access to the mass media were 25.5% more likely to utilise skilled assistance compared with women in the reference category (OR = 1.255; CI: 1.055–1.494). Similarly, women who had car/truck were 43.8% more likely to use skilled assistance compared with women who had no means of transportation (OR = 1.438; CI: 1.055–1.960).

Community literacy level exerted significant influence on the likelihood of using skilled assistance. Women who live in communities with high proportion of women who cannot read or write at all were 65.4% less likely to utilise skilled assistance compared with women in communities with low proportion of women who cannot read or write at all (OR = 0.346; CI: 0.208–0.575). Also, community poverty level revealed significant influence on the odds of skilled assistance. Women in communities with high proportion of women in poorest wealth group were 59.8% less likely to use skilled assistance during delivery compared with women in communities with low proportion of women in poorest wealth group (OR = 0.402; CI: 0.241–0.670). Women in communities where high proportion of women perceived distance to health facility as a big problem were more likely to use skilled assistance during delivery compared with women in the reference category (OR = 1.815; CI: 1.374–2.397). Women in southern region of Nigeria were almost twice more likely to use skilled assistance compared with women in northern region of the country (OR = 1.818; CI: 1.265–2.611). The three selected control variables showed significant influence on the likelihood of using skilled assistance during delivery. The odds of using skilled assistance during delivery increased progressively as household wealth group improved. Women who had four or more antenatal care visits were almost three times more likely to utilise skilled assistance during delivery compared with women who had no antenatal care visits (OR = 2.602; CI: 1.803–3.756). Women whose first antenatal visit took place either in the second or third trimester were less likely to use skilled assistance during delivery compared with women whose first antenatal visit took place in the first trimester of pregnancy.

Table 4 presents the random effects of the mixed-effects models. As shown in the table and using the significance of the LR test, all the models fitted showed a good fit. In the absence of individual-level and community-level characteristics, the result of the ICC in the empty model reveal that the use of skilled assistance was highly identical among women in the community (ICC = 0.705). When only individual variables were included in Model 1, the ICC reduced to 0.515 to indicate that higher proportion of variation in the use of skilled assistance was attributable to community-level characteristics (ICC = 0.515). This proportion further

reduces to 0.381 in Model 2. With the combination of individual-level and community-level characteristics in Model 3, the variation in the use of skilled assistance attributable to community-level characteristics remained substantial (ICC = 0.359) indicating that more than one-third of the women in the communities had identical use of skilled assistance during delivery. In the full model, more than a quarter of variation in the use of skilled assistance during delivery were attributable to community-level characteristics (ICC = 0.286).

Discussion

This study examined individual-level and community-level characteristics associated with assistance during delivery in rural Nigeria. It improves research attention on skilled delivery in the rural areas which in spite of poor health infrastructure is usually the area with higher incidences of pregnancies and child deliveries in Nigeria [2, 8, 9]. The study not only compliment existing studies that have explicitly examined associated factors of assistance during delivery in rural areas [30–33], it also analysed community-level influence on the use of assistance during delivery in rural areas of Nigeria compared with previous rural studies that investigated mainly individual-level characteristics [34–38]. The study provided additional support for the socio-ecological model [50] by confirming the significance of factors operating at both individual and community levels, and thus consistent with previous studies that stressed the importance of community factors in initiatives to improve human health behaviour particularly health-seeking behaviour [45–49]. Based on this finding, it is plausible to assert that factors affecting utilisation of skilled assistance during delivery in rural areas of Nigeria operates at multiple levels, which require that initiatives seeking to boost utilisation of skilled assistance during delivery should endeavour to identify and address the important factors at each distinct level of the social environment.

The study found that utilisation of skilled assistance at delivery is very poor in the rural areas of Nigeria. Though, the 23.0% prevalence of skilled assistance found in the study was higher than the 13.0% reported in an earlier study in Nigeria [53], it corroborates prevalence reported in both the 2008 and 2013 NDHS [8, 9]. There are two possible reasons for poor utilisation of skilled

Table 4 Random Effects showing influence of community characteristics on use of skilled assistance during delivery

Parameter	Empty Model	Model 1	Model 2	Model 3	Model 4
Community level variance (SE)	7.850 (0.925)	3.488 (0.449)	2.023 (0.258)	1.840 (0.243)	1.320 (0.177)
Log likelihood	− 5028	− 4698.3	− 4761.8	− 4550.8	− 4229.6
LR test	$\chi^2 = 4192.2; p < 0.001$	$\chi^2 = 1231.1; p < 0.001$	$\chi^2 = 1024.3; p < 0.001$	$\chi^2 = 781.2; p < 0.001$	$\chi^2 = 571.9; p < 0.001$
ICC	0.705	0.515	0.381	0.359	0.286

assistance at delivery in rural Nigeria. The first reason may relate to poor health infrastructure in rural areas of the country which made unskilled health providers more accessible to rural women [2]. In many rural and remote areas of the country, there are no Primary Health Care (PHC) centres, and where the PHCs are available, many of the health personnel including skilled birth attendants are usually unwilling to reside in the rural communities [13]. The implementation of the MSS was expected to improve maternity care in the rural areas of Nigeria, but it is yet to yield significant positive results due to challenges such as retention of health personnel in rural areas, availability and training of midwives, and lack of political will by States and Local government in the country [14]. Also, where PHCs are available, several adjoining communities may have to depend on its services. This usually creates distance barrier to some of the communities and may affect utilisation. This implies that utilisation of skilled delivery may likely improve in the rural areas if more health centres are provided with qualified health personnel. As evident in the study, though a high proportion of the women perceived distance to health facility as a big problem, but they reported a higher use of skilled assistance than the proportion who perceived distance to health facility as not a big problem which indicates that distance to health facility may not be as important as the availability of health facilities and accessibility to desired services. It is therefore important that government at all tiers of the Nigerian federation should improve public investment on the provision of more health facilities for rural dwellers. In the interim, the staff strength at existing rural health facilities could be expanded by the recruitment of more qualified health personnel especially those already trained in delivery care.

The second reason that may account for poor use of skilled assistance among rural women is the socio-demographic condition of the women. As found in the study, educational attainment was poor among the women, the majority of them were multiparous, had no autonomy on their healthcare, and belong to poorest household wealth group. Such social conditions have been found in earlier studies [2, 51, 53] to promote non-use of maternal healthcare services. Beyond the provision of healthcare centres in rural areas, it is imperative that more concerted efforts be made to improve the socio-economic conditions of rural women. This could be achieved through more rural development efforts such as the creation of more roads to enhance economic activities of rural women, and strengthening existing rural empowerment programmes. The advocacy for free Maternal and Child Health (MCH) services [56] should be given fresh impetus in the country to encourage more States of the federation to implement free MCH services particularly for rural families. This will

reduce the economic burden of healthcare among rural women. Where free MCH services are not feasible, rural women could be assisted to improve their use of skilled delivery through the design and implementation of more CCT programme already piloted in some States of the country [57].

Hence, individual characteristics of women cannot be ignored in interventions to improve utilisation of skilled assistance during delivery. Existing initiatives should endeavour to focus more on three specific characteristics, namely, education, autonomy on healthcare decision, and religion. Education is central to all efforts aiming to improve use of skilled delivery in the rural areas because in spite of the effectiveness of existing interventions, utilisation may remain low in the absence of widespread awareness of the dangers of unskilled delivery. Also, several socio-cultural practices such as unequal power relations between male and female partners, and lack of male involvement in maternal healthcare [19] that undermine prompt health-seeking behaviour are best confronted through the provision of accurate information, communication and education on maternal and child health issues. It is thus important that the current IMNCH strategy reposition its information and communication initiative through massive public health education messages using the mass media particularly the radio which are more widely used in the rural areas.

This should be complimented by promoting women autonomy in the communities. Men in the communities should be mobilised through public campaigns to encourage women to have sole autonomy on issues affecting their reproductive life. Also, there should be more interventions to focus on Muslim women. As evident in this study and consistent with findings in similar previous studies [63, 65], there is unequal likelihood of maternal healthcare services utilisation among Christian and Muslim women. This may indicate that the different religions have different practices that impact women's perception and use of services. This differences in religious beliefs as it relates to maternal health should not only be fully understood by health policy planners, it is also important that religion be made an important component of future maternal healthcare interventions in line with the submission of several scholars on the subject [61, 62, 64, 70].

The study further found that community-level characteristics are crucial for improvement of the use of skilled assistance at delivery in the rural areas. This necessitates more community-based maternal healthcare interventions in rural Nigeria to increase the coverage of the existing community-based programme of the IMNCH Strategy [2]. Community-based interventions are more important in the rural areas because women in the rural communities tend to have identical perception and use of accessible health services. Findings from the study provided evidence that community-level factors such as community poverty or literacy levels have important effects on use of skilled assistance during delivery. Hence, existing community-based intervention such as the community extension workers programme [2] needs to be strengthened in the country. Finally, the antenatal care programme should be appropriately perceived as a veritable means of reaching rural women about other services within the continuum of maternal and child healthcare. In many rural communities and as found in this study, high proportions of women had no antenatal care visits. Also, among those who reported antenatal care visits, more than one-third of the visits took place in the third trimester of pregnancy. Such visitations may not be as a result of seeking adequate antenatal information and counselling, but more likely to be a response to complications or health challenges. Thus, there should be renewed efforts to strengthen the antenatal care programme not only in terms of expanding its coverage to all rural communities to enhance visits in the first trimester of pregnancy, but to also ensure that women who visited health facility for antenatal care are followed up, retained in the continuum to ensure facility deliveries and use of skilled attendants during delivery, and ultimately to reduce rate of drop out from maternity care [31, 54].

This study cannot claim to have established a cause-effect relationship between the explanatory and outcome variables of the study due to the cross-sectional nature of the data analysed. The study however buttress existing observation that both individual-level and community-level characteristics have important implications for the use of maternal healthcare services among women. Likewise, the socio-ecological theory could not be applied in its original form because the data analysed did not provide sufficient information required to capture all its theoretical constructs. It is not impossible that a different pattern of relationship between the variables may be observed if all the theoretical constructs are derivable. Future studies on the subject matter may therefore consider the use of primary data to enhance availability of all needed information.

Conclusions

This study provided additional empirical evidence that utilisation of maternal healthcare services particularly skilled delivery service is influenced by individual-level characteristics such as maternal education, parity, religion, and healthcare decision, and community-level characteristics such as community poverty level, and community literacy level. The study provided evidence that to a significant extent, individual-level and community-level characteristics are associated with assistance during delivery in rural Nigeria. Initiatives seeking to reduce

rural-urban inequity in skilled delivery should endeavour to identify and address the important factors at the individual and community levels of the social environment.

Abbreviations
DHS: Demographic and Health Survey; FMoH: Federal Ministry of Health; MSS: Midwives Service Scheme; NDHS: Nigeria Demographic and Health Survey; PRB: Population Reference Bureau; WHO: World Health Organization

Acknowledgements
The author expresses gratitude to the National Population Commission (NPC) [Nigeria], ICF International and MEASURE DHS Project for granting prompt authorisation to analyse the data.

Authors contribution
BLS developed the concept, carried out the statistical analyses, and interpreted the results. RAY reviewed literature. Both authors discussed the results, and read through the manuscript for intellectual content. Both authors read and approved the final manuscript.

Author information
BLS has a PhD in Demography and Social Statistics from Obafemi Awolowo University, Ile-Ife, Nigeria. His research interests are fertility, contraception, and women's health issues. He is a Senior Lecturer. RAY is a postgraduate student in the Department.

Competing interests
The authors declares that they have no competing interests.

References
1. Population Reference Bureau. 2017 World Population Data Sheet with a special focus on Youth. https://assets.prb.org/pdf17/2017_World_Population.pdf. Accessed 27 May 2018.
2. Federal Ministry of Health. Saving newborn lives in Nigeria: Newborn health in the context of the Integrated Maternal, Newborn and Child Health Strategy. 2nd ed. Abuja: Federal Ministry of Health, Save the Children, Jhpiego; 2011.
3. Mafimisebi TE, Oguntade AE. Health Infrastructure Inequality and Rural-Urban Utilization of Orthodox and Traditional Medicines in Farming Households: A Case Study of Ekiti State, Nigeria. 2011. https://doi.org/10.5772/19798. Accessed 20 July 2017.
4. Adewuyi EO, Zhao Y, Auta A, Lamichhane R. Prevalence and factors associated with non-utilization of healthcare facility for childbirth in rural and urban Nigeria: analysis of a national population-based survey. Scand J Public Health. 2017:1–8. https://doi.org/10.1177/1403494817705562.
5. Limwattananon S, Tangcharoensathien V, Sirilak S. Trends and inequities in where women delivered their babies in 25 low-income countries: evidence from demographic and health surveys. Reprod Health Matters. 2011;19(37): 75–85. https://doi.org/10.1016/S0968-8080(11)37564-7.

6. Bobo FT, Yesuf EA, Woldie M. Inequities in utilization of reproductive and maternal health services in Ethiopia. Int J Equity Health. 2017;16:105. https://doi.org/10.1186/s12939-017-0602-2.

7. Crowe S, Utley M, Costello A, Pagel C. How many births in sub-Saharan Africa and South Asia will not be attended by a skilled birth attendant between 2011 and 2015? BMC Pregnancy Childbirth. 2012;12(4). https://doi.org/10.1186/1471-2393-12-4.

8. National Population Commission (NPC) [Nigeria] & ICF International. Nigeria Demographic and Health Survey. Abuja, Nigeria, and Rockville, Maryland. USA: NPC and ICF International; 2008. p. 2009.

9. National Population Commission (NPC) [Nigeria] & ICF International. Nigeria Demographic and Health Survey. Abuja, Nigeria, and Rockville, Maryland. USA: NPC and ICF International; 2013. p. 2014.

10. Nkwo PO, Lawani LO, Ezugwu EC, Iyoke CA, Ubesie AC, Onoh RC. Correlates of poor perinatal outcomes in non-hospital births in the context of weak health system: the Nigerian experience. BMC Pregnancy Childbirth. 2014;14(341). https://doi.org/10.1186/1471-2393-14-341.

11. Koblinsky M, Matthews Z, Hussein J, Mavalankar D, Mridha MK, Anwar I, et al. Going to scale with professional skilled care. Lancet. 2006;3. https://doi.org/10.1016/S0140-6736(06)69382-3.

12. Adegoke AA, van den Broek N. Skilled birth attendance-lessons learnt. BJOG. 2009;116(Suppl. 1):33–40. https://doi.org/10.1111/j.1471-0528.2009.02336.x.

13. Ebuehi OM, Campbell PC. Attraction and retention of qualified health workers to rural areas in Nigeria: a case study of four LGAs in Ogun state. Nigeria Rural Remote Health. 2011;11:1515.

14. Abimbola S, Okoli U, Olubajo O, Abdullahi MJ, Pate MA. The midwives service scheme in Nigeria. PLoS Med. 2012;9(5):e1001211. https://doi.org/10.1371/journal.pmed.1001211.

15. Ossai EN, Azuogu BN, Uwakwe KA, Anyanwagu UC, Ibiok NC, Ekeke N. Are medical students satisfied with rural community posting? A survey among final year students in medical schools of south-East Nigeria. Rural Remote Health. 2016;16:3632.

16. Rourke JWHO. Recommendations to improve retention of rural and remote health workers - important for all countries. Rural Remote Health. 2010;10:1654.

17. Guerra Arias M, Nove A, Michel-Schuldt M, de Bernis L. Current and future availability of and need for human resources for sexual, reproductive, maternal and newborn health in 41 countries in sub-Saharan Africa. Int J Equity Health. 2017;16:69. https://doi.org/10.1186/s12939-017-0569-z.

18. Adjiwanou V, LeGrand T. Gender inequality and the use of maternal healthcare services in rural sub-Saharan Africa. Health Place 2014; 29:67–78, http://dx.doi.org/https://doi.org/10.1016/j.healthplace.2014.06.001

19. Morgan R, Tetui M, Kananura RM, Ekirapa-Kiracho E, George AS. Gender dynamics affecting maternal health and health care access and use in Uganda. Health Policy Plan. 2017;32:v13–21. https://doi.org/10.1093/heapol/czx011.

20. Ahmed S, Creanga AA, Gillespie DG, Tsui AO. Economic status, education and empowerment: implications for maternal health service utilization in developing countries. PLoS One. 2010;5(6):e11190. https://doi.org/10.1371/journal.pone.0011190.

21. Obiyan MO, Kumar A. Socioeconomic inequalities in the use of maternal health Care Services in Nigeria: trends between 1990 and 2008. SAGE Open. 2015:1–11. https://doi.org/10.1177/2158244015614070.

22. Solanke BL. Association between intimate partner violence and utilisation of maternal health services in Nigeria. Afr Popul Stud. 2014;28(2 Suppl):933–45 https://doi.org/10.11564/28-0-547.

23. Ononokpono DN, Azfredrick EC. Intimate partner violence and the utilization of maternal health Care Services in Nigeria. Health Care Women Int. 2014;35:973–89. https://doi.org/10.1080/07399332.2014.924939.

24. Worku AG, Yalew AW, Afework MF. Factors affecting utilization of skilled maternal care in Northwest Ethiopia: a multilevel analysis. BMC Int Health Hum Rights. 2013;13(20). https://doi.org/10.1186/1472-698X-13-20.

25. Singh PK, Kumar C, Rai RK, Singh L. Factors associated with maternal healthcare services utilization in nine high focus states in India: a multilevel analysis based on 14385 communities in 292 districts. Health Policy Plan. 2014;29:542–59. https://doi.org/10.1093/heapol/czt039.

26. Jat TR, Ng N, San Sebastian M. Factors affecting the use of maternal health services in Madhya Pradesh state of India: a multilevel analysis. Int J Equity Health. 2011;10:59 https://doi.org/10.1186/1475-9276-10-59.

27. Yadav A, Kesarwani R. Effect of individual and community factors on maternal health care service use in India: a multilevel approach. J Biosoc Sci. 2016;48:1–19. https://doi.org/10.1017/S0021932015000048.

28. Babalola S, Fatusi A. Determinants of use of maternal health services in Nigeria – looking beyond individual and household factors. BMC Pregnancy Childbirth. 2009;9:43. https://doi.org/10.1186/1471-2393-9-43.

29. Babalola SO. Factors associated with use of maternal health services in Haiti: a multilevel analysis. Rev Panam Salud Publica. 2014;36(1):1–9.

30. Yanagisawa S, Oum S, Wakai S. Determinants of skilled birth attendance in rural Cambodia. Tropical Med Int Health. 2006;11(2):238–51. https://doi.org/10.1111/j.1365-3156.2005.01547.x.

31. Magoma M, Requejo J, Campbell OMR, Cousens S, Filippi V. High ANC coverage and low skilled attendance in a rural Tanzanian district: a case for implementing a birth plan intervention. BMC Pregnancy Childbirth. 2010;10(13). https://doi.org/10.1186/1471-2393-10-13.

32. Crissman HP, Engmann CE, Adanu RM, Nimako D, Crespo K, Moyer CA. Shifting norms: pregnant women's perspectives on skilled birth attendance and facility–based delivery in rural Ghana. Afr J Reprod Health. 2013;17(1):15–26.

33. Adamu YM, Salihu HM. Barriers to the use of antenatal and obstetric care services in rural Kano, Nigeria. J Obstet Gynaecol. 2002;22(6):600–3. https://doi.org/10.1080/0144361021000020349.

34. Adjiwanou V, LeGrand T. Does antenatal care matter in the use of skilled birth attendance in rural Africa: a multi-country analysis. Soc Sci Med. 2013;86:26–34 https://doi.org/10.1016/j.socscimed.2013.02.047.

35. Vidler M, Ramadurg U, Charantimath U, Katageri G, Karadiguddi C, Sawchuck D, et al. Utilization of maternal health care services and their determinants in Karnataka state. India Reproductive Health. 2016;13(Suppl 1):37. https://doi.org/10.1186/s12978-016-0138-8.

36. Sakeah E, Doctor HV, McCloskey L, Bernstein J, Yeboah-Antwi K, Mills S. Using the community-based health planning and services program to promote skilled delivery in rural Ghana: socio-demographic factors that influence women utilization of skilled attendants at birth in northern Ghana. BMC Public Health. 2014;14:344. https://doi.org/10.1186/1471-2458-14-344.

37. Ejembi CL, Alti-Muazu M, Chirdan O, Ezeh HO, Sheidu S, Dahiru T. Utilisation of maternal health services by rural Hausa women in Zaria environs, northern Nigeria: has primary health care made a difference? J Comm Med Prim Health Care. 2004;16(2):47–54.

38. Osubor KM, Fatusi AO, Chiwuzie JC. Maternal health-seeking behavior and associated factors in a rural Nigerian community. Matern Child Health J. 2006;10(2):159–69. https://doi.org/10.1007/s10995-005-0037-z.

39. Ebuehi OM, Akintujoye IA. Perception and utilization of traditional birth attendants by pregnant women attending primary health care clinics in a rural local government area in Ogun state, Nigeria. Int J Womens Health 2012; 4:25–34. https://doi.org/10.2147/IJWH.S23173

40. Emelumadu OF, Ukegbu AU, Ezeama NN, Kanu OO, Ifeadike CO, Onyeonoro UU. Socio-demographic determinants of maternal health-care service utilization among rural women in Anambra state, south East Nigeria. Ann Med Health Sci Res. 2014;4:374–82. https://doi.org/10.4103/2141-9248.133463.

41. Oguntunde O, Aina O, Ibrahim MS, Umar HS, Antenatal Care PP. Skilled birth attendance in three communities in Kaduna state. Nigeria Afr J Reprod Health. 2010;14(3):89–96.

42. Ononokpono DN, Odimegwu CO, Imasiku E, Adedini S. Contextual determinants of maternal health care service utilization in Nigeria. Women Health. 2013;53(7):647–68. https://doi.org/10.1080/03630242.2013.826319.

43. Aremu O, Lawoko S, Dalal K. Neighborhood socioeconomic disadvantage, individual wealth status and patterns of delivery care utilization in Nigeria: a multilevel discrete choice analysis. Int J Womens Health. 2011; 3:167–174. https://doi.org/10.2147/IJWH.S21783

44. Ononokpono DN, Odimegwu CO. Determinants of maternal health care utilization in Nigeria: a multilevel approach. Pan Afr Med J. 2014;17(Supp 1):2. https://doi.org/10.11694/pamj.supp.2014.17.1.3596.

45. Lippman SA, Leslie HH, Neilands TB, Twine R, Grignon JS, MacPhail C, et al. Context matters: community social cohesion and health behaviors in two south African areas. HEALTH PLACE 2018; 50:98–104. https://doi.org/10.1016/j.healthplace.2017.12.009

46. Elmusharaf K, Byrne E, O'Donovan D. Strategies to increase demand for maternal health services in resource-limited settings: challenges to be addressed. BMC Public Health. 2015;15:870. https://doi.org/10.1186/s12889-015-2222-3.

47. Chikhungun LC, Madise NJ, Padmadas SS. How important are community characteristics in influencing children's nutritional status? Evidence from Malawi population-based household and community surveys. Health Place. 2014; 30:187–195. https://doi.org/10.1016/j.healthplace.2014.09.006

48. Akinyemi JO, Adedini SA, Odimegwu CO. Individual v. community-level measures of women's decision-making involvement and child survival in Nigeria. S Afr J Child Health. 2017;11(1):26–32. https://doi.org/10.7196/SAJCH.2017.v11i1.1148.

49. Ngome E, Odimegwu C. The social context of adolescent women's use of modern contraceptives in Zimbabwe: a multilevel analysis. Reprod Health. 2014;11(64). https://doi.org/10.1186/1742-4755-11-64.

50. McLeroy KR, Bibeau D, Steckler A, Glanz K. An ecological perspective on health promotion programs. Health Educ Q. 1988;15:351–77.

51. Yaya S, Bishwajit G, Uthman OA, Amouzou A. Why some women fail to give birth at health facilities: a comparative study between Ethiopia and Nigeria. PLoS One 2018; 13(5): e0196896. https://doi.org/10.1371/journal.pone.0196896

52. Adinma ED, Adinma JIB, Obionu CC, Asuzu MC. Effect of government-community healthcare co-financing on maternal and child healthcare in Nigeria. West Afr J Med. 2011;30(1):35–41.

53. Doctor HV, Findley SE, Ager A, Cometto G, Afenyadu GY, Adamu F, Green C. Using community-based research to shape the design and delivery of maternal health services in northern Nigeria. Reprod Health Matters. 2012;20(39):104–12. https://doi.org/10.1016/S0968-8080(12)39615-8.

54. Akinyemi JO, Afolabi RF, Awolude OA. Patterns and determinants of dropout from maternity care continuum in Nigeria. BMC Pregnancy Childbirth. 2016;16:282. https://doi.org/10.1186/s12884-016-1083-9.

55. Adewuyi EO, Auta A, Khanal V, Bamidele OD, Akuoko CP, Adefemi K, et al. Prevalence and factors associated with underutilization of antenatal care services in Nigeria: a comparative study of rural and urban residences based on the 2013 Nigeria demographic and health survey. PLoS One 2018;13(5): e0197324. https://doi.org/10.1371/journal.pone.0197324

56. Okonofua F, Lambo E, Okeibunor J, Agholor K. Advocacy for free maternal and child health care in Nigeria—results and outcomes. Health Policy. 2011;99:131–8. https://doi.org/10.1016/j.healthpol.2010.07.013.

57. Okoli U, Morris L, Oshin A, Pate MA, Aigbe C, Muhammad A. Conditional cash transfer schemes in Nigeria: potential gains for maternal and child health service uptake in a national pilot programme. BMC Pregnancy Childbirth. 2014;14(408). https://doi.org/10.1186/s12884-014-0408-9.

58. Onyeneho NG, Amazigo UV, Njepuome NA, Nwaorgu OC, Okeibunor JC. Perception and utilization of public health services in Southeast Nigeria: implication for health care in communities with different degrees of urbanization. Int J Equity Health. 2016;15:12. https://doi.org/10.1186/s12939-016-0294-z.

59. Odeyemi IAO. Community-based health insurance programmes and the national health insurance scheme of Nigeria: challenges to uptake and integration. Int J Equity Health. 2014;13:20. https://doi.org/10.1186/1475-9276-13-20.

60. Utz B, Siddiqui G, Adegoke A, vAN Den Broek N. Definitions and roles of a skilled birth attendant: a mapping exercise from four south-Asian countries. Acta Obstet Gynecol Scand. 2013;92:1063–9. https://doi.org/10.1111/aogs.12166.

61. Gitsels–van der Wal JT, Manniën J, Gitsels LA, Reinders HS, Verhoeven PS, Ghaly MM, et al. Prenatal screening for congenital anomalies: exploring midwives' perceptions of counselling clients with religious backgrounds. BMC Pregnancy Childbirth. 2014;14(237). https://doi.org/10.1186/1471-2393-14-237.

62. Aziato L, Odai PNA, Omenyo CN. Religious beliefs and practices in pregnancy and labour: an inductive qualitative study among post-partum women in Ghana. BMC Pregnancy Childbirth. 2016;16:138. https://doi.org/10.1186/s12884-016-0920-1.

63. Doku D, Neupane S, Doku PN. Factors associated with reproductive health care utilization among Ghanaian women. BMC Int Health and Hum Rights. 2012;12(29). https://doi.org/10.1186/1472-698X-12-29.

64. Ganle JK. Why Muslim women in northern Ghana do not use skilled maternal healthcare services at health facilities: a qualitative study. BMC Int Health and Hum Rights. 2015;15:10. https://doi.org/10.1186/s12914-015-0048-9.

65. Solanke BL, Oladosu OA, Akinlo A, Olanisebe SO. Religion as a social determinant of maternal health care service utilisation in Nigeria. Afr Popul Stud 2015; 29(2):1868–1881. https://doi.org/10.11564/29-2-761.

66. Rai RK, Singh PK, Singh L. Utilization of maternal health care services among married adolescent women: insights from the Nigeria demographic and health survey, 2008. Womens Health Issues. 2012;22(4):e407–14. https://doi.org/10.1016/j.whi.2012.05.001.

67. O'Brien RM. A caution regarding rules of thumb for variance inflation factors. Qual Quant. 2007;41:673–90. https://doi.org/10.1007/s11135-006-9018-6.

68. Akinwande O, Dikko HG, Samson A. Variance inflation factor: as a condition for the inclusion of suppressor variable(s) in regression analysis. Open J Statistics 2015; 5:754–767. https://doi.org/10.4236/ojs.2015.57075

69. StataCorp. Stata: Release 12. Statistical Software. College Station, TX: StataCorp LP; 2011.

70. Adanikin AI, Onwudiegwu U, Akintayo AA. Reshaping maternal services in Nigeria: any need for spiritual care? BMC Pregnancy Childbirth. 2014;14(196). https://doi.org/10.1186/1471-2393-14-196.

25

Perinatal outcomes in twin pregnancies complicated by maternal morbidity: evidence from the WHO Multicountry Survey on Maternal and Newborn Health

Danielly S. Santana[1], Carla Silveira[1], Maria L. Costa[1], Renato T. Souza[1], Fernanda G. Surita[1], João P. Souza[2], Syeda Batool Mazhar[3], Kapila Jayaratne[4], Zahida Qureshi[5], Maria H. Sousa[6], Joshua P. Vogel[2], José G. Cecatti[1]* and on behalf of the WHO Multi-Country Survey on Maternal and Newborn Health Research Network

Abstract

Background: Twin pregnancy was associated with significantly higher rates of adverse neonatal and perinatal outcomes, especially for the second twin. In addition, the maternal complications (potentially life-threatening conditions-PLTC, maternal near miss-MNM, and maternal mortality-MM) are directly related to twin pregnancy and independently associated with adverse perinatal outcome. The objective of the preset study is to evaluate perinatal outcomes associated with twin pregnancies, stratified by severe maternal morbidity and order of birth.

Methods: Secondary analysis of the WHO Multicountry Survey on Maternal and Newborn Health (WHOMCS), a cross-sectional study implemented in 29 countries. Data from 8568 twin deliveries were compared with 308,127 singleton deliveries. The occurrence of adverse perinatal outcomes and maternal complications were assessed. Factors independently associated with adverse perinatal outcomes were reported with adjusted PR (Prevalence Ratio) and 95%CI.

Results: The occurrence of severe maternal morbidity and maternal death was significantly higher among twin compared to singleton pregnancies in all regions. Twin deliveries were associated with higher rates of preterm delivery (37.1%), Apgar scores less than 7 at 5th minute (7.8 and 10.1% respectively for first and second twins), low birth weight (53.2% for the first and 61.1% for the second twin), stillbirth (3.6% for the first and 5.7% for the second twin), early neonatal death (3.5% for the first and 5.2% for the second twin), admission to NICU (23.6% for the first and 29.3% for the second twin) and any adverse perinatal outcomes (67% for the first twin and 72.3% for the second). Outcomes were consistently worse for the second twin across all outcomes. Poisson multiple regression analysis identified several factors independently associated with an adverse perinatal outcome, including both maternal complications and twin pregnancy.

Conclusion: Twin pregnancy is significantly associated with severe maternal morbidity and with worse perinatal outcomes, especially for the second twin.

Keywords: Twin pregnancy, Perinatal outcome, Maternal morbidity

* Correspondence: cecatti@unicamp.br
[1]Department of Obstetrics and Gynecology, University of Campinas, Alexander Fleming Street, 101, Campinas, SP 13083-891, Brazil
Full list of author information is available at the end of the article

Background

Every year more than 10 million infants die before their fifth birthday and 8 million even before their first year of life. Over 6.3 million perinatal death occurred worldwide, in the year 2000, most of them in developing countries [1]. Global efforts and strategies have been aimed at reducing these numbers, including the fourth Millennium Development Goal and the new Sustainable Development Goals, which include ending preventable deaths of newborns and children under 5 years of age in its third goal [2, 3]. However, it is important to understand the magnitude of perinatal and neonatal morbidity and mortality to address their determinants [1].

Among the obstetric conditions known to increase the risk of perinatal mortality, twin pregnancy is a well-recognized factor [4–6] Twin pregnancy results from a complex interaction of genetic and environmental determinants (maternal age, parity, family history of multiple pregnancies, habits, social conditions) occurring in approximately 2–4% of livebirths and interestingly, rates are highest in some parts of Africa where care is often poorest [7–10]. However, its incidence increased more than 70% globally in the last three decades mainly in high and middle-income countries due to the use of assisted reproductive technologies [8, 9, 11, 12]. Twin pregnancy is associated with a number of obstetric complications, some of them with serious perinatal consequences, especially for the second twin [10, 13]. The rate of perinatal mortality can be up to six times higher in twin compared to singleton pregnancies, largely due to higher rates of preterm delivery and fetal growth restriction seen in twin pregnancies [4, 5, 10]. Preterm birth and birth weight are also significant determinants of morbidity and mortality into infancy and childhood [5].

The risk of maternal mortality is approximately 2.5 times higher in twin than in singleton pregnancies [8]. Maternal death (MD) is understood as the last stage of a continuum of increasingly severe morbidity, which may occur in pregnancy and is preceded by any potentially life-threatening conditions (PLTC) and by maternal near miss (MNM) [14]. Research has been interested in the relationship of twin pregnancies and severe maternal morbidity. A secondary analysis was recently conducted using data from the WHO Global Survey on Maternal and Perinatal Health (2004–2008), where twin pregnancy was a significant, independent risk factor for maternal and perinatal morbidity and mortality compared to singleton pregnancies [6]. A more recent secondary analysis from the WHO Multicountry Survey on Maternal and Newborn Health (WHOMCS, 2010–2011) explored the association of twin pregnancy with adverse maternal outcomes using the MNM criteria, reporting a 3 times higher risk of MNM and a 4 times higher risk of MD among twin pregnancy than in singleton [15]. These analyses, however, did not explore or report on any associations with adverse perinatal outcomes.

The current study aims to asses in the WHOMCS database the prevalence of potentially life-threatening conditions, maternal near miss and maternal death between twin and singleton pregnancies by regions. Then, considering the birth order, to evaluate the prevalence of perinatal outcomes (preterm births, Apgar Score at 5th min < 7, fetal death, neonatal death, perinatal death, neonatal intensive care unit admission, adequacy of weight for gestational age) between singleton versus twin. In addition, it aims to identify sociodemographic, obstetric characteristics and the occurrence of maternal complications in singleton and twin deliveries associated with any adverse perinatal outcome.

Methods

The WHOMCS was a cross-sectional study performed to assess the maternal and perinatal morbidity and mortality in 359 institutions from 29 countries (Afghanistan, Angola, Argentina, Brazil, Cambodia, China, Democratic Republic of the Congo, Ecuador, India, Japan, Jordan, Kenya, Lebanon, Mexico, Mongolia, Nepal, Nicaragua, Niger, Nigeria, Pakistan, Palestine, Paraguay, Peru, Philippines, Qatar, Sri Lanka, Thailand, Uganda, Vietnam), from May 2010 to December 2011. This is a secondary analysis of the database from this worldwide network. Methodological details of the WHOMCS have been previously published elsewhere [16, 17].

Briefly, the survey was conducted in a network of health facilities in Latin America, Africa, Asia and the Middle East, the same that had previously participated in the WHO Global Survey on Maternal and Perinatal Health (2004–2008) [18]. Countries, provinces, and health facilities were randomly selected through a stratified multistage cluster sampling strategy. Countries in each region were selected with a probability proportional to population size. In each country, three sub-regions were also selected: the capital plus two other randomly selected provinces. In each province, seven health facilities with at least 1000 deliveries annually and full capacity for performing caesarean sections were randomly selected. Data was collected from two to four months depending on the annual number of deliveries in each institution. The coordination of the study was of World Health Organization in Geneva; each region had a regional coordinator; each country had a country coordinator; each province had province coordinator, and each facility had a local coordinator who was responsible for selecting some health professional staff to collect data.

Trained data collectors identified eligible subjects in participating facilities. Eligible participants were all women who gave birth during the data collection period in the participating facilities with their respective newborns and all women who were admitted with a severe maternal outcome (maternal death or maternal near miss) up to seven postpartum days, independently of gestational age and delivery status. Data were collected from the time of admission to death, discharge or 7 days postpartum/post-abortion (whichever came first), irrespective of gestational age and type of delivery. Adverse outcomes occurring after discharge or during a subsequent readmission were not reported.

A paper form was developed with the following variables, maternal and newborns individual data, data related to pregnancy outcomes, severe complications and their management and characteristics of each health facility. This paper form was reviewed by other researchers and pre-tested on a convenient sample of records and clinical settings; the final version was translated to the main language of each participating country. The medical records were reviewed and the data was completed in the paper form, after that, it was entered into a web-based data management system developed for this purpose; the regional data managers monitored the data flow and the quality of data using data validation and progress reports automatically generated by the system. All instructions regarding eligibility criteria, identification, sociodemographic and obstetric characteristics, maternal complications, neonatal complications, and characteristics of deliveries were standardized in a

manual of operations used for training and study operationalization. The training also included workshops at country and facility level and a pilot phase to test the complete data management process.

The study protocol was approved by the WHO Ethical Review Committee and by relevant Institutional Review Boards in participating countries and institutions. The WHOMCS was a study of anonymized data, extracted from medical records (with no contact with women) and therefore individual consent was not required.

At the end of the data collection, 316,695 deliveries were included with complete information on pregnancy outcomes [17]. For this analysis, twin deliveries were compared with singleton deliveries. To define the study groups, 1839 pregnancies with the following conditions were excluded: pregnancies resulting in abortion or ectopic pregnancy; neonate weighing less than 500 g or with no information on birthweight; less than 22 weeks of gestation; and missing data on termination of pregnancy, final mode of delivery or abortion, and total number of neonates delivered. Analyses were based on 8568 twins and 308,127 singletons (Fig. 1).

Statistical analysis

The occurrence of maternal outcomes (potentially life-threatening conditions, maternal near miss, maternal death and no complications, according to the WHO

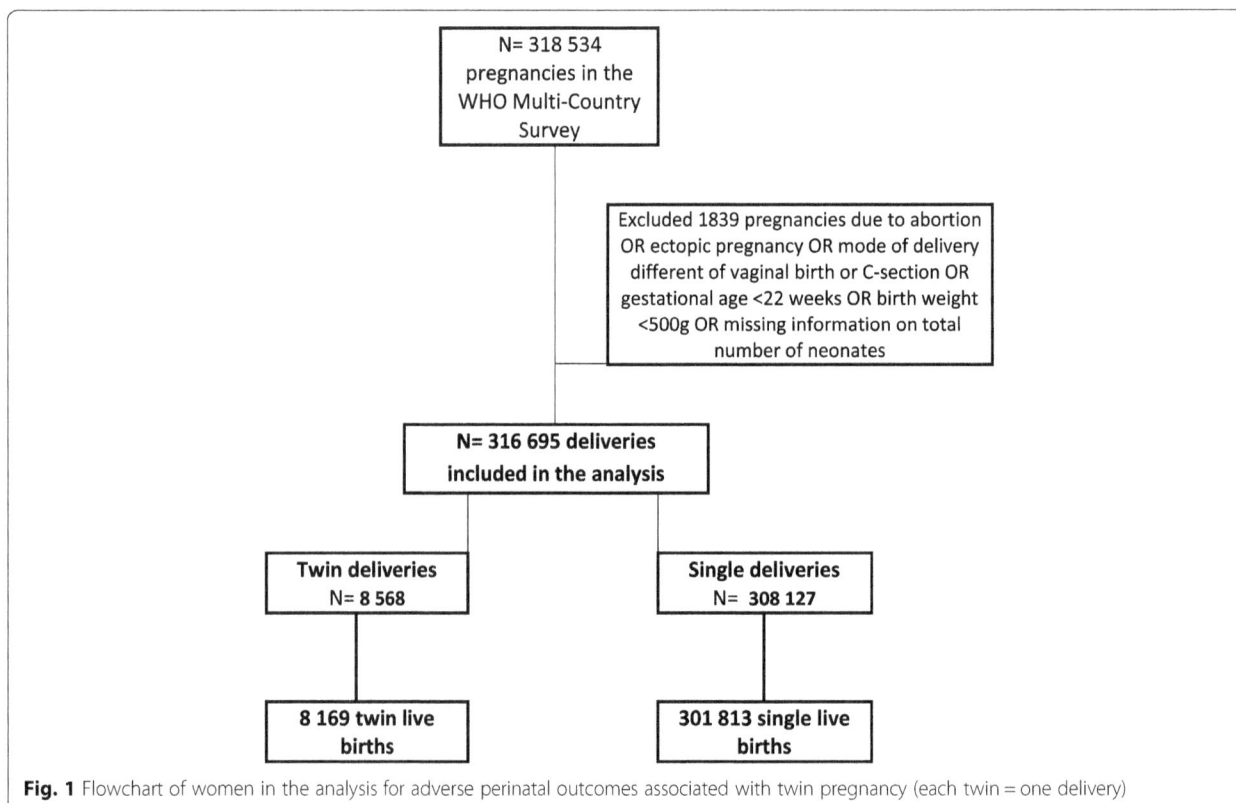

Fig. 1 Flowchart of women in the analysis for adverse perinatal outcomes associated with twin pregnancy (each twin = one delivery)

definitions and criteria [14]– Fig. 2) was assessed by continent for twin and singleton pregnancies. For this step, women were the unit of analysis. Statistical significance of differences between twins and singletons was assessed by χ^2 tests. The diagnostic criteria used to characterize women with potentially life-threatening conditions, maternal near miss and maternal death are those recommended by WHO (Fig. 2) [14, 17].

For assessing perinatal outcomes, the unit of analysis was neonates (regardless of vital status at birth). Each newborn corresponds to one delivery, so pregnancy resulting in two newborns is considered as two deliveries. We used several perinatal outcomes: Apgar score less than 7 at 5 min, fetal death (the death of a fetus from 22 completed weeks or 500 g until before birth), early neonatal death (intra-hospital neonatal death in first week of life, occurring prior to discharge), late fetal death (the death of a fetus from 28 weeks until before birth), perinatal death (early neonatal death plus fetal death), preterm birth (birth before 37 weeks gestation), neonatal intensive care unit admission (NICU), and small-for-gestational-age (defined as the weight at child-birth below the 10th percentile for the correspondent gestational age). In addition, we developed two composite outcomes– acute adverse perinatal outcome (AcAPO: Apgar score less than 7 at 5 min, or perinatal death, or neonatal intensive care unit admission) and any adverse

perinatal outcome (APO: Apgar score less than 7 at 5 min, or perinatal death, or neonatal intensive care unit admission, or small-for-gestational-age). All perinatal outcomes were separately reported for the first and the second twins, using Prevalence Ratios adjusted by the cluster design effect (PR_{adj}). Comparisons were performed in three steps to assess if they differed by birth order: first twins versus singletons; second twins versus singletons; and second versus first twins. The adequacy of weight for gestational age in the present analysis was evaluated based on Fenton growth chart [19]. The Fenton growth chart is based on the growth target recommended for preterm infants, has specific graphics for girls and boys, and the chart is designed to allow tracing how children are measured, this growth chart was chosen due to the high prevalence of preterm birth in the present study [19].

Differences in sociodemographic, obstetric characteristics and maternal complications (PLTC, MNM, and MD) among twins or singletons according to the occurrence of any adverse perinatal outcome were estimated using χ^2 test.

Finally, a Poisson multiple regression analysis was performed to identify factors independently associated with adverse perinatal outcomes. For that, a regression model was built using acute adverse perinatal outcome and any adverse perinatal outcome as the main outcomes and all

PLTC Potentially Life-Threatening Conditions			
Hemorrhagic disorders	Hypertensive disorders	Other systemic disorders	Severe management indicators
Abruptio placentae	Severe pre-eclampsia	Endometritis	Blood transfusion
Accreta/increta/percreta placenta	Eclampsia	Pulmonary oedema	Central venous access
Ectopic pregnancy	Severe Hypertension	Respiratory failure	Hysterectomy
Postpartum haemorrhage	Hypertensive encephalopathy	Seizures	ICU admission
Ruptured uterus	HELLP syndrome	Sepsis	Prolonged hospital stay (7 days)
		Shock	Non-anaesthetic intubation
		Thrombocytopenia <100.000	Return to operating room
		Thyroid crisis	Surgical intervention

MNM Maternal Near Miss		
Clinical criteria	Laboratory based criteria	Management based criteria
Acute cyanosis	Oxygen saturation <90% for ≥60 minutes	Use of continuous vasoactive drugs
Gasping		Hysterectomy following infection or
Respiratory rate >40 or <6/min	PaO_2/FiO_2 <200 mmHg	hemorrhage
Shock	Creatinine ≥ 300μmol/l or ≥ 3,5mg/dl	Transfusion of ≥5 units red cell transfusion
Oliguria non-responsive to fluids or diuretics	Bilirubin > 100μmol/l or 6,0 mg/dl	Intubation and ventilation for ≥60 minutes not related to anesthesia
Clotting failure	pH <7,1	Dialysis for acute renal failure
Loss of consciousness lasting ≥12 h	Lactate >5	Cardio-pulmonary resuscitation (CPR)
Loss of consciousness and absence of pulse/heart beat	Acute thrombocytopenia (<50.000 platelets)	
Stroke	Loss of consciousness and the presence of glucose and Ketoacids in urine	
Uncontrollable fit/total paralysis		
Jaundice in the presence of pre-eclampsia		

MD Maternal Death: Death of a woman while pregnant or within 42 days of termination of pregnancy

Fig. 2 Definitions of severe maternal complications according to the World Health Organization [14]. Portions reprinted from Say L, Souza JP, Pattinson RC; WHO working group on Maternal Mortality and Morbidity classifications. Maternal near miss—towards a standard tool for monitoring quality of maternal health care. Best Pract Res Clin Obstet Gynaecol 2009; 23:287–96, with permission from Elsevier. *HELLP* hemolysis, elevated liver enzymes, low platelet count, *ICU* intensive care unit, *CPR* cardiopulmonary resuscitation

other variables as predictors, including the information on the pregnancy being twin or singleton, and the occurrence of maternal complications. The resultant Prevalence Ratios were therefore adjusted not only for the survey design but also for all other predictors (PR_{adj}). Results were considered significant when the estimated *p*-values were below 0.05. All statistical procedures were performed using SPSS (Version 20.0) and Stata (Release 7) programs. Results were reported in accordance with the STROBE statement [20].

Results

Among the 318,534 women initially enrolled in the WHOMCS, 312,867 women and 316,695 deliveries remained after the exclusion criteria were applied, 4756 (1.5%) of them with twin pregnancies corresponding to 8568 deliveries of neonates (Fig. 1). Table 1 shows the occurrence of potentially life-threatening conditions, maternal near miss and maternal death by region comparatively between twin and singleton pregnancies. All regions showed significantly higher occurrence of maternal complications and maternal death for twin pregnancies. Rates were consistently higher for the African and Asian regions than for Latin America.

Table 2 shows that twin deliveries were associated with higher rates of preterm birth (< 37 weeks), early preterm birth (< 34 weeks), low birth weight, small for gestational age, and Apgar score less than 7. For all perinatal outcomes, rates were significantly higher for twins compared to singletons, and also for the second twin compared to the first twin (Fig. 3).

The occurrence of any adverse perinatal outcome (APO) was more frequent among twin deliveries in women between 18 and 35 years (87,1%), with lower maternal education (55,3% with 0–9 years of education), higher parity, with a partner, in preterm birth, whose delivery was through an elective C-section. The gestational age at delivery for singleton pregnancies was 37 weeks or more in about 90% of cases, while in twin pregnancies this prevalence was approximately 65%. In addition, all maternal morbid conditions were more frequent among twins than singletons and more associated with any APO (Table 3).

The factors independently identified as protective for acute or any adverse perinatal outcome were the higher gestational age at birth, vaginal delivery, parity ≥1 and maternal age (Table 4). Any maternal complications (PLTC, MNM and MD) and twin pregnancy were both identified as the main factors associated with a higher risk of APO.

Discussion

Twin pregnancy has increased risks of preterm labor, spontaneous preterm birth, premature rupture of membranes, neonatal and perinatal morbidity and mortality [5, 10, 21, 22]. The occurrence of any potentially life-threatening conditions, maternal near miss or maternal death was twice as high or more, in twin pregnancies; they had complications in 15.3% while singleton pregnancies had only in 6.8%. Results were reasonably consistent across geographical regions. These outcomes were the object of study in at least another two articles with data from World Health Organization detailing the relationship between twin pregnancy and severe maternal morbidity [6, 15]. No explanations were found to variable rates of adverse maternal outcomes in twin pregnancies in different countries with similar income, however it may relate to differences in the quality of available care and local complication patterns [6, 15].

The reported preterm birth rates among twins are very similar to that found in other studies, ranging from 31% [6, 22] to 44% [23], but some reporting up to 63% [24]. Early preterm births are less frequent than late (34–36 weeks), as Vogel et al. reported in the WHO Global Survey, with 11.9% of preterm birth below 34 completed weeks [6]. Higher early preterm rates are important, as they are associated with higher neonatal morbidity and perinatal death rates, mainly due to respiratory complications [6, 23, 25, 26].

Low birth weight is also more frequent among twin pregnancies. A previous study found that this risk was 8.3 times higher than in singletons, with a mean birth weight of 2300 g [24], higher than that observed in our study (5 times higher). This risk is associated with the increase in Apgar score at 5th minute < 7 and death during the first year of life [22–24, 27]. Adequacy of weight

Table 1 PLTC, MNM and MD for twin and singleton pregnancies by region. WHO Multicountry Survey, 2010–2011

Region	Twin pregnancies				Singleton pregnancies				*p*-value
	NC (%)	PLTC (%)	MNM (%)	MD (%)	NC (%)	PLTC (%)	MNM (%)	MD (%)	
Africa	1219 (84·2)	196 (13·5)	27 (1·9)	5 (0·3)	67,547 (93·3)	4181 (5·8)	495 (0·7)	139 (0·2)	< 0·001
Asia	2078 (85·8)	299 (12·4)	32 (1·3)	12 (0·5)	161,118 (94·2)	9129 (5·3)	686 (0·4)	131 (0·1)	< 0·001
Latin America	735 (82·8)	141 (15·9)	11 (1·2)	1 (0·1)	58,412 (90·3)	5935 (9·2)	314 (0·5)	24 (< 0·1)	< 0·001
TOTAL	4032 (84·8)	636 (13·4)	70 (1·5)	18 (0·4)	287,077 (93·2)	19,245 (6·2)	1495 (0·5)	294 (0·1)	< 0·001

MD maternal death, *MNM* maternal near miss, *NC* No complication, *PLTC* potentially life-threatening condition
P value referring to the comparison between no complication/any complication in twin vs singleton

Table 2 Perinatal outcomes in twin and singleton deliveries (unity of analysis are neonates). WHO Multicountry Survey, 2010–2011

Perinatal outcomes	Twin deliveries n (%)		Singleton deliveries n (%)	Total n (%)	PR$_{adj}$ (95% CI)		
Gestational age at delivery [a]							
< 34 weeks	1098 (13·0)		7337 (2·4)	8435 (2·7)	**6·77 (5·99–7·66)**		
34–36 weeks	2035 (24·1)		14,791 (4·9)	16,826 (5·4)	**5·57 (5·03–6·17)**		
≥ 37 weeks	5312 (62·9)		282,801 (92·7)	288,113 (91·9)	Ref.		
Birth weight [b]	**1st twin**	**2nd twin**			**1st vs Single**	**2nd vs Single**	**2nd vs 1st**
< 2500 g	2495 (53·2)	2299 (61·1)	32,480 (10·6)	37,274 (11·8)	**5·03 (4·59–5·52)**	**5·78 (5·41–6·17)**	**1·15 (1·06–1·24)**
≥ 2500 g	2193 (46·8)	1464 (38·9)	274,665 (89·4)	278,322 (88·2)	Ref.	Ref.	Ref.
Adequacy of weight for GA [c]							
SGA	2385 (51·7)	2043 (55·2)	77,855 (25·7)	82,283 (26·4)	**2·01 (1·88–2·15)**	**2·15 (2·03–2·28)**	**1·07 (1·01–1·13)**
No SGA	2232 (48·3)	1658 (44·8)	225,285 (74·3)	229,175 (73·6)	Ref.	Ref.	Ref.
Apgar Score at 5th min [d]							
< 7	352 (7·8)	364 (10·1)	7928 (2·6)	8644 (2·8)	**2·97 (2·49–3·54)**	**3·85 (3·20–4·63)**	**1·29 (1·12–1·50)**
7–10	4142 (92·2)	3227 (89·9)	292,805 (97·4)	300,174 (97·2)	Ref.	Ref.	Ref.
Fetal and neonatal outcomes							
Fetal death [e]	169 (3·6)	215 (5·7)	6151 (2·0)	6535 (2·1)	**1·79 (1·52–2·11)**	**2·83 (2·48–3·23)**	**1·58 (1·35–1·86)**
Early neonatal death [f]	160 (3·5)	189 (5·2)	2636 (0·9)	2985 (1·0)	**4·03 (3·29–4·94)**	**5·99 (4·93–7·29)**	**1·49 (1·26–1·76)**
Late fetal death [g]	130 (2·7)	165 (4·3)	5241 (1·7)	5536 (1·7)	**1·62 (1·35–1·94)**	**2·55 (2·21–2·94)**	**1·58 (1·30–1·92)**
Perinatal death [h]	328 (7·0)	381 (10·0)	8706 (2·8)	9415 (3·0)	**2·46 (2·21–2·73)**	**3·55 (3·21–3·90)**	**1·44 (1·14–1·32)**
Preterm births [a]	1634 (35·0)	1492 (39·8)	22,128 (7·3)	25,254 (8·1)	**4·82 (4·36–5·33)**	**5·48 (5·05–5·94)**	**1·14 (1·05–1·23)**
NICU admission [i]	1073 (23·6)	1059 (29·3)	19,468 (6·4)	21,600 (7·0)	**3·65 (3·23–4·14)**	**4·54 (4·14–4·99)**	**1·24 (1·12–1·38)**
Acute Adverse Perinatal Outcome (AcAPO) [j]	1395 (29·9)	1390 (36·8)	30,006 (9·8)	32,791 (10·4)	**3·06 (2·77–3·38)**	**3·76 (3·47–4·08)**	**1·23 (1·11–1·32)**
Any Adverse Perinatal Outcome (APO) [k]	3101 (67·0)	2709 (72·3)	98,128 (32·4)	103,938 (33·3)	**2·07 (1·96–2·19)**	**2·24 (2·14–2·34)**	**1·08 (1·03–1·13)**
Total	**4733**	**3811[l]**	**308,127**	**316,671**			

Chi-square test adjusted for the cluster design effect
Missing information for a: 3320; b: 1075; c: 5213; d: 7853; e: 178; f: 6761; g: 159; h: 375; i: 6638; j: 1508; k: 4712 neonates
Values in bold mean they are statistically significant ($p < 0.05$)
AcAPO Acute Adverse Perinatal Outcome (Apgar score at 5th min < 7 OR Perinatal death OR NICU admission)
APO any Adverse Perinatal Outcome (Apgar score at 5th min < 7 OR Perinatal death OR NICU admission OR SGA)
[l]There is no available information for the second or higher twin for the countries Paraguay, Peru, Philippines, Qatar, Thailand, Vietnam and Uganda

for gestational age better assesses the size of the fetus for a given gestational age (compared to birth weight alone). This is particularly useful in populations where preterm birth rates are high. A fetus that is small for gestational age is more likely to experience perinatal morbidity and mortality and adverse effects in adult life [28]. Few studies have evaluated this outcome among twin deliveries, but associations between twin pregnancies and higher rates of small-for-gestational-age have been reported [28, 29]. For these estimations, we used the curves of Fenton et al. [19] because we believed that it was more appropriate to be used when the prevalence of preterm birth is very high, as is the case among twin pregnancies in this population. However, due to the number of cases to have such estimates, it was not feasible to have such assessment performed using different nomograms for comparison.

The risk for low 5th minute Apgar score was three times higher for twin pregnancy (either for the first or second twin) than for singletons. Additionally, it was 1.3 times higher for the second when both twins were compared. This significantly lower Apgar score for the second twin is always taken into consideration in discussions about the best mode of delivery for twin pregnancies and the time interval between first and second twin, although not justifying an indication for a systematic Cesarean section for twin pregnancies [6, 30–32]. The higher rates of admission to a neonatal intensive care unit we found have also been reported by previous studies on the topic [6, 31].

Prevalence of fetal death of one of the twins varies from 0,5-6,8% with the worst result for monochorionic pregnancy presenting a high prevalence for this condition (50–70%) and risk for the surviving fetus including

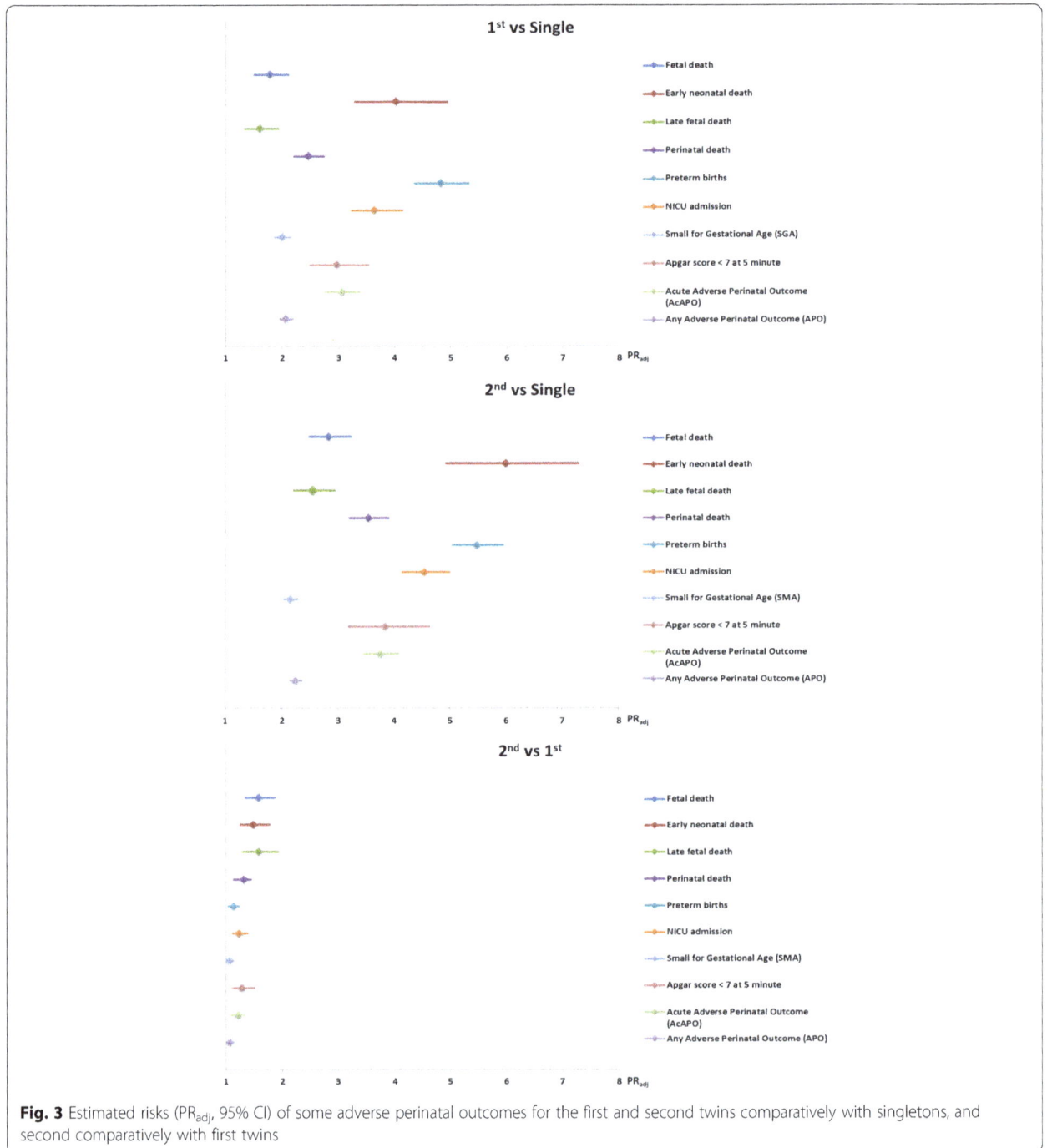

Fig. 3 Estimated risks (PR_adj, 95% CI) of some adverse perinatal outcomes for the first and second twins comparatively with singletons, and second comparatively with first twins

the fetal death of this co-twin, neurological morbidity and iatrogenic preterm delivery [33, 34]. In the current study, we have not data on chorionicity, however fetal death (death after 28 weeks) occurred over 1.5 times (3.6%) for the first twin and almost 3 times (5.7%) for the second twin when compared to singletons (2.0%).

Perinatal death has been described as up to four times higher in twin pregnancies than in singletons, mainly due to preterm birth, fetal growth restriction, low Apgar scores and extremely low birth weight [5, 6, 23, 25]. In our study, it was found to be 2.5 times higher for the first twin and 3.5 for the second one. This difference between both twins has already been described [31]. In the current study, we also observed a higher risk for fetal and early neonatal death, supporting previous findings from other studies [6, 31].

Cesarean section, including that performed electively, was the most common mode of delivery in twin

Table 3 Sociodemographic and obstetric conditions among twin and single deliveries according to the occurrence of any Adverse Perinatal Outcome (APO). WHO Multicountry Survey, 2010–2011

Perinatal outcomes	Twin deliveries n (%)		Singleton deliveries n (%)		Total	p-value*
	APO	No APO	APO	No APO		
Maternal age[a]						< 0.001
< 18	49 (1.6)	22 (1.4)	3987 (4.1)	6971 (3.4)	11,029	
18–35	2693 (87.1)	1296 (85.0)	86,375 (88.3)	179,196 (87.6)	269,560	
> 35	349 (11.3)	206 (13.5)	7510 (7.7)	18,420 (9.0)	26,485	
Maternal education (years)[b]						< 0.001
0–4	694 (24.6)	259 (18.1)	21,295 (23.4)	34,647 (18.3)	56,895	
5–9	865 (30.7)	414 (28.9)	29,664 (32.6)	57,190 (30.3)	88,133	
> 10	1263 (44.8)	758 (53.0)	40,025 (44.0)	97,219 (51.4)	139,265	
Parity[c]						< 0.001
0	1121 (36.3)	401 (26.3)	47,293 (48.3)	81,773 (39.9)	130,588	
1–2	1306 (42.3)	793 (52.1)	37,017 (37.8)	88,631 (43.3)	127,747	
> 2	661 (21.4)	329 (21.6)	13,681 (14.0)	34,487 (16.8)	49,158	
Marital status[d]						0.013
With no partner	251 (8.2)	91 (6.0)	10,898 (11.2)	19,766 (9.7)	31,006	
With partner	2825 (91.8)	1422 (94.0)	86,434 (88.8)	183,915 (90.3)	274,596	
Gestational age at delivery[e]						< 0.001
< 34 weeks	488 (15.8)	74 (4.8)	5966 (6.1)	1329 (0.6)	7857	
34–36 weeks	619 (20.1)	435 (28.5)	5850 (6.0)	8838 (4.3)	15,742	
≥ 37 weeks	1972 (64.0)	1017 (66.6)	86,010 (87.9)	195,007 (95.0)	284,006	
Onset of labour[f]						< 0.001
Spontaneous	3902 (67.2)	1611 (62.9)	74,825 (76.4)	159,268 (77.7)	239,606	
Induced	455 (7.8)	162 (6.3)	11,572 (11.8)	20,638 (10.1)	32,827	
Elective C-section	1446 (24.9)	787 (30.7)	11,561 (11.8)	25,054 (12.2)	38,848	
Mode of delivery[g]						< 0.001
Vaginal birth	1575 (50.8)	691 (45.3)	70,422 (71.8)	146,340 (71.3)	219,028	
Cesarean section	1525 (49.2)	835 (54.7)	27,701 (28.2)	58,834 (28.7)	88,895	
Maternal complications[h]						< 0.001
No complications	2606 (84.1)	1312 (86.0)	88,416 (90.1)	194,250 (94.7)	286,584	
PLTC	425 (13.7)	200 (13.1)	8567 (8.7)	10,365 (5.1)	19,557	
MNM	53 (1.7)	13 (0.9)	921 (0.9)	507 (0.2)	1494	
MD	16 (0.5)	1 (0.1)	221 (0.2)	52 (0.0)	290	
Total	5810	2562	98,128	205,178	311,678	
	8372		303,306			

*design-based p-value
Missing information for: a: 9597; b: 32378; c: 9178; d: 11069; e: 9066; f: 5390; g: 8748; and h: 8746 cases
APO any Adverse Perinatal Outcome (Apgar score at 5th min < 7 OR Perinatal death OR NICU admission OR SGA)
MD maternal death, MNM maternal near miss, PLTC potentially life-threatening condition

pregnancy in the present study. The debate on the best mode of delivery is extensive, especially considering higher adverse outcomes for the second twin, and that neither labor nor vaginal delivery is associated with worse perinatal outcomes, since the first twin is in cephalic presentation. There is currently no indication for a policy of planned cesarean delivery, although still some controversies frequently arise among professionals [11, 12, 30, 35, 36].

In the current analysis higher rates of maternal complications are directly related to twin pregnancy (15.9% in twins with APO, 14.1% in twins with no APO and 9.8% in singletons with APO and 5.3% in singletons with no APO). This reinforces some recent studies identifying

Table 4 Factors independently associated with Acute Adverse Perinatal Outcome (AcAPO) and with any Adverse Perinatal Outcome (APO) by Poisson multiple regression analysis. WHO Multicountry Survey, 2010–2011

Model/ Variables	PR_{adj}	95% CI	p
AcAPO [n = 283,549]			
Gestational age at delivery (weeks)	0.81	0.80–0.82	< 0.001
Maternal complications (PLTC, MNM, MD)	1.88	1.76–2.02	< 0.001
Group (Twin)	1.50	1.40–1.61	< 0.001
Mode of delivery (Vaginal)	0.64	0.58–0.70	< 0.001
Parity (≥1)	0.86	0.81–0.91	< 0.001
Marital status (With no partner)	1.43	1.12–1.83	0.004
Maternal education (Up to nine years)	1.18	1.04–1.33	0.011
Maternal age (years)	1.006	1.001–1.011	0.014
APO [n = 283,393]			
Group (Twin)	1.87	1.78–1.97	< 0.001
Maternal complications (PLTC, SMM, MD)	1.39	1.32–1.46	< 0.001
Parity (≥1)	0.82	0.80–0.85	< 0.001
Gestational age at delivery (weeks)	0.96	0.95–0.97	< 0.001
Maternal education (Up to nine years)	1.23	1.15–1.32	< 0.001
Maternal age (years)	0.99	0.986–0.994	< 0.001

AcAPO Acute Adverse Perinatal Outcome (Apgar score at 5th min < 7 OR Perinatal death OR NICU admission)
APO any Adverse Perinatal Outcome (Apgar score at 5th min < 7 OR Perinatal death OR NICU admission OR SGA)
PR_{adj} = prevalence ratio adjusted for cluster effect; 95% CI: 95% confidence interval for prevalence ratio
Poisson multiple regression analysis, controlled by: Group (Single:0; Twin: 1); Age (years); Maternal education (Up to nine years: 1; > 10 years: 0); Parity (0/≥1: 1); Marital status (With no partner: 1/With partner: 0); Gestational age at delivery (weeks); Onset of labor (Spontaneous: 0; Other: 1); Mode of delivery (Vaginal: 1; C-section: 0); Maternal complications (No complication: 0/PLTC, MNM, MD: 1)

twin pregnancy as a risk factor for the occurrence of severe maternal morbidity. In a WHO Global Survey analysis, Vogel et al. reported a 1.85 higher risk of occurrence of a severe maternal outcome (maternal death, admission to an intensive care unit, blood transfusion or hysterectomy) between twin pregnancies compared to singletons [6]. Using the new WHO diagnostic criteria for severe maternal conditions, another recent study from our group using the same database identified that twin pregnancies increased twofold the risk of occurrence of PLTC, threefold the risk of MNM and fourfold of occurrence of MD compared with singleton pregnancies [15]. These differences reinforce that twin pregnancy is associated with worse outcomes for both newborns and women. Whether this justifies the need for a more specialized care for women with a twin pregnancy, not only aiming at a good perinatal outcome but also for the maternal outcome, is not completely understood and deserves more specific studies [5, 6, 12, 15, 37].

In the multivariate analysis, both twin pregnancy and maternal complications (PLTC, MNM and MD) still appear as factors independently associated with acute or any adverse perinatal outcome. As already argued, a twin pregnancy is associated with a number of perinatal complications either acute or chronic. However, the relationship between adverse perinatal outcomes and severe maternal conditions reinforces that when the woman

develops an adverse condition, the fetus suffers direct consequences (growth restriction and stillbirth) or indirectly by the need of interrupting pregnancy before term, with all the consequences of being preterm. In view of these results and knowing that twin pregnancy is not a modified condition but maternal complications are preventable conditions through improvement of the quality of obstetric care theattention to the pregnant woman is able to modify the perinatal outcomes associated with a twin pregnancy.

There were a few limitations to our study. We had no data on the chorionicity and pregnancies archived by ART/FIV for twin pregnancies – what could be associated with perinatal outcomes. In addition, there is no information at all on ethnicity and BMI of the women, what could also be associated with both twin pregnancy and perinatal outcomes. This was a big international multicenter study that for collecting information on all deliveries during a period of time should use a very short questionnaire to facilitate data collection. Considering twin pregnancy was not the main objective of the study, these variables were not included. Despite all quality control procedures some inconsistency could occur unnoticed from data collected from each individual women with a paper form until the feeding of the electronic database, either by the reviewer or by the system. The reported patterns probably relate more to Low- and

Middle-Income Countries settings as a result of the included countries, and therefore the generalization of results for High-Income countries may be limited. In addition, this WHOMCS was mainly performed in secondary and tertiary facilities functioning as referral hospitals with a probable over-representation of maternal complications and maternal/perinatal deaths and considering that the results are based on the facility, countries with low health-facility coverage will be underrepresented, in those facilities the results will probably be lower mainly to severe maternal morbidity. These data might not be representative of maternal outcomes and coverage of essential interventions in smaller facilities or in the community, with variations among countries. In addition, the data collection included only women and newborns up to seven days postpartum or abortion with that cases progressed to maternal and neonatal complications beyond this period may be lost.

On the other hand, we could also highlight some strengths of the current study. The WHOMCS is a large, multi-country database and based on information collected in a standardized way; outcome data on more than 8000 twins were captured, and results obtained identify worse perinatal outcomes for twins, especially for the second and the association between severe maternal morbidity and twin pregnancy. These findings allow the understanding that twin pregnancy is not only associated with obstetric complications but also maternal death. In the clinical practice, these results could assist in the implementation of protocols for identification of risk conditions and maternal and perinatal care.

Conclusion

In this analysis, twin pregnancy was associated with significantly higher rates of adverse neonatal and perinatal outcomes. Our results confirm previous observations of increased perinatal mortality and morbidity; outcomes for the second twin were generally poorer than for the first twin. Despite the limitations discussed above, for being a multicenter study, ours finding confirm the necessary identification of higher risk cases and referral to high complexity facilities with capacity for quality prenatal care and intensive care for newborns. Further studies on the topic would be welcome in the future, especially to assess whether specialized obstetric and neonatal care is able to reduce the occurrence of some complications, thus improving maternal and perinatal outcomes.

Abbreviations

AcAPO: Acute adverse perinatal outcome; APO: Any adverse perinatal outcome; MD: Maternal death; MM: Maternal mortality; MNM: Maternal near miss; NICU: Neonatal intensive care unit; PLTC: Potentially life-threatening conditions; PR: Prevalence Ratio; WHO: World Health Organization

Acknowledgements

We thank all members of the WHO Multi-Country Survey on Maternal and Newborn Health Research Network, including regional and country coordinators, facility coordinators, data collectors, and all staff of the participating facilities who made the survey possible. This manuscript represents the views of the named authors only, and not the position of their institutions or organizations.

Funding

Study supported by the UNDP/UNFPA/UNICEF/WHO/World Bank Special Programme of Research, Development and Research Training in Human Reproduction (HRP), World Health Organization (WHO), United States Agency for International Development (USAID), the Ministry of Health, Labour and Welfare of Japan, and Gynuity Health Projects. Specifically for this analysis, a sponsorship from the University of Campinas was provided (Faepex, grant 11014). Funding agencies played no other role nor influenced data analysis, interpretation of results and writing the manuscript.

Author's contributions

Conceived and designed the experiments: DSS, JGC, FGS, CS, MLC, JPS. Performed the experiments: JGC, CS, MLC, JPS, SBM, KJ, ZQ, JPV. Analyzed the data: DSS, JGC, MHS, RTS. Contributed reagents/materials/analysis tools: DSS, JGC, FGS, CS, MLC, JPS, SBM, KJ, ZQ, JPV, RTS. Wrote the paper: DSS, JGC, FGS, MLC. Final review of manuscript and agreement: all the authors.

Competing interests

Prof. Fernanda G Surita is an Associate Editor of BMC Pregnancy and Childbirth. The authors declare that they have no competing interests.

Author details

[1]Department of Obstetrics and Gynecology, University of Campinas, Alexander Fleming Street, 101, Campinas, SP 13083-891, Brazil. [2]UNDP/UNFPA/UNICEF/WHO/World Bank Special Programme of Research, Development and Research Training in Human Reproduction (HRP), Department of Reproductive Health and Research, World Health Organization, Geneva, Switzerland. [3]Pakistan Institute of Medical Sciences, Islamabad, Pakistan. [4]Maternal & Child Morbidity & Mortality Surveillance Unit, Family Health Bureau, Ministry of Health, Colombo, Sri Lanka. [5]Department of Obstetrics and Gynecology, University of Nairobi, Nairobi, Kenya. [6]Department of Public Health, Jundiai Medical School, Jundiai, Brazil.

References

1. World Health Organization. Neonatal and perinatal mortality: country, regional and global estimates. 2006. http://apps.who.int/iris/bitstream/10665/43444/1/9241563206_eng.pdf . Access on 2nd Apr. 2016.
2. United Nations. The Millennium Development Goals Report 2015. http://www.un.org/millenniumgoals/2015_MDG_Report/pdf/MDG%202015%20rev%20(July%201).pdf . Access on 2nd Apr. 2016.
3. United Nations. Sustain Dev Goals: 17 goals to transform our world. 2015. http://www.un.org/sustainabledevelopment/health. Access on 2nd Apr. 2016.

4. Rao A, Sairam S, Shehata H. Obstetric complications of twin pregnancies. Best Pract Res Clin Obstet Gynaecol. 2004;18(4):557–76.

5. Rizwan N, Abbasi RM, Mughal R. Maternal morbidity and perinatal outcome with twin pregnancy. J Ayub Med Coll Abbottabad. 2010;22(2):105–7.

6. Vogel JP, Torloni MR, Seuc A, Betrán AP, Widmer M, Souza JP, et al. Maternal and perinatal outcomes of twin pregnancy in 23 low- and middle-income countries. PLoS One. 2013;8(8):e70549.

7. Smits J, Monden C. Twinning accros the developing world. PLoS One. 2011; 6(9):e25239.

8. National Institute for Health and Clinical Excellence. Multiple prenancy. The management of twin and triplet pregnancies in the antenatal period. NICE clinical Guideline. 2011. http://guidance.nice.org.uk/cg129 . Accessed 2 Apr 2016.

9. Bortolus R, Parazzini F, Chatenoud L, Benzi G, Bianchi MM, Marini A. The epidemiology of multiple births. Human Reprod Update. 1999;5(2):179–87.

10. Ananth CV, Chauhan SP. Epidemiology of twinning in developed countries. Semin Perinatol. 2012;36(3):156–61.

11. Young BC, Wylie BJ. Effects of twin gestation on maternal morbidity. Semin Perinatol. 2012;36(3):162–8.

12. Walker MC, Murphy KE, Pan S, Yang Q, Wen SW. Adverse maternal outcomes in multifetal pregnancies. BJOG. 2004;111:1294–6.

13. Smith GCS, Fleming KM, White IR. Birth order of twins and risk of perinatal death related to delivery in England, Northern Ireland, and Wales, 1994-2003: retrospective cohort study. BMJ. 2007;334(7593):576.

14. Say L, Souza JP, Pattinson RC. WHO working group on maternal mortality and morbidity classifications. Maternal near miss – towards a standard tool for monitoring quality of maternal health care. Best Pract Res Clin Obstet Gynaecol. 2009;23(3):287–96.

15. Santana DS, Cecatti JG, Surita FG, Silveira C, Costa ML, Souza JP, et al. Twin pregnancy and severe maternal outcomes. The World Health Organization Multicountry Survey on Maternal and Newborn Health. Obst Gynecol. 2016; 127(4):631–41.

16. Souza JP, Gülmezoglu AM, Carroli G, Lumbiganon P, Qureshi Z. WHOMCS research group. The World Health Organization multicountry survey on maternal and newborn health: study protocol. BMC Health Serv Res. 2011;11:286.

17. Souza JP, Gülmezoglu AM, Vogel J, Carroli G, Lumbiganon P, Qureshi Z, et al. Moving beyond essential interventions for reduction of maternal mortality (the WHO multicountry survey on maternal and newborn health): a cross-sectional study. Lancet. 2013;381(9879):1747–55.

18. Shah A, Faundes A, Machoki M, Bataglia V, Amokrane F, Donner A, et al. Methodological considerations in implementing the WHO global survey for monitoring maternal and perinatal health. Bull World Health Organ. 2008; 86(2):126–31.

19. Fenton TR, Kim JH. A systematic review and meta-analysis to revise the Fenton growth chart for preterm infants. BMC Pediatr. 2013;13:59.

20. Von Elm E, Altman DG, Egger M, Pocock SJ, Gøtzsche PC, Vandenbroucke JP, Initiative STROBE. The strengthening the reporting of observational studies in epidemiology (STROBE) statement: guidelines for reporting observational studies. Lancet. 2007;370(9596):1453–7.

21. Bangal VB, Patel SM, Khairmar DN. Study of maternal and fetal outcomes in twin gestation at tertiary care teaching hospital. Int J Biomed Advance Res. 2012;3(10):758–62.

22. Qazi G. Obstetric and perinatal outcome of multiple pregnancy. J Coll Physicians Surg Pak. 2011;21(3):142–5.

23. Nwankwo TO, Aniebue UU, Ezenkwele E, Nwafor MI. Pregnancy outcome and factors affecting vaginal delivery of twin at University of Nigeria Teaching Hospital, Enugu. Niger J Clin Pract. 2013;16(4):490–5.

24. Assunção RA, Liao AW, Brizot ML, Krebs VL, Zugaib M. Perinatal outcome of twin pregnancies delivered in a teaching hospital. Rev Assoc Med Bras. 2010;56(4):447–51.

25. Werder E, Mendola P, Männistö, O'Loughlin J, Laughon SK. Effect of maternal chronic disease on obstetric complications in twin pregnancies in a United States cohort. Fertil Steril 2013; 100(1): 142–149.

26. Tunçalp O, Souza JP, Hindin MJ, Santos CA, Oliveira TH, Vogel JP, et al. On behalf of the WHO multicountry survey on maternal and newborn Health Research network. Education and severe maternal outcomes in developing countries: a multicountry cross-sectional study. BJOG. 2014;121(Suppl. 1):57–65.

27. Fonseca CR, Strufaldi MW, Carvalho LR, Puccini RF. Risk factors for low birth weight in Botucatu city, SP state, Brazil: a study conducted in the public health system from 2004 to 2008. BMC Res Notes. 2012;5:60.

28. Wen SW, Tan H, Yang O, Walker M. Prediction of small for gestational age by logistic regression in twins. Aust N Z J Obstet Gynaecol. 2005;45(5):399–404.

29. Inde Y, Satomi M, Miyake H, Suzuki S. Neonatal small for gestational age status as a favorable factor for the complete vaginal delivery of both fetuses in Japanese dichorionic twins. J Obstet Gynaecol Res. 2011;37(7):843–50.

30. Barrett JF, Hannah ME, Hutton EK, Willan AR, Allen AC, Armson BA, et al. Twin birth study collaborative group. A randomized trial of planned cesarean or vaginal delivery for twin pregnancy. N Engl J Med. 2013;369(14):1295–305.

31. Jacquemyn Y, Martens G, Ruyssinck G, Michiels I, Van Overmeire B. A matched cohort comparison of the outcome of twin versus singleton pregnancies in Flanders, Belgium. Twin Res. 2003;6(1):7–11.

32. Lindroos L, Elfvin A, Ladfors L, Wennerholm B. The effect of twin-to-twin delivery time intervals on neonatal outcome for second twins. BMC Pregnancy and Childbirth. 2018;18:36.

33. Southwest Thames Obstetric Research Collaborative. (STORK). Prospective risk of late stillbirth in monochorionic twins: a regional cohort study. Ultrasound Obstet Gynecol. 2012;39:500–4.

34. Fernandes-Vale E, Dias J, Belandina G, Cahilhe A. Single fetal death in monochorionic twin pregnancy: co-twin prgnosis and neonatal outcome. Acta Medica Port. 2017;30(2):148–51.

35. Liu AL, Yung WK, Yeung HN, Lai SF, Lam MT, Lai FK, et al. Factors influencing the mode of delivery and associated pregnancy outcomes for twins: a retrospective cohort study in a public hospital. Hong Kong Med. 2012;18(2):99–107.

36. Asztalos EV, Hannah ME, Hutton EK, Willan AR, Allen AC, Armson BA, et al. Twin birth study: 2-year neurodevelopmental follow-up of the randomized trial of planned caesarean or planned vaginal delivery for twin pregnancy. Am J Obstet Gynecol. 2016;214(3):371.e1–371.

37. Dodd JM, Dowswell T, Crowther CA. Specialised antenatal clinics for women with a multiple pregnancy for improving maternal and infant outcomes. Cochrane Database Syst Rev. 2015;11:CD005300.

26

Magnitude and factors associated with anemia among pregnant women attending antenatal care in public health centers in central zone of Tigray region, northern Ethiopia: a cross sectional study

Teklit Grum[1*], Ermyas Brhane[2], Solomon Hintsa[3] and Gizienesh Kahsay[1]

Abstract

Introduction: Anemia is defined as a low blood hemoglobin concentration (< 11 mg/dl). It is a global public health problem especially in pregnant women and is associated with higher risk for both maternal and perinatal mortality and morbidity. In developing countries, like Ethiopia where anemia is common, determining the magnitude and identifying factors that are associated with anemia is necessary to control it.

Methods: Facility based cross sectional study design were conducted among 638 pregnant women attending antenatal care in public health centers in central zone of Tigray region, Northern Ethiopia from November 1/2017 to January 30/2018 using stratified multi stage sampling method. The data was collected through interviewing the pregnant women face to face after getting informed consent using structured and pre-tested questionnaire. The data was coded and entered in to Epi-info 7 then exported to Stata 14 for cleaning and further analysis. Both Bivariable and multi variable logistic regression model was used in the data analysis.

Results: The overall magnitude of anemia (hemoglobin level < 11 mg/dl) were found that 16.88% (95% CI: 13.95%, 19.8%). Factors which were significantly associated with anemia in the multivariable analysis were: history of malaria attack 1 year prior to study period (AOR – 4.73, 95% CI: 2.64, 8.46), women who had history of excessive menstrual bleeding (AOR = 3.94, 95% CI: 2.11, 7.35), unplanned pregnancy (AOR = 2.5, 95% CI: 1.4, 4.42) and three times or less meal frequency (AOR = 1.89, 95% CI: 1.02, 3.5).

Conclusion: The magnitude of anemia among pregnant were found that 16.88%. Malaria attack, excessive menstrual bleeding, pregnancy planning and meal frequency were found that significantly associated with anemia in the multivariable analysis. Pregnant women are recommended to increase meal frequency. Health providers should give attention to pregnant women who had history of malaria attack, excessive menstrual bleeding and women whose pregnancy were not planned.

Keywords: Anemia, Pregnant women, Ethiopia

* Correspondence: teklitvip@gmail.com
[1]Department of Reproductive Health, College of Health sciences, Aksum University, Aksum, Ethiopia
Full list of author information is available at the end of the article

Introduction

Anemia is defined as a low blood hemoglobin concentration [1]. It is a global public health problem affecting people in all age groups with major consequences for human health as well as social and economic development [1–3]. Anemia is a common health problem in pregnant women which is wider in developing countries than developed countries. As a result, it is associated with higher risk of low birth weight and both maternal and perinatal mortality and morbidity [4–7].

In developing countries, pregnant women are prone to anemia due to low socioeconomic conditions. The poor nutritional intake, repeated infections, frequent pregnancies and low health-seeking behaviors are associated with anemia [5, 8].

Since anemia is more common in child bearing women especially during pregnancy in Ethiopia, national nutritional strategies are formulated to reduce as part of the health sector transformation plan [9]. In countries like Ethiopia where anemia due to nutritional deficiencies mainly related to iron deficiency are the major causes [10, 11], identifying factors that are associated with anemia is necessary to control it. So, this study is aimed at assessing the magnitude and factors associated with anemia in pregnant women attending antenatal care.

Methods

Study design

Facility based cross sectional study design was conducted.

Study area and period

The study was conducted in central zone of Tigray region, Northern Ethiopia from November 1/2017 to January 30/2018. Central zone of Tigray is one of the six zones found in Tigray region. According to the 2007 census, Central zone of Tigray has 12 districts with estimated population of 1,500,000. Out of these population 750,000 are females and 750,000 are males. Central zone of Tigray has 66 health facilities (one referral hospital, 3 general hospitals, 6 primary hospitals and 56 health centers). The antenatal care (ANC) coverage of zone administration is 90%.

Source population

All pregnant women who attend ANC in public health centers in central zone of Tigray region during the study period.

Study population

All pregnant women who attend ANC at randomly selected public health centers in central zone of Tigray region during the study period.

Inclusion and exclusion criteria

Inclusion criteria

Pregnant women who attend 1st ANC visit and above at the same health center. Hence hemoglobin level of pregnant women was taken from base line assessment during 1st ANC visit as routine activities before starting any intervention.

Exclusion criteria

Women who attend 1st ANC other than the selected health center.

Sample size determination

The sample size was calculated using single proportion formula using epinfo-7 from study conducted in north west Ethiopia where the proportion of women with anemia was 25.2% [12].

Therefore, the total sample size was calculated using the assumption of marginal error 0.05, and 95% confidence interval. Based on these assumptions, the sample size was estimated as 290. After multiplying by 2 for design effect and adding 10% of non-respondents, the final sample size was determined as 638 study subjects.

Sampling procedures

Stratified multi stage sampling method was used to select health centers found in the central zone of Tigray region. During the selection of health centers, we stratified them as rural and urban. Two health centers each were randomly selected from 3 randomly selected woreda and one health center from urban in the central zone were included in the study. Proportion to sample size allocation was used to allocate the number of pregnant women from each health facilities by taking 3 months case load pregnant women on ANC visit. Systematic random sampling technique was used to get the study units.

Data collection procedure and tools

The data was collected through interviewing the pregnant women face to face after getting informed consent using structured and pre-tested questionnaire. The questionnaire was originally developed in English and then translate into Tigrigna (local language). Later on it was translated back to English to ensure its consistency. Finally, it was prepared in Local language (Tigrigna language) to collect data. In addition to that chart review was conducted to extract hemoglobin level at ANC 1st visit and another necessary data from ANC longitudinal register. During data collection, two BSC Degree and 7 diploma holder in nursing were hired as supervisors and data collectors respectively.

Data analysis

The data was coded and entered in to Epi-info 7 then exported to Stata 14 for cleaning and further analysis. Both Bivariable and multi variable logistic regression model was used in the data analysis. The assumption of logistic regression model fitness was checked using Hosmer and Lemeshow goodness of fit test statistics. Variables with P-value < 0.05 in the Bivariable logistic regression analysis was considered for inclusion in the multivariable logistic regression analysis to control the effect of confounders.

Variables which were significantly associated with the outcome variable were declared when adjusted odds ratio (AOR) with 95% confidence interval was significant in the multivariable analysis at P-value< 0.05.

Data quality

Three days intensive training were given to data collectors and supervisors on the data collection tools and collection procedures by the principal investigator.

Daily supervision of data collectors were made at each health centers during the study period by the supervisors and principal investigator. The collected data were carefully checked for completeness and consistency. Any confusion on the data collection procedure and responses were handled timely.

Results

Socio-demographic and economic characteristics of study participants

A total of 634 pregnant women were interviewed with the response rate of 99%. The average mean age of study participants was 26.99 years with standard deviation (SD) of 5.99. The majority of age group belongs to 20–34 years which accounts 487(76.81%). Nearly all 609(96.06%) of study participants were with orthodox religion. Regarding to marital status, 13(2.05%) of study participants were not married whereas 552(87.07%) were married. Eighty five (13.41%) of participants were with housewife occupation and 277(43.69%) of the study participants were with primary educational level. Four hundred fifteen (65.46%) of the study participant's household size were 1–4 and about a quarter of study participants 127(25.08%) were with second wealth quintile (Table 1).

Out of the total study participants, 175(27.6%) were nulliparous and 79(16.92%) had history of abortion. Fifty seven (12.42%) and 37(8.06%) of the study participants were with less than 2 years birth interval and had history of still birth respectively. Regarding to history of malaria attack 1 year prior to this study period, 112(17.67%) of the study subjects had history of malaria. Most of the participants 542(85.49%) and 582(91.8%) had no history of excessive menstrual bleeding and pregnancy related complications respectively. Only 132(20.82%) of study

Table 1 Socio-demographic and economic characteristics of pregnant women attending ANC in public health centers in central zone of Tigray region, northern Ethiopia, 2018

Variables	Frequency	Percentage
Age in years		
15–20	55	8.68
20–34	487	76.81
≥35	92	14.51
Mean = 26.99 (SD = 5.99)		
Religion		
Orthodox	609	96.06
Muslim	25	3.94
Marital status		
Not married	13	2.05
Married	552	87.07
Divorced	20	3.15
Separated	46	7.26
Others	3	0.47
Occupation		
House wife	85	13.41
Farmer	399	62.93
Merchant	89	14.04
Employee	43	6.78
Others	18	2.84
Level of education		
No formal education	173	27.29
Primary	277	43.69
Secondary	126	19.87
Diploma and above	58	9.15
Household size		
1–4	415	65.46
5–7	181	28.55
≥8	38	5.99
Wealth quintile		
Lowest	127	20.03
Second	159	25.08
Middle	181	28.55
Fourth	60	9.46
Highest	107	16.88

subjects were with planned pregnancy. Almost half 315(49.68%) of the participants were with MUAC less than 23 cm.

The magnitude of anemia (hemoglobin level < 11 mg/dl) were found that 16.88% (95% CI: 13.95%, 19.8%). The mean hemoglobin level of study participants were 12.3 (SD ± 1.33). Most of the pregnant women 489 (77.13%)

who attend their first ANC were at the 3–6 months of gestational age (Table 2).

The meal frequency of study participants with greater than three times per day were 252(39.75%). Majority 541(85.33%) of the total participants were reported that they consume food made from cereals and grains daily. Besides, 179(28.23%) of the total participants didn't take

tea or coffee. Concerning to fruit and green leafy vegetables intake, only 11(1.74%) and 40(6.31%) of the total study participants reported with daily intake respectively (Table 3).

Socio-demographic factors like; age of women, religion, marital status, occupation, household size and

Table 2 Obstetric history characteristics of pregnant women attending ANC in public health centers in central zone of Tigray region, northern Ethiopia, 2018

Variables	Frequency	Percentage
Parity		
Nulliparous	175	27.60
1–4	391	61.67
≥5	68	10.73
Ever had abortion		
No	388	83.08
Yes	79	16.92
Birth interval		
< 2 years	57	12.42
≥2 years	402	87.58
Had ever still birth		
No	422	91.94
Yes	37	8.06
Have got malaria in previous year		
No	522	82.33
Yes	112	17.67
Had excessive menstrual bleeding		
No	542	85.49
Yes	92	14.51
Had pregnancy related complication		
No	582	91.80
Yes	52	8.20
Planned pregnancy		
No	132	20.82
Yes	502	79.18
Nutritional status (MUAC)		
< 23 cm	315	49.68
≥23 cm	319	50.32
Hemoglobin level		
< 11 mg/dl	107	16.88
≥11 mg/dl	527	83.12
Mean 12.38(SD ± 1.33)		
HGB level by gestational age (Average HGB level)		
< 3 Months Mean = 12.2(SD ± 1.63)	19	3
3–6 Months Mean = 12.22(SD ± 1.29)	489	77.13
> 6 Months Mean = 12.13(SD ± 1.41)	126	19.87

Table 3 Dietary factors characteristics of pregnant women attending ANC in public health centers in central zone of Tigray region, northern Ethiopia, 2018

Variables	Frequency	Percentage
Meal frequency		
≤3times per day	382	60.25
>3times per day	252	39.75
Eating food made from cereals, grains		
Daily	541	85.33
Weekly	84	13.25
Monthly or above	9	1.42
Drinking tea or coffee		
No	179	28.23
Before meal	73	11.51
Within 1 h	249	39.27
After 1 h	133	20.98
Fruit intake		
No	291	45.9
Daily	11	1.74
Weekly	266	41.96
Monthly or above	66	10.41
Green leafy vegetables intake		
No	91	14.35
Daily	40	6.31
Weekly	463	73.03
Monthly or above	40	6.31
Dairy products/ milk product intake		
No	297	46.85
Daily	58	9.15
Weekly	211	33.28
Monthly or above	68	10.73
Meat intake		
No	100	15.77
Daily	16	2.52
Weekly	172	27.13
Monthly or above	346	54.57
Egg intake		
No	132	20.82
Daily	62	9.78
Weekly	343	54.10
Monthly or above	97	15.30

wealth quintile were not significantly associated with the anemia in Bivariable analysis at *P*-value < 0.05. Similarly, parity of women, history of abortion, birth interval, history of still birth and nutritional status were not significantly associated with anemia in Bivariable analysis. Regarding to dietary intake, variables which were not significantly associated with anemia in Bivariable analysis at *P*-value < 0.05 were; eating food made from cereals and grains, drinking tea or coffee, fruit intake, green leafy vegetables intake, dairy products/ milk product intake, meat intake and egg intake.

Variables which were significantly associated with anemia in Bivariable analysis but remains insignificant in multivariable analysis were; women's level of education, birth interval and had pregnancy related complication. However, history of malaria attack 1 year prior to study period, women who had history of excessive menstrual bleeding, planned pregnancy and meal frequency were significantly associated with anemia in the multivariable analysis. Women with history of malaria attack were

significantly associated with anemia comparing to women who had no malaria attack (AOR = 4.73, 95% CI: 2.64, 8.46). Comparing to women who had no history of excessive menstrual bleeding, anemia was 3.94 times higher in women with history of excessive menstrual bleeding (AOR = 394, 95% CI: 2.11, 7.35). Similarly anemia was higher in pregnant women who had no pregnancy planning (AOR = 2.5, 95% CI: 1.4, 4.42) comparing to their counter parts. Meal frequency less than or equal to 3 times per day was also significantly associated with anemia (AOR = 1.89, 95% CI: 1.02, 3.5) (Table 4).

Discussion

We conducted study aimed on determining magnitude of anemia and factors associated with it. Out of 634 pregnant women included in the study, 107 (16.88%) were found to be anemic with 95% CI of 13.95 to 19.8% which is lower that studies conducted in Woldia (39.1%) [13], Gode town (56.8%) [11], Butajira (27.6%) [5],

Table 4 Bivariable and multivariable analysis of factors associated with anemia among pregnant women attending ANC in public health centers of central zone of Tigray region, northern Ethiopia, 2018

Variables	Anemia		COR (95%, CI)	AOR (95%, CI)
	Yes	No		
Women's level of education				
No formal education	39(36.45%)	134(25.43%)	1	1
Primary	35(32.71%)	242(45.92%)	2.01(1.22, 3.33)*	1.53(0.81, 2.89)
Secondary	20(18.69%)	106(20.11%)	1.54(0.89, 2.8)	0.98(0.43, 2.25)
Diploma and above	13(12.15%)	45(8.54%)	1.01(0.49, 2.06)	0.52(0.17, 1.61)
Birth interval				
< 2 years	16(20.78%)	41(10.73%)	2.2(1.2, 4.13)*	0.57(0.27,1.2)
≥2 years	61(79.22%)	341(89.27%)	1	1
Malaria attack in last 1 year				
No	64(59.81%)	458(86.91%)	1	1
Yes	43(40.19%)	69(13.09%)	4.46(2.8, 7.1)*	4.73(2.64, 8.46)*
Had excessive menstrual bleeding				
No	69(64.49%)	473(89.75%)	1	1
Yes	38(35.51%)	54(10.25%)	4.82(2.0, 7.84)*	3.94(2.11,7.35)*
Had pregnancy related complication				
No	93(86.92%)	489(92.79%)	1	1
Yes	14(13.08%)	38(7.21%)	1.94(1.01, 3.72)*	1.87(0.77, 4.54)*
Planned pregnancy				
No	38(35.51%)	94(17.84%)	2.54(1.61, 4.0)	2.5(1.4,4.42)*
Yes	69(64.49%)	433(82.16%)		1
Meal frequency				
≤3 times per day	74(69.16%)	308(58.44%)	1.6(1.02, 2.49)	1.89(1.02, 3.5)*
>3times per day	33(30.84%)	219(41.56%)	1	1

COR Crude Odds Ratio, *AOR* Adjusted Odds Ratio
*p-Value < 0.05

Nekemt (52%) [14], Mizan Tepi (23.5%) [15], Dera (30.5%) [4] and North West Tigray (36.1%) [16], but similar with the study conducted in Mekelle (19.3%) [10]. Overall magnitude of anemia in pregnant women is currently decreasing due to multi-sectorial interventions like increasing health access and economy in the country through time but still it remains a public health problem.

In this finding, pregnant women who had history of malaria attack in the last 1 year prior to study period were found that significantly associated with anemia (AOR = 4.73, 95% CI: 2.64, 8.46). This finding is similar with the study conducted in North Western zone of Tigray [16], in Dera District, South Gondar Zone [4] and Sunyani Municipal Hospital, Ghana [17] among pregnant women which declared that malaria attack was significantly associated with anemia. This could be explained that parasitic infections especially malaria results destruction of red blood cells [2].

In this study pregnant women with history of excessive menstrual bleeding were 3.94 times more likely to be anemic than those who had normal menstrual bleeding. A study conducted in Mizan Tepi University Teaching Hospital, South West Ethiopia [15] were also reported that heavy menstrual bleeding was significantly associated with anemia. This may be due to low iron reserves following excess bleeding during menstruation period.

Planned pregnancy was found that significantly associated with anemia. Anemia was 2.5 times higher in pregnant women whose pregnancy was not planned (AOR = 2.5, 95% CI: 1.4, 4.42). Women with their planned pregnancy may prepare prior or early in pregnancy on nutritional intake.

Meal frequency with 3 times or less per day was associated with anemia (AOR = 1.89, 95% CI: 1.02, 3.5). This study is consistent with Studies conducted in Mekelle town [10] and in North West of Tigray [16]. This implies increased meal frequency during pregnancy needs to fulfill the nutrients demand of pregnant women.

Conclusion

The magnitude of anemia among pregnant were found that 16.88. Factors that were independently significant with anemia were; history of malaria attack, excessive menstrual bleeding, pregnancy which was not planned and three or less meal frequency per a day. It is recommended that pregnant women should increase meal frequency. Health providers should give attention to pregnant women who had history of malaria attack, excessive menstrual bleeding and women whose pregnancy were not planned to control malaria in pregnancy.

Abbreviations

ANC: Antenatal care; AOR: Adjusted odds ratio; CI: Confidence interval; CM: Centimeter; COR: Crude odds ratio; HGB: Hemoglobin; MUAC: Middle upper arm circumference; SD: Standard deviation

Acknowledgments

We would like to thank Aksum University for financial support of this study. Our thanks goes to directors of public health centers for their cooperation. Finally, we would like to thank the study subjects, data collectors and supervisors for their voluntariness in participating this study.

Funding

This research has been funded through college of Health sciences, Aksum University.

Authors' contributions

TG have contributed in the design, data analysis, write up and manuscript development. EB, SH contributed in data collection and analysis. GK contributed to editing and revising of the final manuscript. All authors read and approved the final manuscript.

Competing interests

The authors declare that they have no competing interests.

Author details

[1]Department of Reproductive Health, College of Health sciences, Aksum University, Aksum, Ethiopia. [2]Department of Human Nutrition, College of Health sciences, Aksum University, Aksum, Ethiopia. [3]Department of Epidemiology and Biostatistics, College of Health sciences, Aksum University, Aksum, Ethiopia.

References

1.   United Nations Children's Fund. United Nations University and World Health Organization. Iron Deficiency Anaemia Assessment, Prevention and Control A guide for programme managers. Geneva 2001.

2.   WHO and UNICEF. Focusing on anaemia towards an integrated approach for effective anaemia control. Geneva: World health organization; 2004.

3.   World Health Organization. The global prevalence of anaemia. Geneva: World health organization; 2011.

4.   Derso T, Abera Z, Tariku A. Magnitude and associated factors of anemia among pregnant women in Dera District: a cross-sectional study in Northwest Ethiopia. BMC Res Notes. 2017;10:359.

5.   Getahun W, Belachew T, Wolide AD. Burden and associated factors of anemia among pregnant women attending antenatal care in southern Ethiopia: cross sectional study. BMC Res Notes. 2017;10:276.

6.   Lelissa D, Yilma M, Shewalem W, Abraha A, Worku M, Ambachew H, et al. Prevalence of Anemia among women receiving antenatal Care at Boditii Health Center, southern Ethiopia. Clin Med Res. 2015;4(3):79–86.

7.   Zillmer K, Pokharel A, Spielman K, Kershaw M, Ayele K, Kidane Y, et al. Predictors of anemia in pregnant women residing in rural areas of the Oromiya region of Ethiopia. BMC Nutr. 2017;3(65).

8.   Tadesse SE, Seid O, G/Mariam Y, Fekadu A, Wasihun Y, Endris K, et al. Determinants of anemia among pregnant mothers attending antenatal care

in Dessie town health facilities, northern central Ethiopia, unmatched case -control study. Plose One. 2017;12(3):e0173173.

9. Federal Democratic Republic of Ethiopia Ministry of Health. Health Sector Transformation Plan 2015/16–2019/20. Addis Ababa: Federal democratic republic of Ethiopia ministry of health; 2015.

10. Abriha A, Yesuf ME, Wassie MM. Prevalence and associated factors of anemia among pregnant women of Mekelle town: a cross sectional study. BMC Res Notes. 2014;7:888.

11. Alene KA, Dohe AM. Prevalence of Anemia and Associated Factors among Pregnant Women in an Urban Area of Eastern Ethiopia. Cairo: Hindawi Publishing Corporation; 2014.

12. Asrie F. Prevalence of anemia and its associated factors among pregnant women receiving antenatal care at Aymiba Health Center, northwest Ethiopia. J Blood Med. 2017;8:35–40.

13. Brhanie TW, Sisay H. Prevalence of Iron deficiency Anemia and determinants among pregnant women attending antenatal Care at Woldia Hospital, Ethiopia. J Nutr Dis Ther. 2016;6(4).

14. Mihiretie H, Fufa M, Mitiku A, Bacha C, Getahun D, Kejela M, et al. Magnitude of Anemia and Associated Factors among Pregnant Women Attending Antenatal Care in Nekemte Health Center, Nekemte, Ethiopia. Med Microbiol Diag. 2015;4(3).

15. Zekarias B, Meleko A, Hayder A, Nigatu A, Yetagessu T. Prevalence of Anemia and its associated factors among pregnant WomenAttending antenatal care (ANC) in Mizan Tepi University teaching hospital, South West Ethiopia. Health Sci J. 2017;11(5,529).

16. Gebre A, Mulugeta A. Prevalence of Anemia and associated factors among pregnant women in North Western zone of Tigray, northern Ethiopia: a cross-sectional study. J Nutr Metab. 2015;2015.

17. Anlaakuu P, Anto F. Anaemia in pregnancy and associated factors: a cross sectional study of antenatal attendants at the Sunyani municipal hospital, Ghana. BMC Res Notes. 2017;10:402.

Permissions

Contributors

Sven Cnattingius
Clinical Epidemiology Unit, Department of Medicine, Karolinska Institute, Solna, Sweden

Siavash Maghsoudlou
Clinical Epidemiology Unit, Department of Medicine, Karolinska Institute, Solna, Sweden
Department of Obstetrics and Gynecology, McMaster University, 1280 Main Street West, room 3N52F, Hamilton, ON L8S 4K1, Canada

Scott Montgomery
Clinical Epidemiology Unit, Department of Medicine, Karolinska Institute, Solna, Sweden
Clinical Epidemiology and Biostatistics, School of Medical Sciences, Örebro University, Örebro, Sweden
Department of Epidemiology and Public Health, University College London, London, UK

Anna-Karin Wikström
Clinical Epidemiology Unit, Department of Medicine, Karolinska Institute, Solna, Sweden
Department of Clinical Sciences, Karolinska Institute, Danderyd Hospital, Stockholm, Sweden

Mohsen Aarabi
Faculty of Medicine, Mazandaran University of Medical Sciences, Sari, Iran

Shahriar Semnani
Faculty of Medicine, Golestan University of Medical Sciences, Gorgan, Iran

Shahram Bahmanyar
Clinical Epidemiology Unit and Centre for Pharmacoepidemiology, Department of Medicine, Karolinska Institute, Solna, Sweden

Donna B. Mak
Communicable Disease Control Directorate, Department of Health, Shenton Park, Western Australia
School of Medicine, University of Notre Dame, Fremantle, Western Australia

Annette K. Regan
Communicable Disease Control Directorate, Department of Health, Shenton Park, Western Australia
School of Public Health, Curtin University Bentley, Western Australia

Dieu T. Vo
Communicable Disease Control Directorate, Department of Health, Shenton Park, Western Australia
School of Population Health, University of Western Australia, Crawley, Western Australia

Paul V. Effler
Communicable Disease Control Directorate, Department of Health, Shenton Park, Western Australia
School of Pathology andLaboratory Medicine, University of Western Australia, Crawley, Western Australia

Maryam Sina, Freya MacMillan, Tinashe Dune, Navodya Balasuriya, Nouran Khouri, Ngan Nguyen, Vasyngpong Jongvisal, Xiang Hui Lay and David Simmons
Western Sydney University, Sydney, NSW 2751, Australia

Stefan Kohler
Heidelberg Institute of Global Health, Heidelberg University, Heidelberg,Germany
Division of Global Health, Department of Public Health Sciences, Karolinska Institutet, Stockholm, Sweden

Kristi Sidney Annerstedt and Ayesha De Costa
Division of Global Health, Department of Public Health Sciences, Karolinska Institutet, Stockholm, Sweden

Vishal Diwan
Division of Global Health, Department of Public Health Sciences, Karolinska Institutet, Stockholm, Sweden
Department of Public Health and Environment, R. D. Gardi Medical College, Ujjain, India
International Centre for Health Research, Ujjain Charitable Trust Hospital and Research Centre, Ujjain, India

Bharat Randive
Department of Public Health and Environment, R. D. Gardi Medical College, Ujjain, India
Epidemiology and Global Health, Department of Public Health and Clinical Medicine, Umeå University, Umeå, Sweden

Lars Lindholm
Epidemiology and Global Health, Department of Public Health and Clinical Medicine, Umeå University, Umeå, Sweden

Kranti Vora
Indian Institute of Public Health, Ahmedabad, India

Claudia Schoenborn and Myriam De Spiegelaere
1Research centre in Health Policies and Health Systems, Ecole de Santé Publique, Université Libre de Bruxelles (ULB), Route de Lennik 808, 1070Bruxelles, Belgium

Mouctar Sow
Research centre in Health Policies and Health Systems, Ecole de Santé Publique, Université Libre de Bruxelles (ULB), Route de Lennik 808, 1070Bruxelles, Belgium

Department of social and preventive medicine Ecole de Santé Publique, Université de Montréal, Montréal, Québec H3N 1X9, Canada

Judith Racape
Research centre in Epidemiology, Biostatistics and Clinical research, Ecole de Santé Publique, Université Libre de Bruxelles(ULB), CP598. Route de Lennik 808, 1070 Bruxelles, Belgium

Samir Buainain Kassar
Health Sciences University of Alagoas (UNCISAL), Maceió, Brazil

Telmo Henrique Barbosa de Lima
Health Sciences University of Alagoas (UNCISAL), Maceió, Brazil
Health Sciences, Federal University of São Paulo (UNIFESP), São Paulo, Brazil
Maternidade Santa Mônica, Maceió, Brazil

Leila Katz
Postgraduate Program, Fernando Figueira Institute of Integral Medicine (IMIP), Obstetric Intensive Care Unit, IMIP, Recife, Brazil

Melania Maria Amorim
Postgraduate Program, Fernando Figueira Institute of Integral Medicine (IMIP), Obstetric Intensive Care Unit, IMIP, Recife, Brazil
Federal University of Campina Grande (UFCG), Campina Grande, Brazil

Justina Kacerauskiene Meile Minkauskiene, Egle Bartuseviciene, Dalia R. Railaite, Arnoldas Bartusevicius, Mindaugas Kliucinskas, Ruta J. Nadisauskiene and Kastytis Smigelskas
Lithuanian University of Health Sciences, Eiveniu str. 2, 50167 Kaunas, Lithuania

Tahir Mahmood
Victoria Hospital, Kirkcaldy, Fife KY2 5AH, Scotland, UK

Kornelija Maciuliene
Vilnius Maternity Hospital, Tyzenhauzu str. 18A, 02106 Vilnius, Lithuania

Grazina Drasutiene and Diana Ramasauskaite
Vilnius University Hospital Santaros Klinikos, Santariskiu str. 2, 08661 Vilnius, Lithuania

Alfred Kwesi Manyeh
Dodowa Health Research Centre, Dodowa, Accra, Ghana
Division of Epidemiology and Biostatistics, School of Public Health, University of the Witwatersrand, Parktown, Johannesburg, South Africa

Alberta Amu, David Etsey Akpakli and John Williams
Dodowa Health Research Centre, Dodowa, Accra, Ghana
Ghana Health Service, Accra, Ghana

Margarete Gyapong
Dodowa Health Research Centre, Dodowa, Accra, Ghana
Centre for Health Policy and Implementation Research, Institute for Health Research, University of Health and Allied Sciences, Volta Region, Ho, Ghana

Kayvan Bozorgmehr, Louise Biddle and Joachim Szecsenyi
Department of General Practice and Health Services Research, University Hospital Heidelberg, Marsilius Arkaden, INF 130.3, 69120 Heidelberg, Germany

Stella Preussler
Institute for Medical Biometry and Informatics, University Hospital Heidelberg, Heidelberg, Germany

Andreas Mueller
Clinic of Gynaecology, Karlsruhe City Hospital, Karlsruhe, Germany

Rakesh Parashar
Health Systems, USAID-VRIDDHI/ IPE Global, New Delhi, India

Anadi Gupt
Maternal Health, Department of Health and Family Welfare, Government of Himachal Pradesh, Shimla, India

Devina Bajpayee
Maternal and Newborn Health, USAID-VRIDDHI/IPE Global, New Delhi, India

Anil Gupta
USAID-VRIDDHI/IPE Global, Shimla, Himachal Pradesh, India

Rohan Thakur
USAID-VRIDDHI/IPE Global, Mandi, Himachal Pradesh, India

Ankur Sangwan
USAID-VRIDDHI/IPE Global, Kinnaur, Himachal Pradesh, India

Anuradha Sharma and Deshraj Sharma
Department of Health and Family Welfare, Government of Himachal Pradesh, Mandi, Himachal Pradesh, India

Sachin Gupta
Maternal and Child Health, USAID-India, New Delhi, India

Dinesh Baswal
Maternal Health, Ministry of Health and Family Welfare, Government of India, New Delhi, India

Gunjan Taneja and Rajeev Gera
USAID-VRIDDHI/IPE Global, New Delhi, India

Eveline Thobias Konje
Department of Biostatistics and Epidemiology, School of Public Health,Catholic University of Health and Allied Sciences, Bugando Area, Mwanza, Tanzania
Department of Community Health Sciences, Cumming School of Medicine, University of Calgary, 3280 Hospital Drive, NW, Calgary, AB, Canada

Jennifer Hatfield and Reginald S. Sauve
Department of Community Health Sciences, Cumming School of Medicine, University of Calgary, 3280 Hospital Drive, NW, Calgary, AB, Canada

Margret Dewey
Department of Community Health Sciences, Cumming School of Medicine, University of Calgary, 3280 Hospital Drive, NW, Calgary, AB, Canada
Department of Paediatrics, University of Calgary, 2888 Shaganappi Tr. NW, Calgary, AB, Canada
Owerko Centre at the Alberta Children's Hospital Research Institute, Cumming School of Medicine, University of Calgary, 2500 University Dr. NW, Calgary, AB, Canada

Moke Tito Nyambita Magoma
Options Tanzania Ltd 76 Ali Hassan, Mwinyi Road, Dar es Salaam, Tanzania

Susan Kuhn
Department of Paediatrics, University of Calgary, 2888 Shaganappi Tr. NW, Calgary, AB, Canada

Kıymet Yeşilçiçek Çalik
Obstetrics and Gynaecology Nursing Department, Karadeniz Technical University, Faculty of HealthScience, University District, Farabi Street, Ortahisar, Trabzon, Turkey

Özlem Karabulutlu
Department of Midwifery, Kafkas University, Faculty of Health Sciences, Kars, Turkey

Canan Yavuz
Midwife, Tekirdağ Community Health Center, Tekirdağ, Turkey

Bettina Böttcher, Belal Aldabbour and Fadel Naim Naim
Faculty of Medicine, Islamic University of Gaza, Gaza strip, Gaza, Palestine

Nasser Abu-El-Noor and Yousef Aljeesh
Faculty of Nursing, Islamic University of Gaza, Gaza Strip, Gaza, Palestine

Camila Caram-Deelder and Johanna G van der Bom
Center for Clinical Transfusion Research, Sanquin Research, Plesmanlaan 1a – 5th floor, 2333, BZ, Leiden, The Netherlands
Department of Clinical Epidemiology, Leiden University Medical Center, Albinusdreef 2, 2333, ZA, Leiden, The Netherlands

Ada Gillissen and Dacia D C A Henriquez
Center for Clinical Transfusion Research, Sanquin Research, Plesmanlaan 1a – 5th floor, 2333, BZ, Leiden, The Netherlands
Department of Clinical Epidemiology, Leiden University Medical Center, Albinusdreef 2, 2333, ZA, Leiden, The Netherlands
Department of Obstetrics, Leiden University Medical Center, Albinusdreef 2, 2333, ZA, Leiden, The Netherlands

Thomas van den Akker
Department of Obstetrics, Leiden University Medical Center, Albinusdreef 2, 2333, ZA, Leiden, The Netherlands
National Perinatal Epidemiology Unit, University of Oxford, University of Oxford, Old Road Campus, Oxford OX3 7LF, UK

Jos J M van Roosmalen
Department of Obstetrics, Leiden University Medical Center, Albinusdreef 2, 2333, ZA, Leiden, The Netherlands
3584, EA, Utrecht, The Netherlands. 6Athena Institute, VU University Amsterdam, De Boelelaan 1105, 1081, HV, Amsterdam, The Netherlands

Kitty W M Bloemenkamp
Department of Obstetrics, Birth Centre Wilhelmina's Children Hospital, University Medical Center Utrecht, Lundlaan

Jeroen Eikenboom
Department of Internal Medicine, Division of Thrombosis and Haemostasis, Leiden University Medical Center, Leiden, the Netherlands

Jocelyn D. Glazier1, Dexter J. L. Hayes, Sabiha Hussain1, Stephen W. D'Souza and Alexander E. P. Heazell1
Maternal and Fetal Health Research Centre, Division of Developmental Biology and Medicine, Faculty of Biology, Medicine and Health, University of Manchester, 5th Floor (Research), St Mary's Hospital, Oxford Road, Manchester M13 9WL, UK

Joanne Whitcombe
Trust Library, Central Manchester University Hospitals NHS Foundation Trust, Education South, Oxford Road, Manchester M13 9WL, UK

Nick Ashton
Division of Cardiovascular Sciences, Faculty of Biology, Medicine and Health, University of Manchester, 3rd Floor Core Technology Facility, 46 Grafton Street, Manchester M13 9NT, UK

Saffie Colley
Ministry of Health and Social Welfare, West Africa, Banjul, The Gambia

Chien-Huei Kao and Meeiling Gau
Graduate Institute of Nurse-Midwifery National Taipei University and Health Sciences, 365 Ming-Te Road, Taipei 112, Taiwan

Su-Fen Cheng
Graduate Institute of Nursing, National Taipei University and Health Sciences, 365 Ming-Te Road, Taipei 112, Taiwan

Tih P. Muffih
Cameroon Baptist Convention Health
Service (CBCHS), Tiko, Health
Services Complex, Mutengene, South
West Region, Cameroon

Pascal N. Atanga
Cameroon Baptist Convention Health
Service (CBCHS), Tiko, Health
Services Complex, Mutengene, South
West Region, Cameroon
Department of Public Health
and Hygiene, Faculty of Health
Sciences, University of Buea, Buea,
Cameroon
Centre for InternationalHealth (CIH),
University of Munich (LMU), Munich,
Germany

Peter N. Fon
Department of Public Health
and Hygiene, Faculty of Health
Sciences, University of Buea, Buea,
Cameroon

Michael Hoelscher
Centre for InternationalHealth (CIH),
University of Munich (LMU), Munich,
Germany
Division of Infectious Diseases and
Tropical Medicine, Medical Centre
of the University of Munich (LMU),
Munich, Germany
German Centre for Infection Research
(DZIF), Partner Site Munich, Munich,
Germany

Harrison T. Ndetan
Department of Epidemiology and
Biostatistics, University Texas Health
Northeast, School of Community and
Rural Health, Tyler, USA
Department of Biostatistics and
Epidemiology, School of Public
Health, University of North Texas
Health Science Center, Fort Worth,
TX, USA

Eric A. Achidi
Faculty of Science, University of
Buea, Buea, Cameroon

Henry D. Meriki
Department of Microbiology and
Parasitology,Faculty of Sciences,
University of Buea, Buea, Cameroon

Laboratory Department, Regional
Hospital Buea, Buea, Cameroon

Arne Kroidl
Division of Infectious Diseases and
Tropical Medicine, Medical Centre
of the University of Munich (LMU),
Munich, Germany
German Centre for Infection Research
(DZIF), Partner Site Munich, Munich,
Germany

**Nkwati Michel Maboh, Susan Etta
Maeya, Lerry Dibo Ndumbe, Pauline
Bessem Nyenti, Obale Armstrong
and Derick Etiendem**
Department of Nursing, School of
Health Sciences, Biaka University
Institute of Buea-Cameroon, Buea,
Cameroon

Aminkeng Zawuo Leke
Department of Nursing, School of
Health Sciences, Biaka University
Institute of Buea-Cameroon, Buea,
Cameroon
Office of the Deputy Vice Chancellor
i/c Research/Cooperation/Quality,
Biaka Universit Institute of Buea,
Buea, Cameroon

**Helen Dolk, Maria Loane, and
Karen Casson**
Centre for Maternal, Fetal and Infant
Research, Institute for Nursing and
Health Research, Ulster University,
Shore Rd Newtownabbey, BT370QB
Ulster, Ireland

**Maureen I. Heaman and Kellie R.
Thiessen**
College of Nursing, Rady Faculty
of Health Sciences, University of
Manitoba, 89 Curry Place, Winnipeg,
MB R3T 2N2, Canada

**Patricia J. Martens Marni D.
Brownell and Mariette J. Chartier**
Department of Community Health
Sciences, Max Rady College of
Medicine, Rady Faculty of Health
Sciences, University of Manitoba, S113
- 750 Bannatyne Avenue, Winnipeg,
MB R3E 0W3, Canada
Manitoba Centre for Health Policy,
University of Manitoba, 408-727
McDermot Avenue, Winnipeg, MB
R3E 3P5, Canada

Shelley A. Derksen
Manitoba Centre for Health Policy,
University of Manitoba, 408-727
McDermot Avenue, Winnipeg, MB
R3E 3P5, Canada

Michael E. Helewa
Department of Obstetrics, Gynecology
and Reproductive Sciences, Max Rady
College of Medicine, Rady Faculty
of Health Sciences, University of
Manitoba, WR120-735 Notre Dame
Avenue, Winnipeg, MB R3E 0L8,
Canada

**Wenjing Ding, Lieqiang Zhong,
Yuhang Long, Zhuyu Li, Cong Sun,
Yanxin Wu, Hanqing Chen, Haitian
Chen and Zilian Wang**
1Department of Obstetrics and
Gynaecology, The First Affiliated
Hospital of Sun Yat-sen University,
Guangzhou, China

Wai-Kit Ming
Department of Obstetrics and
Gynaecology, The First Affiliated
Hospital of Sun Yat-sen University,
Guangzhou, China
Harvard Medical School, Harvard
University, Boston, MA, USA
Division of Pharmacoepidemiology
and Pharmacoeconomics, Brigham
and Women's Hospital, Boston, MA,
USA

Casper J. P. Zhang
School of Public Health, The
University of Hong Kong, Hong
Kong, China

**Melania Elena Pop-Tudoseand and
Ioan Victor Pop**
Department of Medical Genetics,
"Iuliu Hațieganu" University of
Medicine and Pharmacy, Pasteur
Louis Street No.6, 400349 Cluj-
Napoca, Romania

Petru Armean
Department of Specific Disciplines,
Faculty of Midwifery and Nursing,
"Carol Davila" University of
Medicine and Pharmacy, Bucharest,
Romania

Dana Popescu-Spineni
Department of Specific Disciplines, Faculty of Midwifery and Nursing, "Carol Davila" University of Medicine and Pharmacy, Bucharest, Romania "Francisc I. Rainer" Anthropology Research Centre, Bucharest, Romania

Melissa C. Morgan
Department of Pediatrics, University of California San Francisco, 550 16th Street, San Francisco, CA 94158, USA
Institute for Global Health Sciences, University of California San Francisco, 550 16th Street, San Francisco, CA 94158, USA
Maternal, Adolescent, Reproductive, and Child Health Centre, London School of Hygiene and Tropical Medicine, Keppel Street, London WC1E 7HT, UK

Dilys M. Walker
Institute for Global Health Sciences, University of California San Francisco, 550 16th Street, San Francisco, CA 94158, USA
Pronto International, 5419 Greenwood Avenue North, Seattle, WA 98103, USA
Department of Obstetrics, Gynecology, and Reproductive Sciences, University of California SanFrancisco, 1001 Potrero Ave, San Francisco, CA 94110, USA

Jessica Dyer
Pronto International, 5419 Greenwood Avenue North, Seattle, WA 98103, USA

Aranzazu Abril
Médecins Sans Frontières, Nou de la Rambla 26, 08001 Barcelona, Spain

Amelia Christmas
Pronto International; State RMNCH+A Unit, C-16 Krishi Nagar, A.G. Colony, Patna, Bihar 80002, India

Tanmay Mahapatra and Aritra Das
CARE India, 14 Patliputra Colony, Patna, Bihar 800013, India

Dawud Muhammed Ahmed
Obstetrics and Gynecology, Bahir Dar University, College of Medicine and Health Sciences, Bahir Dar, Ethiopia

Tesfaye Setegn Mengistu
Bahir Dar University College of Medicine and Health Sciences, Bahir Dar, Amhara Regional State, Ethiopia

Aemiro Getu Endalamaw
Marie Stops International Ethiopia, Bahir Dar, Ethiopia

Bola Lukman Solanke and Semiu Adebayo Rahman
Department of Demography and Social Statistics, Faculty of Social Sciences, Obafemi Awolowo University, Ile-Ife, Nigeria

Danielly S. Santana, Carla Silveira, Maria L. Costa, Renato T. Souza, Fernanda G. Surita and José G. Cecatti
Department of Obstetrics and Gynecology, University of Campinas, Alexander Fleming Street, 101, Campinas, SP 13083-891, Brazil

João P. Souza and Joshua P. Vogel
UNDP/ UNFPA/UNICEF/WHO/ World Bank Special Programme of Research Development and Research Training in Human Reproduction (HRP), Department of Reproductive Health and Research, World Health Organization, Geneva, Switzerland

Syeda Batool Mazhar
Pakistan Institute of Medical Sciences, Islamabad, Pakistan

Kapila Jayaratne
Maternal and Child Morbidity and Mortality Surveillance Unit, Family Health Bureau, Ministry of Health, Colombo, Sri Lanka

Zahida Qureshi
Department of Obstetrics and Gynecology, University of Nairobi, Nairobi, Kenya

Maria H. Sousa
Department of Public Health, Jundiai Medical School, Jundiai, Brazil

Teklit Grum and Gizienesh Kahsay
Department of Reproductive Health, College of Health sciences, Aksum University, Aksum, Ethiopia

Ermyas Brhane
Department of Human Nutrition, College of Health sciences, Aksum University, Aksum, Ethiopia

Solomon Hintsa
Department of Epidemiology and Biostatistics, College of Health sciences, Aksum University, Aksum, Ethiopia.

Index

www.ingramcontent.com/pod-product-compliance
Lightning Source LLC
Chambersburg PA
CBHW061330190326
41458CB00011B/3949